Scientific Basis
of Urology

Scientific Basis of Urology

Edited by

Anthony R. Mundy

Professor of Urology, Institute of Urology and Nephrology,
London, UK

John M. Fitzpatrick

Professor of Surgery, Surgical Professorial Unit,
University College Dublin, Ireland

David E. Neal

Professor of Surgery, Department of Surgery, School of Surgical and Reproductive Sciences,
University of Newcastle upon Tyne, UK

Nicholas J. R. George

Consultant Urologist, Withington Hospital, Manchester, UK

I S I S
MEDICAL
MEDIA

© 1999 by Isis Medical Media Ltd.
59 St. Aldates
Oxford OX1 1ST, UK

First published 1999

British Library Cataloguing in Publication Data.
A catalogue record for this title is available from
the British Library.

ISBN 1 899066 21 7

Mundy, A. R. (Anthony)
Scientific Basis of Urology
Anthony R. Mundy, John M. Fitzpatrick, David E. Neal and Nicholas J. R. George (eds)

Always refer to the manufacturer's Prescribing
Information before prescribing drugs cited in this book.

Additional technical writing and editorial
services provided by Robert Reford (Oxford)

Typeset by
J&L Composition Ltd., UK

Image reproduction
Track Direct, London, UK

Isis Medical Media staff
Commissioning Editor: John Harrison
Senior Editorial Controller: Catherine Rickards
Production Controller: Geoff Holdsworth

Printed and bound by
Artegrafica, Italy

Distributed in the USA by
Books International Inc., P. O. Box 605,
Herndon, VA 20172, USA

Distributed in the rest of the world by
Plymbridge Distributors Ltd., Estover Road,
Plymouth, PL6 7PY, UK

Contents

List of contributors

John P. Blandy
Emeritus Professor of Urology, University of London at the Royal London Hospital; Consulting Surgeon to St. Peter's Hospital, London, UK

Steven C. Clifford
Department of Pathology, University of Cambridge, Tennis Court Road, Cambridge CB2 1QP, UK and Division of Medical and Molecular Genetics, Department of Paediatrics and Child Health, University of Birmingham Medical School, Edgbaston, Birmingham B15 2TT, UK

Anne C. Cunningham
Senior Lecturer in Immunology, School of Health Sciences, University of Sunderland, Wharncliffe Street, Sunderland SR2 3SD, UK

Gillian M. Duchesne
Associate Professor, Radiation Oncology, Peter MacCallum Cancer Institute, Locked Bag 1, A'Beckett Street, Melbourne, Victoria 8006, Australia

Mark Emberton
Senior Lecturer in Oncological Urology and Honorary Consultant Urologist, Institute of Urology and Nephrology, 48 Riding House Street, London W1N 7PN, UK

John M. Fitzpatrick
Professor of Surgery, University College Dublin, Surgical Professorial Unit, 47 Eccles Street, Dublin 7, Ireland

Nicholas J. R. George
Senior Lecturer/Consultant Urologist, University Hospital of South Manchester, Withington Hospital, West Didsbury, Manchester M20 2LR, UK

Freddie C. Hamdy
Senior Lecturer in Urological Surgery, Department of Surgery, The Medical School, University of Newcastle, Newcastle-upon-Tyne NE2 4HH, UK

Stephen J. Harland
Senior Lecturer in Medical Oncology, Institute of Urology and Nephrology, University College London, UK

George B. Haycock
Professor of Paediatrics, Department of Paediatrics, Guy's Hospital, St. Thomas Street, London SE1 9RT, UK

Nicholas J. Hegarty
Surgical Professorial Unit, University College Dublin, 47 Eccles Street, Dublin 7, Ireland

Paul G. Horgan
Lecturer in Surgery, University College Dublin, 47 Eccles Street, Dublin 7, Ireland

Mark I. Johnson
Department of Surgery, School of Surgical Sciences, The Medical School, University of Newcastle, Newcastle-upon-Tyne NE2 4HH, UK

John A. Kirby
Senior Lecturer in Transplant Immunology, Department of Surgery, The Medical School, University of Newcastle, Newcastle-upon-Tyne NE2 4HH, UK

T. R. Leyshon Griffiths
Department of Surgery, School of Surgical Sciences, The Medical School, University of Newcastle, Newcastle-upon-Tyne NE2 4HH, UK

Thomas H. Lynch
Senior Registrar in Urology, Mater Misericordiae Hospital and University College Dublin, 47 Eccles Street, Dublin, Ireland

Eamonn R. Maher
Department of Pathology, University of Cambridge, Tennis Court Road, Cambridge CB2 1QP, UK and Division of Medical and Molecular Genetics, Department of Paediatrics and Child Health, University of Birmingham Medical School, Edgbaston, Birmingham B15 2TT, UK

Julie A. Morris
Senior Medical Statistician, Department of Medical Statistics, University Hospital of South Manchester, Withington Hospital, Nell Lane, Manchester M20 8LR, UK

Anthony R. Mundy
Professor of Urology, Institute of Urology and Nephrology, 48 Riding House Street, London W1P 7PN, UK

David E. Neal
Department of Surgery, School of Surgical Sciences, The Medical School, University of Newcastle, Newcastle-upon-Tyne NE2 4HH, UK

Guy H. Neild
Professor of Nephrology, Institute of Urology and Nephrology, Middlesex Hospital, Mortimer Street, London W1N 8AA, UK

M. Constance Parkinson
Consultant Histopathologist, University College London Hospitals Trust and Institute of Urology U.C.L., Rockefeller Building, University Street, London WC1E 6JJ, UK

John P. Pryor
Consultant Uroandrologist, The Lister Hospital, Chelsea Bridge Road, London SW1 8RH, UK and Reader, Institute of Urology and Nephrology, Middlesex Hospital, University College London, UK

Craig N. Robson
Lecturer in Urological Sciences, Department of Surgery, School of Surgical Sciences, The Medical School, University of Newcastle, Newcastle-upon-Tyne NE2 4HH, UK

Rosemary L. Ryall
Professor of Urological Research and Chief Medical Scientist, Department of Surgery, Flinders Medical Centre, Bedford Park, SA 5042, Australia

Martin O. Savage
Professor of Paediatric Endocrinology, St. Bartholomew's Hospital, West Smithfield, London EC1A 7BE, UK

C. Sultan
Professor of Paediatric Endocrinology, Endocrinologie/Gynécologie Pédiatrique, Service de Pédiatric l'Hôpital A. de Villeneuve, 34259 Montpellier, France

David F. M. Thomas
Consultant Paediatric Urologist, Department of Paediatric Surgery, Clinical Sciences Building, St. James's University Hospital and General Infirmary, Leeds LS9 7TF, UK

Suzanne N. Venn
Institute of Urology and Nephrology, 48 Riding House Street, London W1N 7PN, UK

Leonie S. Young
Surgical Professorial Unit, University College Dublin, 47 Eccles Street, Dublin 7, Ireland

Preface

For even the most junior urological trainee learning the basic medical sciences is all but a distant memory. Since then the sciences have changed as knowledge has advanced and whole new disciplines have developed. The focus of a urological trainee is, in any case, fundamentally different from a student just beginning his or her medical education who must have a grounding in order to be equipped to comprehend the whole field of medicine and surgery in the ensuing few years of undergraduate medical training. So, even discounting all that a trainee urologist has forgotten, there is a great deal of new knowledge to acquire and a specifically urological perspective from which to view that knowledge.

Five years ago the Editors were asked to organise an annual course on 'The Scientific Basis of Urology'. The aim was to address basic science in urology from just this perspective and to take account of the recent changes in the scope and format of medical and surgical undergraduate and postgraduate examinations, as a result of which the student and subsequently the trainee is no longer expected to have such a detailed knowledge of these subjects as used to be expected. This annual course is sponsored by the *British Association of Urological Surgeons* and the *British Journal of Urology* and is regarded nowadays as mandatory for all urological trainees during the first two years of training. It is evidence of how highly we regard the importance of a grounding in basic science for training in clinical urology.

This book arose from the course, although some of the authors have not taught on the course, some of the course teachers are not authors here, and the titles of the chapters in this book do not match closely with the titles of the lectures on the course. This is because we have tried to make the scientific material more clinically relevant with a wider audience in mind. In this way we hope to make this book interesting to all practising urologists, although we should stress that although many of the chapters address specific disease conditions the authors cover only the scientific aspects. Details of diagnosis and treatment will have to be sought elsewhere. Equally, this book does not aim to be comprehensive. We have tried to keep it to a size that a reader, with an average attention span, might expect to read in its entirety rather than let the book expand to a size that would confine it to a dusty shelf. Indeed some of the more basic 'basic sciences' have been skated over to a degree that the purist might find objectionable. We have aimed the text, however, at the specifically urological audience who, we think, wants to be able to understand these particular topics without necessarily acquiring any great depth of knowledge. Hence, also, the use of recommended reading lists in such chapters rather than the more traditional list of references.

The Editors have all learnt a great deal from the exercise of preparing the annual courses and now from the preparation of this book. For those who have attended the courses and have nagged us (incessantly) for the book during its preparation – here it is, and thank you for giving us the opportunity to benefit from the whole teaching process as well.

A. R. Mundy
London, 22nd December, 1998

An introduction to cell biology

A. R. Mundy

Introduction

For many urologists, the mere mention of the words cell and molecular biology is sufficient to induce a state of anxiety. It is a recent and changing science with an unfamiliar and often confusing jargon. Nonetheless, even these same urologists appreciate that it is impossible to escape the subject altogether if one is to understand many of the recent developments in urology, especially in the field of urological oncology.

The aim of this chapter is to present the subject from a specifically urological viewpoint so that the reader might be better able to understand some of the discussion in later chapters of this volume. Some of the more important or key terms are highlighted in italic to draw attention to them as they may be unfamiliar to some. Also, suggested reading material is given at the end of the chapter, rather than using specific references in the text as is usual as these are unlikely to be helpful to the clinical urologist.

This first chapter deals with events outside the nucleus while Chapter 2 deals with the nucleus and cell division. The purpose of this chapter is to describe the mechanisms that hold cells, and therefore tissues, together and how cells communicate, and so provide the basis for understanding, for example, how organs can distend and collapse as the bladder does during filling and emptying; how the mechanisms that hold cells together can be broken down in tumour invasion; and how different cells communicate at a local level as in the stromal–epithelial interaction in benign prostatic hyperplasia or in the development of neoplasia. In essence, the purpose is to outline those aspects of cellular structure and function that are important when considering the relationship between one cell and another and between cells and the extracellular matrix. The interface in both instances is the cell membrane.

The cell membrane

The cell membrane and the membranes of intracellular organelles all have a very similar structure (Figure 1.1), although there is considerable variation in detail from cell to cell in different tissues. The principal components are lipids and proteins. Forty per cent to 80% of the cell membrane is lipid and 50% is phospholipid. The protein content is much more variable – anything from a $0.2:1$ protein to lipid ratio in cells in the central nervous system, in which electrical insulation is important, to a $3.2:1$ ratio in mitochondrial membranes, where metabolic activity is particularly high. Cell membranes essentially depend on lipids for their structure and on proteins for their function. These proteins are of two types. There are integral proteins that span the full thickness of the cell membrane from the exterior to the cytosol, such as the transmembrane signalling proteins; and there are peripheral proteins that are adherent to the cytosolic aspect of the cell membrane, such as the structural proteins related to the cytoskeleton.

The phospholipids that form the cell membrane are arranged in two layers, with a hydrophilic head and a hydrophobic tail. The hydrophilic head faces outwards to the exterior on the outer leaflet and

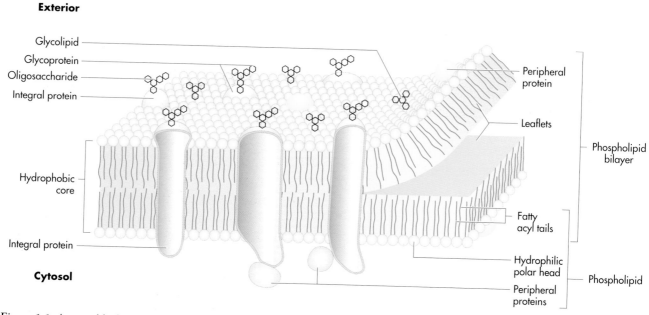

Figure 1.1 *A typical biological membrane. Two leaflets of phospholipids are orientated with their hydrophilic polar heads like the bread of a sandwich and the fatty acyl tails like the filling of a sandwich. Integral proteins span the full thickness of the lipid bilayer and peripheral proteins attach onto them (generally) on the cytosolic aspect of the cell membrane. Sugars are generally located as oligosaccharide glycoproteins or glycolipids bound to the external aspect of the integral proteins. (Modified from Darnell J, Lodish H, Baltimore D. Molecular cell biology, second edition. New York: Scientific American Books, 1990.)*

inwards to the cytosol on the inner leaflet, and the hydrophobic tails of the phospholipids of both leaflets face inwards to the centre of the membrane. This orientation in the form of a 'lipid sandwich' is particularly important when considering transmembrane signalling and membrane transport in general – How do molecules get through the lipid layer?

It is important to appreciate that the membrane is fluid – it is a viscous gel. This means that the proteins and phospholipids can move around within the membrane gel; indeed, they can move very rapidly in some instances.

The phospholipids of the cell membrane are variable and numerous, but the principal ones in most cell membranes are: phosphatidylcholine, phosphatidylinositol, phosphatidylethanolamine and phosphatidylserine. Although principally subserving a structural role, some of these molecules take part in important functional activities, as described below. Not all metabolic function is related to the protein component.

The sugar component of the cell membrane is small. The vast majority of sugars are related to the external aspect of the cell membrane or to the internal aspect of organelles. Outside the cell, these are mostly oligosaccharides, glycoproteins or glycolipids (which are discussed in more detail below).

Membrane transport

Transport may be passive or active. Passive transport processes do not require energy; examples include the diffusion of gases such as oxygen and carbon dioxide and of small uncharged molecules down a concentration gradient, and of water down an osmotic gradient.

Diffusion of specific molecules such as glucose and certain amino acids – molecules that either are too big to diffuse or for which a speedier process is needed – may be *facilitated* by *multipass transmembrane proteins*.

Sometimes, the transport of one molecule across a membrane by a facilitator molecule is linked, or *coupled*, to the movement of another (Figure 1.2). If both molecules move in the same direction, the co-transport molecule is known as a symport; if the movement of the two molecules is in opposite directions, the co-transport molecule is called an antiport.

Active transport consumes energy, usually generated by the hydrolysis of adenosine triphosphate (ATP). Sodium–potassium adenosine triphosphatase (ATPase) is a multipass transmembrane protein (Figure 1.3) enzyme that exchanges sodium for potassium so as to maintain intracellular potassium at 20 to 40 times its extracellular concentration and extracellular sodium at 10 to 20 times its intracellular concentration (Figure 1.4). Similar ATPases pump calcium out of cells or into intracellular stores.

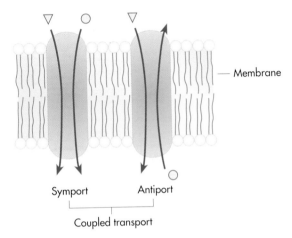

Figure 1.2 *Coupled transport. (Modified from Darnell J, Lodish H, Baltimore D. Molecular cell biology, second edition. New York: Scientific American Books, 1990.)*

The hydrophobic phospholipid membrane is virtually impermeable to ions in aqueous solution. Various systems exist to allow ionic movement to occur. These include *permeases* such as the ATPase enzymes described above. An important mechanism is provided by transmembrane proteins that form aqueous ion channels across the lipid bilayer. They allow ion transport at high speed without expending energy, but although they influence the speed of flow, they do not affect the direction of flow, which is always down a concentration gradient. These transmembrane ion channels are important in transmitting nerve impulses and in muscle contraction. They are all glycoproteins and they all work such that when they are stimulated they undergo a *conformational change* (Figure 1.5) so that a central pore is created through the molecule from one side of the cell membrane to the other, with a hydrophilic lining to allow the passage of water-soluble ions (Figure 1.6).

Stimuli for the conformational change include:

- a change in voltage,
- the binding of another molecule – known as a *ligand* – to the original molecule,
- mechanical deformation (in some cells),
- gap junction activation (described below).

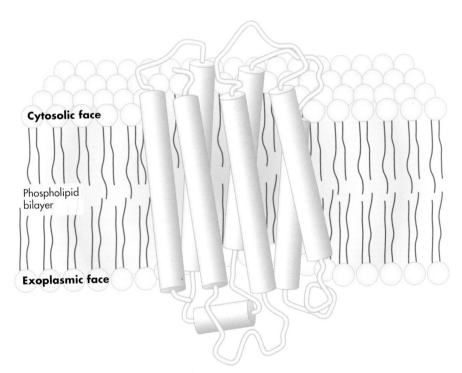

Figure 1.3 *The general structure of a multipass transmembrane protein. The transmembrane helices are here represented as cylinders spanning the phospholipid bilayer. (Modified from Darnell J, Lodish H, Baltimore D. Molecular cell biology, second edition. New York: Scientific American Books, 1990.)*

Extracellular space

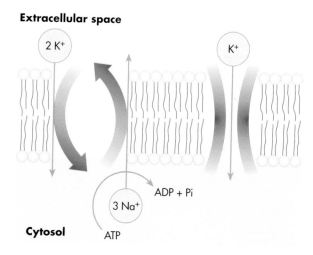

Cytosol

Figure 1.4 *Two classes of membrane transport proteins. On the left, active transport mediated by sodium/potassium ATPase; on the right, passive transport through potassium channel-forming proteins. (Modified from Goodman SR. Medical cell biology. Philadelphia: JB Lippincott Company, 1994.)*

Extracellular space

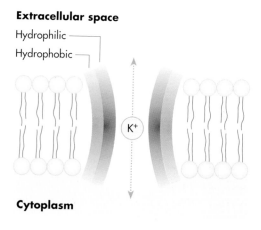

Cytoplasm

Figure 1.6 *An aqueous channel-forming protein. The hydrophilic portion of the molecule lines the pore and the hydrophobic portion is interposed between the hydrophilic lining and the surrounding membrane lipid. (Modified from Goodman SR. Medical cell biology. Philadelphia: JB Lippincott Company, 1994.)*

Extracellular space

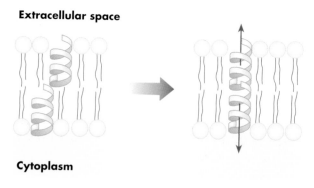

Cytoplasm

Figure 1.5 *A transmembrane channel developing as two peptides dimerise head to head (in this case) to span the lipid bilayer. (Modified from Sawyer DB, Koepp ER, Andersen O. Biochemistry 1989; 28: 6571.)*

Opening and closing the protein channel is called *gating* (Figure 1.7) and so there are *voltage-gated channels*, *ligand-gated channels* and *mechanically-gated channels* and different channels exist both for different stimuli and for different ions.

These ion channels make cells electrically excitable. Cells maintain slightly more negative than positive ions in the cytosol and slightly more positive than negative ions in the extracellular fluid. This causes a voltage difference across the lipid membrane, which is a poor conductor because of its lipid content and therefore allows the voltage difference to exist. This *resting membrane potential* – largely caused by

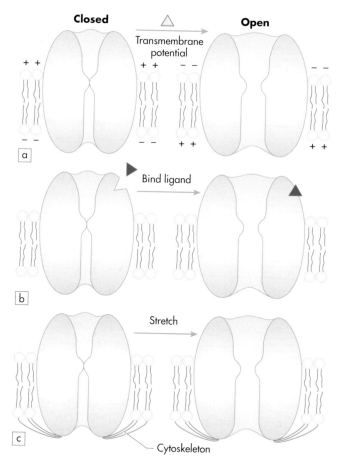

Figure 1.7 *Diagrammatic view of three different types of ion channels stimulated by different gating mechanisms. (a) Voltage-gated ion channel. (b) Ligand-gated receptor. (c) Mechanically gated channel. (Modified from Kandel ER, Schwartz JH, Jessell TM. Principles of neural science, third edition. New York: Elsevier, 1991.)*

sodium–potassium ATPase – is the driving force for many biochemical processes.

The cytoskeleton

The cytoskeleton has an important role in maintaining the integrity of the cell membrane and is also involved in cell–cell and cell–matrix adhesions. It stops major deformation of the cell membrane when contraction of the cell pulls on the inner aspect of the cell membrane or when distension, adhesion and other forces pull on the outside of the cell membrane.

Within the cell there is a meshwork of filaments of different types that run from one side of the cell to the other, mainly the thin filaments and intermediate filaments. On the inner aspect of the cell membrane there is a scaffolding of proteins that supports the cell membrane in the way that rafters support a roof or poles support the canvas of a tent (Figure 1.8). This scaffolding is called the *spectrin membrane skeleton* as spectrin is its principal component. It maintains the shape and stability of the cell membrane and was first identified in red blood cells, where it is most elaborately developed. It is now known to be ubiquitous.

There are three main types of filaments involved in the cytoskeleton: microtubules, thin filaments and intermediate filaments. Thick filaments, which are principally myosin, are contractile rather than structural and are only found in significant concentrations in muscle cells. The principal thin filament is actin, which is also mainly known for its contractile role in muscle cells but is an essential structural component of the cytoskeleton of most cells. The intermediate filaments are the most variable in composition, with different types in smooth muscle, fibroblasts and epithelia. Microtubules that are composed of tubulin are principally important in intracellular transport, especially in neurons and in the activity of villi and cilia.

Microfilaments
Microfilaments include actin, tropomyosin and caldesmon. The most important is actin, which forms 5% to 30% of the total protein content of non-

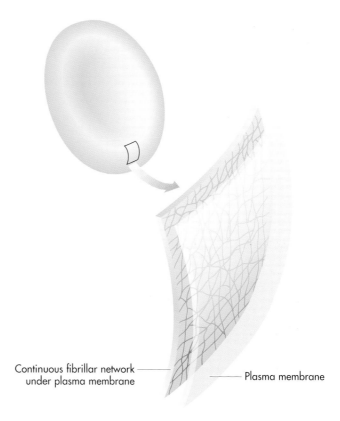

Continuous fibrillar network under plasma membrane — Plasma membrane

Figure 1.8 The membrane cytoskeleton in relation to the plasma membrane, in this case in a red blood cell. A continuous fibrillar network of spectrin molecules links to integral membrane proteins on the under aspect of the plasma membrane. (Modified from Darnell J, Lodish H, Baltimore D. Molecular cell biology, second edition. New York: Scientific American Books, 1990.)

muscle cells. It is a globular and contractile protein component of the cytoskeleton and its role in the cell can be compared to the muscular element of the musculoskeletal system of the body as a whole. It links to the membrane scaffolding system and to adjacent cells or extracellular proteins, as described below; it forms the contraction ring that separates the two daughter cells in cell division; and it controls the gel–sol state of cytoplasm and so allows cells to change their shape or move.

Intermediate filaments
These, by comparison, correspond to the ligaments in the musculoskeletal system of the human body. They are heterogeneous fibrous proteins that bind one cell to another or to the extracellular membrane (as do the microfilaments) by means of transmembrane *linker* proteins or protein complexes. The best known of the

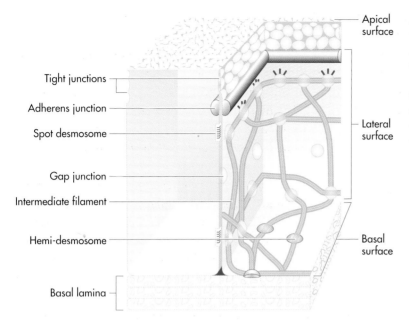

Tight junctions

Adherens junction

Spot desmosome

Gap junction

Intermediate filament

Hemi-desmosome

Basal lamina

Apical surface

Lateral surface

Basal surface

Figure 1.9 *The principal types of cell junctions: tight junctions at the apices of cells, adherens junctions below, spot desmosomes between cells, and desmosomes between cells and the basal lamina, all interlinked by intermediate filaments. Gap junctions join adjacent cells. (Modified from Darnell J, Lodish H, Baltimore D. Molecular cell biology, second edition. New York: Scientific American Books, 1990.)*

intermediate filaments are keratin in epithelial cells, vimentin in fibroblasts, and desmin which coexists with vimentin in smooth muscle cells.

Cell to cell adhesion

Cell to cell adhesion is mediated by different types of *junctions*. The mains ones are: tight junctions, anchoring junctions (or desmosomes) and communicating (or gap) junctions (Figure 1.9). These junctions are usually proteinaceous and their integrity is commonly calcium dependent. There are various *adhesion molecules*, which again are mainly proteinaceous and calcium dependent in their action, of which the best known are the *cadherins*. These are the glue that holds the junctions together. In epithelia, the principal adhesion molecule is *E-cadherin* (also known as uvomorulin). In different cell types there are different cadherins and there are also adhesion molecules that are not calcium dependent in their action, but proteinaceous and calcium-dependent adhesion is the general rule in the urinary tract.

Tight junctions

At a tight junction, adjacent cell membranes actually fuse together (Figure 1.10). Tight junctions are usually close to the apex of cells, particularly in epithelial cell

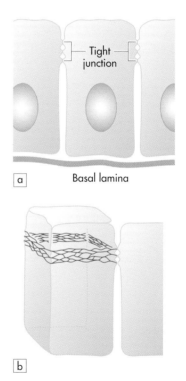

Tight junction

Basal lamina

a

b

Figure 1.10 *A tight junction. (a) The cross-sectional appearance. (b) The circumferential disposition of a tight junction. (Modified from Goodman SR. Medical cell biology. Philadelphia: JB Lippincott Company, 1994.)*

layers, where they form and maintain a watertight seal. They are therefore prominent in a system such as bladder epithelium, where they help avoid backward flux of urinary constituents into the blood stream thereby reversing the effects of renal function. Equally important is the integrity of the intestinal epithelium, for similar reasons, and here tight junctions are also prominent. Tight junctions are formed by calcium-dependent, single-span, transmembrane linker glycoproteins, like cadherins, and the more there are, the more impermeable the junction.

Anchoring junctions

Anchoring junctions are the means by which the cytoskeleton connects, via transmembrane linker proteins and calcium-dependent adhesive molecules, to the cytoskeleton of other cells or to the extracellular matrix. There are two main types of anchoring junctions: one is related to the microfilaments of the cytoskeleton and the other to the intermediate filaments of the cytoskeleton. In each main type there are two subtypes, depending on whether the junctional complex relates to another cell or to the extracellular matrix (Figures 1.11 and 1.12 and Table 1.1).

Microfilamentous junctions with adjacent cells
The microfilament actin commonly produces a band of adhesion around the inside of epithelial cells, close to the apex of the cell and just below the tight junctions mentioned above. This belt of actin filaments circling the periphery of the inside of the cell membrane is commonly known as a *belt desmosome* and depends on cadherins to anchor it to the adjacent cell.

Microfilamentous junctions with the extracellular matrix
Actin links to the extracellular matrix by means of a system of linker proteins that connects the actin to extracellular *fibronectin*, which is an important adhesive glycoprotein in the extracellular matrix (Figure 1.13). In this linker protein complex is another type of cell adhesion molecule, which – like the cadherins – is calcium dependent, called an *integrin*. The integrins are a family of cell adhesion molecules of which one type helps bind cytoskeletal actin to matrix fibronectin. Another type is involved in the binding of

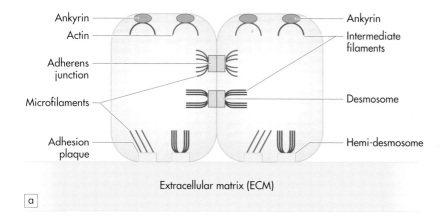

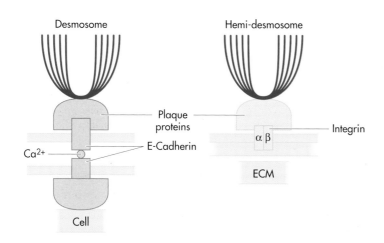

Figure 1.11 *(a,b) The features of desmosomes (between cells) and hemi-desmosomes (between cells and the basement membrane). (Modified from Darnell J, Lodish H, Baltimore D. Molecular cell biology, second edition. New York: Scientific American Books, 1990.)*

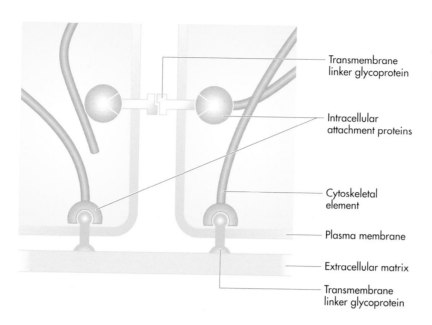

Transmembrane linker glycoprotein

Intracellular attachment proteins

Cytoskeletal element

Plasma membrane

Extracellular matrix

Transmembrane linker glycoprotein

Figure 1.12 *The principal features of adherens junctions: their morphological disposition. (Modified from Goodman SR. Medical cell biology. Philadelphia: JB Lippincott Company, 1994.)*

Table 1.1 The principal features of adherens junctions for each of the main types

Junctional complex	Type	Cytoskeletal element	Transmembrane linker glycoprotein	Intracellular attachment protein
Adhesion belt/ zonula adherens	Cell–cell	Microfilament	Cadherins	Catenins
Focal contacts/ adhesion plaques	Cell–matrix	Microfilament	Fibronectin receptor	Vinculin, talin, and α-actinin
Desmosome/ macula adherens	Cell–cell	Intermediate filament	Desmocollins and desmogleins	Plakoglobin and desmoplakins
Hemi-desmosome	Cell–matrix	Intermediate filament	Laminin receptor	?

Modified from Goodman SR. Medical cell biology. Philadelphia: JB Lippincott Company, 1994.

intermediate filaments to other protein fibres in the extracellular matrix.

Intermediate filamentous junctions with adjacent cells
Intermediate filaments communicate with the intermediate filaments of adjacent cells by means of *spot desmosomes*. These have been likened to 'spot welds' or rivets and are relatively fixed, as are belt desmosomes and tight junctions.

Intermediate filamentous junctions with the extracellular matrix
Intermediate filamentous anchoring junctions to the extracellular matrix are called *hemi-desmosomes*.

Here, the linker protein that joins the intermediate filament to the extracellular matrix is called *laminin*, and the specific protein in the extracellular matrix that laminin links to is type IV collagen in the basement membrane. The laminin receptor complex is another integrin. These anchoring junctions to the basement membrane and to the other proteins of the extracellular matrix are less fixed than anchoring junctions or spot desmosomes between adjacent cells, and the microfilamentous junctions to fibronectin are particularly mobile to allow cell movement in growth and repair and during inflammatory and immune responses. Adhesions should not be thought of as producing rigidity.

Communicating junctions

These are sometimes called *gap junctions*. Gap junctions are composed of protein subunits that connect the inside of one cell, across an 'intercellular gap', to the inside of the adjacent cell across both cell membranes (Figure 1.14). They behave as transmembrane ion channels, which undergo conformational change with the appropriate stimulus to give a central pore (Figure 1.14b), as described above. In this way, small molecules can move between cells and allow them to communicate with each other. This may also account for so-called 'cable properties' in the transmission of electrical impulses in excitable cells such as nerve and smooth muscle.

Because most of these adhesions are proteinaceous and calcium dependent, they are vulnerable to fluctuating extracellular calcium and to proteases – hence the importance of proteases and metalloproteases (which bind a metal as a catalyst), and collagenases in tumour invasion.

The extracellular matrix

The extracellular matrix used to be thought of as an essentially inert ground substance in which cells lay, connecting one cell type to another and one tissue to the next. It is nothing of the sort. Other than providing structural support, it is extremely important in growth, differentiation, nutrition and repair.

There are three principal components of the extracellular matrix: fibrous proteins, especially collagen; the glycosaminoglycans and proteoglycans; and the adhesive glycoproteins, especially laminin and fibronectin, mentioned above.

Collagen

Collagen gives the extracellular matrix tensile strength to resist stretch. It is the single most abundant protein in the animal kingdom and there are at least 12 types, all of which, except Type IV, are fibrous and generally disposed in a cable structure. Types I, II and III are the most abundant. Type II is a particularly important component of cartilage. Types I and III go together

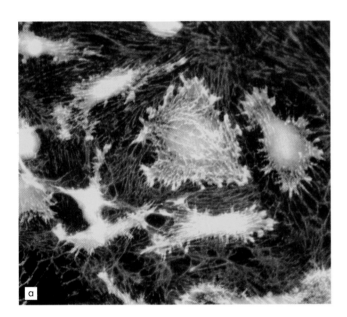

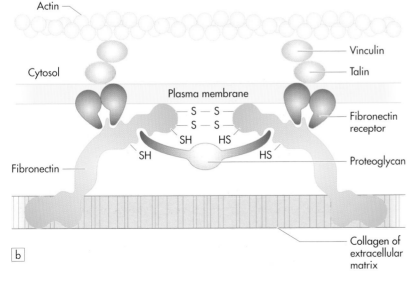

Figure 1.13 (a) *Histochemical illustration of the interrelationship between intracellular actin (stained yellow) and extracellular fibronectin (stained red). (b) The transmembrane linker protein complex. (Modified from Darnell J, Lodish H, Baltimore D. Molecular cell biology, second edition. New York: Scientific American Books, 1990.)*

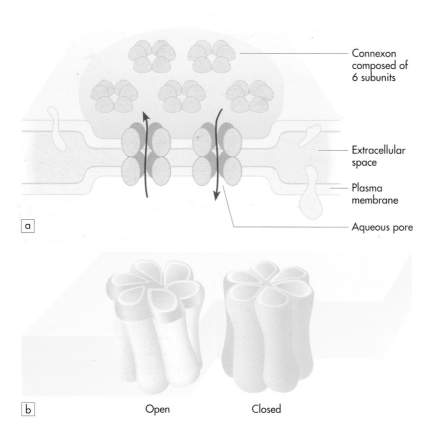

Connexon composed of 6 subunits

Extracellular space

Plasma membrane

Aqueous pore

a

b   Open   Closed

Figure 1.14 *A gap junction: (a) to show the general format, and (b) to show how conformational change of the connexon subunits allows the formation of a transcellular porous channel between neighbouring cells. (Modified from Darnell J, Lodish H, Baltimore D. Molecular cell biology, second edition. New York: Scientific American Books, 1990.)*

and are almost ubiquitous as the main interstitial types in general connective tissue.

Type IV collagen is the main component of the basal lamina. It forms a mesh, which looks like chicken wire and which gives the basal lamina its structure (Figure 1.15). The basal lamina acts as a sheet to which epithelial cells are fixed by means of the specific receptor protein laminin and to which the fibrous proteins and other components of the underlying connective tissue are connected (Figure 1.16).

Glycosaminoglycans and proteoglycans

The principal glycosaminoglycan is *hyaluronic acid*. This is a very long compound composed of repeating disaccharide molecules. Although the most widespread of the glycosaminoglycans, it is different from the remainder, which are sulphated and linked to proteins to form the proteoglycans. These other glycosaminoglycans are chondroitin sulphate, dermatan sulphate, keratan sulphate, heparan sulphate and heparin. Like hyaluronic acid, the other glycosaminoglycans consist of repeating disaccharide molecules, but they are also highly negatively charged. This

means that they tend to attract water and can thereby fill a lot of space in comparison with their actual size. Proteoglycans have the appearance of a bottlebrush in which the core protein is the handle and the glycosaminoglycans are the bristles. They help to anchor cells to matrix fibres, binding to types I and II collagen and to fibronectin. In turn, proteoglycans often bind to hyaluronic acid, also 'bottlebrush' fashion, giving two levels of organisation of these molecules (Figure 1.17).

Like collagen, the glycosaminoglycans provide structural support to the extracellular matrix, but whereas collagen gives tensile strength to resist stretch, the glycosaminoglycans help resist shearing strains and compression. Cartilage is obviously the best example. The glycosaminoglycans tend to keep cells apart and, by virtue of this and their lattice-like structure, they allow the rapid diffusion of nutrients, waste products and signalling molecules through the extracellular matrix. This filtering role is particularly prominent in the kidney, where those of the extracellular matrix are largely responsible for glomerular filtration. Many of them, particularly heparan sulphate

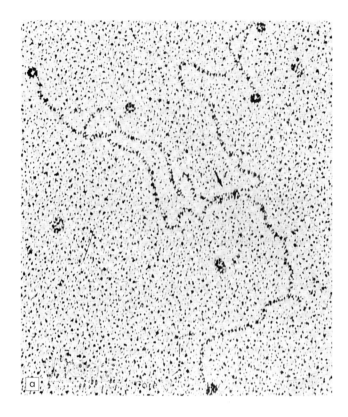

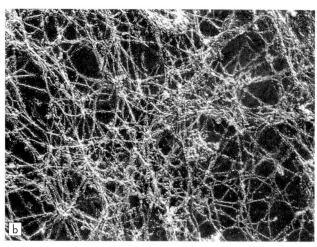

Figure 1.15 (a) The general appearance of a type IV collagen molecule. (b) The general appearance of type IV collagen molecules bound together – like a chicken-wire mesh – to form basement membrane. (Modified from Darnell J, Lodish H, Baltimore D. Molecular cell biology, second edition. New York: Scientific American Books, 1990.)

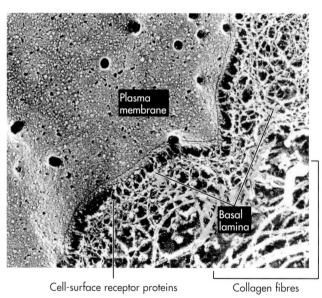

Figure 1.16 The relationship between a cell and the type IV collagen fibres of the basal lamina. (Modified from Darnell J, Lodish H, Baltimore D. Molecular cell biology, second edition. New York: Scientific American Books, 1990.)

and heparin, bind and activate various growth factors (see below), especially *fibroblast growth factor*. In this role, they act both to protect the so-called *heparin binding growth factors* (of which fibroblast growth factor is the best example) against degradation by sequestering them away from the reach of proteolytic enzymes, and also as co-factors to facilitate binding to high-affinity receptors on the cell membrane.

Adhesive glycoproteins

The two main adhesive glycoproteins are laminin and fibronectin. Laminin binds Type IV collagen of the basal lamina to the plasma membrane and to the intermediate filaments of the cytoskeleton through cell-surface laminin receptors and also by means of receptors on both components for heparan sulphate. Fibronectin binds to everything except Type IV collagen, principally to actin in the cytoskeleton using cell-surface fibronectin receptors and transmembrane linker proteins as an intermediary. Fibronectin also binds to fibrous collagen and other extracellular matrix proteins.

Both these glycoproteins help maintain the structural integrity of the extracellular matrix, but they also facilitate the movement of nutrients and waste products and in addition allow cell movement in growth, repair and during inflammatory and immune responses. The fibronectin receptor, in particular,

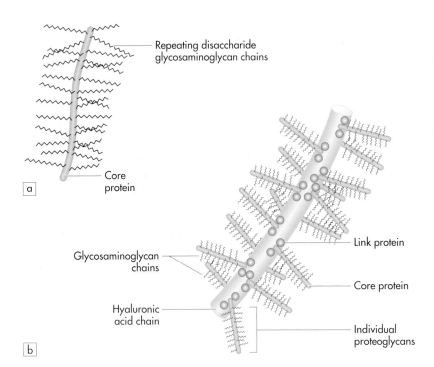

Figure 1.17 *A proteoglycan showing (a) the 'bottlebrush' structure, with glycosaminoglycan chains as the 'bristles' attached to the core protein, and (b) the further 'bottlebrush' structure with individual proteoglycans, as in (a), attached to the central hyaluronic acid chain. (Modified from Alberts B, Bray D, Lewis J et al. Molecular biology of the cell, second edition. New York: Garland Publishing, 1989.)*

allows mobility so that inflammatory and immune cells (for example) can reach out pseudopodia to make contact with fibronectin and then pull themselves along fibronectin fibres to reach their destination by virtue of the mobility of connections made both on the cell membrane and on the fibronectin fibre. In a similar way, fibronectin promotes cell migration during embryogenesis and healing by providing tracks along which the cells can migrate.

Glycoproteins on the cell surface are also important in immune reactivity (described in Chapter 24).

The basement membrane

Viewed under the electron microscope, the basal lamina consists of two layers: the lamina rara, which consists of laminin and the proteoglycans that are interposed between the cell membrane itself; and the lamina densa, which is the two-dimensional reticulum of Type IV collagen. The lamina lucida (or rara) and lamina densa together form the basal lamina, but in many circumstances there is a third layer – the lamina reticularis – which is the underlying connective tissue component. These three laminae together constitute the basement membrane (Figure 1.18).

The basement membrane, in addition to providing

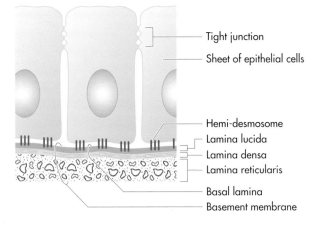

Figure 1.18 *The structural organisation of the basal lamina and the basement membrane. (Modified from Alberts B, Bray D, Lewis J et al. Molecular biology of the cell, second edition. New York: Garland Publishing, 1989.)*

a means by which nutrient, waste and signalling molecules can be transported and cell migration can occur (as described above), is also important in cellular differentiation. In embryogenesis in particular, the mesenchyme – the basal lamina, extracellular matrix and mesodermal cells – is essential. Without the underlying dermal mesenchyme, the overlying 'skin' cannot differentiate into nails, hairs or the cornea, nor can it simply differentiate into thin skin or thick skin. Cunha's studies on prostatic epithelium show that even differentiated epithelium can be 'redifferentiated' in the presence of embryonic mesenchyme; in his experiments, mature bladder epithelium in the presence of male urogenital sinus mesenchyme developed into prostatic epithelium (Figure 1.19).

Similarly, without attachment to fibronectin, smooth muscle cells change from their differentiated phenotype, which contracts, to an undifferentiated proliferative phenotype. For similar reasons, explanted cells grown in vitro tend to group together so that a mixed group of kidney cells, liver cells and other cells will separate out into groups of specific types even when the cell types come from different species. In part, this is because of growth factor binding to the basal lamina and other components of the extracellular matrix, but there are undoubtedly other factors and the details are as yet unknown.

Cell to cell communication

Reference has been made already to cellular adhesion mechanisms and, through the medium of the extracellular matrix, to some of the mechanisms of cell migration. Reference has also been made to the possibility of cell to cell communication through gap (communicating) junctions. Cells also communicate together, locally, by so-called *autocrine* or *paracrine* mechanisms (Figure 1.20). In autocrine signalling, a cell is stimulated through receptors on its cell membrane by signalling molecules it has produced and secreted itself. In paracrine signalling, the same molecules diffuse out into the extracellular space and extracellular matrix and act on cell surface receptors of the cells close by. The best and most specialised example of paracrine signalling is across the neuromuscular junction, but in general the features are very similar to those of endocrine signalling but over very much smaller distances and by means of compounds produced by all cells rather than by highly specialised 'glands'.

Cell to cell signalling

Gap junctions and adhesive junctions are not considered any further here and only brief reference is made to neurotransmission as this is discussed in a later chapter. The main point of this section is to discuss how the huge range of extracellular stimuli act across the cell membrane to regulate enzymes or genes with a similarly wide range of outcomes. The mechanism is

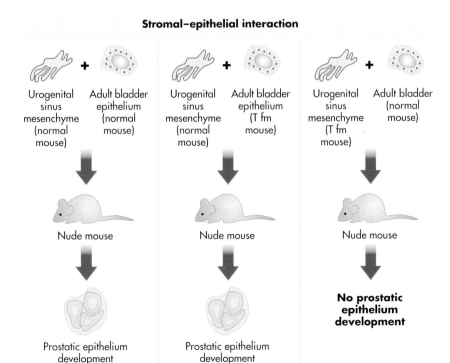

Stromal–epithelial interaction

Figure 1.19 Cunha's experiments. Three experiments are illustrated to show that normally functioning urogenital sinus mesenchyme induces the differentiation or redifferentiation of epithelium so that it develops into prostatic epithelium. Tfm = testicular feminisation syndrome (mice with androgen receptor deficiency).

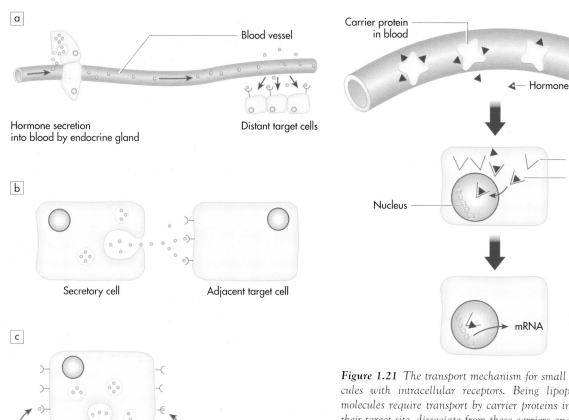

Figure 1.20 The differences between (a) endocrine, (b) paracrine and (c) autocrine signalling. ° Extracellular signal; Υ receptor.

Figure 1.21 *The transport mechanism for small lipid-soluble molecules with intracellular receptors. Being lipophilic, these small molecules require transport by carrier proteins in the blood but, at their target site, dissociate from these carriers and diffuse across the cell membrane with ease. In the cytosol they bind to their specific receptors and the receptor–hormone complex then acts on nuclear DNA. (Modified from Darnell J, Lodish H, Baltimore D. Molecular cell biology, second edition. New York: Scientific American Books, 1990.)*

surprisingly simple. The very numerous extracellular stimuli have an equally large range of receptors on the cell surface but the transmembrane signalling and intracellular transmission systems of these signals are very much fewer in number. With the exception of the steroid hormones and a few other substances that are lipid soluble and can therefore cross the cell membrane with ease (Figure 1.21), most of the remaining signals are transmitted by water-soluble molecules that bind to very specific receptors on the cell surface. There are thousands of these specific receptors, but they transmit their signals through to the interior of the cell by only a few transmembrane signalling mechanisms, which in turn activate just a few intracellular second messenger systems (Figure 1.22). These *second messenger systems* activate proteins, most of which are enzymes, generally by a process of *phosphorylation*.

Phosphorylation involves the activity of protein *kinases* that transfer phosphate groups (usually from ATP) onto the substrate protein, thereby activating it. This activity is in turn 'switched off' by specific *phosphatases* that remove the phosphate group, thereby greatly reducing the activity of the protein/enzyme. Whether the end result of an extracellular signal is gene activation in the nucleus or extracellular secretion from vesicles in the cytoplasm, protein phosphorylation by an appropriate kinase and dephosphorylation by an appropriate phosphatase are the most common end result of signal transduction (Figure 1.23).

Extracellular stimuli

There is a vast range of extracellular stimuli that excite human cells, from light falling on the retina to a sperm cell penetrating an ovum, but the majority fall into

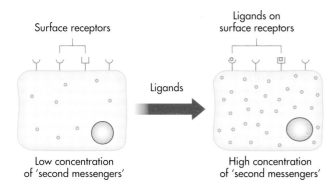

one of two types. The commonest are large, hydrophilic molecules that react directly and with high affinity to cell surface receptors, which in turn activate second messengers in the cytosol, which in turn leads to the intracellular changes characteristic of that particular stimulus.

Secondly, there are small, lipophilic molecules, typically the steroid hormones, that diffuse through the plasma membrane and bind to receptors within the cytosol or the nucleus. These molecules generally act to control the transcription of DNA or the stability of mRNA. Typically, the steroid receptor molecule is in two parts that are hinged so that the receptor becomes folded in on itself, thus concealing the DNA-binding *domain* of the receptor (Figure 1.24). This closed-hinge position is maintained by a steroid inhibitor protein such as a heat shock protein. When the relevant steroid binds to the hormone binding site on the hormone binding domain of the receptor, this

Figure 1.22 *The transport mechanism for large water-soluble molecules by means of cell surface receptors and second messenger systems. These do not need carrier proteins in the blood because they are water soluble, but for the same reason cannot cross the cell membrane – hence the need for the surface receptor/second messenger system. (Modified from Darnell J, Lodish H, Baltimore D. Molecular cell biology, second edition. New York: Scientific American Books, 1990.)*

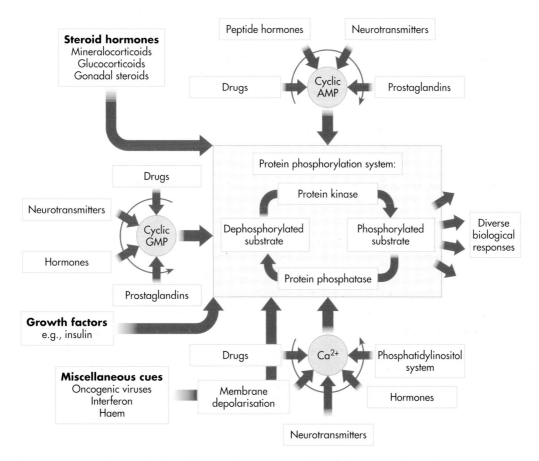

Figure 1.23 *The importance of phosphorylation and dephosphorylation in cellular mechanisms. (Modified from Goodman SR. Medical cell biology. Philadelphia: JB Lippincott Company, 1994.)*

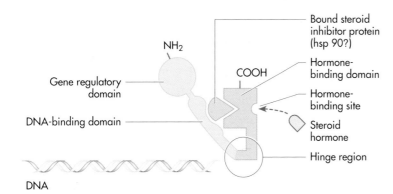

Figure 1.24 *A steroid hormone receptor and receptor activation (i). (Modified from Goodman SR. Medical cell biology. Philadelphia: JB Lippincott Company, 1994.)*

causes the steroid inhibitor protein to be displaced and the hinge opens (i.e. there is a conformational change), so that the receptor molecule opens up, exposing the DNA-binding domain so that it can bind to DNA – to the so-called hormone-responsive element – to initiate transcription (Figure 1.25).

Cell surface receptors

Much more commonly, extracellular stimuli are in the form of larger hydrophilic molecules that, because they are hydrophilic, cannot cross the lipid cell membrane in the way that steroid hormones can. These need to have a system for transmembrane signal transduction to the interior; this system begins with the cell surface receptor.

Receptors come in two main types. The first and simpler type is a single molecule with three functional components or *domains*. The first, or external, domain is an outward-facing recognition site; the second is the transmembrane domain in the middle, which traverses the cell membrane; and the third, or cytosolic, domain is the inward-facing component of the molecule on the interior of the cell, which initiates a mechanism for the onward transmission of the stimulus to the interior (Figure 1.26). This mechanism for onward transmission may be to open a channel for ions to pass through to the interior, as in the case of a *ligand-gated ion channel* like the nicotinic acetylcholine receptor (Figure 1.27), or it may be a kinase (referred to above), which acts by phosphorylating a substrate protein. An example of this latter type of receptor is one with *tyrosine kinase* activity such as the *epidermal growth factor receptor* (Figure 1.28).

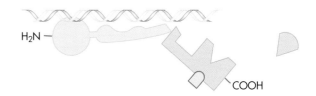

Figure 1.25 *A steroid hormone receptor and receptor activation (ii). Binding of the steroid hormone causes the receptor to 'open up' at its hinge region, allowing it to bind to its appropriate DNA binding site. (Modified from Goodman SR. Medical cell biology. Philadelphia: JB Lippincott Company, 1994.)*

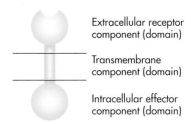

Figure 1.26 *Stylised form of a simple type of transmembrane receptor. (Modified from Darnell J, Lodish H, Baltimore D. Molecular cell biology, second edition. New York: Scientific American Books, 1990.)*

The other main type of receptor system is a relay system in which, rather than having a single receptor molecule to change the extracellular stimulus to an intracellular stimulus, there is a relay consisting of a receptor protein molecule, a coupling protein and an effector protein (Figure 1.29) These receptor proteins, many of the coupling proteins and some of the effector proteins are integral cell membrane proteins referred to earlier in this chapter. In effect, each of the three domains of the simpler receptor system described in the last paragraph is here represented by a separate protein molecule.

In this type of system, the receptor protein is in an

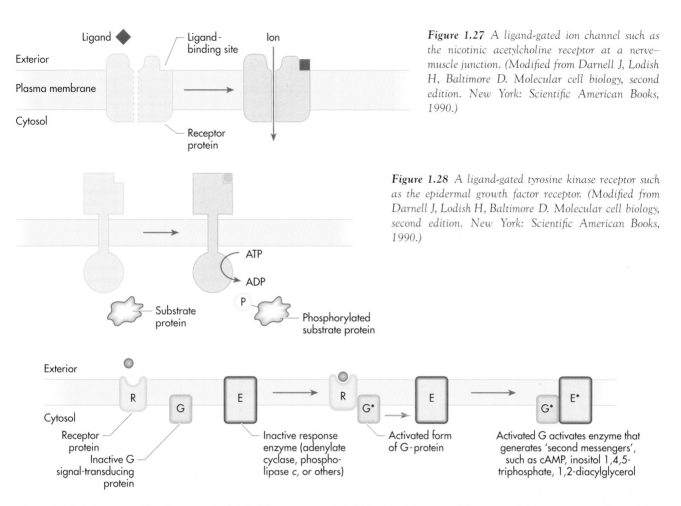

Figure 1.27 *A ligand-gated ion channel such as the nicotinic acetylcholine receptor at a nerve–muscle junction. (Modified from Darnell J, Lodish H, Baltimore D. Molecular cell biology, second edition. New York: Scientific American Books, 1990.)*

Figure 1.28 *A ligand-gated tyrosine kinase receptor such as the epidermal growth factor receptor. (Modified from Darnell J, Lodish H, Baltimore D. Molecular cell biology, second edition. New York: Scientific American Books, 1990.)*

Figure 1.29 *A G-protein-linked receptor. (Modified from Darnell J, Lodish H, Baltimore D. Molecular cell biology, second edition. New York: Scientific American Books, 1990.)*

inactive state until it binds its highly specific stimulatory molecule (the ligand), which it binds with high affinity. Ligand binding activates the receptor, which allows it to activate its specific coupling protein (Figure 1.30). Because the plasma membrane is a fluid gel and because the integral proteins of the cell membrane, including receptor proteins, are mobile, the ligand–receptor complex can activate several coupling proteins. This is the first step in amplifying the stimulus. Many of the coupling proteins are known as *G-proteins* because they have guanosine triphosphatase (GTPase) enzymic activity. The G-protein has three subunits, one of which – the alpha subunit – has a guanosine diphosphate (GDP) molecule bound to it in the inactive state. Binding (coupling) of the ligand–receptor complex to the G-protein catalyses the conversion of intracellular guanosine triphosphate (GTP) to GDP.

This enzymatic conversion of GTP to GDP transfers a phosphate molecule from the intracellular GTP molecule onto the GDP molecule of the alpha subunit of the G-protein, which activates this alpha subunit by converting its own GDP molecule to GTP, thus causing it to separate off from the combined beta-gamma subunit of the G-protein and bind to the effector protein, to which it remains bound until its GTP molecule is hydrolysed back to GDP. When this happens, the alpha subunit of the G-protein dissociates from the effector molecule and recombines with the beta-gamma subunit to restore the G-protein to its unified, inactive state. It is this latter phenomenon that gives this relay system the additional feature of self-limiting duration. The system is only active in stimulating the effector protein for the short period that the alpha subunit of the G-protein is

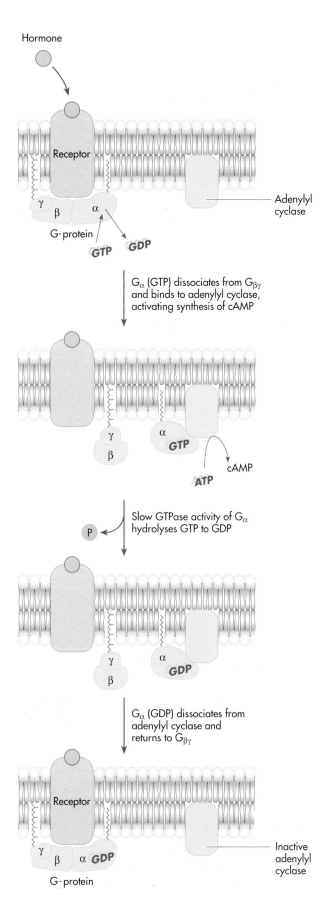

Hormone

Receptor

G-protein

GTP   GDP

Adenylyl cyclase

G$_\alpha$ (GTP) dissociates from G$_{\beta\gamma}$ and binds to adenylyl cyclase, activating synthesis of cAMP

γ

α
GTP

β

cAMP

ATP

Slow GTPase activity of G$_\alpha$ hydrolyses GTP to GDP

P

γ

α
GDP

β

G$_\alpha$ (GDP) dissociates from adenylyl cyclase and returns to G$_{\beta\gamma}$

Receptor

γ

β   α GDP

Inactive adenylyl cyclase

G-protein

activated by having its GDP molecule phosphorylated to GTP. As soon as the GTP reverts to GDP, the system switches itself off.

To recapitulate, the three features of this system are:

1. as with all types of receptor, there exists a common system for onward transmission of a stimulus in which only the receptor molecule needs to be specialised for its own particular ligand;
2. there is an in-built mechanism for amplification of the signal to guarantee a significant cellular response to the initiating signal;
3. there is a mechanism for switching the signal off so that the whole process is self-limiting.

From these observations, one can readily extrapolate the three ways in which the mechanism can break down in a disease such as cancer:

1. if the ligand-binding process goes wrong, becoming persistent rather than transient;
2. if the amplification process goes wrong, again becoming persistent rather than transient;
3. if the switch-off mechanism goes wrong, so that it remains switched on.

There are various different types of *G-protein-coupled receptors*. In some, the effector protein is the enzyme *adenylyl cyclase*. When this is the case, the G-protein may be stimulatory, activating the adenylyl cyclase enzyme, or inhibitory, having the opposite effect (Figure 1.31). In such cases, we have the same effector molecule – adenylyl cyclase – but a different type of G-protein switching it on and off. Examples of receptors that activate adenylyl cyclase are the beta-1 and beta-2 adrenergic receptors. The alpha-2 adrenergic receptor inhibits it. The action of the adenylyl cyclase enzyme is to break down ATP to cyclic adenosine monophosphate (cyclic AMP or cAMP). Cyclic AMP in turn initiates chemical reactions that are specific to the cell type, in which role it is functioning as a second messenger molecule.

Sometimes, the effector protein in a G-protein-coupled receptor is an ion channel such as the hyper-

Figure 1.30 *Activation of a G-protein-linked receptor, in this case an adrenoceptor in which the effector is adenylyl cyclase. (Garrett RH, Grisham CM. Molecular aspects of cell biology. Fort Worth: Harcourt Brace College Publishers, 1995.)*

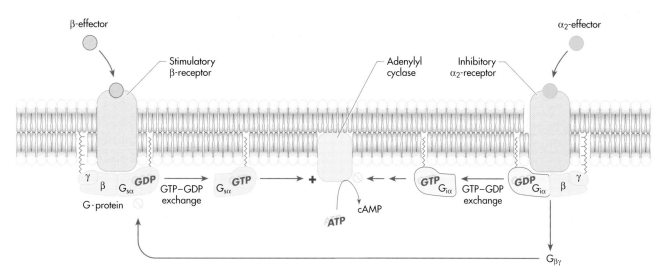

Figure 1.31 *Effector activity – in this case adenylyl cyclase activity – can be modulated by the interplay of stimulatory (Gs) and inhibitory (Gi) G-proteins, in this case the β-receptor and α₂-receptor, respectively. (Garrett RH, Grisham CM. Molecular aspects of cell biology. Fort Worth: Harcourt Brace College Publishers, 1995.)*

polarising potassium channel opened by the M2 muscarinic receptor. In this circumstance, the alpha subunit of the activated G-protein binds to the effector molecule, which then undergoes a conformational change so that it develops a central pore through which potassium ions flow from one side of the cell membrane to the other.

Many receptors, including the muscarinic receptor, have several simultaneous and complementary effects (Figure 1.32)

Another important effector molecule is the enzyme *phospholipase C* (Figure 1.33). This molecule breaks down phosphatidylinositol 4,5-biphosphate (PIP₂), which is derived from one of the membrane phospholipids, phosphatidylinositol, referred to at the beginning of this chapter. Splitting PIP₂ liberates two molecules, both of which are second messengers. The first is *inositol 1,4,5-triphosphate* (IP₃), which is active within the cytosol as a second messenger, and the second is *1,2-diacylglycerol* (DAG), which remains membrane bound in its role as a second messenger. IP₃ acts to release calcium, which is itself a second messenger, from intracellular stores.

All of these second messenger systems – cyclic AMP, cyclic guanosine monophosphate (GMP), DAG, IP₃, and calcium – have many different effects but in any particular system those effects are governed by the type of cell that is stimulated. Calcium, for

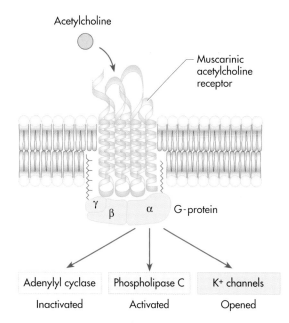

Figure 1.32. *Various actions of the muscarinic acetylcholine receptor. (Garrett RH, Grisham CM. Molecular aspects of cell biology. Fort Worth: Harcourt Brace College Publishers, 1995.)*

example, will make muscle cells contract, the epithelial cells of the salivary glands secrete, and the cells of the islets of Langerhans in the pancreas produce insulin, to give but a few examples. Cyclic AMP will cause the breakdown of glycogen in liver cells, where its action is stimulatory, and will cause smooth muscle cells to relax, in which case its action is

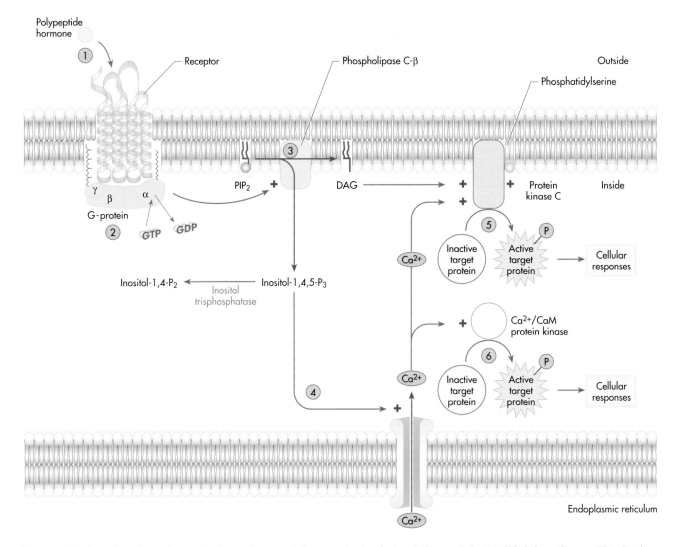

Figure 1.33 *IP$_3$-mediated signal transduction pathway and the central role of phospholipase C-β. (Modified from Garrett RH, Grisham CM. Molecular aspects of cell biology. Fort Worth: Harcourt Brace College Publishers, 1995.) (1) The receptor is activated by ligand binding. (2) This activates its G-protein, which in turn activates (3) phospholipase C-β. This has two effects: firstly (4), the production of inositol-1,4, 5-triphosphate which binds to calcium channel receptors on the endoplasmic reticulum to cause the liberation of calcium (Ca^{2+}). The second action of phospholipase C-β is to stimulate by means of diacylglycerol (DAG), in conjunction with calcium. (5) Protein kinase C activates its particular target proteins, and calcium bound with calmodulin activates its own target proteins (6), and both produce appropriate cellular responses.*

inhibitory. Thus, a very small number of second messenger systems can produce different effects according to the cell type that they are being generated in.

The reader should also bear in mind that examples are largely being chosen to illustrate the subject from a urological perspective. In a book with a different readership in mind, different examples would be given and the emphasis would be placed on the second messengers, receptor types and extracellular stimuli appropriate to that alternative perspective.

Inositol triphosphate and calcium

These are two very important second messengers, particularly with respect to detrusor smooth muscle as rises in intracellular calcium are the basis of detrusor smooth muscle contraction. The liberation of IP$_3$ from PIP$_2$ in the cell membrane by the action of phospholiphase C following activation of phospholiphase C by its appropriate G-protein in response to ligand binding of the receptor molecule has already been described. In the case of detrusor contraction, the ligand is acetylcholine and the receptor molecule is the M3 muscarinic receptor. The IP_3 thus liberated binds to receptor proteins on intracellular calcium stores. These receptors are ligand-gated ion channels that release stored intracellular calcium into the cytosol. As with other second messenger systems, the binding of IP_3 to its receptor is highly specific but of short duration and lasts only until the IP_3 is metabolised to inactive IP_2. Whilst the IP_3 is bound to its receptor, calcium is released from intracellular stores into the cytoplasm. When IP_3 is converted to IP_2, the calcium channel closes off and the IP_2 is recycled to IP_3.

To replenish intracellular calcium stores and also further to increase intracellular calcium, some IP_3 is metabolised to IP_4, which opens cell membrane calcium channels from the inside. These let calcium in from outside the cell.

In addition to its own actions, calcium activates the DAG liberated in the same chemical reaction that produced its 'parent' IP_3 but which has been left in the cell membrane. DAG in turn activates a protein kinase – protein kinase C – which produces an array of intracellular responses by phosphorylating various substrate proteins (see below and also Figure 1.33).

The calcium liberated into the cytosol is bound to a protein called *calmodulin* and it is the calcium–calmodulin complex, thereby activated (Figure 1.34), that produces the effect rather than calcium itself in most instances. In smooth muscle, calcium–calmodulin produces contraction, but the reader should remember that in other systems calcium–calmodulin produces other effects, as referred to above.

The system of smooth muscle contraction is described in Chapter 6 (Figure 1.35). It should be noted at this stage that this excitatory system that starts with IP_3 in smooth muscle is inhibited by adenylyl cyclase and cAMP in the same system, and so we see another feature of the second messenger system – that almost all of the second messengers are interrelated to modulate the final response of the cell. Not only is each signal transduction system specific, amplifying and self-regulatory, but stimulatory and inhibitory systems interact at several points to produce a finely tuned response. A description or illustration in a book is two dimensional and generally shows just one reaction taking place. In real life, most

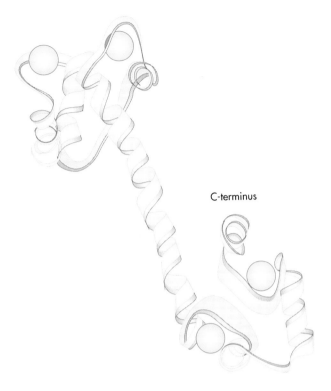

C-terminus

Figure 1.34 Structure of calmodulin as deduced from crystallographic analysis of the calcium–calmodulin complex. The blue spheres are bound calcium ions. (Modified from Darnell J, Lodish H, Baltimore D. Molecular cell biology, second edition. New York: Scientific American Books, 1990.)

reactions depend upon a critical amount of stimulus producing the appropriate response by producing the relevant intracellular changes at the right time and for the correct duration. The system described here does just this. To recapitulate with an example: when a single neuronal impulse travels down a terminal nerve ending to the detrusor, an aliquot of about 5000 acetylcholine molecules is liberated from the axonal terminus at each neuromuscular junction to bind with the same number of receptor molecules on the smooth muscle cell membrane. This process is repeated as long as nerve impulses are being generated. Because the muscarinic receptor protein is mobile within the cell membrane, each ligand–receptor complex within the neuromuscular junction activates several G-proteins, maybe a dozen or so, before the acetylcholine is displaced or metabolised. Each activated G-protein probably only activates one phospholipase C molecule, but until the alpha subunit of the G-protein is deactivated again, each phospholipase C

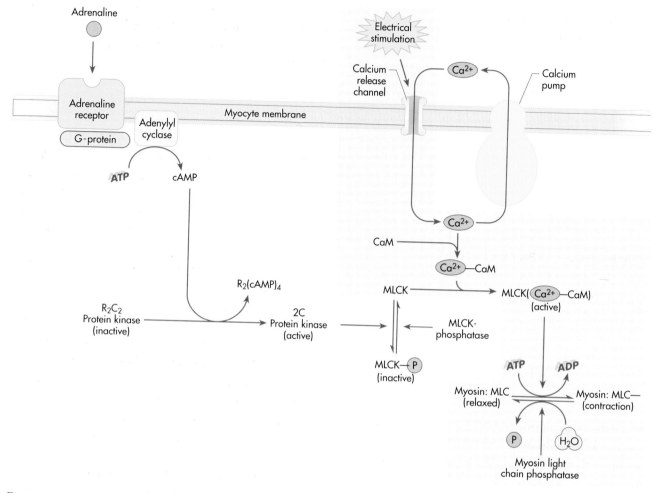

Figure 1.35 *The biochemical basis of smooth muscle contraction. CaM = calmodulin. MLCK = myosin light-chain kinase. (Modified from Garrett RH, Grisham CM. Molecular aspects of cell biology. Fort Worth: Harcourt Brace College Publishers, 1995.)*

molecule will catalyse the breakdown of several molecules of PIP_2 – again, maybe a dozen or more. Each PIP_2 molecule liberates a molecule of IP_3 (and a molecule of DAG) which in turn liberate a considerable number of calcium ions and activate several molecules of protein kinase C, respectively. The calcium liberated in the former reaction helps to potentiate the activation of the protein kinase C in the latter reaction and the liberation of calcium not only produces its own effect – contraction – through further intracellular activity, but also opens membrane calcium channels to let more calcium in, to potentiate the response and to refurbish the intracellular calcium stores.

One factor that makes calcium so important as an intracellular ion is its presence in the cytosol in such low concentrations. Whereas there are ten-fold to 20-fold differences in sodium concentration and 30-fold to 40-fold differences in potassium concentration across the cell membrane, there is a 10 000-fold difference in calcium ion concentration across the cell membrane keeping the intracellular calcium concentration at around 1 micromolar. This concentration is so low that even a few calcium ions released into the cytosol will make a large difference in the concentration. The calcium concentration is kept so low by active pumping of calcium either out of the cytosol and out of the cell altogether through the cell membrane, or out of the cytosol and into intracellular calcium stores where it is sequestered and bound to the sequestering protein *caldesmon* (as described above).

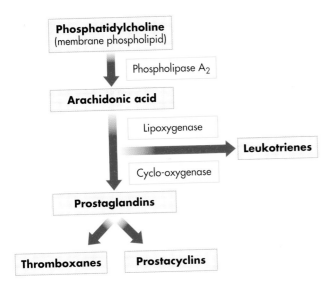

Figure 1.36 The eicosanoids and their derivation from arachidonic acid.

Other compounds derived from membrane phospholipids

The reader will appreciate the importance of the enzyme phospholipase C and the products of its reaction with the membrane phospholipid phosphatidylinositol. Another important phospholipase enzyme – phospholipase A_2 – also acts on membrane phospholipids, in response to a wide range of stimuli, to produce the *eicosanoids*. The eicosanoids are three groups of compounds: the *prostaglandins*, the *thromboxanes* and the *leukotrienes* (Figure 1.36). The parent molecule produced by the action of phospholipase A2 is *arachidonic acid*, which is a polyunsaturated fatty acid. The eicosanoids are all lipid-soluble, freely diffusible, oxygenated molecules with effects, in general terms, that are associated with inflammation, injury and nociception.

The prostaglandins are the best-known products of the arachidonic acid cascade. They are lipid-soluble molecules that are unusual in that they bind to cell surface receptors rather than diffuse through the cell membrane like other small, lipophilic molecules such as the steroid hormones. There are 16 prostaglandins in nine classes designated PGA to PGI, although the latter are generally known as the prostacyclins. The prostaglandins and thromboxanes, which are prosta-

glandin derivatives, are synthesised and secreted continuously by many cells. They act locally in both an autocrine and a paracrine fashion and are broken down by enzymes in the extracellular fluid.

Tyrosine kinase receptors

These have already been referred to as a fairly simple form of signal transduction system in which the same molecule has an extracellular domain for receptor binding, a transmembrane component and an intracellular domain that acts as a tyrosine kinase to phosphorylate tyrosine residues on substrate protein. These are very unusual: most residues on intracellular proteins that generate a second messenger response are either serine or threonine residues; tyrosine residues are unusual. They are of particular interest, though, because they are the principal receptors for the so-called *growth factors*. The intracellular response to the tyrosine kinase receptors is not entirely clear but involves the *ras* protein, which is a sort of G-protein, and *raf* protein, which is activated by reaction with the *ras* protein to activate intermediaries which in turn activate the so-called *mitogen-activated protein kinase* (MAP kinase), which phosphorylates a number of transcription factors including the *fos*, *myc* and *jun* proteins to initiate gene transcription (see below).

Thus, whereas most of the other receptors described produce an intracytoplasmic response appropriate to the cell type, such as contraction or secretion, the tyrosine kinase receptors tend to lead to cell division – they are *mitogenic*.

Growth factors

There is a large number of known growth factors and this number has been growing exponentially in recent years. There is a wide variety of different chemical types of growth factors, all of which include among their actions the ability to stimulate cell proliferation, which may be the only feature they have in common. It is important to appreciate that all growth factors have other effects besides stimulation of cell proliferation and that they are no more related than members of a football team who put on the same shirt once a week when they actually play football.

Growth factors were initially identified in serum as the factors necessary to grow cells in culture – hence their collective name – where growth refers to expansion of number rather than increase in size. It has always been known that serum is necessary to allow cells to replicate in culture rather than just survive, and because plasma does not have the same effect, it was assumed that the relevant factor(s) was liberated from platelets during the process of clotting. As a result, one of the first growth factors to be identified was called *platelet-derived growth factor* (PDGF). Insulin was also known to be necessary for the growth of cells in culture. Slowly, other factors were identified so that it is now possible to grow certain cell types with individual growth factor ingredients specific to that cell type rather than adding whole serum (although this is much cheaper and simpler).

The various growth factors are wildly dissimilar in many ways, but it was observed that groups of two or three or more often produced a similar sort of response, and so growth factors became grouped into families. Most growth factors in a family have molecules which are three-dimensionally similar and it is thought that this three-dimensional similarity means that there are chemical or physico-chemical regions on the molecules that produce the functional effect and give similarity in action to members of the same family group. Thus, in the *epidermal growth factor* (EGF) family (EGF being one of the first growth factors to be identified), *transforming growth factor alpha* (TGFα) has similar actions and a similar three-dimensional structure to EGF (Figure 1.37).

It should also be noted that the names given to these growth factors relate to the effect originally observed rather than to their current family grouping or to any other effects that they may have. Thus, for example, it was observed that two factors were acting in a particular experiment to cause cells to grow in the centre of an agar gel without any physical attachment, a condition which hitherto had been thought to be necessary for cell growth. Because the factors had caused the cells to be 'transformed' in this way, they were called TGFα and TGFβ. It later became clear that TGFα and TGFβ had completely different properties,

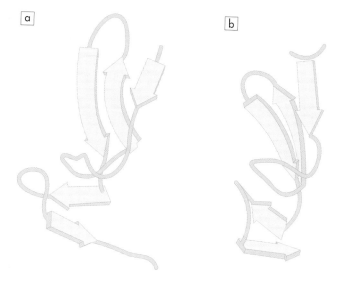

Figure 1.37 *The three-dimensional similarity of (a) epidermal growth factor (EFG) and (b) transforming growth factor alpha (TGFα). (Redrawn from Heath JK. Growth factors. Oxford: IRL Press, 1993.)*

and are accordingly classified in completely different families, but together shared the common factor of causing transformation in that particular experimental design. Hence, some of the confusion about growth factors.

One of the other confusing points about the subject of growth factors is that in a normal individual we tend to regard tissues as essentially static and fail sometimes to appreciate that there is cell death and cell division producing a net turnover of zero to achieve that static effect. Cell growth is not necessarily associated with neoplasia. Growth factors are therefore important in health. They are, of course, particularly important in healing, inflammation, the immune response and more so still in embryogenesis, in which they have been particularly widely studied, especially in the nervous system.

The growth factor families that are discussed later on in this volume include the EGF family, the fibroblast growth factor (FGF) family, the TGFβ family, the insulin-like growth factor (IGF) family and the PDGF family. The characteristic feature of all of these is that they are polypeptides that are produced locally in tiny concentrations and act in an autocrine fashion on the cells that produced them or in a paracrine fashion on their neighbouring cells. Different growth factors may be produced by different cells in a tissue or by the same cells under differing circumstances, and another characteristic feature is that there tend to be several factors that act to limit their release or the response to their release and thereby control their actions.

A final problem is that we understand comparatively little about them. Our knowledge is largely based on a collection of isolated facts in experimental models. To give the best idea of how growth factors

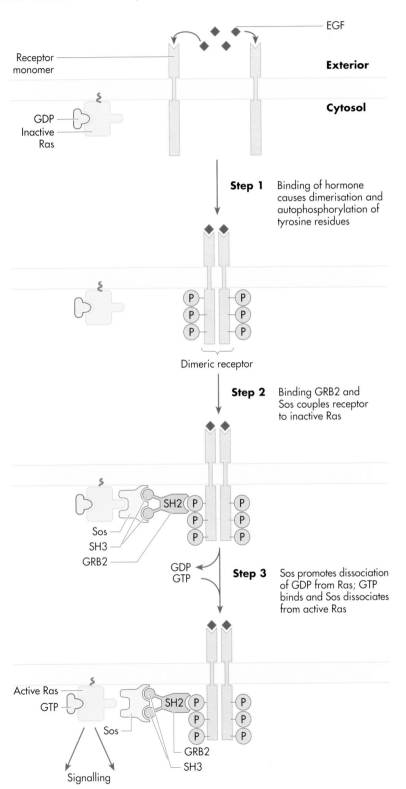

Step 1 Binding of hormone causes dimerisation and autophosphorylation of tyrosine residues

Step 2 Binding GRB2 and Sos couples receptor to inactive Ras

Step 3 Sos promotes dissociation of GDP from Ras; GTP binds and Sos dissociates from active Ras

Figure 1.38 *The activation of ras following the binding of EGF by means of the intermediates GRB2 and Sos. (Modified from Darnell J, Lodish H, Baltimore D. Molecular cell biology, second edition. New York: Scientific American Books, 1990.)*

work, one has to slip from urology to haematology and observe haemopoiesis, in which a number of growth factors act to produce a co-ordinated proliferation of multiple cell types derived from a set of common precursor cells in a series of steps. The system of haemopoiesis is itself by no means fully understood, but it is clear that specificity of action on each cell type is the key to the system as different

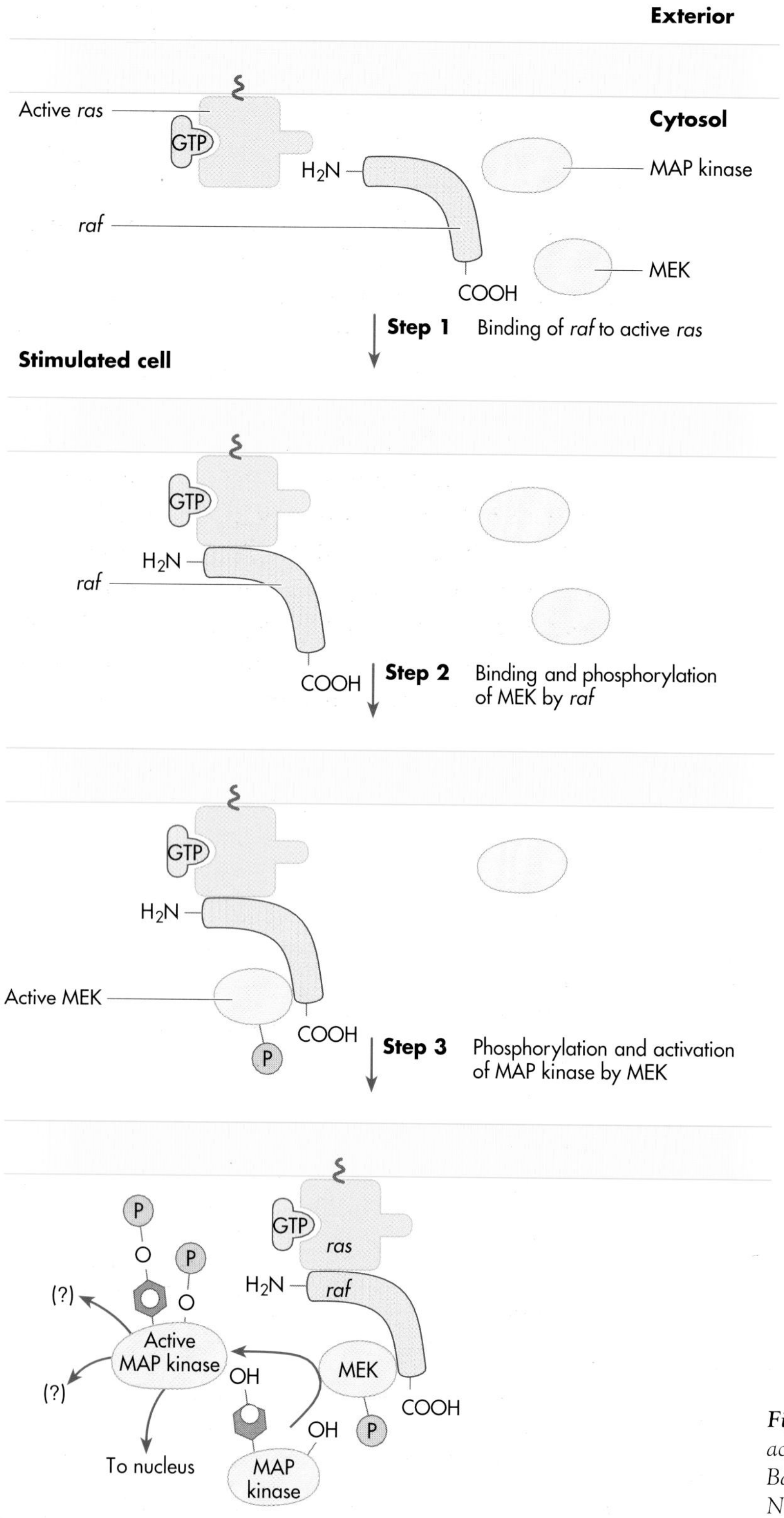

Figure 1.39 Activation of raf and MAP kinase by activated ras. (Modified from Darnell J, Lodish H, Baltimore D. Molecular cell biology, second edition. New York: Scientific American Books, 1990.)

growth factors act at different stages to produce the different responses that end up in a perfectly co-ordinated system. Presumably, other organs are subject to equally complex and possibly hierarchical controls

involving a large number of growth factors released in sequence to act in specific ways at specific times to produce the required end result. In this way, the apparently multiple and seemingly unrelated actions of many of the growth factors in vitro may be carefully controlled in vivo in terms of their release, effects and duration of response.

It is clearly important that mechanisms exist to control the release and effect of these potent agents. EGF and TGFα are localised in their effects because their precursor molecules are transmembrane proteins that are therefore fixed in position. EGF is still more localised in its action because it is only produced in a very small number of organs, principally the submaxillary gland and the kidney, although once secreted it can have effects elsewhere such as, in the case of renal EGF, in the remainder of the urinary tract. TGFα, which is from the same family and has very similar effects, is more widely distributed.

The activity of the FGF family is restricted in its effects in a different way. Some members of the FGF family are not secreted and can only be released by cell death, so although they are almost ubiquitous, their effects are tightly controlled by circumstances. Even

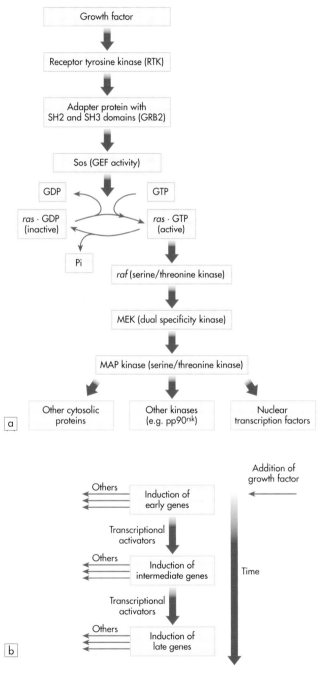

Figure 1.40 (a) An overview of the growth factor/tyrosine kinase cascade. (Modified from Darnell J, Lodish H, Baltimore D. Molecular cell biology, second edition. New York: Scientific American Books, 1990.) (b) Activation of nuclear transcription factors illustrating the sequence of activation. (Taken from Heath JK. Growth factors. Oxford: IRL Press, 1993.)

Table 1.2 The growth factor/tyrosine kinase cascade: the relevant genes activated and their function

Genes	Function
Early	
c-fos	
Krox-20	
Krox-24	Transcription factors
Fra-1	
c-myc	
Intermediate	
Collagenase	Metalloprotease
JE	Cytokine
Cathepsin L	Protease
Osteopontin	Extracellular matrix protein
Fibronectin	Extracellular matrix protein
TIMP	Protease inhibitor
Late	
Dihydrofolate reductase	Nucleotide metabolism
Histone H4	Chromatin structure
Thymidine kinase	Nucleotide metabolism

From Heath JK. Growth factors. Oxford: IRL Press, 1993.

then, basic FGF is only active when bound to heparin in the extracellular matrix, which thereby not only activates it but also sequesters it from enzymic degradation. Furthermore, the effects of various members of the FGF family are different at different times of life – acidic FGF is active in early life and basic FGF later on.

Whereas most growth factors stimulate cellular proliferation, the members of the TGFβ family are different. They are secreted in an inactive or 'latent' form that must be activated – another example of growth factor control. They generally modulate the activity of other growth factors and are often inhibitory, but are nonetheless capable of inducing anchorage-independent growth – the property known as transformation referred to above, which gives the family its name.

The receptors for the various growth factors confer cell-type specificity on the growth factors and their intracellular effects. Tyrosine kinase receptors have been referred to already and the EGF, PDGF, FGF and IGF receptors are all of this type. They stimulate transcription through the ras and raf proteins, mitogen-activated protein kinase and the various nuclear transcription factors such as the fos, jun and myc proteins, which activate genes in a time-dependent sequence leading to the synthesis of DNA and the passage of the cell through the cell cycle, ultimately to cell division (see below). The mechanism by which this happens is important to understand because it illustrates how precisely the system has to function to produce its intended effects and so illustrates how it might be therapeutically manipulated – for example, in the treatment of cancer.

Using the EGF receptor as an example, the first step is the binding of the ligand (EGF) to the receptor (Figure 1.38), which in the inactive state is a monomer, causing adjacent monomers to dimerise, that is, to form pairs. Dimerisation of the receptor monomers causes autophosphorylation of tyrosine residues on the cytosolic domain of the receptor molecule, thereby activating the molecule. The next step is the activation of the ras protein, which requires two events: firstly the GDP on the inactive ras molecule must be replaced by GTP, which is done by a guanine nucleotide exchange factor, in this case a molecule called Sos, which itself requires an adapter protein (GRB2) to bind it to the cystosolic domain of the EGF receptor; and, secondly, the ras molecule must be bound to the inner aspect of the cell membrane by a biochemical bonding to membrane phospholipids called farnesylation. If farnesylation could be inhibited, preventing the localisation of ras to the inner aspect of the cell membrane, then activation of ras and its mitogenic effects could be inhibited.

The activated ras molecule then binds and thereby activates raf, which must also occur in relation to the cell membrane. raf then binds and phosphorylates a mitogen-activated protein (MAP) kinase called MEK, which in turn activates another mitogen-activation protein kinase that is actually called MAP kinase (Figure 1.39). MAP kinase is a serine/threonine kinase that phosphorylates transcription factors in the nucleus such as fos, jun and myc, which in turn leads to gene transcription, as described in the next chapter (Figure 1.40 and Table 1.2).

Another substrate of tyrosine kinase, other than the G-protein-like ras protein, is a particular type of phospholipase C that generates inositol triphosphate and diacylglycerol leading to the activation of protein kinase C. Protein kinase C is a serine/threonine kinase and a potent mitogen, although its substrates and mode of action are unclear. It is also not clear what part, if any, inositol triphosphate has in the mitogenic process.

Specific growth factors are discussed in later chapters with regard to specific circumstances.

Further reading

Garrett RH, Grisham CM. Molecular aspects of cell biology. Fort Worth: Harcourt Brace College Publishers, 1995

Goodman SR. Medical cell biology. Philadelphia: JB Lippincott Company, 1994

Heath JK. Growth factors. Oxford: IRL Press, 1993

Lodish H, Baltimore D, Berk A, Zipursky SL, Matsudaira P, Darnell J. Molecular cell biology. New York: Scientific American Books, 1995

The cell and cell division

2

D. E. Neal

Structure of the cell

The cell membrane

The cell membrane confines the contents of the cell and consists of a continuous bilayer of phospholipid with the polar hydrophilic ends forming the outer and inner layers and the hydrophobic tails forming the central core of the bilayer. The hydrophilic heads on the two sides of the cell membrane are of different composition, those on the outside often being modified by glycosylation, a process that involves the addition of various sugar residues. Embedded in this lipid bilayer are proteins whose function can be classified as follows.

- Signal transduction (mediating the action of external ligands, e.g. growth, factors, neurotransmitters). These receptor proteins cross the cell membrane and may have intrinsic enzyme functions (e.g. the tyrosine kinase activity of the receptor for epidermal growth factor [EGF]) or may be linked to other proteins such as G-proteins (e.g. the muscarinic acetylcholine receptor) (Figure 2.1).
- Cell–cell or cell–matrix contact. Specialised junctions between cells and between cells and the intercellular matrix occur that involve transmembrane proteins such as integrins and cadherins. These proteins interact on the outside with molecules such as fibronectin and on the inside with molecules such as catenin, talin and vinculin, which act as intermediate links to the cell skeleton, which is made of actin fibres. These proteins form specialised cellular contacts such as desmosomes and tight junctions.

- Carrier proteins. These are involved in the transport of small molecules and ions across the cell membrane, e.g. glucose, the sodium/potassium pump or the multidrug resistance pump. These proteins may be energy dependent or passive; if they are active, they are usually utilise adenosine triphosphate (ATP). The carrier proteins will often transport other molecules at the same time in the opposite direction (Figure 2.2).
- Channel proteins. These are involved in the transport of ions across the cell membrane. They function in a passive way and effectively are hydrophilic pores; they function more efficiently than carrier proteins and can carry ions more than 1000-fold faster. They are selective for certain ions and may be closed or open. The stimuli for opening these channels may be electrical current, ligand binding (e.g. nicotinic acetylcholine) or mechanical deformation.

Intracellular organelles: rough and smooth endoplasmic reticulum, Golgi apparatus, nuclear membranes

The endoplasmic reticulum compartmentalises the cell into functionally distinct units (Figure 2.3). They are extensive, having a surface area 10–25-fold greater than the cell membrane itself. Intracellular proteins are synthesised on free cytosolic ribosomes and remain in the cytoplasm. Proteins for export begin their life by being synthesised on ribosomes that have special signalling molecules that dock with receptors on the endoplasmic reticulum (ER), Golgi apparatus, lysosomes etc., which mediate transport to their final destination.

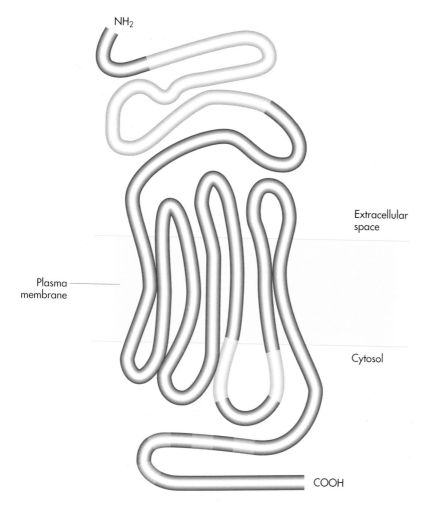

NH$_2$

Extracellular space

Plasma membrane

Cytosol

COOH

Figure 2.1 *A schematic drawing of a G-protein-linked receptor. Receptors that bind protein ligands have a large extracellular ligand-binding domain formed by the part of the polypeptide chain. Receptors for small ligands such as adrenaline have small extracellular domains, and the ligand-binding site is usually deep within the plane of the membrane, formed by amino acids from several of the transmembrane segments. The parts of the intracellular domains that are mainly responsible for binding to trimeric G-proteins are shown in orange, while those that become phosphorylated during receptor desensitisation (discussed later) are shown in red.*

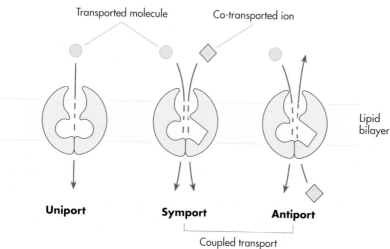

Transported molecule   Co-transported ion

Lipid bilayer

Uniport   **Symport**   **Antiport**

Coupled transport

Figure 2.2 *Three types of carrier-mediated transport. The schematic diagram shows carrier proteins functioning as uniports, symports and antiports.*

Endoplasmic reticulum

The ER is convoluted and may occupy up to 10% of the cell volume. It plays a central role in protein and lipid biosynthesis and is the site for the synthesis of proteins and lipids that are destined to be incorpo-rated in other cell organelles such as mitochondria (Figure 2.4).

Ribosomes are found free in the cytosol or attached to the ER (rough ER) when a ribosome is making a protein destined for export. In this latter cir-

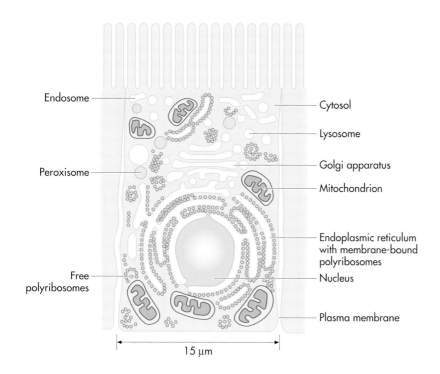

Figure 2.3 *The major intracellular compartments of an animal cell. The cytosol, endoplasmic reticulum, Golgi apparatus, nucleus, mitochondrion, endosome, lysosome and peroxisome are distinct compartments isolated from the rest of the cell by at least one selectively permeable membrane.*

cumstance, a signalling molecule targets the ribosome with its mRNA, and then binds to the ER into which it secretes its protein (Figure 2.5).

Smooth ER is abundant in some cells. It is involved in the storage of calcium and may have a vital role in the contraction of smooth muscle cells; together with the Golgi apparatus, it is involved in the synthesis of lipoproteins. In the liver and some other cells, it contains the cytochrome p450 enzymes that detoxify lipid-soluble drugs by converting them into water-soluble forms.

Golgi apparatus

This is a system of flattened sacs that lie in continuity with the ER and that is involved in sorting, packaging and modifying macromolecules for secretion or for delivery to other intracellular organelles (Figure 2.6). It consists of a stack of four to six flattened cisternae with an entry (*cis*) and exit (*trans*) surface. Glycosylation of proteins such as mucin takes place in the Golgi apparatus. Other proteins are sorted for differential transport to certain organelles; for instance, acid hydrolase is transported from here to the lysosomes and, if the cell synthesises hormones or neurotransmitters, these are excreted by small smooth vesicles budding off from the Golgi apparatus before

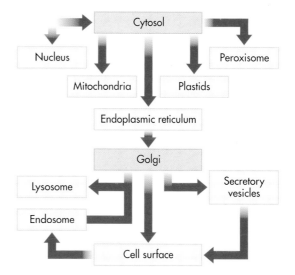

Figure 2.4 *The intracellular compartments of the eukaryotic cell involved in the biosynthetic secretory and endocytic pathways. Each compartment encloses a space that is topologically equivalent to the outside of the cell, and they all communicate with one another by means of transport vesicles. In the biosynthetic secretory pathway, protein molecules are transported from the endoplasmic reticulum (ER) to the plasma membrane or (via late endosomes) to lysosomes. In the endocytic pathway, molecules are ingested in vesicles derived from the plasma membrane and delivered to early endosomes and then (via late endosomes) to lysosomes. Many endocytosed molecules are retrieved from early endosomes and returned to the cell surface for re-use; similarly, some molecules are retrieved from the late endosome and returned to the Golgi apparatus, and some are retrieved from the Golgi apparatus and returned to the ER.*

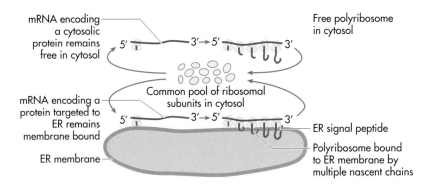

Figure 2.5 *Free and membrane bound ribosomes. A common pool of ribosomes is used to synthesise both the proteins that stay in the cytosol and those that are transported into the endoplasmic reticulum (ER). It is the ER signal peptide on a newly formed polypeptide chain that directs the engaged ribosome to the ER membrane. The mRNA molecule may remain permanently bound to the ER as part of a polyribosome, while the ribosomes that move along it are recycled; at the end of each round of protein synthesis, the ribosomal subunits are released and rejoin the common pool in the cytosol.*

transport to the cell membrane where exocytosis takes place.

The mitochondrion

Mitochondria are the power-houses of the cell and are responsible for the production of most of the high-energy phosphate intermediates such as ATP. They are present in virtually all cells and mediate oxidative respiration in which pyruvate is converted to carbon dioxide and water with the production of about 30 molecules of ATP. Mitochondria consist of an outer membrane and a convoluted inner membrane

containing the inner space, or matrix, which is packed with hundreds of enzymes. Acetyl coenzyme A (CoA) is the central intermediate produced by fatty acid oxidation and glycolysis (Figure 2.7), and the citric acid cycle takes place in the mitochondrion (Figure 2.8). In the mitochondrion, high-energy electrons from NADH and $FADH_2$ are passed to oxygen during oxidative phosphorylation by the respiratory chain which is situated on the inner membrane of the mitochondrion (Figure 2.9). There are three large enzyme groups embedded in the inner membrane (Figure 2.10):

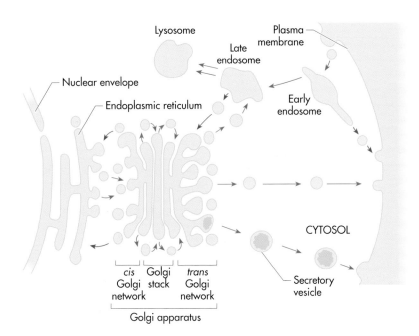

Figure 2.6 *The Golgi apparatus.*

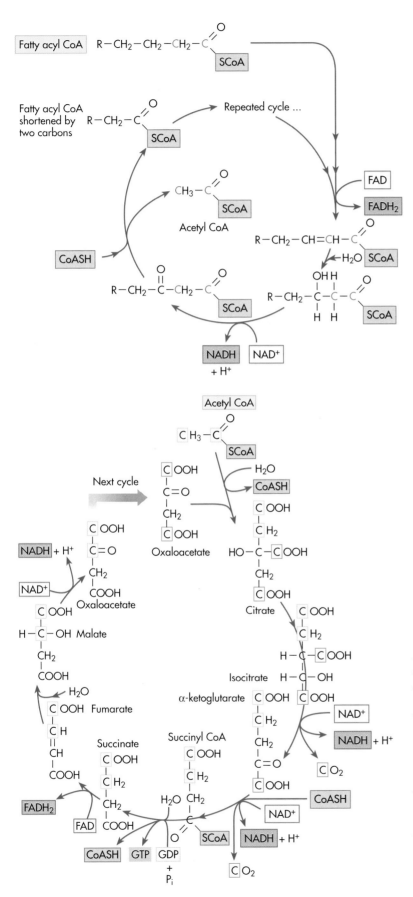

Figure 2.7 *The fatty acid oxidation cycle. The cycle is catalysed by a series of four enzymes in the mitochondrial matrix. Each turn of the cycle shortens the fatty acid chain by two carbons (shown in red), as indicated, and generates one molecule of acetyl CoA and one molecule each of NADH and $FADH_2$. The NADH is freely soluble in the matrix. The $FADH_2$, in contrast, remains tightly bound to the enzyme fatty acyl-CoA dehydrogenase; its two electrons will be rapidly transferred to the respiratory chain in the mitochondrial inner membrane, regenerating FAD.*

Figure 2.8 *The citric acid cycle. The intermediates are shown as their free acids, although the carboxyl groups are actually ionised. Each of the indicated steps is catalysed by a different enzyme located in the mitochondrial matrix. The two carbons from acetyl CoA that enter this turn of the cycle (shadowed in red) will be converted to CO_2 in subsequent turns of the cycle: it is the two carbons shadowed in blue that are converted to CO_2 in this cycle. Three molecules of NADH are formed. The GTP molecule produced can be converted to ATP by the exchange reaction GTP + ADP → GDP + ATP. The molecule of $FADH_2$ formed remains protein bound as part of the succinate dehydrogenase complex in the mitochondrial inner membrane; this complex feeds the electrons acquired by $FADH_2$ directly to ubiquinone (see Figure 2.9).*

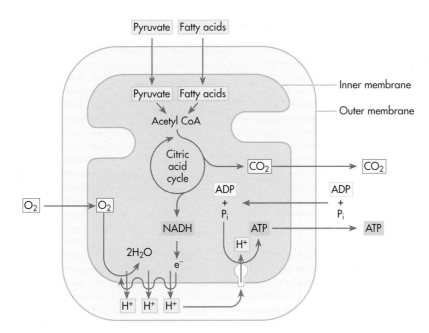

Figure 2.9 A summary of mitochondrial energy metabolism. Pyruvate and fatty acids enter the mitochondrion, are broken down to acetyl CoA, and are then metabolised by the citric acid cycle, which produces NADH (and FADH₂, which is not shown). In the process of oxidative phosphorylation, high-energy electrons from NADH (and FADH₂) are then passed to oxygen by means of the respiratory chain in the inner membrane, producing ATP by a chemi-osmotic mechanism.

NADH generated by glycolysis in the cytosol also passes electrons to the respiratory chain (not shown). Because NADH cannot pass across the mitochondrial inner membrane, the electron transfer from cytosolic NADH must be accomplished indirectly by means of one of several 'shuttle' systems that transport another reduced compound into the mitochondrion. After being oxidised, this compound is returned to the cytosol, where it is reduced by NADH again.

NADH dehydrogenase complex, which contains a flavin and ubiquinone;

cytochrome b-c₁ complex, which contains three haems and iron-sulphur protein;

cytochrome oxidase complex, which contains two cytochromes and copper.

It is thought that ATP is formed by a process of chemi-osmotic coupling. The passage of electrons down each of the three parts of the respiratory chain results in H⁺ being pumped into the intermembrane space of the mitochondrion to set up an electrochemical proton gradient. The subsequent backflow of H⁺

into the matrix provides the energy to drive the enzyme ATP synthase.

Mitochondrial DNA

Mitochondria and chloroplasts contain DNA that encodes structural and functional proteins which permit the mitochondrion to divide during cell division. Mitochondrial DNA utilises pathways that are biochemically distinct from those of nuclear DNA. For instance, protein synthesis mediated by nuclear DNA in the cytoplasm is blocked by cyclohexidine, whereas that in the mitochondrion is blocked by chloramphenicol, erythromycin and tetracycline. Mito-

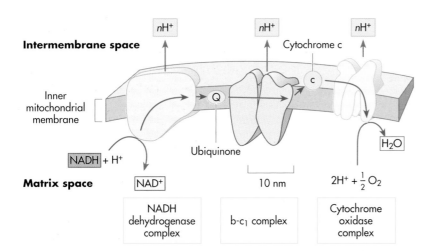

Figure 2.10 The path of electrons through the three respiratory enzyme complexes. The size and shape of each complex are shown, as determined from images of two-dimensional crystals (crystalline sheets) viewed in the electron microscope at various tilt angles. During the transfer of two electrons from NADH to oxygen (red arrows), ubiquinone and cytochrome c serve as carriers between the complexes.

chondria are not synthesised de novo, but arise from division of the organelle that occurs during mitosis and is driven by mitochondrial DNA. Mitochondrial DNA is a circular structure like that of bacteria, and in mammalian cells contains around 16.5 kilobase pairs. It synthesises two ribosomal RNAs, 22 transfer RNAs (tRNAs) and 13 peptides. Unlike nuclear DNA, most of the nucleotides are direct coding sequences with little or no space left for regulatory codons. On looking at the genetic code, the codon sequence is relaxed, allowing many tRNA molecules to recognise any one of four nucleotides in the third, or 'wobble', position. In addition, in humans, three of the 64 codons have different meanings from the standard codons (Table 2.1).

Because mitochondrial inheritance is cytoplasmic, one would expect mitochondria to be inherited from the maternal side as the sperm has little cytoplasm. It is thought that both mitochondria and chloroplasts evolved from endosymbiotic bacteria more than a billion years ago. However, over time, some mitochondrial genes have been transferred to nuclear DNA, for instance lipoproteins in the mitochondrial membranes are synthesised from nuclear genes and modified in the cell's Golgi apparatus.

The nucleus

This is the most striking organelle in the cell. It is separated from the rest of the cell by the nuclear membrane, which consists of a lipid bilayer fenestrated by multiple nuclear pores. Inside the nucleus is the nucleolus, which is the factory that produces ribosomes. All chromosomal DNA is held in the nucleus, but it is associated with an equal mass of histone proteins. The dense nucleolus is the site for the assembly of ribosomes.

Arrangement of DNA

Each DNA molecule in the nucleus is packaged as a chromosome, which in essence is an enormously long molecule arranged as two strands of a double helix. There are 23 pairs of chromosomes (22 autosomes and one sex chromosome: X or Y), which contain about 6×10^9 nucleotide pairs. Each DNA molecule has not only to be able to code for many different proteins (Figure 2.11), but also has to be able to replicate itself reliably during mitosis and to repair itself when damaged by chemicals or radiation. At the ends of each chromosome are the telomeres and at the centre is the centromere, which serves to anchor the chromosome via the kinetochore to the mitotic spindle during cell division. Not all DNA in the chromosomes is used to produce mRNA; indeed, most of it is arranged into regulatory elements (non-coding sequences), introns or junk DNA, so-called because its function is not yet understood.

Histone proteins

These proteins allow formal packaging of DNA in the nucleus. Without them, DNA in mammalian cells would not be arranged in a regular way and cell division and gene transcription would not be possible. They are small proteins with a large amount of dibasic amino acids such as arginine and lysine that bind to DNA because of their positive charges. There are five types: the H1 histones and the nucleosomal histones (H2A, H2B, H3 and H4), which are highly evolutionarily conserved. The nucleosomal histones are responsible for the coiling of DNA into nucleosomes (Figure 2.12), which are essential to the accommodation of DNA into the nucleus. It is thought that nucleosome histones are preferentially bound to areas of DNA that are AT rich. These proteins can be prevented from binding by the attachment of inhibitory proteins. Nucleosomes are themselves packed together even more tightly by H1 histone proteins.

Figure 2.13 shows how DNA within chromosomes is ordered. DNA that is actively being transcribed into

Table 2.1 Differences between nuclear and mitochondrial coding

Codon	Standard	Mitochondrial
UGA	STOP	Trp (tryptophan)
AUA	Ile (isoleucine)	Met (methionine)
AGA/AGG	Arg (arginine)	STOP

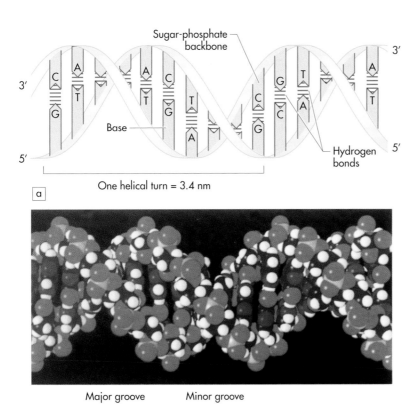

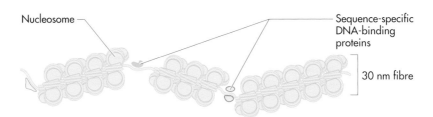

Figure 2.11 *The DNA double helix. In a DNA molecule, two antiparallel strands that are complementary in their nucleotide sequence are paired in a right-handed double helix with about ten nucleotide pairs per helical turn. A schematic representation (a) and a space-filling model (b).*

Figure 2.12 *Nucleosome-free regions in 30 nm fibres. A schematic section of chromatin illustrating the interruption of its regular nucleosomal structure by short regions where the chromosomal DNA is unusually vulnerable to digestion by DNase I. At each of these nuclease-hypersensitive sites, a nucleosome appears to have been excluded from the DNA by one or more sequence-specific DNA-binding proteins.*

mRNA is unfolded, but is at its most condensed during mitosis, when individual chromosomes can be recognised by their specific banded structure.

DNA replication

Replication of DNA requires that it is unwound at so-called replication forks, each strand acting as a template for synthesis. DNA polymerase α is used on the lagging strand and DNA polymerase δ on the leading strand (Figure 2.14). Both sections are synthesised in the 5′ (five prime in speech) to the 3′ (three prime) direction (on the new strand); the lagging strand is initially synthesised as short segments called Okazaki segments. In humans, each molecule of DNA (the full length of the chromosome) is so long that several replication forks are required; these are often clustered together in areas of DNA that are transcriptionally active. For example, in women whose second X chromosome is condensed as heterochromatin (Barr body), the active X chromosome replicates throughout each S phase, which lasts for about eight hours, whereas the heterochromatin replicates only late in S phase. During mitosis, a huge amount of histone protein has to be synthesised (histone protein forms an equal mass to DNA), and in humans there are 20 replicated sets of histone protein genes arranged as tandem repeats on several chromosomes; each set of which contains all five histone proteins.

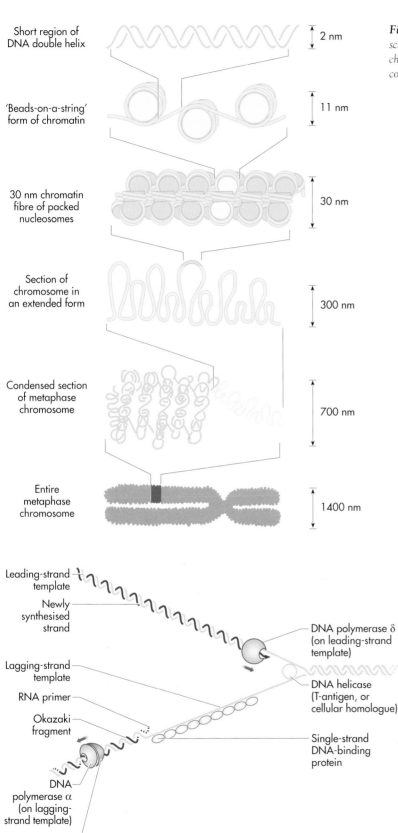

Short region of DNA double helix — 2 nm

'Beads-on-a-string' form of chromatin — 11 nm

30 nm chromatin fibre of packed nucleosomes — 30 nm

Section of chromosome in an extended form — 300 nm

Condensed section of metaphase chromosome — 700 nm

Entire metaphase chromosome — 1400 nm

Leading-strand template
Newly synthesised strand
Lagging-strand template
RNA primer
Okazaki fragment
DNA polymerase α (on lagging-strand template)
DNA primase

DNA polymerase δ (on leading-strand template)
DNA helicase (T-antigen, or cellular homologue)
Single-strand DNA-binding protein

Figure 2.13 *A model of chromatin packing. This schematic drawing shows some of the many orders of chromatin packing postulated to give rise to the highly condensed mitotic chromosome.*

Figure 2.14 *A mammalian replication fork. The mammalian fork replicates in two different ways. First, it makes use of two DNA polymerases, one for the leading strand and one for the lagging strand. It seems likely that the leading-strand polymerase is designed to keep a tight hold on the DNA, whereas that on the lagging strand must be able to release the template and then rebind each time that a new Okazaki fragment is synthesised. Second, the mammalian DNA primase is a subunit of the lagging-strand DNA polymerase, while that of bacteria is associated with the DNA helicase.*

DNA replication errors

Errors can arise during DNA replication owing to the insertion of the wrong base or the insertion of a run of microsatellite repeats (replication errors). These are normally repaired by nucleotide excision enzymes or replication error repair enzymes respectively.

Telomeres and telomerase

Because of its structure and the way that it synthesises nucleotides, DNA polymerase cannot replicate the very ends of chromosomes that are modified into special regions called telomeres. In many species, these telomeres consist of tandem repeats rich in G (in humans this is GGGTTA). This region is replicated by a special enzyme called telomerase, which recognises the GGGTTA sequence. Because there is no complementary DNA strand to replicate, telomerase uses an RNA template that is structurally part of the telomerase as a temporary extension for replication of the other strand. After several rounds of extension, one strand is longer and therefore can be used in turn as a template for replication of the second strand by DNA polymerase. It is thought that the telomeres shorten after each round of cell division and that this may limit the lifespan of a cell (senescence). Some malignant tumours are known to have high levels of telomerase, which may mean that the cell can divide without the lengths of the telomeres being a limiting factor.

Cell division and senescence

Senescence

Normal human cells cannot go on dividing for ever in tissue culture; eventually they senesce and will not divide further in response to mitogens. This process is accompanied by loss of telomerase, a failure to phosphorylate the retinoblastoma protein in response to mitogens, and high levels of p21 (WAF1) and p16, which are cyclin-dependent kinase inhibitors that profoundly inhibit cell division.

Cell division

Cell division involves duplication of DNA, mitosis (nuclear division) and cytokinesis (division of the cytoplasm). Following replication of DNA, the cen-

trosome divides to form the mitotic spindle; the chromosomes condense and align in the centre of the cell, where they are pulled apart by the mitotic spindle.

Mitosis (Figure 2.15): the 'M' phase

Prophase
The chromatin condenses into chromosomes that have duplicated and hence are formed of sister chromatids held together by the centromere. The centrosome divides to form the mitotic spindle. The nucleolus disperses.

Prometaphase
The nuclear membrane disrupts. The kinetochores begin to form. These are specialised proteins attached

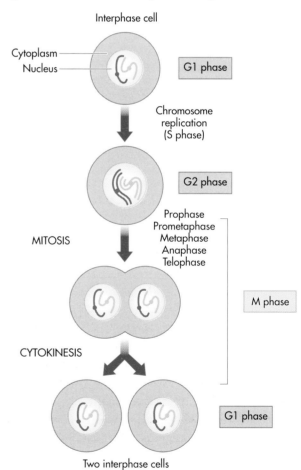

Figure 2.15 *The four successive phases of a standard eukaryotic cell cycle. During interphase, the cell grows continuously; during M phase, it divides. DNA replication is confined to the part of interphase known as S phase. G1 phase is the gap between M phase and S phase; G2 is the gap between S phase and M phase.*

to the centromere to which the microtubule proteins of the spindle pole bind. Patients with scleroderma form autoantibodies to kinetochore protein.

Metaphase

The chromosomes are aligned at the metaphase plate at the centre of the cell.

Anaphase

The paired kinetochores suddenly separate, allowing the chromosomes to be separate and to be pulled towards each spindle pole in a matter of minutes. Contraction of the microtubules pulls the chromosomes towards the spindle pole.

Telophase

The nuclear membrane begins to reform and the microtubules disappear. The nucleolus reappears.

Cytokinesis

The cytoplasm separates at a specialised contractile ring situated in the centre of the cell, which actively nips off the cytoplasm into two parts.

The cell cycle

In the adult human, cells are continuously being lost by the process of planned programmed cell death (apoptosis). Some cells do not divide at all, although they can be destroyed (neurons and skeletal muscle fibres); some divide slowly; whereas others have to divide rapidly (e.g. cells in the bone marrow and lining of the gut). During cell division, DNA is replicated and the reproduction of intracellular organelles takes place. Replication of DNA takes place during a specific part of mitosis known as the S phase. G2 is the period of rest before the prophase part of M phase starts. The G1 phase occupies the period between the completion of the previous mitosis and the S phase; however, some mature cells enter a specialised period of rest, G0, which can last for months or years.

The proportion of dividing cells can be measured by a number of different tests. Administration of radiolabelled thymidine or of bromo-deoxyuridine can allow labelling of cells in S phase to be demon-strated by the use of photographic plates or mono-clonal antibodies respectively. Other antibodies can be used to measure the Ki67 antigen (Ki67 or MIB1) and proliferating cell nuclear antigen, which are expressed during particular parts of the cell cycle. These are useful in measuring cell proliferation within tumours. The amount of DNA within a population of cells can be estimated by the use of fluorescent stains such as ethidium bromide plus a fluorescence-activated cell sorter.

The control of cell division

This process is tightly controlled at certain critical points of the cell cycle, known as cell cycle checkpoints, at which certain brakes can be applied to stop the process if conditions are unfavourable (Figure 2.16). Checkpoints are found at the G1/S transition (the start checkpoint); another is found at G2/M. Most studies have concentrated on the G2/M transition (the mitosis checkpoint). This cell cycle control mechanism is based on two series of proteins: the cyclin-dependent protein kinases (cdks), which phosphorylate a series of downstream proteins on serine and threonine residues, and the cyclins, which, along with other regulatory proteins, bind to cdks to inhibit their activity. Different cyclins are synthesised during different parts of the cell cycle (mitotic cyclins and G1 cyclins; Figure 2.17). In mammalian cells, there are at least six types of cyclin (A, B, C, D, E and F). Entry into mitosis is stimulated by activation of a cdk by mitotic cyclin; in amphibians, this is known as maturation promotion factor (MPF) and consists of cyclin and a cyclin-dependent kinase called cdc2; another is known as cdc4. Repetitive synthesis and degradation of cyclins are associated with the cell cycle. Activation of MPF drives mitosis; degradation of cyclin then allows the cell to enter S phase. As shall be seen later, there is a set of proteins that can inhibit cdk known as cyclin-dependent kinase inhibitors (cdki) or inhibitors of cyclin-dependent kinases (INKs). The activity of the cdk can therefore be abruptly switched on and off during different parts of the cell cycle.

In part, this is controlled by synthesis and degradation of the cyclins, but it is also affected by phosphorylation of the cdk on two sites (Figure 2.18),

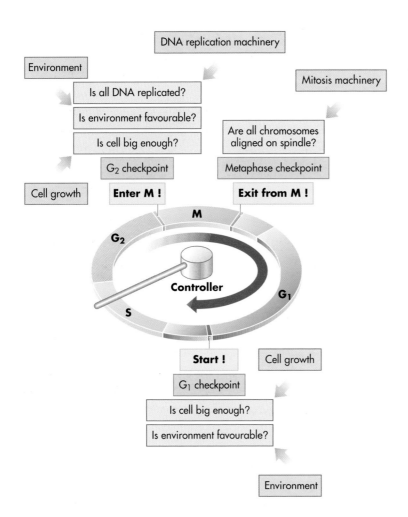

Figure 2.16 *Checkpoints and inputs of regulatory information to the cell-cycle control system. Feedback from downstream processes and signals from the environment can prevent the control system from passing through certain specific checkpoints. The most prominent checkpoints are where the control system activates the triggers shown in yellow boxes.*

which is controlled by two phosphatases known as Wee 1 and MO15. Removal of one of the phosphate residues by means of another phosphatase (cdc25) is then needed for activation of MPF. It is thought that the MPF can activate itself autocatalytically, which results in a steady rise in its levels during the cell cycle until the critical point when an explosive increase in activity takes place and drives the cell irretrievably into M phase. Cdc2 is associated with the G1/S and the G2/M transition, and cdc4 and cdc6 are associated with start, but are bound to different cyclins (cyclin B at mitosis and cyclins E and A at start at G1/S). The Kip/cip family of cyclin-dependent kinases, which includes p21, p27 and p57, is capable of binding to and inhibiting most cyclin–cdk complexes. The expression of these cdk inhibitors is often dependent on upstream events that are activated by physiological signals such as DNA damage, serum deprivation or contact inhibition. In contrast, the INK4 family of

cdk inhibitors, including p15, p16, p18 and p19, bind to and inactivate D-type cyclins.

Growth factors and the control of the cell cycle

In mammalian cells, peptide growth factors are potent inducers of cell division. These include platelet-derived growth factor (PDGF), EGF, insulin and insulin-like growth factors I and II (IGF-I and IGF-II), acidic and basic fibroblast growth factors (a-FGF and b-FGF), transforming growth factor α (TGFα, which binds to the EGF receptor) and transforming growth factor β (TGFβ, which is structurally unrelated to TGFα and is generally inhibitory). Many of these growth factors act as proto-oncogenes.

These growth factors act over very short distances and may act on the cells that produce them (autocrine action) or on neighbouring cell types (paracrine action). Many are found in serum, which is one reason why serum is required to maintain cells in culture. High-affinity receptors for these growth factors are found on the cell membrane, and in culture cells compete for growth factors. As well as requiring growth factors for cell division, many cells require signals

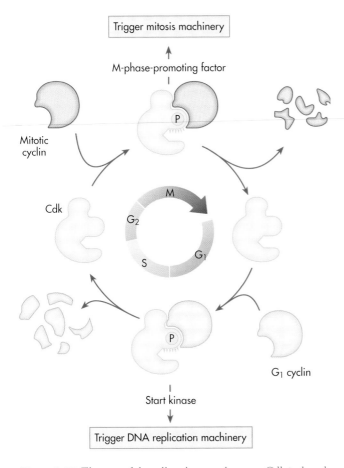

Figure 2.17 *The core of the cell-cycle control system. Cdk is thought to associate successively with different cyclins to trigger downstream processes of the cycle. Cdk activity is terminated by cyclin degradation.*

produced by intercellular contact and adherence (anchorage) mediated by means of adhesion molecules before they divide (anchorage-dependent growth).

Many growth factor receptors contain an endogenous tyrosine kinase that is activated by ligand binding (Figure 2.19). These receptors interact with proto-oncogenes such as G-proteins (e.g. *ras*) because tyrosine phosphorylation of the receptors facilitates binding of intermediate proteins with so-called SH2 domains, which then link with other proteins (SOS, GRB2), which then activate the Ras pathway. Phosphorylation of downstream protein by growth factor receptors activates several early response genes that are stimulated within a few minutes of adding growth factor. Delayed response gene activation, in contrast, requires protein synthesis. Many early response genes activated by growth factor receptors control gene transcription and include *myc*, *jun* and *fos*, which are known to be crucial for gene transcription. *myc*, in particular, is thought to be closely linked to activation of cell division.

Apoptosis

In many tissues, such as the haematopoietic system and the lining of the gut, cell proliferation and cell division are balanced by a process of planned cell death, the control of which is every bit as important as that involved in cell division. Programmed cell death also occurs in tumours, but the control of it is disrupted.

Apoptosis is a carefully orchestrated event in

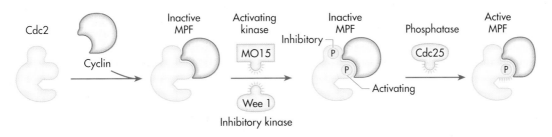

Figure 2.18 *Genesis of maturation promotion factor (MPF) activity. Cdc2 becomes associated with cyclin as the level of cyclin gradually increases; this enables Cdc2 to be phosphorylated by an activating kinase on an 'activating' site as well as by Wee 1 kinase on Cdc2's catalytic site. The latter phosphorylation inhibits Cdc2 activity until this phosphate group is removed by the Cdc25 phosphatase. Active MPF is thought to stimulate its own activation by activating Cdc25 and inhibiting Wee 1, either directly or indirectly.*

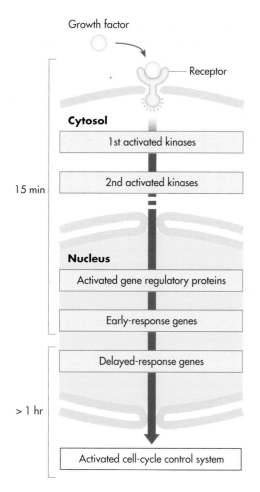

Growth factor

Receptor

Cytosol

1st activated kinases

2nd activated kinases

15 min

Nucleus

Activated gene regulatory proteins

Early-response genes

Delayed-response genes

> 1 hr

Activated cell-cycle control system

Figure 2.19 *Typical signalling pathway for stimulation of cell proliferation by a growth factor. This greatly simplified diagram shows some of the major steps. It omits many of the intermediate steps in the relay system.*

Several genes are involved in this process. For example, in thymic cells damaged by radiation, *p53* is up-regulated, which increases the level of p21 (an inhibitor of cyclin-dependent kinase), which slows down cell division, placing the cell in G1 arrest, allowing DNA repair to take place. It is thought that *p21* is not directly concerned with the onset of apoptosis. In some cell types, such DNA damage initiates apoptosis which is also associated with up-regulation of p53. There is a number of known proteins that can promote apoptosis. These include the bax family which binds and is inhibited by *bcl2*. Homodimers of bax (which is up-regulated by *p53*) bring on apoptosis. The bcl-2 protein binds and inactivates bax preventing homodimerisation, thereby preventing apoptosis. Some types of apoptosis are not activated through *p53*. It is thought that the end point of apoptosis is the activation of a set of ICE-like cysteine proteases.

Aberrant expression of *p53* and up-regulation of *bcl2* will decrease the rate of apoptosis (although this is often higher in tumours with mutated *p53* and up-regulated *bcl2* because other mechanisms of apoptosis are activated). The point is that, in many tumours, DNA damage and the presence of mutated tumour suppressors and oncogenes will stimulate cell division, which will be in excess of the rate of apoptosis, so continued deregulated proliferation will probably lead to more DNA mutations occurring with each cell cycle.

Structure of DNA and RNA

The structure of DNA and RNA is based on nucleic acids. Nucleic acids are made of three compounds:

1. bases: nitrogenous ring compounds called purines (adenine and guanine) or pyrimidines (cytosine, thymine [DNA], or uracil [RNA]);
2. pentose sugars: of which there are two types – ribose (β-D-ribose: RNA) and deoxyribose (β-D-2-deoxyribose: DNA);
3. phosphate: the phosphate bond is attached to the 5′ C hydroxyl group and in a nucleic acid it bonds to the 3′ C position of the adjacent sugar residue.

which the cell is programmed to die. The nucleus becomes shrunken and pyknotic, and the cytoplasm shrinks. The nucleus is sometimes extruded and may be engulfed by neighbouring cells. No inflammatory reaction is excited by the process, which is characterised by disintegration of the nuclear envelope and marked condensation of DNA into chromatin. On electrophoresis, the DNA assumes a characteristic banding pattern, implying that it is being cut by endonuclease enzymes. Nearby macrophages recognise the apoptotic cell and begin to engulf and digest it. How this recognition process is mediated is unclear. The macrophages do not secrete inflammatory cytokines and chemokines, so inflammation does not occur: apoptosis is quite different from necrosis.

Definitions of these molecules include:

nucleoside: this is defined as a base plus a sugar (adenosine, guanosine, cytidine, thymidine or uridine);

nucleotide: this is defined as a base plus a sugar plus a phosphate (Figure 2.20). In addition to being the building blocks of DNA and RNA, nucleotides are used as high-energy intermediates, e.g. ATP; in combination with other structures to form enzymes (coenzyme A) and as signalling molecules, e.g. cyclic AMP.

RNA forms a single chain, whereas DNA forms a double helix held together by hydrogen bonding between bases on opposing strands. The individual nucleotides are held together by phosphate linkages between sugar residues, the individual bases being suspended from the other end of the sugar residue. The sequence of bases forms the basis for all genetic information and is organised as a series of triplets that code for individual amino acids. The hydrogen bonding between bases on opposing strands is not random, and on opposite sides of DNA the following bases are always matched as complementary pairs (or Watson–Crick base pairs):

G with C,
A with T (or A with U in RNA).

The triplet code for DNA and the corresponding amino acids are shown in Tables 2.2 and 2.3. A section

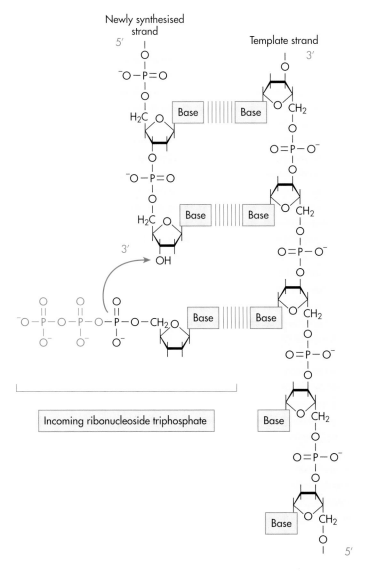

Figure 2.20 DNA synthesis. The addition of a deoxyribonucleotide to the 3' end of a polynucleotide chain is the fundamental reaction by which DNA is synthesised. As shown, base-pairing between this incoming deoxyribonucleotide and an existing strand of DNA (the template strand) guides the formation of a new strand of DNA with a complementary nucleotide sequence.

Table 2.2 The genetic code

1st position – 5′ end	U	C	A	G	3rd position – 3′ end
U	Phe	Ser	Tyr	Cys	U
	Phe	Ser	Tyr	Cys	C
	Leu	Ser	STOP	STOP	A
	Leu	Ser	STOP	Trp	G
C	Leu	Pro	His	Arg	U
	Leu	Pro	His	Arg	C
	Leu	Pro	Gln	Arg	A
	Leu	Pro	Gln	Arg	G
A	Ile	Thr	Asn	Ser	U
	Ile	Thr	Asn	Ser	C
	Ile	Thr	Lys	Arg	A
	Met	Thr	Lys	Arg	G
G	Val	Ala	Asp	Gly	U
	Val	Ala	Asp	Gly	C
	Val	Ala	Glu	Gly	A
	Val	Ala	Glu	Gly	G

of DNA can be read in a number of different 'reading frames', depending upon which particular nucleotide is the start of the reading frame.

The double helix formed by DNA occupies 3.4 nm for one complete turn, which contains ten nucleotide pairs per turn and has a major and a minor groove. A single strand of DNA acting as a template will induce the formation of a second complementary strand if there are the appropriate nucleoside trisphosphates and DNA polymerase present in solution. Errors

introduced by such complementary replication will induce a 'point mutation' where a single inappropriate base is inserted.

Basic genetic mechanisms

Genes

Certain sections of DNA are arranged into genes, which are defined as lengths of DNA that produce

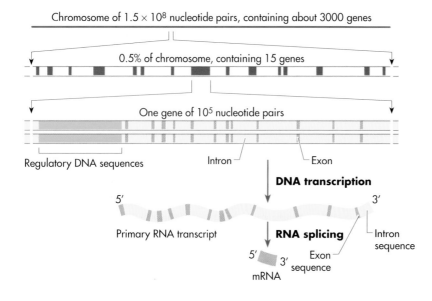

Figure 2.21 The organisation of genes on a typical vertebrate chromosome. Proteins that bind to the DNA in regulatory regions determine whether a gene is transcribed; although often located on the 5′ side of a gene, as shown here, regulatory regions can also be located in introns, in exons, or on the 3′ side of a gene. Intron sequences are removed from primary RNA transcripts to produce messenger RNA (mRNA) molecules. The figure given here for the number of genes per chromosome is a minimal estimate.

Table 2.3 Amino acids and their symbols

Letter	Symbols	Amino acid	Codons
A	Ala	Alanine	GCA, GCC, GCG, GCU
C	Cys	Cysteine	UGC, UGU
D	Asp	Aspartic acid	GAC, GAU
E	Glu	Glutamic acid	GAA, GAU
F	Phe	Phenylalanine	UUC, UUU
G	Gly	Glycine	GGA, GGC, GGG, GGU
H	His	Histidine	CAC, CAU
I	Ile	Isoleucine	AUA, AUC, AUU
K	Lys	Lysine	AAA, AAG
L	Leu	Leucine	UUA, UUG, CUA, CUC, CUG, CUU
M	Met	Methionine	AUG
N	Asn	Asparagine	AAC, AAU
P	Pro	Proline	CCA, CCC, CCG, CCU
Q	Gln	Glutamine	CAA, CAG
R	Arg	Arginine	AGA, AGG, CGA, CGC, CGG, CGU
S	Ser	Serine	AGC, AGU, UCA, UCC, UCG, UCU
T	Thr	Threonine	ACA, ACC, ACG, ACU
V	Val	Valine	GUA, GUC, GUG, GUU
W	Trp	Tryptophan	UGG
X	Tyr	Tryosine	UAC, UAU

specific mRNA and protein, although this definition is not quite correct because in some organisms several species of RNA may be produced from one gene and spliced variants of mRNA in higher organisms are commonly tissue specific (e.g. splice variants for FGF receptors). The size of genes varies a great deal, depending partly on the size of the protein to be produced (Table 2.4). Even within a gene sequence, although all of it is transcribed as primary RNA, not all sections are exported as mature RNA. The gene is arranged into exons, which are exported from the nucleus as mature mRNA, and introns, which are excised from the primary transcript mRNA (Figure 2.21) by means of RNA splicing and degraded in the nucleus.

Each gene produces messenger RNA (mRNA) and most genes (except those encoding ribosomal and tRNA) eventually produce proteins, some of which control the synthesis and modification of other compounds such as nucleic acids, lipids and carbohydrates. Less than 1% of DNA is transcribed into mature mRNA. Proteins have myriad functions,

Table 2.4 The size of some human genes

Protein	Gene size (kb)	mRNA size (kb)	No. of introns
β globulin	1.5	0.6	2
Insulin	1.7	0.4	2
Protein kinase C	11	1.4	7
Albumin	25	2.1	14
Catalase	34	1.6	12
LDL receptor	45	5.5	17
Factor VIII	186	9	25
Thyroglobulin	300	8.7	36
Dystrophin	>2000	17	>50

ranging from structural proteins such as actins right through to those that precisely control the rate of gene transcription.

mRNA synthesis

The first step in this process is the synthesis of primary or heterogenous mRNA (hnRNA), which is initiated by RNA polymerase type II, a large multi-unit enzyme. This enzyme binds to the promoter unit of the gene which is to be transcribed in conjunction with several other proteins called transcription factors.

The promoter region contains the site at which transcription factors bind and which is rich in TATA sequences (the so-called TATA box); it is situated about 25 nucleotides upstream of the start site of the gene. An AUG codon (methionine) always represents the start of each gene. RNA polymerase opens up the double-stranded helix and RNA is synthesised by the polymerase, moving from the 3' to the 5' direction of DNA (i.e. the RNA is extended from the 5' to the 3' direction; Figure 2.22). This elongation continues until the polymerase reaches a stop signal (UAA; UAG). Thirty nucleotides are added per second, so a chain of 5000 nucleotides will take about three minutes to make. Each strand of the double helix could, in theory, be used to copy into RNA, but in any one section of DNA only one strand is used, although in any one chromosome different strands are used in different parts.

There are three types of RNA polymerase (types I, II and III). Type I RNA polymerase makes large ribosomal RNA, type III makes tRNA and the small 5S ribosomal RNA. Type II RNA polymerase is responsible for the synthesis of the other types of RNA. Both ends of mRNA are modified. The 5' end is 'capped' by a methylated G nucleotide, whereas a polyadenylated (poly-A) tail is added to the 3' end. The 5' cap plays an important part in protein synthesis and protects the mRNA from degradation. The

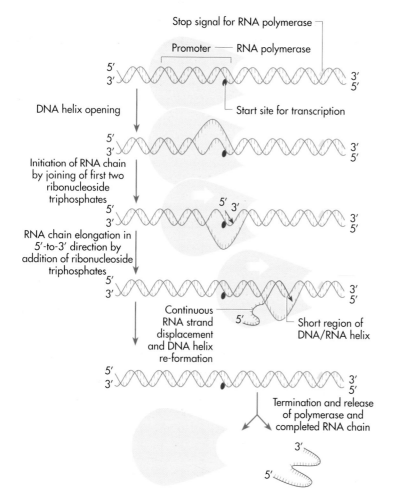

Figure 2.22 *The synthesis of an RNA molecule by RNA polymerase. The enzyme binds to the promoter sequence on the DNA and begins its synthesis at a start site within the promoter. It completes its synthesis at a stop (termination) signal, whereupon both the polymerase and its completed RNA chain are released. During RNA chain elongation, polymerisation rates average about 30 nucleotides per second at 37 °C. Therefore, an RNA chain of 5000 nucleotides takes about three minutes to complete.*

poly-A tail aids the export of mRNA; it may stabilise mRNA in the cytoplasm and it serves as a recognition signal for the ribosome. The primary RNA transcript from the gene is known as heterogeneous RNA (hnRNA), most of which is rapidly destroyed by removal and splicing of the remaining mRNA. The presence of the poly-A tail allows purification of the mRNA from other types of RNA, which is useful in purifying mRNA for studies.

Introns and exons: mRNA processing

Early evidence for the presence of introns was the finding that mature RNA was relatively short, and when in experiments it was annealed to DNA containing the gene of interest, it was found that the DNA formed several large loops, only short sections of DNA being adherent to mRNA. Primary mRNA transcribed from the loops of DNA not bound to the mature mRNA does not form part of mature mRNA and is excised as introns. hnRNA, which is the primary transcript of the gene, is much longer than the mature mRNA; although it has the 5′ cap and poly-A tail, it also contains several introns. The hnRNA in the nucleus is coated with proteins and small nuclear ribonucleoproteins (snRNP), which are somewhat

similar to ribosomes but much smaller (250 kDa compared with 4500 kDa); they are crucial to the excision of introns. Patients with systemic lupus erythematosus form autoantibodies against one or more snRNPs. As pointed out in Table 2.4, introns form much the largest part of hnRNA and of the genome itself. Introns can accumulate several mutations without necessarily affecting protein function (i.e. they comprise so-called junk DNA). However, point mutations near the exon/intron junction can have disastrous effects on protein function if they result in introns not being removed (e.g. thalassaemia) and in the formation of longer sections of mRNA and therefore of new types of protein. Spliceosomes are formed by aggregation of several snRNPs, ATP and other proteins onto the exon/intron junction. They remove the intron as a 'lariat' or noose-like structure (Figure 2.23). Most genes contain several introns. Following excision of introns, the exons are then spliced together to form mature mRNA, which is then exported from the nucleus via the nuclear pores.

In the formation of some proteins, differential RNA splicing is the norm and can produce different forms of RNA and hence different proteins. This is achieved by differential binding of distinct repressors

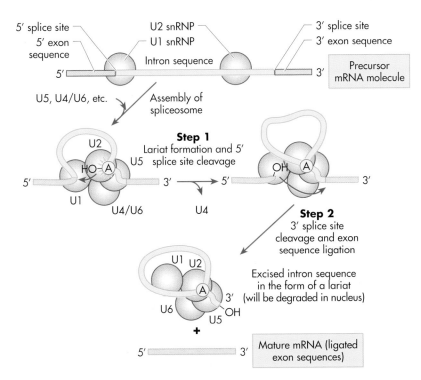

Figure 2.23 The RNA-splicing mechanism. RNA splicing is catalysed by a spliceosome formed from the assembly of U1, U2, U5 and U4/U6 snRNPs (shown as green circles) plus other components (not shown). After assembly of the spliceosome, the reaction occurs in two steps: in step 1, the branch-point A nucleotide in the intron sequence, which is located close to the 3′ splice site, attacks the 5′ splice site and cleaves it; the cut 5′ end of the intron sequence thereby becomes covalently linked to this A nucleotide, forming the branched nucleotide. In step 2, the 3′-OH end of the first exon sequence, which was created in the first step, adds to the beginning of the second exon sequence, cleaving the RNA molecule at the 3′ splice site; the two exon sequences are thereby joined to each other and the intron sequence is released as a lariat. The spliceosome complex sediments at 60S, indicating that it is nearly as large as a ribosome. These splicing reactions occur in the nucleus and generate mRNA molecules from primary RNA transcripts (mRNA precursor molecules).

or activators to the primary RNA transcript which can alter the splice site and therefore alter the exact structure of the final mature mRNA. This occurs with the FGF receptors, which have several different spliced variants and different affinities for various members of the FGF family.

Control of transcription

Various proteins bind to the promoter regions of genes to act as promoters and repressors. These can be classified into the following types.

Helix-turn-helix proteins. These are comprised solely of amino acids and have a structure that facilitates binding into the major groove of DNA. Their binding may block transcription or, conversely, may force bending of the DNA molecule facilitating transcription. The homeo-domain proteins are a type of helix-turn-helix protein which are involved in sequential embryonic development. Each of these homeo-domain proteins contains an identical section of 60 amino acids.

Zinc finger proteins. Some transcription factors are rich in histidine and cysteine residues which can bind zinc, thereby bending the protein into a finger-like shape. Steroid hormone receptors also contain several zinc fingers and are thought to function as transcription factors.

Proteins with a leucine zipper motif. Certain α protein chains can form Y-shaped dimers which can attach to DNA. The two chains are held together by interactions between hydrophobic regions that are rich in leucine.

Helix-loop-helix proteins. These form structures similar to leucine zippers.

These protein regulators of gene transcription can turn genes on or off, depending on how they link with other transcription factors and RNA polymerase. It is also clear that many gene regulatory proteins act at a distance upstream or downstream from the gene itself (Figure 2.24). These gene regulatory proteins can have their function changed by increased de-novo synthesis when needed, by ligand binding, by phosphorylation or by combination with a second agent.

In addition to these specific transcription factors, general transcription factors are also required. Several proto-oncogenes are transcription factors. Fos and jun combine when phosphorylated to form the AP-1 protein, which functions as a transcription factor. Several growth factors interact through ras to activate mitogen-activated protein (MAP) kinase which phosphorylates a protein called Elk-1, which itself activates the transcription of fos.

Modification of DNA can alter transcription

DNA that is tightly packaged around nucleosomes or the type that is packaged into heterochromatin is not easily transcribed. Condensation of the second X chromosome in women may affect the maternal or paternal copy at random, but small zones of neighbouring cells in tissues will have the same X chromosome inactivated as a mosaic pattern. Another method of inactivating genes is heavy methylation of cytosine bases, which can result in inactivation of either the maternal or the paternal copies of particular

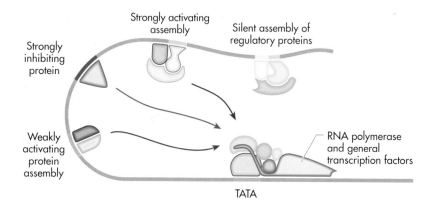

Figure 2.24 *Integration at a promoter. Multiple sets of gene regulatory proteins can work together to influence a promoter, as they do in the eve stripe 2 module. It is not yet understood in detail how the integration of multiple inputs is achieved.*

genes. For instance, only the paternal IGF-II gene is active; the maternal copy is inactivated or 'imprinted' throughout the whole body. Recent data have suggested that some tumour suppressor genes can be inactivated – not through mutations or deletions as is the case of retinoblastoma or p53, but through heavy methylation (e.g. the *MTS* gene which encodes the p16 protein).

Post-transcriptional modifications in mRNA stability

Another method of controlling how much protein is produced by mRNA is by altering the stability of mRNA, which is normally a nascent molecule with a half-life of around 30 minutes to 10 hours. Some mRNAs have lengths of AU-rich non-coding sequences at the 3′ end that stimulate the removal

of the poly-A tail, making the mRNA more stable. Some steroid hormones also increase the stability of certain mRNA molecules. Modification of the mRNA molecule can be mediated by proteins or, in some instances, by RNA sequences that have intrinsic enzymic activity (i.e. they are RNA-ases). Post-translational modifications in peptide chains can also lead to increased protein stability and increased duration of action.

Ribosomal RNA

During cell division, a large number of new ribosomes is required and, because the amplification process involved in protein synthesis (mRNA being translated into many protein molecules) is not available, most cells contain tandemly arranged multiple copies of ribosomal genes (around 200 per cell) on

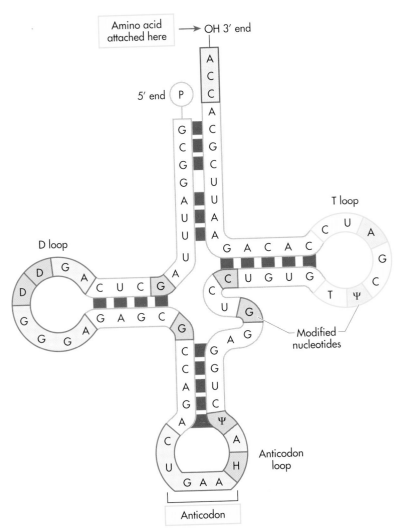

Figure 2.25 *The 'cloverleaf' structure of tRNA. This is a view of a molecule after it has been partially unfolded. There are many different tRNA molecules, including at least one for each kind of amino acid. Although they differ in nucleotide sequence, they all have the three stem loops shown plus an amino acid-accepting arm. The particular tRNA molecule shown binds phenylalanine and is therefore denoted tRNA^{Phe}. In all tRNA molecules, the amino acid is attached to the A residue of a CCA sequence at the 3′ end of the molecule. Complementary base-pairings are shown by red bars.*

five pairs of different chromosomes. A tandem repeat is formed when duplicated DNA segments are joined head to tail. The initial ribosomal RNA (rRNA) transcript is 13 000 nucleotides long and is cut into three to form the 28S rRNA (5000 nucleotides), the 18S rRNA (2000 nucleotides) and the 5.8S rRNA (160 nucleotides) components of the ribosome. The 5S component of the large ribosomal subunit is transcribed separately by RNA polymerase III and there are 2000 copies of the 5S rRNA genes arranged as a single cluster.

Packaging of ribosomal RNA occurs in the nucleolus, into which protrude several large loops of DNA containing the tandem repeats for rRNA which are known as nucleolar organiser regions. Here, rRNA is transcribed by RNA polymerase I.

Protein synthesis

When the mature mRNA reaches the cytoplasm after passing through the nuclear pores, it becomes attached to ribosomes which catalyse the production of a peptide chain. Each amino acid is brought to the ribosome by its own specific small molecule of RNA – tRNA (Figure 2.25) – which has an 'anti-codon' at its base which corresponds to the codon for that particular amino acid. Specific enzymes couple specific amino acids to their particular tRNA molecule after the amino acid is activated by the attachment of AMP (an adenylated amino acid). The tRNA connected to its amino acid is referred to as an amino-acyl tRNA because of the bond between the amino acid and the tRNA. These mechanisms ensure that the right amino acid is brought by the correct tRNA to its specified position within the peptide chain. The genetic code is degenerate because most amino acids are coded for by more than one triplet, so that there is more than one tRNA for each amino acid and a single tRNA can bind with more than one codon. Many amino acids require that the codon is accurate only in its first two positions (see Table 2.2) and will tolerate 'wobble' in the third position. Each incoming amino acid is attached to the carboxy end of the growing peptide chain.

Each ribosome consists of two major parts: the 60S and 40S subunits. The large 60S subunit comprises three separate parts: a 28S rRNA, a 5.5S rRNA and a 5S rRNA (Figure 2.26). These two subunits dock separately (the small subunit attaches first) on the mRNA at the AUG start codon (Figure 2.27) and dock separately when the stop codon (UAG) is reached (Figure 2.28). Identification of the initiation site is important because, in principle, the mRNA can be read in any one of three reading frames, depending on the exact start site. Initiation factors assemble with the methionine tRNA at the start site before translation occurs.

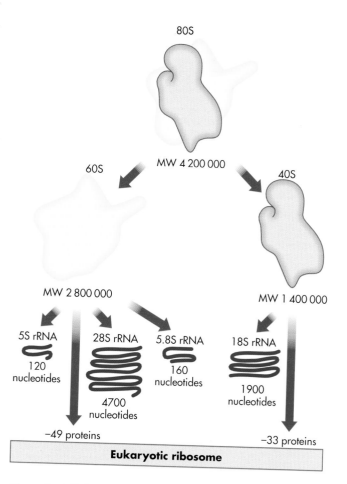

Figure 2.26 Eukaryotic ribosomes. Ribosomal components are commonly designated by their 'S values', which indicate their rate of sedimentation in an ultracentrifuge. Despite the differences in the number and size of their rRNA and protein components, both types of ribosomes have nearly the same structure and they function in very similar ways. Although the 18S and 28S rRNAs of the eukaryotic ribosome contain many extra nucleotides not present in their bacterial counterparts, these nucleotides are present as multiple insertions that are thought to protrude as loops and leave the basic structure of each rRNA largely unchanged.

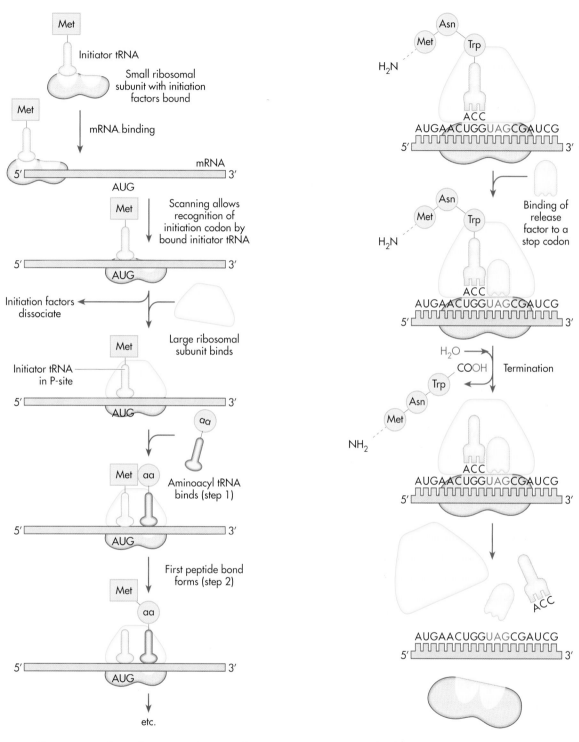

Figure 2.27 *The initiation phase of protein synthesis in eukaryotes.*

Figure 2.28 *The final phase of protein synthesis. The binding of release factor to a stop codon terminates translation. The completed polypeptide is released, and the ribosome dissociates into its two separate subunits.*

Usually, there are several ribosomes attached to each mRNA molecule so that at any one time there are several peptide chains in various stages of completion of synthesis. About 50% of the weight of the ribosome is RNA; the remainder is comprised of several types of proteins. Initially, it was thought that these proteins carried out the catalytic reactions of the RNA, but it is now suggested that the RNA itself has these properties and the function of the proteins is to modify these enzymatic functions. The ribosome has three binding sites for RNA, one for mRNA, one for incoming tRNA (A site), and the other for outgoing tRNA and peptide chain (P site). On binding of an incoming tRNA, the amino-acyl-RNA bond is lysed and a peptide bond is formed between the new amino acid and the peptide chain. The peptidyl-RNA in the A site is then moved to the P site by means of an energy-dependent reaction (GTP driven) which frees up the A site for a new amino acid.

Obviously, recognition of the correct amino acid attached to the correct tRNA molecule is important. Firstly, the attachment of the amino acid to the tRNA is specific and, if an incorrect amino acid is bound to the amino-acyl synthetase enzyme, it is removed by hydrolysis. Secondly, the tRNA is attached to the mRNA as a complex with elongation factors which prevent the amino acid immediately undergoing attachment to the peptide chain; there is a short delay which allows an incorrect tRNA to exit from the codon.

It should be noted that the control of the levels of protein formation is achieved by:

1. control over gene transcription;
2. controlling the speed of mRNA degradation;
3. controlling post-translational peptide and altering protein stability.

For instance, up-regulation of *p53* in epidermal cells following exposure to sunlight is achieved by increasing the stability of protein which has already been made.

Further reading

Garrett RH, Grisham CM. Molecular aspects of cell biology. Fort Worth: Harcourt Brace College Publishers, 1995

Goodman SR. Medical cell biology. Philadelphia: JB Lippincott Company, 1994

Heath JK. Growth factors. Oxford: IRL Press, 1993

Lodish H, Baltimore D, Berk A, Zipursky SL, Matsudaira P, Darnell J. Molecular cell biology. New York: Scientific American Books, 1995

The nature of renal function

3

G. B. Haycock

Homeostasis

Homeostasis was originally defined as maintenance of the constancy of the internal environment. The 'internal environment' is the fluid that bathes the cells, the extracellular fluid (ECF). In modern language, therefore, homeostasis is the regulation of the volume and composition of the ECF. The kidney is the pre-eminent organ of homeostasis, although the lungs, gut and skin also contribute to it. One component of homeostasis is excretion of the products of metabolism: failure of excretion leads to accumulation of these products, with progressive pollution of the ECF. A second component is conservation of ECF solutes (mainly nutrients) that are too valuable to be allowed to escape into the urine. The third component is constant adjustment of the urinary excretion rate of water and inorganic solutes to maintain their concentrations in the ECF within the normal range, in the face of unpredictably changing input from the diet and from other body water compartments. This last might be called homeostasis proper. In order to achieve it, the kidney must:

sense small changes in ECF volume or in the concentration of any of its many constituents, before such changes become serious;
respond by altering the volume or composition of the urine so as to correct the tendency to abnormality.

This is achieved by negative feedback: a rise in the ECF concentration of, say, potassium leads to an increase in its excretion rate, with a consequent return of the ECF concentration to normal; whereas a fall in the concentration leads to a decrease in excretion rate, defending the ECF against hypokalaemia. The kidney's capacity to alter the volume of urine and the concentration of its constituent solutes is very large. For instance, an adult can vary daily urine volume between a minimum of a few centilitres and a maximum of more than 20 litres, while the urinary concentration of the major ECF cation, sodium, can vary by at least three orders of magnitude.

The concept of external balance

Homeostasis requires (in the non-growing organism) that net input of any substance into the ECF be exactly equal to net output from it. In health, body composition remains constant because output, mainly via the kidney, can be varied continuously in response to changes in input. The net external balance (NEB) for any substance is the algebraic difference between input and output over any specified period of time, i.e.:

$$NEB = input - output \qquad (1)$$

Balance may be positive (input > output), negative (output > input) or zero (input = output). Normally, NEB for all non-metabolised substances is zero, except in growing individuals in whom it is continuously positive. Because the main determinant of input is food intake, an obvious survival advantage enjoyed by an animal with a large reserve of renal function is the ability to eat a varied diet. As renal function is lost, dietary freedom becomes constrained. In advanced renal failure, survival is only possible on a rigorously controlled diet, reversing the normal physiological state of affairs: homeostasis is achieved by adjusting intake to match a relatively constant urinary output.

Growth and renal function

The size of the kidneys, and therefore their functional capacity, increases with the growth of the body as a whole. Between the age of two years and maturity, glomerular filtration rate (GFR) and renal blood flow are approximately proportional to body surface area (BSA) [1]. Average GFR in the healthy human is about 120 ml/min per 1.73 m^2 BSA (range 90–150).† The association between renal function and BSA is empirical, and probably does not reflect any underlying physiological principle. Others have argued that it should be standardised to ECF volume [3] or weight [4]; the latter undoubtedly gives a better fit than BSA in newborn infants (Figure 3.1).

Whatever standardising factor is applied, renal function is low at birth and during the first few months of extrauterine life, even corrected for body size. Despite this, normal infants thrive and show no clinical or biochemical evidence of failure of excre-

tion or homeostasis. This can be explained by the fact that the infant is growing very rapidly at this stage, increasing body weight by up to 5% per week. This results in a strongly positive NEB for most nutrients, particularly since they are supplied by the baby's normal diet (human milk) in quantities that provide only just enough energy, protein and minerals to support normal growth and activity. The residue remaining for excretion is therefore very small: growth provides the infant with a 'third kidney' [5]. A major advantage to the infant of constraining glomerular filtration at a low level is conservation of energy. Approximately 99% of filtered sodium is absorbed, with its attendant anions, in the renal tubule. This is an active process (see below) and accounts for almost all of the energy expenditure of the kidney. The additional energy cost of reabsorbing the sodium filtered at an 'adult' level of glomerular filtration would be prohibitive, given the marginal sufficiency provided by human milk as referred to above [6, 7]. The negative aspect of the low GFR of the newborn is its lack of reserve. If growth is interrupted for any reason (e.g. intercurrent infection), or if an unphysiological diet is given (e.g. unmodified cow's milk), the solute load presented for excretion can overwhelm the kidney, leading to a form of acute renal insufficiency with resulting metabolic

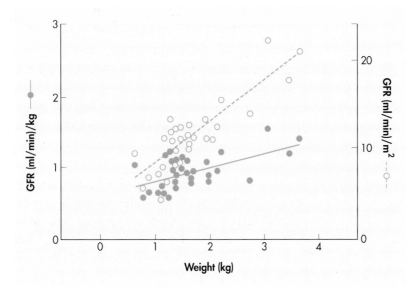

Figure 3.1 *The relationship between glomerular filtration rate (GFR) corrected for body surface area (interrupted line) and weight (continuous line) in newborn infants. Within the range studied, glomerular filtration rate per m^2 increases threefold, while glomerular filtration rate per kg less than doubles. (Reproduced by permission from Coulthard and Hey [4].)*

† In a rational world, the ridiculous figure of 1.73 m^2, taken as the surface area of the 'average adult' [2], would be consigned to the waste-paper basket and physiological values would be nominalised to 1 m^2. The average GFR would then be expressed as 70 ml/min/m^2 (range 50–90).

imbalance. This is exemplified by the syndrome of late metabolic acidosis of prematurity [8, 9].

The concept of renal clearance

It follows from the above that, in a steady state, the composition of the urine is determined by dietary and metabolic input to the ECF and not by renal function: individuals with a GFR of 100 ml/min and 10 ml/min, respectively, will produce identical urine if they are eating identical diets. Because the function of the kidneys is to regulate the ECF, one way of quantifying renal function is to measure the rate of processing of ECF (plasma). For any substance (x) present in both plasma and urine, it is simple to calculate the volume of plasma containing the quantity of x excreted in the urine in a specified period of time. This volume is the renal clearance of x, the volume of plasma (not urine) cleared of x per unit of time [10, 11].

Renal clearance is given by the formula:

$$C_x = \frac{U_x \times V}{P_x} \qquad (2)$$

where C, U and P represent clearance, urine and plasma concentrations respectively and V is the urine flow rate. C is expressed in the same units as those chosen to express V (e.g. ml/min, l/day).

In the special case of a substance which is freely filtered by the glomerulus, such that its concentration in plasma water and glomerular filtrate are the same, and which is not secreted or reabsorbed by the tubule or metabolised by the kidney, the filtration rate of x (F_x) must equal its excretion rate (E_x). The renal clearance of such a substance is equal to the GFR. No endogenous substance has been described that fulfils these criteria exactly. Inulin, a starch-like polymer of fructose, does fulfil them, and is therefore an ideal marker for measurement of GFR. The chelating agents EDTA and DTPA, which can be labelled with radioisotopes for easy assay in plasma and urine, and the radio contrast chemical sodium iothalamate, are excellent alternatives. Creatinine is an ideal marker for GFR in the dog; unfortunately, in humans it is secreted by the tubule, to a small extent when renal function is normal but to a considerably greater extent when renal

function is reduced [12]. Despite this limitation, a carefully performed creatinine clearance test is an adequate measure of GFR for most clinical purposes [13].

Any substance whose clearance is greater than GFR must be secreted by the tubule. Conversely, any freely filtered substance with a clearance less than GFR must be reabsorbed by the tubule. Dividing C_x by GFR gives the fractional excretion of x (FE_x). If creatinine clearance (C_{cr}) is taken as the GFR:

$$FE_x (\%) = \left(\frac{U_x \times P_{cr}}{U_{cr} \times P_x} \right) \times 100 \qquad (3)$$

Note that it is not necessary to measure V to calculate FE_x: a random, simultaneously obtained blood and urine sample is all that is required.

A substance that is completely cleared by the kidney, i.e. its concentration in renal venous plasma is zero, has a clearance equal to renal plasma flow (RPF). The organic anions para-aminohippurate (PAH) and ortho-aminohippurate (hippuran) are almost ideal markers for the measurement of RPF in most circumstances. An exception is in the newborn, in whom renal extraction of PAH is incomplete [14]. Dividing GFR by RPF gives the filtration fraction (FF), the proportion of renal arterial plasma removed from the circulation as glomerular filtrate:

$$FF = \frac{GFR}{RPF} = \frac{C_{inulin}}{C_{PAH}} = \frac{U/P_{inulin}}{U/P_{PAH}} \qquad (4)$$

Typical normal values (after infancy) for GFR, RPF and FF are 120 ml/min per 1.73 m^2, 600 ml/min per 1.73 m^2, and 0.2 respectively.

Functional segmentation of the nephron

Each nephron consists of a glomerulus and its attached tubule (Figure 3.2). The tubule is divided into two major segments: the proximal and distal tubules. The proximal tubule is further divided into the early (S$_1$) and late (S$_2$) proximal convoluted tubule, the proximal straight tubule (pars recta, S$_3$) and the loop of Henle. About 90% of the human nephron population have short loops of Henle that descend only into the outer medulla before bending and returning towards the surface of the cortex. The

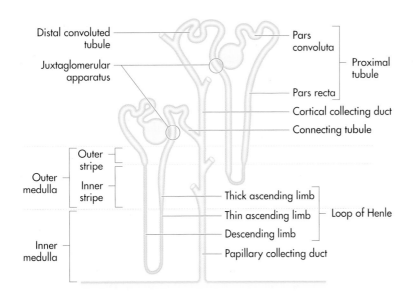

Distal convoluted tubule

Juxtaglomerular apparatus

Pars convoluta

Pars recta

Proximal tubule

Cortical collecting duct

Connecting tubule

Outer medulla

Outer stripe

Inner stripe

Inner medulla

Thick ascending limb

Thin ascending limb

Descending limb

Papillary collecting duct

Loop of Henle

Figure 3.2 Schematic representation of two nephrons, one of which is a juxtamedullary nephron (long loop of Henle) and one a superficial cortical nephron (short loop of Henle). Neither the relative lengths of the different nephron segments nor the dimensions of the various cortical and medullary layers is drawn to scale.

remaining 10% have long loops of Henle that descend deep into the inner medulla and bend at or near the papillary tip. These are the tubules that arise from those glomeruli situated in the deepest layer of the cortex, the juxtamedullary nephrons; they form an important part of the mechanism for urinary concentration and dilution. The parts of the loop that extend into the inner medulla are thin walled and called the thin descending and thin ascending limbs of the loop, respectively. The cortical part of the ascending limb is relatively thick walled and is referred to as the thick ascending limb (TAL). The TAL of both types of nephron passes through the vascular pole of its own glomerulus, where it is intimately related to both the afferent and the efferent arterioles in a structure called the juxtaglomerular apparatus (JGA) [15]. The JGA marks the functional division between the proximal and distal tubules.

The distal tubule is also divided into the distal convoluted tubule, connecting tubule, cortical collecting duct and medullary collecting duct. The different segments of the nephron are identifiable not only by their anatomical relationships but also by the ultrastructural and histochemical characteristics of their epithelia. Details may be found in relevant anatomical and pathological studies [16–20].

The function of the glomerulus

The glomerulus is a microscopic network of specialised capillaries that act as a size-selective and electrical charge-selective ultrafilter, retaining large molecules such as proteins within the lumen while allowing the passage of small molecules (water, electrolytes and other crystalloid solutes) into Bowman's space. The concentration of these solutes in glomerular filtrate is almost identical with that in plasma, with a small correction for the Gibbs–Donnan effect (due to the fact that negatively charged proteins are in much higher concentration within the capillary lumen than in glomerular filtrate). Ultrafiltration is a passive process, and the concentrations of small solutes in glomerular filtrate depend entirely on their concentrations in plasma. Glomerular filtrate is therefore a precursor of urine, the final composition of which is extensively modified by tubular reabsorption and secretion. Some important waste products of protein metabolism such as urea and creatinine are mainly excreted by glomerular filtration. Although the excretion rate of these compounds is maintained at reduced levels of GFR, this is at the cost of sustained elevation of their plasma concentrations.

The function of the proximal tubule

Pars convoluta and pars recta
Two-thirds of the volume of the glomerular filtrate is reabsorbed in the proximal tubule [21]. The nature of the reabsorptive process can be summarised as follows:

It is isotonic.

Some solutes (bicarbonate, glucose, amino acids) are preferentially reabsorbed in the initial segments of the proximal tubule, leading to their almost complete removal from the tubular fluid and a rise in the concentration of chloride (Cl^-).

It is energy and oxygen dependent.

Some solutes (e.g. inulin, creatinine and urea) are reabsorbed little or not at all, and are therefore markedly concentrated with respect to plasma by the end of the proximal tubule.

Organic anions such as PAH and penicillin are actively secreted in this segment. The fluid delivered into the loop of Henle is therefore:

isotonic with plasma;

chloride rich and bicarbonate poor;

at a pH lower than that of plasma;

more concentrated than plasma with respect to those substances (urea, creatinine, inulin) excreted solely or principally by glomerular filtration. The ratio of the tubular fluid inulin concentration to the plasma inulin concentration ($TF:P_{inulin}$) at any point along the tubule is a measure of the volume of filtrate that has been absorbed at that point.

Loop of Henle

Net reabsorption continues in the loop so that about 85% of filtered sodium and 70% of filtered water have been reabsorbed at entry into the distal tubule. The major function of the loop is concentration and dilution of urine; reabsorption in this segment is therefore no longer isotonic.

Concentration and dilution of urine are both powered by the same energy-dependent process: absorption of salt without water in the TAL. This results in the fluid entering the distal tubule being hypotonic with respect to plasma, irrespective of whether the final urine is concentrated or dilute at the time. It also generates hypertonicity in the interstitium surrounding the TAL. This hypertonicity is amplified by countercurrent exchange and multiplication in the loops of Henle and vasa recta, leading to the establishment of an osmotic gradient in the medulla with the highest osmolality at the papillary tip. In the presence of antidiuretic hormone (ADH),

the collecting duct becomes permeable to water, which is osmotically extracted from the lumen by the hypertonic medulla, leading to the formation of concentrated urine.

The function of the distal tubule

The distal tubule adjusts the composition of the final urine by selectively reabsorbing or secreting individual solutes according to the need of the moment. For example, reabsorption of Na from the tubular fluid is virtually complete in Na depletion, whereas in Na repletion exactly sufficient Na escapes reabsorption to balance dietary input. Many substances (e.g. Na, Cl, calcium, phosphate) are normally filtered in amounts greatly exceeding dietary input and the excretion rate is regulated by varying the amount reabsorbed. Other important substances, notably hydrogen ions and potassium, generally enter the distal tubule in very small amounts and the rate of excretion depends mainly on varying the rate of active secretion into the tubular fluid. The rate of water excretion is determined by ADH, which increases the water permeability of the collecting duct and thus regulates the rate of osmotic reabsorption of water into the hypertonic medullary and papillary interstitium.

Glomerular filtration

The glomerular filtration rate (GFR) is determined by the interaction of the physical forces driving filtration and the permeability of the filtration barrier (the glomerular capillary wall) to water and small solutes. The composition of the filtrate in health is that of a protein-free ultrafiltrate of plasma, due to the almost complete impermeability of the glomerular capillaries to protein.

The glomerular capillary wall

Structure

The glomerular capillary wall has three layers: a lining endothelium composed of thin, fenestrated polygonal squames, a basement membrane, and an outer epithelium consisting of cells (podocytes), each of which possesses a central body from which radiate fern-like foot processes (pedicels) that interdigitate with those of adjacent cells. In section, the transected foot processes appear as islands of cytoplasm intimately attached to the basement membrane and connected to one another by a fine membrane. The view afforded by scanning electron microscopy shows these islands to be sections through alternating processes from adjacent cells [22, 23]. The basement membrane is a hydrated proteoglycan gel with a thickness of about 3200 Å in the adult [24] and rather less in the infant [25]. Ultrastructural examination reveals a central, relatively electron dense lamina densa, sandwiched between a lamina rara interna and a lamina rara externa (although this appearance may be a fixation artefact). The thin squames of the endothelium contain numerous fenestrae of 700 Å diameter [26]. This differentiates them from the endothelium of capillaries in other tissues. All three layers take up cationic stains, indicating that they are negatively charged [27].

Location of the filtration barrier

All three layers of the glomerular capillary wall probably contribute to the retention of macromolecules in the capillary lumen. Ultrastructural studies using macromolecular tracers of different sizes and electrical charge [27–29] suggest that very large molecules are completely excluded from the basement membrane, whereas smaller ones penetrate it to varying degrees. Small quantities of molecules of approximately the size of albumin appear to traverse the basement membrane but are retained at the filtration slits between the epithelial foot processes [30]. The electrical charge, as well as the size, of molecules is an important determinant of their ability to cross the capillary wall into Bowman's space [31, 32]. Proteinuric states are associated with loss of negative charge from one or more layers of the capillary wall [33]. It is widely accepted that the escape of large amounts of protein from the plasma into the glomerular filtrate is prevented partly by the physical structure of the proteoglycan mesh of the basement membrane and partly by its electronegativity. The small amount of albumin that crosses the membrane is further contained by the polyanionic coat surrounding the epithelial cells and extending to the filtration slits between them. The relative importance of charge selectivity and size selectivity is still controversial, however [34].

Dynamics of glomerular filtration

Starling forces

Glomerular filtration is driven by the balance between the hydrostatic pressure gradient between capillary and Bowman's space, generated by myocardial contraction, and the oncotic pressure (colloid osmotic pressure) gradient generated by the protein concentration gradient between the same two compartments. Hydrostatic pressure favours, and oncotic pressure opposes, filtration. These forces are referred to as Starling forces [35]. Starling forces govern the movement of fluid between the intravascular and extravascular compartments of the extracellular fluid throughout the body as a whole, glomerular filtration being a special example of their application. The net ultrafiltration pressure (P_{UF}) is therefore the algebraic sum of the hydrostatic (P) and oncotic (Π) pressure gradients between capillary (C) and Bowman's space (BS):

$$P_{UF} = (P_C - P_{BS}) - (\Pi_C - \Pi_{BS}) \qquad (5)$$

Since Π_{BS} is insignificant:

$$P_{UF} = P_C - P_{BS} - \Pi_C \qquad (6)$$

P must be higher at the arterial than at the venous end of the glomerular capillary plexus, or blood would not flow. The pressure drop is small, however, since the glomerular capillaries are low-resistance vessels between two high-resistance components (the afferent and efferent arterioles). As plasma passes through the glomerulus, filtration occurs and the plasma proteins are progressively concentrated towards the venous end by the removal of water. The force opposing filtration (Π_C) therefore increases. The combination of falling P and rising Π causes P_{UF} to diminish towards the venous end of the capillary [36, 37]. These pressures have been directly measured in several species. At least in the Munich–Wistar rat and the squirrel monkey, P_{UF} at the venous end of the circuit is zero [38, 39]. This means that filtration actually stops before the efferent arteriole is reached, a condition referred to as filtration equilibrium. A normalised plot of filtration pressure gradients can therefore be drawn (Figure 3.3). The mean ultrafiltration pressure is shown as the integrated area between the curves for P and Π. For technical reasons, it is not possible in filtration

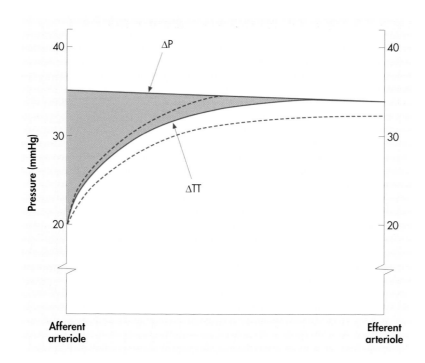

Figure 3.3 *Hydrostatic (P) and oncotic (Π) pressure profiles along an idealised glomerular capillary. As plasma traverses the capillary bed from afferent to efferent arteriole, removal of fluid by filtration causes the plasma protein concentration to rise, with a consequent increase in ΔΠ. In filtration equilibrium (unbroken lines), ΔΠ rises to equal ΔP, and filtration stops, before the efferent arteriole is reached. An infinite number of lines (e.g. upper interrupted line) can be drawn that yield filtration equilibrium: these curves cannot be distinguished by measurement of P and Π in preglomerular and postglomerular vessels. As flow increases, the point of intersection of ΔP and ΔΠ moves to the right, eventually producing filtration disequilibrium (lower interrupted line). In filtration disequilibrium, measurement of afferent and efferent arteriolar pressure allows a unique ΔΠ curve to be plotted from which Kf can be calculated. The shaded area represents P_{UF}. (Modified from Deen et al. [40].)*

equilibrium to measure at what point along the notional distance between afferent and efferent arteriole equilibrium is achieved. If all other variables are held constant, and plasma flow is increased or decreased, this point will move to the right or the left, respectively; there is an infinite family of curves yielding pressure equilibrium at the efferent arteriole. Under these conditions, filtration fraction is constant, and:

$$GFR \propto GPF \qquad (7)$$

i.e., GFR is plasma flow (GPF) dependent [38]. It is not known whether filtration equilibrium is the normal condition in humans.

The ultrafiltration coefficient

At any given P_{UF}, filtration rate is inversely proportional to the resistance offered by the filtering membrane. The reciprocal of this resistance is the ultrafiltration coefficient (Kf). Kf is the product of the surface area of the membrane (S) and its hydraulic permeability or conductivity (k), the latter being expressed as rate of flow (Q) per unit S per unit P_{UF}:

$$k = Q \times S^{-1} \times P_{UF}^{-1} \qquad (8)$$

Although S can be estimated morphometrically, it is difficult or impossible to measure effective S, the area

participating in filtration at any given time. In the absence of a reliable value for S, k cannot be calculated. The composite term Kf is therefore preferred for most purposes [40, 41]. Thus:

$$GFR = P_{UF} \times k \times S = P_{UF} \times Kf \qquad (9)$$

In filtration equilibrium, Kf is not limiting to GFR and cannot be calculated from experimental measurements. When filtration disequilibrium is induced by massive volume expansion, Kf becomes rate limiting and a unique value can be calculated for it from measurements of hydrostatic and oncotic pressures in the afferent and efferent arterioles and in Bowman's space, and single nephron GFR. In the Munich–Wistar rat, Deen *et al.* [40] arrived at a value for single nephron Kf of 0.08 nl/s per mmHg. Navar *et al.* [41] obtained an identical value in the dog, a species in which filtration equilibrium is not present. Depending on the value taken for S, this yields a estimate for k in the range 25–50 nl/s per mmHg per cm^2 [42, 43]. This is 10–100 times higher than that found in capillaries from other tissues [44, 45] enabling filtrate to be formed at a very high rate despite rather low values for P_{UF} (<10 mmHg). It is evident from Equation 9 that GFR may change as a result of changes in factors affecting one or more of the components of P_{UF}

(changes of glomerular plasma flow, plasma albumin concentration or urinary tract obstruction), changes in S (reduction of nephron numbers) or changes in k (diffuse glomerular disease). More than one of these may be involved in progressive renal disease.

Regulation of glomerular filtration

Factors affecting P_{UF}

As discussed above (see Equation 7), GFR is plasma flow dependent if:

filtration equilibrium exists;
$\Delta P - \Delta \Pi$ at the afferent arteriole does not change;
Kf is constant.

Under physiological conditions, these requirements are probably met, at least approximately. Plasma flow is determined by arterial pressure and renal vascular resistance, which resides mostly in the afferent and efferent glomerular arterioles [36]. Angiotensin II (AII) and norepinephrine (noradrenaline, NE) constrict both afferent and efferent arterioles [46]; these hormones are released in ECF volume contraction and other conditions in which arterial filling, and therefore renal perfusion pressure, is reduced. Efferent arteriolar constriction raises P_C, and therefore P_{UF}, more than it reduces glomerular blood flow, leading to maintenance of GFR by an increase in FF (Equation 4). Conversely, vasodilators such as prostaglandins E2 and I2 (prostacyclin) and bradykinin, despite a lowering of arterial blood pressure, cause renal plasma flow to rise due to dilatation of both afferent and efferent arterioles [47, 48]. Here again, GFR remains relatively constant with an associated fall in FF. It is likely that both vasodilator and vasoconstrictor hormones also affect Kf (see below). Obstruction to the flow of urine causes reduction or abolition of glomerular filtration due to a rise in P_{BS} (Equations 5 and 6).

Factors affecting Kf

The mesangial cells that support the glomerular capillaries are contractile [49]. Their contraction causes constriction of the capillaries, with a resulting fall in S and therefore Kf [50]. AII, NE and prostaglandins all alter Kf to the degree necessary to offset their effects on P_{UF}; in other words, the glomerular haemodynamic response to vasoactive substances is nicely balanced by changes in Kf, maintaining GFR approximately constant. Both AII and ADH cause cultured mesangial cells to contract, and this may be a physiologically important effect in vivo.

Autoregulation

In common with other vital organs, the kidney is capable of regulating its own blood flow, even in an artificial perfusion system in which systemic humoral and nervous controlling factors cannot operate. Micropuncture studies in rats show this to be due to differential constriction of the afferent and efferent arterioles [51]. Analysis of the determinants of GFR in this model system suggests that the damping effect on it is mediated in part by autoregulation of plasma flow and partly by compensatory changes in P_C, producing parallel changes in P_{UF}. As mentioned in the previous section, a role for mesangial cell contraction in autoregulation is likely, probably by altering Kf; locally produced AII may be involved in this process. Autoregulation fails at extremes of blood pressure. In malignant hypertension, the exposure of the kidney to excessive pressure leads acutely to disturbance of the mechanisms coupling GFR to tubular reabsorption, causing the phenomenon of pressure natriuresis. When blood pressure falls below the autoregulatory range, RPF and GFR fall and prerenal failure develops.

Proximal tubular function

About two-thirds of filtered salt and water is reabsorbed in the proximal tubule. Other solutes, including glucose, amino acids, bicarbonate and low molecular weight proteins, are almost completely reclaimed in this tubule segment, as is about 90% of filtered inorganic phosphate. Epithelial transport of all of these is linked to sodium transport and dependent on it for its energy supply.

Salt and water reabsorption in the proximal tubule

Sodium reabsorption

The proximal tubular epithelial cells are arranged in a single layer lining the cylindrical basement membrane. They exhibit polarity: the membranes on opposite sides of the cells have different characteristics. The part of the cell membrane that faces the tubular lumen is called the apical membrane; the part that faces the basement membrane and the intercellular space is the basolateral membrane. Adjacent cells are attached to one another at the tight junction, which separates the apical from the basolateral membranes (Figure 3.4).

The enzyme sodium, potassium adenosine triphosphatase (Na$^+$, K$^+$-ATPase, commonly known as the sodium pump) is located in the basolateral membrane. Powered by energy released by the hydrolysis of ATP, it transports sodium out of the cell interior and potassium into it, with a stoichiometry of 3Na$^+$:2K$^+$. This process is called primary active transport. A consequence of the action of Na$^+$, K$^+$-ATPase is a very low intracellular sodium concentration, establishing a

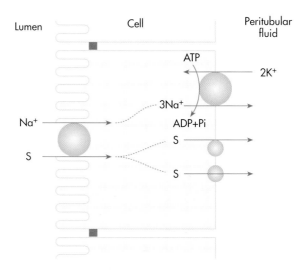

Figure 3.4 *Schematic view of a proximal tubular cell. The brush border of the apical membrane (left) is depicted as a wavy line. The basolateral membrane (right and lining the intercellular space) is separated from the apical membrane by the tight junction (black squares). S represents any substance that enters the cell across the apical membrane by secondary active transport via Na–S co-transporter. The enzyme Na$^+$, K$^+$-ATPase (upper right) maintains a steep gradient for sodium across the apical membrane by constantly extruding Na$^+$ across the basolateral membrane.*

steep concentration gradient between the tubular fluid and the cell interior that favours sodium entry across the apical membrane. This membrane is impermeable to sodium, but contains proteins of several different types that act as specialised sodium channels. Each of these not only allows sodium entry but also transports another solute into or out of the cell. This is called secondary active transport, because the energy driving it is provided indirectly by Na$^+$, K$^+$-ATPase at a site remote from the transport process itself. Inhibition of Na$^+$, K$^+$-ATPase by ouabain blocks sodium reabsorption in all nephron segments [52, 53].

One of these proteins is a member of a group of transporters called Na$^+$, H$^+$-antiporters, known as NHE3 [54]. Antiporters are so called because they transport sodium and hydrogen ions (protons) in opposite directions. Sodium entry therefore leads to alkalinisation of the cell interior and acidification of the tubular fluid. By an indirect process described later in this chapter, this effectively causes reabsorption of bicarbonate in an amount chemically equivalent to the amount of sodium entering via the antiporter. This takes place early in the proximal tubule, and because bicarbonate, in common with other solutes described below, is reabsorbed in preference to chloride [55–58], the concentration of chloride in the tubular fluid increases to a level substantially higher than that in the peritubular fluid [59]. Chloride therefore moves down its concentration gradient from tubular fluid to peritubular space, partly by simple diffusion across the tight junction (which is not really chemically tight) and partly via chloride channels in the apical and basolateral membranes. Diffusion across the tight junction, bypassing the cell interior, is referred to as reabsorption via the paracellular shunt pathway. Because chloride is an anion, its removal from the luminal to the peritubular aspects of the tubule generates an electrical voltage, lumen positive, across the epithelium that acts as a further driving force for sodium reabsorption [57]. At least some of this also occurs through the paracellular shunt pathway.

Other apical membrane proteins transport sodium and another solute (the co-transportate) in the same direction, and are called co-transporters. For example, the sodium–glucose co-transporter is activated when one sodium ion and one glucose molecule attach to specific receptors on the protein on the luminal side of the membrane. The molecule then either rotates in the membrane or alters its configuration in such a way that the sodium and glucose are transferred to the cytoplasmic side of the apical membrane, where they are released. Other co-transporters include a sodium–phosphate transporter and a whole set of specific transporters for different amino acids. The general mode of operation of secondary active transport in the apical membrane of the proximal tubule is schematised in Figure 3.4. It should be realised that both the antiporter and the co-transporters are potentially bidirectional. It is only the maintenance of the steep concentration gradient favouring sodium entry, resulting from sodium removal by Na^+, K^+-ATPase, that causes them to transport protons out of the cell and the various co-transportates in. The antiporter and several of the apical membrane co-transporter proteins have now been sequenced and the corresponding genes mapped and cloned.

Water reabsorption in the proximal tubule

Water is reabsorbed by osmosis, diffusing down the osmotic gradient established by solute reabsorption. The epithelium is sufficiently permeable to water that osmotic equilibration is virtually instantaneous, and the osmolality of the tubular fluid at all points in the proximal tubule is not measurably different from that of plasma. An unknown, but probably substantial, proportion of water reabsorption takes place through the paracellular shunt pathway and provides yet another mechanism promoting sodium reabsorption. Active transport of sodium across the basolateral membrane into the lateral intercellular spaces leads to a small, transient osmotic water gradient favouring water reabsorption across the tight junction. The resulting water flux causes salt to be transported passively by a process known as convection or solvent drag, given that the tight junction is permeable to sodium and chloride [60]. The relative importance of transcellular and paracellular reabsorption of sodium and water is still uncertain.

The effect of physical forces on proximal tubular reabsorption

Water and solute reabsorbed from the tubular lumen is returned to the blood in the peritubular capillary plexus, which is perfused by blood draining from glomerular efferent arterioles. The peritubular capillaries are therefore in series with and downstream from the glomerulus. The rate of reabsorption of tubular fluid is governed by the Starling forces across the peritubular capillary wall [61]. The importance of the peritubular oncotic pressure in this process has been demonstrated both by micropuncture in the intact animal [62] and by studies in the isolated, perfused rabbit proximal tubule [63]. The effect of changes in peritubular hydrostatic pressure is less clear. Since the protein concentration of postglomerular plasma is proportional to the filtration fraction (Equation 4), it follows that changes in glomerular function may induce secondary changes in proximal tubular reabsorption rate; this may be important in the maintenance of glomerulotubular balance (see below).

Proximal tubular reabsorption of other solutes

Glucose

Glucose is reabsorbed by co-transport with sodium, chiefly in the early proximal tubule [58]. Glucose is not merely acting as an energy source for sodium transport, because the non-metabolised analogue α-methyl-D-glucoside can be substituted for it [56], but its transport is dependent on sodium reabsorption. Glucose and sodium enter the cell together by secondary active transport via the sodium–glucose co-transporter. This transporter is saturable, and when the filtered load of glucose exceeds its maximal transporting capacity (Tm), the excess is excreted in the urine. The relationship between glucose filtration, reabsorption and excretion is shown in Figure 3.5. Glycosuria occurs in hyperglycaemia (as in diabetes mellitus) because the filtered load of glucose exceeds the Tm of the transport system. Glycosuria due to abnormalities of the tubular glucose transport system (renal glycosuria) occurs when the renal threshold for glucose is less than the normal blood glucose concentration.

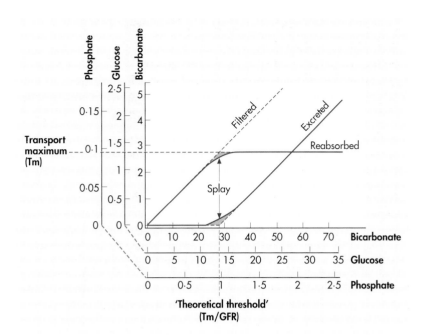

Figure 3.5 *Curves of filtration, excretion and re-absorption of three solutes re-absorbed actively from glomerular filtrate, plotted against plasma concentration of the solute. Values on the abscissa are plasma concentration (mmol/l); those on the ordinate are the quantities filtered, excreted and reabsorbed respectively (mmol/100 ml GFR).*

Phosphate

The majority of filtered phosphate is reabsorbed, with sodium, in the early proximal tubule [64, 65]. Studies of phosphate excretion at different plasma phosphate concentrations show that the ion is handled in a manner similar to glucose, i.e. by a saturable transport system with a Tm and a threshold [66] and hence a similar set of titration curves can be drawn (Figure 3.5). In contrast to glucose, some degree of phosphaturia is normally present because dietary phosphate in excess of requirement must be excreted. Thus, the normal plasma phosphate concentration is just above the threshold value, and is indeed defined by it, whereas in health the plasma glucose concentration is always well below the renal threshold.

Amino acids

Amino acids are reabsorbed with sodium in the same general manner as glucose and phosphate. At least five transport proteins exist, each co-transporting sodium and one of the major subclasses of amino acids with high specificity [67, 68]. The normal plasma concentrations of all the amino acids are below threshold in health, so that normal urine contains virtually no amino acids of any kind. Several inherited defects of sodium–amino acid co-transport systems have been described. By far the commonest is cystinuria, due to abnormalities of the protein that transports sodium with cystine and the dibasic amino acids (arginine, lysine and ornithine).

Proteins

Several low molecular weight proteins are present in normal plasma in measurable concentrations. Examples are α-1 microglobulin, β-2 microglobulin and retinol-binding protein (RBP). Because they are smaller than the size barrier of the glomerular ultra-filter, significant amounts are present in glomerular filtrate and enter the proximal tubule, where they are reabsorbed by pinocytosis into the tubular epithelial cells, where they are digested to their component amino acids and returned to the body protein pool [69, 70]. They are therefore virtually absent from normal urine. Proximal tubular dysfunction, however, leads to a urinary leak of these proteins and a characteristic pattern of low molecular weight proteinuria known as tubular proteinuria [71]. Measurement of urinary excretion of β-2 microglobulin and RBP, usually expressed as fractional excretion rates, is a useful means of distinguishing between renal disease of glomerular and non-glomerular (tubulo-interstitial) origin.

Only very small amounts of albumin and other large plasma proteins normally pass the glomerular filter. These are essentially completely reabsorbed by a mechanism similar to that for low molecular weight proteins [72]. At low filtered loads, the system behaves as a high-affinity, low-capacity transporter with virtually complete clearance of albumin from the tubular fluid, whereas at high filtered loads, this mechanism becomes saturated and a high-capacity, low-affinity mode operates so that reabsorption continues to rise with increasing load, but about one-third of the filtered albumin escapes reabsorption and appears in the urine [73]. In such conditions of glomerular proteinuria, the urinary albumin excretion rate is always considerably less than the amount filtered and catabolised. This probably explains why proteinuria of nutritionally trivial amounts (<10 g/day) may cause hypoalbuminaemia in some cases of the nephrotic syndrome.

Proximal tubular secretion of organic anions
Many organic substances, anionic at physiological pH, are actively secreted by the proximal tubule [74]. These include endogenous substances such as hippurate and exogenous substances such as penicillin, probenecid and derivatives of hippuric acid such as ortho- and para-aminohippurate (hippuran and PAH). The renal clearance of these compounds exceeds GFR and in the case of hippuran and PAH, at least, extraction may be practically complete. The secretory site is the proximal convoluted tubule, especially the middle and late segments. The small amount of PAH that escapes secretion is accounted for by blood perfusing the deepest (juxtamedullary) nephrons, in which the postglomerular blood flows directly into the medullary vasa recta system without passing through the cortical peritubular capillary plexus, bypassing the secretory site [19]. In the adult, only about 10% of nephrons are of this type, so the underestimation of renal plasma flow by PAH clearance is small. In the newborn infant, in contrast, the superficial cortical nephrons (the last to be formed) function little or not at all, and the juxtamedullary nephrons provide the lion's share of renal function. Clearance of PAH and similar substances is therefore an unreliable measure of renal plasma flow in babies and newborn animals. PAH secretion is saturable and Tm limited [11]; below the renal threshold, excretion increases in parallel with rising plasma concentration, whereas above this value there is no further rise in excretion. A similar,

but separate, transport system exists for the secretion of organic cations.

Glomerulo-tubular balance

Delivery of fluid to the distal tubule is, by definition, the difference between GFR and proximal tubular reabsorption rate. Since the rate of distal fluid delivery is an important determinant of distal tubular function, and therefore of homeostasis, it is important that glomerular and proximal tubular functions are coupled together. This coupling is known as glomerulo-tubular balance (GTB); changes in GFR are partially offset by parallel and proportional changes in proximal tubular reabsorption [75]. GTB has been shown experimentally to exist: when GFR is manipulated by altering renal perfusion pressure, changes in proximal tubular reabsorption take place as the theory predicts [76]. At least three mechanisms are involved.

Peritubular physical forces
The protein concentration in postglomerular plasma is determined by arterial plasma protein concentration and filtration fraction. If GFR increases without a parallel increase in plasma flow, filtration fraction rises and peritubular capillary oncotic pressure is increased. This alters the balance of Starling forces in the peritubular environment in a direction that favours reabsorption. Conversely, a fall in GFR and filtration fraction leads to a reduction in the pressure gradient for reabsorption [77]. The oncotic pressure of the peritubular capillary plasma has been shown to be a powerful, and possibly rate-limiting, factor in proximal tubular reabsorption [62].

Filtration of preferentially reabsorbed substances
Sodium is reabsorbed in the early proximal tubule with bicarbonate, phosphate, amino acids, lactate and citrate in preference to chloride; glucose is also absorbed by co-transport. The more of these substances presented to the tubule, the more sodium (and therefore water) will be reabsorbed. At any plasma concentration, a change in GFR will produce a parallel

and proportionate change in the rate of filtration of these substances, inducing a change in proximal tubular reabsorption rate in the same direction [56]. This effect will be amplified by the secondary effect on downstream, passive sodium reabsorption described in a previous section. Thus, any random fluctuation in GFR will cause secondary changes in both active proximal tubular sodium reabsorption and the peritubular environment, reinforcing one another in the preservation of GTB.

Tubuloglomerular feedback

The ascending limb of the loop of Henle passes through the vascular pole of its own glomerulus, where it is intimately associated with the afferent and efferent arterioles in the JGA [15] (Figure 3.2). There is strong evidence that delivery of some solute, probably chloride, is sensed at the JGA, where it provides the afferent stimulus for regulation of GFR by negative feedback [78]. In experiments in which the loop of Henle was perfused in both orthograde and retrograde directions with solutions of various NaCl concentrations and at various rates, a clear inhibitory effect was seen on RPF and GFR as concentration (or flow rate) was increased [79]. The effect is probably mediated, at least in part, by local production and conversion of angiotensin, producing glomerular vasoconstriction (especially of the efferent arteriole) and increasing vascular resistance [80]. Tubuloglomerular feedback (TGF) may provide an emergency defence against drastic salt and water depletion in tubular injury. If proximal tubular NaCl reabsorption were severely impaired by anoxia or the action of a nephrotoxic drug, the resulting flood of sodium-rich urine would lead rapidly to fatal dehydration and electrolyte depletion unless GFR were to fall by some means. The oliguria of acute renal failure may be seen, in this light, as a life-preserving response rather than an undesirable feature of the syndrome [81]. Recognition that the thick ascending limb (TAL) of the loop of Henle is the most vulnerable part of the nephron to ischaemic injury [82] is entirely consistent with this view, since the TAL is included in the anatomical feedback loop consisting of glomerulus–proximal tubule–loop of Henle–JGA.

Sodium excretion and extracellular fluid volume

Sodium and extracellular fluid volume

The major osmotically active solute in the ECF is sodium chloride; 90% of the sodium in the body, and almost all the chloride, is located in the extracellular compartment. Because the tonicity of body fluids is held within very narrow limits by the regulation of water intake and excretion, it follows that a gain or loss of total body NaCl leads to expansion or contraction of ECF volume. Conversely, ECF volume is the major determinant of sodium excretion rate. Strauss et al. [83] showed that, in subjects on a salt-restricted diet, a tiny increase in ECF volume is followed by an immediate natriuresis and that expansion beyond a certain ideal volume is a stimulus to sodium excretion, the magnitude of this stimulus being proportionate to the amount by which this volume is exceeded. McCance [84] similarly showed that below a critical ECF volume, sodium-free urine was produced, whereas sodium appeared in the urine as soon as this volume was even slightly exceeded. The relationship between ECF volume and sodium excretion is shown in Figure 3.6. It is evident that the stimulus producing the increase in sodium excretion cannot be plasma sodium concentration, which does not change, but ECF volume. How changes in this volume are sensed, and whether it is the total ECF volume or a particular component or function of it that is important, has been the subject of much investigation.

Control of sodium excretion

The control system regulating sodium excretion and, therefore, ECF volume is in three parts: an afferent (sensory) component, which detects a signal indicating the need to excrete or conserve sodium; an effector organ (the kidney); and a means of transmitting the response to the afferent stimulus to the kidney, the efferent (messenger) component.

The afferent stimulus
Both acute (saline loading) and chronic (high dietary sodium intake) volume expansion are natriuretic stimuli. Manoeuvres that expand intrathoracic blood

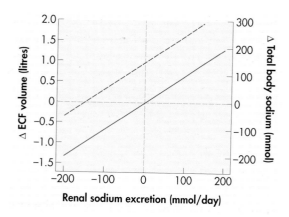

Figure 3.6 *The relationship between extracellular fluid (ECF) volume, total body sodium and urinary sodium excretion rate, assuming that a gain or loss of 1 litre of extracellular fluid corresponds to a gain or loss of 150 mmol sodium and that the extracellular fluid sodium concentration does not change. Negative values for sodium excretion indicate the magnitude of the sodium deficit that must be made up before sodium appears in the urine, which is actually sodium free at points to the left of the vertical zero line. The solid oblique line describes the relationship as derived from recumbent subjects; in the upright position, the point of intercept with the y-axis is displaced upwards, corresponding to sodium retention, but the slope of the relationship is unchanged (interrupted line). (Redrawn from Strauss et al. [83].)*

volume, such as head-out water immersion, are natriuretic even though total ECF volume becomes contracted as natriuresis continues [85]. The magnitude of the response, correlated with left atrial volume, and left atrial stretch receptors probably mediate the effect [86]. Stimulation of carotid sinus baroreceptors by underfilling of the arterial tree, e.g. by hypotension or vasodilatation, is antinatriuretic [87, 88]. Observations in subjects with arteriovenous fistulae indicate that underfilling of the high-pressure (arterial) compartment overrides the effect of overfilling of the low-pressure (venous) compartment, so that the net response is antinatriuretic [89]. Volume or sodium receptors have been postulated in the liver or portal venous system, following the observation that saline infused into the portal vein or ingested orally is more natriuretic than the same amount infused into a peripheral vein [90]. The presence of baroreceptors in the interstitial space is suggested by the differential natriuretic effects of saline infusions of different oncotic pressures [91–93]. The fluid that expands intravascular volume the least and the interstitial compartment the most (isotonic saline) is much more

natriuretic than an equivalent volume of plasma or hyperoncotic albumin. Receptors in the pulmonary interstitium may subserve this function [94]. It has been suggested that receptors in the central nervous system are sensitive to changes in cerebrospinal fluid (CSF) sodium concentration [95]; however, these experiments involved large, supraphysiological alterations of CSF sodium concentration, and the relevance of this observation to changes within the physiological range is not clear.

Changes in the perfusion pressure perceived by the kidney itself, in consequence of changes in arterial blood pressure, lead to changes in urinary sodium excretion both by intrarenal mechanisms and by affecting the rate of renin secretion. It is likely that most or all of these receptors play a part in determining the natriuretic status of the kidney, perhaps via a (hypothetical) integrating mechanism located in the hypothalamus or elsewhere. In general, reduction of effective arterial volume, i.e. underfilling of the arterial tree in relation to its holding capacity, seems to engender a sodium-retaining response sufficient to override conflicting or interfering stimuli from elsewhere.

Renal effector responses

Theoretically, the renal sodium excretion rate could be altered by either changing GFR without an accompanying change in tubular reabsorption, or the reverse. It is almost certain that changes in tubular reabsorption are responsible for physiological regulation of this function. Patients with chronic renal failure are able to remain in external sodium balance on a fixed sodium intake despite progressively falling GFR; an adjustment of tubular reabsorption must have taken place. It has been shown in many experimental models that the natriuretic response to volume expansion is not abolished if GFR is prevented from increasing, or is even artificially decreased [96, 97]. Furthermore, experimental manipulations which produce large increases in GFR are not necessarily natriuretic. For example, in dogs, protein feeding, dexamethasone administration, dopamine infusion and saline infusion all increase GFR by up to 30%: of these, only saline loading is consistently natriuretic [98].

Given that sodium excretion is modulated by changes in tubular reabsorption, the question arises:

which part of the tubule is mainly responsible? Studies of segmental tubular sodium reabsorption favour the distal nephron as the important effector. Natriuresis can be dissociated not only from GFR (see above) but also from absolute and fractional proximal tubular sodium reabsorption [99]. The humoral factors known to influence sodium reabsorption rate (e.g. aldosterone, atrial natriuretic peptide) act mainly on distal nephron segments. In rats, saline loading causes marked changes in sodium reabsorption in the collecting duct [100], amounting in extreme volume expansion to apparent sodium excretion [101]. Also, it appears logical that the most distal part of the nephron is responsible for the final adjustment of the sodium excretion rate in that, by definition, further downstream adjustments are not possible.

It should be emphasised that the response to saline volume expansion is normally a reduction in sodium reabsorption in both the proximal and distal nephron segments, and that the dissociation between these mentioned above was produced by unphysiological experimental manipulations. The fact that the distal parts of the nephron can maintain a degree of sodium homeostasis in the absence of parallel responses in the proximal tubule probably reflects the extreme importance of control of ECF volume; if proximal tubular reabsorption is impaired or abnormal, external balance for sodium can still be maintained.

Intrarenal control of sodium excretion

Sodium excretion is correlated with renal artery pressure [102, 103]. ECF volume is an important determinant of renal artery pressure, with resulting effects on intrarenal haemodynamics. The main resistance vessels in the renal microcirculation are the afferent and efferent glomerular arterioles. The latter are interposed between the glomerular and peritubular capillary plexuses. The hydrostatic pressure in the peritubular capillaries therefore varies in proportion to renal artery pressure and in inverse proportion to renal arteriolar resistance. Volume expansion directly increases perfusion pressure and, partly by inhibition of the renin–angiotensin–aldosterone system (RAAS), reduces arteriolar resistance; volume contraction has the reverse effects. Thus, volume expansion leads to an increase, and volume contraction to a decrease, in

peritubular capillary pressure. The effect of angiotensin II on the renal circulation is complex. It causes both preglomerular (afferent arteriole) and postglomerular (efferent arteriole) vasoconstriction, but the postglomerular effect predominates, largely due to the production of vasodilator prostaglandins in the afferent arteriole that offset the vasoconstrictor action of angiotensin II. Conditions in which the RAAS is stimulated, e.g. volume contraction, therefore increase glomerular capillary pressure, leading to an increase in filtration fraction and an increase in postglomerular plasma oncotic pressure. Suppression of the RAAS (volume expansion) has the opposite effect. In sum, volume expansion causes an increase in hydrostatic pressure and a decrease in oncotic pressure in the peritubular capillaries. This reduces the Starling pressure gradient for fluid reabsorption from the peritubular interstitium and hence from the proximal tubule, favouring natriuresis. Volume expansion initiates the opposite sequence of events and is therefore antinatriuretic. These processes are schematised in Figure 3.7 [104].

Although the above discussion focuses on the proximal tubule, the rate of fluid absorption in the distal nephron is also influenced by Starling forces [91, 97], because the cortical part of the distal tubule is supplied by the same peritubular capillary network that supplies the proximal tubule, and the medullary part by capillaries that receive part of their blood supply from the efferent arterioles of juxtamedullary (deep cortical) nephrons. It has sometimes been argued that physical forces alone are sufficient to explain the regulation of renal sodium excretion, but this hypothesis is rendered untenable by other observations, notably the fact that saline expansion is natriuretic even if renal perfusion pressure is artificially prevented from rising or is even reduced [96]. It follows that extrarenal factors are also involved.

The efferent limb in the regulation of sodium excretion

The fact that sodium excretion is influenced by changes in the apparent volume of ECF subcompartments remote from the kidney indicates not only that volume sensors exist at those sites, but also that some means exists of altering renal sodium excretion in response to the signals received. This message

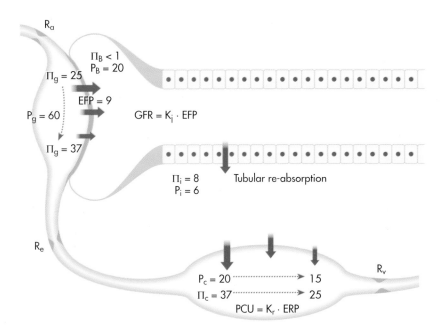

Figure **3.7** *Schematic diagram of the forces responsible for filtration of fluid from the glomerular capillaries and reabsorption of fluid into the peritubular capillaries. The forces are expressed in mmHg and are considered representative of those found in normal humans. (Reproduced by permission from Arendshorst and Navar [104].)*

('increase or decrease sodium excretion') may be transmitted from sensor to effector by a number of efferent pathways. The renal nerve supply contains efferent postganglionic fibres located in the splanchnic nerves; stimulation of these is antinatriuretic [105, 106] while denervation is natriuretic [107]. Alpha-adrenergic endings have been identified in close approximation to proximal and distal tubules as well as to blood vessels [108]; a direct effect on epithelial transport seems likely. Denervation of one kidney causes natriuresis in the ipsilateral and antinatriuresis in the contralateral kidney, suggesting a role also for the afferent fibres in the control of sodium excretion, perhaps by integrating the responses of the two kidneys via reno-renal reflex [109].

Aldosterone

The mineralocorticoid aldosterone is undoubtedly involved in modulating tubular sodium handling. Released in response to activation of the renin–angiotensin system, which in turn is stimulated by volume contraction [110], it acts on the distal convoluted tubule and collecting duct to stimulate sodium reabsorption, where it also promotes secretion of K^+ and H^+ (see below). Although other factors undoubtedly interact with aldosterone and can even override it in the mineralocorticoid escape phenomenon [111],

its importance in sodium homeostasis is illustrated by the finding that adrenalectomised animals, on a fixed replacement dose of mineralocorticoid, achieve sodium balance only at the cost of greatly exaggerated changes in ECF volume, body weight, blood pressure and potassium concentration [112, 113].

Catecholamines

Catecholamines affect sodium excretion, noradrenaline (norepinephrine) being antinatriuretic [114] and dopamine natriuretic [115]. Both α-adrenergic and dopaminergic receptors have been identified in the kidney [116]. It had been suggested that dopamine is an important mediator of sodium excretion, particularly in chronic renal failure [117]; however, it is likely that the major effects of these amines are mediated via their action as locally released neurotransmitters, rather than as circulating hormones proper. The fact that L-dopa, a precursor of dopamine, is natriuretic when infused into the renal artery [118] further supports the view that local synthesis accounts for the origin of most or all of the dopamine present in the kidney. This does not exclude an important role for the amine as a second messenger, i.e. a locally acting vasoactive and natriuretic factor, the activity of which may be increased by other, circulating, substances.

Prostaglandins

The vasodilator prostaglandins PGE2 and PGI2 (prostacyclin) are synthesised within the kidney and are natriuretic. Inhibitors of prostaglandin synthetase such as indomethacin cause RPF and GFR to fall and fractional proximal tubular sodium reabsorption to increase [119, 120]. These effects are partly offset by volume expansion and are greatly exaggerated by volume contraction [121]; the combination of volume contraction and a non-steroidal anti-inflammatory agent may lead to acute renal failure. Angiotensin II stimulates the renal release of prostaglandins: the main physiological role of renal PGs may be to maintain glomerular plasma flow and filtration rate in volume-contracted states, when AII levels are high.

The kallikrein-kinin system

The kinins bradykinin and kallidin are another class of vasodilator and natriuretic substances produced locally within the kidney. They are formed by the action of the proteinase kallikrein, produced in the distal tubule [122], on a circulating precursor. The renin–angiotensin–aldosterone system, prostaglandins and kinins all interact in complex ways. AII and aldosterone both stimulate kallikrein production, while kinins promote prostaglandin synthesis [123]. Angiotensin-converting enzyme (ACE) not only converts angiotensin I (AI) to angiotensin II (AII) but also inactivates bradykinin, and is also known as kininase II. It therefore causes vasoconstriction and antinatriuresis both by AII production and by bradykinin degradation; ACE inhibition has the opposite effects, accounting for the fact that ACE inhibitors lower blood pressure even when the RAAS is not activated. Catecholamines, the RAAS, prostaglandins and kinins can be regarded as components of a complex intrarenal paracrine system that normally act synchronously to regulate and stabilise renal blood flow and GFR in response to changes in extrarenal influences such as ECF volume and circulating hormones.

Natriuretic hormones

Classic studies by de Wardener et al. [96] proved that volume expansion causes natriuresis in dogs even when GFR is artificially constrained and supramaximal doses of mineralocorticoid and vasopressin are given. The design of the experiment excluded all feasible explanations for the natriuresis except the action of a natriuretic hormone. Atlas et al. [124] in the rat, and Flynn & Davies [125] in humans, identified and characterised a new class of peptide hormones now known as atrial natriuretic peptides (ANP), so called because they are synthesised in the cardiac atria and released in response to atrial stretch. Related peptides are produced elsewhere in the body, including the brain, probably in the anterior hypothalamus. Human ANP is composed of 28 amino acids, including a 17-amino acid ring formed by a disulphide bridge. It is formed by cleavage of a 126-amino acid prohormone. At least three other fragments of the same prohormone have hormonal activity and are known respectively as long-acting natriuretic peptide (amino acids 1–30), vessel dilator hormone (31–67) and kaliuretic hormone (79–98). ANP is a systemic and renal vasodilator, and also reduces pulmonary vascular resistance [126]. It acts directly on arteriolar smooth muscle by a pathway not involving prostaglandins or nitric oxide [127]. Its actions on the renal vasculature include dilatation of both arcuate arteries and afferent arterioles [128] and antagonism of mesangial cell contraction induced by both AII and vasopressin [129, 130]. These effects combine to cause an increase in GFR and a reduction in fractional proximal tubular sodium reabsorption, probably due to altered physical (Starling) forces. It also has direct effects on the distal renal tubule, decreasing sodium reabsorption by inhibiting both its entry into the tubular cells through sodium channels in the apical membrane and its exit from the cell across the basolateral membrane by reducing Na^+, K^+-ATPase activity [131]. At the cellular level, the actions of ANP are mediated by cyclic guanosine monophosphate (cGMP) and cGMP-dependent protein kinase [132]. Other actions of ANP include suppression of renin release, inhibition of aldosterone synthesis, and antagonism of AII-mediated vasoconstriction.

There is a compelling logic in atrial distension being an important natriuretic stimulus, because, in most circumstances, atrial stretch is a sensitive indicator of circulating volume. The right atrium is the main source of ANP, which suggests that the observed pulmonary effects of the hormone may be physiologically important. In pathological states such as congestive heart failure, atrial distension may become dissociated from ECF and circulatory volume. It is theorised that ANP release is beneficial in heart failure, both by reducing afterload and by mitigating the salt and water retention characteristic of that condition [133]. It is involved, and may be pre-eminent, in the natriuresis of the syndrome of inappropriate secretion of antidiuretic hormone [134]. Several comprehensive reviews of the biochemistry, physiology and clinical importance of ANP and its congeners have recently been published [131, 135–138]. Its major actions are schematised in Figure 3.8.

The possible existence of other natriuretic hormones, especially a digitalis-like inhibitor of Na$^+$, K$^+$-ATPase, is controversial, although there is some evidence of such a factor. Its physiological role, if any, is unknown.

Sodium reabsorption beyond the proximal tubule

About one-third of filtered sodium is reabsorbed distal to the proximal tubule. As in the proximal tubule, active extrusion of sodium by Na$^+$, K$^+$-ATPase across the basolateral membrane accounts for the exit step of sodium from the cell interior, and also generates a steep concentration gradient across the apical membrane. Entry from tubular fluid to cell interior takes place by secondary active transport down this gradient via a recently described family of Na$^+$-(K$^+$)-Cl$^-$ co-transporters, coded for by genes collectively named *SLC12*, at least three of which are expressed in different segments of the distal nephron [139], and an amiloride-sensitive sodium channel. In contrast to events in the proximal tubule, where reabsorption is isotonic, salt and water reabsorption are dissociated in more distal segments.

The loop of Henle
About 25% of filtered sodium is reabsorbed in the loop of Henle, all of it in the thick ascending limb

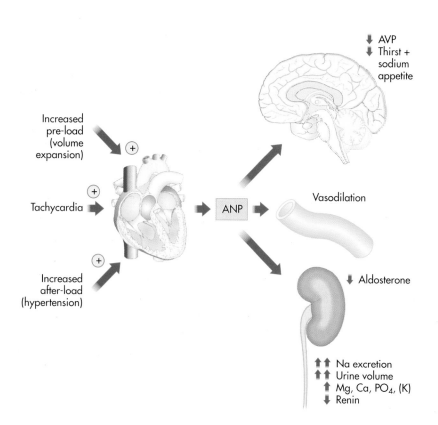

Figure 3.8 *Schematic outline of the major actions of atrial natriuretic peptide(s) (ANP). (Reproduced by permission from Kenyon and Jardine [137].)*

(TAL). Entry into the cell here is effected by the transporter NKCC2 (the correspoding gene is *SLC12A2*, see above), which transports $1Na^+$, $1K^+$ and $2Cl^-$. Since the number of positively and negatively charged ions transported is equal, transport is electroneutral. Ammonia (NH_4^+), if present in the tubular fluid, can substitute for K+. NKCC2 is inhibited by bumetanide and furosemide, which accounts for the diuretic action of these drugs. The gene is located on chromosome 15q, and mutations of it cause classical Bartter's syndrome of hypokalaemic alkalosis and hypercalciuria [140], as had been predicted from the close similarity between Bartter's syndrome and the effect of chronic administration of loop diuretics. The very large amount of sodium reabsorbed by this transport system, and its relatively distal location, accounts for the great pharmacological power of bumetanide and its congeners.

The distal convoluted tubule (DCT)

About 5–8% of filtered sodium is reabsorbed in the DCT. Apical sodium entry in this segment takes place via an electroneutral, thiazide-sensitive Na^+-Cl^- co-transporter (TSC). The gene is *SLC12A3*, located at 16q12–13. Mutations of this gene cause Gitelman's syndrome [141, 142], a variant of Bartter's syndrome distinguished from the classical form by milder clinical course, hypocalciuria and hypomagnesaemia [143]. As would be expected, inhibition of the TSC by thiazide diuretics mimics the features of Gitelman's syndrome precisely. Because much less sodium is reabsorbed by this co-transporter than by NKCC2, thiazides are much weaker diuretics than loop diuretics. However, if a loop diuretic (e.g. furosemide) and a thiazide (e.g. metolazone) are used together, the two effects reinforce one another and massive diuresis results.

The collecting duct

Only 3–5% of filtered sodium enters the cortical collecting duct in most circumstances. However, the filtered load of sodium is so large that this amounts to 750–1250 mmol/day, several times the normal daily intake. Regulation of sodium reabsorption in this terminal nephron segment is therefore crucial to homeostasis, as no further adjustment of urine composition can occur at a more distal site. Sodium enters the cell in this segment via a highly sodium-selective, low-conductance, amiloride-sensitive sodium channel located in the apical membrane of the principal cells [144], commonly abbreviated to ENaC (epithelial sodium channel). Opening of the ENaC is under the control of aldosterone, and therefore volume contraction promotes, and volume expansion inhibits, sodium reabsorption through it. Entry of sodium across the apical membrane, without an accompanying anion, creates a lumen-negative voltage across the epithelium that promotes the movement of H^+ and K^+ in the opposite direction. Blockade of this channel with amiloride therefore leads to H^+ and K^+ retention, as does aldosterone deficiency. The channel consists of three subunits [145], designated α-, β- and γ-ENaC, respectively, coded for by three separate genes. The gene for α-ENaC is on chromosome 12, while those for β- and γ-ENaC are close together on 16p. Very recently, it has been shown that two distinct hereditary diseases are caused by mutations in ENaC genes. Liddle's syndrome, a form of dominantly inherited hypertension with hypokalaemia and suppression of renin and aldosterone, was first shown to be due to mutations in the β-ENaC gene [146] that cause the channel to be constitutively open even in the absence of mineralocorticoid. The consequence is overabsorption of sodium, volume expansion, and increased potassium excretion. In 1996, the same group [147] showed that the syndrome could also be caused by mutations in the gene for γ-ENaC. The rare disorder pseudohypoaldosteronism type 1 (PHA1) is physiologically the mirror image of Liddle's syndrome with salt wasting, hyperkalaemia and acidosis despite high levels of renin and aldosterone. It has been shown to be due to mutations that render ENaC ineffective as a sodium channel. The inheritance of PHA1 is recessive in some pedigrees and dominant in others [148]. Some families with PHA1 have mutations in the α-ENaC gene, others in that for β-ENaC [149]. The three subunits of ENaC have considerable sequence homology and structural similarity, suggesting descent from a common ancestor gene.

Renal control of potassium and hydrogen ion secretion

Potassium excretion

On a normal diet and at normal levels of renal function, the rate of potassium filtration exceeds that of potassium excretion by five- to tenfold. At first sight, this might suggest that excretion is controlled by varying the rate of tubular reabsorption of filtered potassium, as is the case for sodium. In fact, almost all the filtered potassium is reabsorbed in the proximal tubule; potassium excretion depends on distal tubular secretion of the ion.

Proximal tubular potassium reabsorption

The micropuncture studies of Malnic et al. [150] showed that potassium is reabsorbed isotonically throughout the length of the proximal convoluted tubule, a process apparently continued in the proximal straight tubule. The fluid issuing from the loop into the early distal convoluted tubule contains very little potassium (5–15% of the filtered load); this fraction remains constant while urinary potassium excretion varies from minimum to maximum, a 200-fold range. It is therefore logically necessary that changes in potassium excretion are effected at a more distal site. It appears that sodium and potassium are absorbed isotonically and in parallel in the proximal tubule, while avid reabsorption of both continues in the TAL via the transporter NKCC2 (see above).

Potassium transport in the distal tubule and collecting duct

Potassium is secreted in the distal tubule in potassium repletion and reabsorbed in potassium depletion; the latter case is unusual. The major site of potassium secretion is the late distal convoluted tubule and cortical collecting duct (CCD) [151, 152], corresponding to the location of ENaC (see 'Sodium reabsorption in the collecting duct', above). There are two major cell types in the CCD: principal cells and intercalated cells. Potassium secretion is a function of the former, reabsorption of the latter. The driving force for potassium secretion is the lumen-negative voltage resulting from sodium reabsorption [153]. Although perhaps 90% of this potential difference is effaced by sec-ondary, passive chloride reabsorption, the remaining 10% or so is associated with countermovement of potassium and H^+ [154]. Electrophysiological studies indicate that epithelial potassium transport is a complex process involving several component steps [155].

Intracellular potassium concentration is an important modulator of potassium secretion into the tubular lumen. Like all cells, distal tubular cells transport sodium out and potassium in across both basolateral and apical membranes. The apical (luminal) membrane of principal cells, however, allows potassium to leave the cell down its electrochemical gradient by two mechanisms: one is a specific potassium channel and the other a potassium–chloride symporter (cotransporter). A rise in the peritubular (ECF) potassium concentration stimulates Na^+, K^+-ATPase in the basolateral membrane [156], thus increasing potassium entry [157]. The net force driving potassium secretion is therefore made up of two components: a concentration gradient, resulting mainly from intracellular potassium concentration, and an electrical potential gradient, resulting from sodium reabsorption as described above. The electrical driving force is proportional to the rate of sodium reabsorption. This is determined by two main factors. The first is the rate of sodium entry into the CCD: anything that increases distal sodium delivery, such as inhibition of its reabsorption in more proximal segments, stimulates sodium entry into principal cells and hence potassium secretion. The second factor is aldosterone, which increases both sodium entry across the apical membrane via ENaC [158] and sodium–potassium exchange across the basolateral membrane by upregulating Na^+, K^+-ATPase [159].

The interaction between distal sodium delivery and aldosterone is crucially important in the normal control of potassium excretion in response to changes in ECF volume. Volume expansion increases distal sodium delivery by inhibition of reabsorption at more proximal sites, and suppresses activity of the RAAS. The resulting effects on distal sodium reabsorption, and thus on potassium secretion, are mutually opposed and cancel one another. Volume contraction produces opposite effects ($\downarrow$ distal Na delivery, $\uparrow$ aldosterone). Therefore, physiological changes in sodium excretion rate due to changes in

ECF volume do not cause inappropriate secondary effects on potassium excretion. Conditions in which the normal relationship between distal sodium delivery and aldosterone release is disrupted, however, cause predictable disturbances of potassium balance; some examples are given in Table 3.1.

Acute and chronic changes in acid–base status exert important effects on potassium balance. Acute metabolic alkalosis enhances, and metabolic acidosis inhibits, tubular potassium secretion, leading to hypokalaemia and hyperkalaemia, respectively [160]. This is probably secondary to changes in intracellular potassium concentration: alkalosis promotes potassium entry into cells, thus increasing the cell-to-tubular lumen potassium gradient, while acidosis has the opposite effect. The rate of secretion of H^+ may have a further effect on potassium secretion: in acidosis, increased H^+ flux attenuates the potential differ-ence between cell and tubular fluid, reducing the driving force for potassium extrusion. Chronic metabolic acidosis, in contrast to acute, is accompanied by increased potassium secretion and eventual potassium depletion [161]. This is probably due to increased distal delivery of sodium secondary to hyperchloraemia: bicarbonate deficiency inhibits proximal sodium reabsorption by mechanisms discussed in an earlier section [162]. The fact that chronic respiratory acidosis, in which bicarbonate levels are elevated, is not accompanied by potassium wasting lends support to this view. Diuretics that inhibit sodium reabsorption at sites proximal to the CCD cause urinary potassium wasting due to the simultaneous induction of increased distal sodium delivery and hyperaldosteronism secondary to volume contraction. These include loop diuretics such as mercurials [163], furosemide [164] and ethacrynic acid [165], thiazides [166], carbonic anhydrase

Table 3.1 The effects of various conditions on the factors determining renal potassium excretion

Condition	Δ distal sodium delivery	Δ aldosterone	Δ intracellular $[K^+]$	Δ U_KV	Δ P_K
Volume expansion	↑	↓	—	—	—
Volume contraction	↓	↑	—	—	—
K^+ loading	—	—	↑	↑	↓[1]
K^+ depletion	—	—	↓	↓	↑[1]
Acute metabolic acidosis	—	—	↓	↓	↑
Chronic metabolic acidosis	↑	—	—	↑	↓
Metabolic alkalosis	—	—	↑	↑	↓
Mineralocorticoid deficiency	↓	↓	?↓	↓	↑
Mineralocorticoid excess	↑	↑	?↑	↑	↓
Proximal tubulopathies	↑	↑	?↑	↑	↓
Loop diuretics, thiazides	↑	↑	—	↑	↓
K^+-sparing diuretics	↓	↑	?↓	↓	↑

U_KV = urinary potassium excretion rate; P_K = plasma potassium concentration.
[1] Direction of change in U_KV produced in order to restore P_K to normal.
Data from references cited in the text.

inhibitors and osmotic diuretics. Diuretics such as spironolactone [167], triamterene [168] and amiloride [169], that work by inhibiting sodium reabsorption at the potassium secreting site, cause potassium retention and hyperkalaemia.

Hydrogen ion excretion

Volatile and non-volatile acid

The pH of the ECF is regulated within a very narrow range (7.40 ± 0.04), despite a number of perturbing influences. By far the largest of these is the continuous generation of carbonic acid as the end-product of carbohydrate metabolism. Because carbonic acid can be dehydrated to CO_2 and water by the enzyme carbonic anhydrase (CA) in the lung, and the resulting CO_2 excreted in expired air, it is known as volatile acid (VA). Regulation of CO_2 excretion therefore depends on pulmonary function, and its retention or excessive loss results in respiratory acidosis or alkalosis, respectively. In addition, a much smaller amount of non-volatile acid (NVA), acid that cannot be dehydrated to anhydrides in the lung, is generated from other metabolic pathways. The principal components of NVA are:

sulphuric acid, from the combustion of sulphur-containing amino acids;
phosphoric acid, mainly from dietary organic phosphate;
organic acids (OA), such as lactic and aceto-acetic acids, from the incomplete combustion of carbohydrate and fat, respectively.

Organic acids usually form only a small component of NVA but may become important in disease states (diabetic ketoacidosis, lactic acidosis, hereditary organic acidaemias). The amount of sulphuric acid produced depends on the intake of animal protein: strict vegetarians (vegans), who eat no animal products at all, generate predominantly alkaline products of metabolism and therefore excrete alkaline urine. Since, by definition, NVA cannot be excreted via the lungs, it must be excreted by the kidney if the pH of the ECF is not to become progressively, and eventually fatally, lowered. The disproportion between the production rates of VA and NVA is enormous. An adult human

on a mixed Western diet produces about 14 000 mmol of carbonic acid daily, but only about 50–100 mmol of NVA. This fact is dramatically illustrated by the difference in the rates of development of acidosis following total obstruction of the trachea as opposed to total obstruction of the urinary tract.

ECF buffers

A quantity of acid added to plasma or whole blood lowers the pH far less than it would if added to a similar volume of water. This is due to the presence of powerful buffer systems in both plasma and red cells. The most important of the ECF buffers is the carbonic acid–bicarbonate buffer system:

$$pH = 6.1 + \log \frac{[HCO_3^-]}{[H_2CO_3]} \qquad (10)$$

Addition of H^+ depletes $[HCO_3^-]$ by titrating it to H_2CO_3 with a consequent fall in pH. The role of the kidney is to regenerate HCO_3^- (buffer base) by excreting H^+, thus back-titrating or recharging the buffer system. Addition of 1 mol of HCO_3 (as $NaHCO_3$) is equivalent to the excretion of 1 mmol of H+; loss of 1 mmol of HCO_3^- (as in diarrhoea or bicarbonaturia) causes metabolic acidosis quantitatively equivalent to the addition of 1 mol of H^+ (e.g. as HCl) to the ECF.

Reabsorption of filtered bicarbonate

The bicarbonate concentration in glomerular filtrate is the same as that in plasma. At normal GFR (180 l/day) and normal plasma bicarbonate (26 mmol/l) this represents a potential daily loss of more than 4500 mmol of bicarbonate, equivalent to adding 4500 mmol of acid to the ECF. All, or very nearly all, of this filtered bicarbonate must be reabsorbed to prevent severe acidosis. This takes place almost entirely in the proximal tubule [170, 171] according to the scheme shown in Figure 3.9. Note (a) that bicarbonate reabsorption is dependent on H^+ secretion [172]; (b) that it is accompanied by reabsorption of an equivalent amount of sodium; and (c) that the HCO_3^- ion restored to the ECF is synthesised in the proximal tubular cell, and is not the same one that is titrated by secreted H^+ in the tubular lumen. The process is dependent on intracellular CA to provide a source of H^+ and HCO_3^- ions by hydration of CO_2, and intraluminal CA (derived from

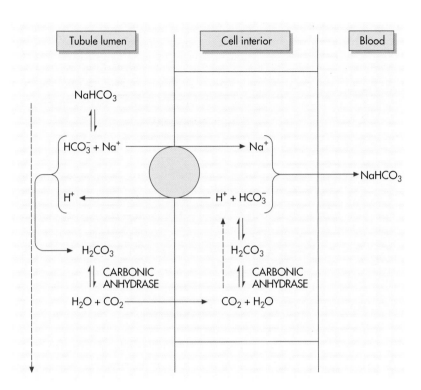

Figure 3.9 *Proximal tubular bicarbonate reabsorption. The process is dependent on intraluminal carbonic anhydrase, present in the proximal but not in the distal tubule.*

the brush border of the apical cell membrane) to remove the H_2CO_3 formed there by dehydration to CO_2 [173]. The high diffusibility of CO_2 [174] leads to its rapid movement down its concentration into the cell, completing the cycle and preventing the intraluminal reaction from coming to equilibrium and stopping.

Titration curves similar to those for glucose and phosphate (Figure 3.6) can be plotted for bicarbonate and a Tm and threshold value identified. An abnormally low threshold defines proximal renal tubular acidosis (RTA), in which urinary acidification capacity is normal but only when the plasma bicarbonate has fallen below the (low) threshold value, i.e. at the cost of sustained metabolic acidosis (Figure 3.10). Proximal RTA is most commonly seen as part of a generalised disorder of proximal tubular function (the Fanconi syndrome), but has been described as an isolated tubular defect in at least two forms [175, 176].

Distal tubular H^+ secretion

Proximal reabsorption of filtered HCO_3^- does not contribute to the excretion of ingested or endogenously formed NVA and is therefore irrelevant to external H^+ balance; it merely prevents acidosis due to

renal HCO_3^- wasting. To achieve acid balance, H^+ must be secreted into the urine in a quantity exactly equivalent to dietary and metabolic input of NVA [177], typically 50–100 mmol/day for an adult. This requires that the pH of the urine be lowered below that of ECF, i.e. the tubule must pump hydrogen ions 'uphill' from high pH (low $[H^+]$) to low pH (high $[H^+]$). This takes place in the distal nephron, particularly the collecting duct [170]. The reaction whereby H^+ is secreted into the lumen in exchange for Na^+, and HCO_3^- returned to the ECF, is the same as that operating in the proximal tubule: intracellular synthesis and ionisation of H_2CO_3 from CO_2 and water. The tubular H^+ pump can sustain a maximum pH gradient of about 10^3 (ECF pH 7.4, urine pH 4.4). One litre of water at pH 4.4 contains only about 0.4 mmol H^+: at a daily urine flow rate of 2–3 litres this is clearly inadequate to achieve H^+ balance. The ability to do so depends on the presence of urinary buffers.

Urinary buffers

The principal buffer in normal urine is inorganic phosphate. The buffering reaction is:

$$H^+ + Na_2HPO_4 \leftrightarrows Na^+ + NaH_2PO_4 \qquad (11)$$

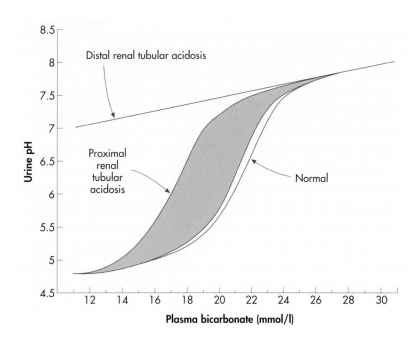

Figure 3.10 *Urine pH plotted against plasma bicarbonate concentration in normal subjects and patients with proximal and distal renal tubular acidosis. In distal renal tubular acidosis, urine pH does not fall significantly below that of plasma, even in severe metabolic acidosis. In proximal renal tubular acidosis, normal acidification is achieved but only at abnormally low plasma bicarbonate concentrations. The curve of the relationship shows the same sigmoid shape as the normal but is diplaced to the left, passing through the shaded area. The more severe the defect of bicarbonate reabsorption, the further left the curve is displaced. (Modified from Rodriguez-Soriano et al. [175].)*

The pK of this reaction is 6.8, leading to the following version of the Henderson–Hasselbalch equation:

$$pH = 6.8 + \log \frac{[NaHPO_4^-]}{[Na_2HPO_4]} \qquad (12)$$

The pK of 6.8 is well suited to the normal ECF pH of 7.4, since maximal buffering will take place within one pH unit of 7.4, i.e. well within the capacity of the H^+ pump.

The other important means of accommodating a large amount of secreted H^+ within the available range of urinary pH is by the formation of ammonium (NH_4^+). This is formed in the urine from secreted pH and ammonia (NH_3), the latter being synthesised from glutamine by the tubular cells. Thus:

$$NH_3 + H^+ + NaCl = NH_4Cl + Na^+ \qquad (13)$$

The Na^+ ion is reabsorbed in exchange for the secreted H^+ and restored to the ECF as $NaHCO_3$. The reactions between secreted H^+ and urinary phosphate and ammonia are illustrated in Figure 3.11. Unlike urinary phosphate excretion, ammonia synthesis can be stepped up in response to increased need to secrete H^+; this is a very important adaptive response to chronic acidosis [178]. The classical (distal) type of RTA is due to inability to lower urinary pH significantly below that of plasma; an acquired form

of distal RTA may be seen in obstructive uropathy [179].

The relationship between H^+ secretion and Na^+ reabsorption

As discussed above, H^+ secretion requires the reabsorption of an equivalent amount of sodium. Conversely, failure of H^+ secretion is associated with impairment of Na^+ reabsorption: patients with proximal and distal RTA have been shown to have proximal and distal Na^+ wasting respectively [180, 181]. It has been suggested that control of H^+ secretion is fundamentally dependent on changes in Na^+ reabsorption at different nephron sites [182].

Divalent cations, phosphate and vitamin D

Renal handling of calcium

Calcium is filtered in amounts greatly exceeding its rate of dietary intake and therefore of excretion; it is reabsorbed in all the actively transporting segments of the tubule by a variety of mechanisms. Reabsorption occurring in the distal tubule is responsive to changes in calcium intake and to other factors known to influence calcium excretion; that in more proximal segments is not.

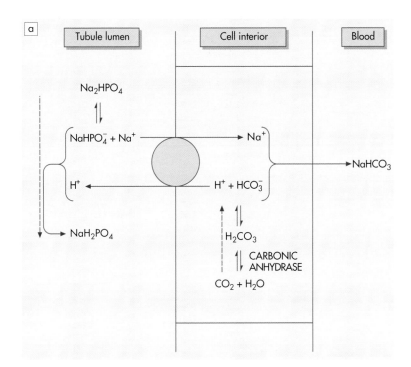

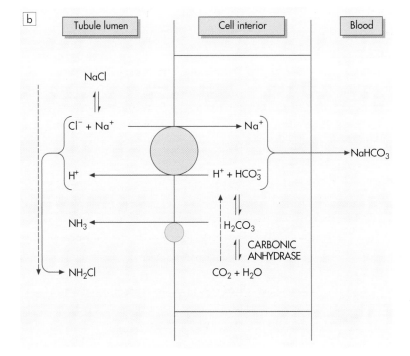

Figure 3.11 *Distal tubular hydrogen ion secretion. (a) Titration of urinary phosphate buffer. (b) Buffering by secreted ammonia.*

Glomerular filtration

Calcium is present in plasma in three forms: protein bound, complexed to anions (principally phosphate), and ionised. The last two together form ultrafilterable calcium (Ca_{UF}). The concentration of calcium in glomerular filtrate is the same as that of plasma Ca_{UF}, approximately 1.58 mmol/l (6.3 mg/dl) [183].

Proximal tubule

Calcium is reabsorbed approximately isotonically in the proximal tubule. A slight rise in tubular fluid concentration occurs in the initial (S1) segment, with little or no change in the remainder of the proximal tubule [184]. Reabsorption is partly passive and dependent on sodium transport, but an active transport system also exists in the basolateral membrane, probably involving sodium–calcium countertransport, i.e. calcium is extruded from the cell as sodium enters [68, 185]. The interdependence of proximal sodium and calcium reabsorption is very close: factors such as changes in ECF volume that affect sodium absorption produce proportionate and parallel changes in calcium absorption [186]. As with sodium, about 60% of filtered calcium is reabsorbed in the proximal tubule [187].

Loop of Henle

Calcium reabsorption continues in parallel with that of sodium in the TAL [187]; factors affecting the delivery of sodium out of the loop produce proportionate changes in calcium delivery. The reabsorption of both is markedly inhibited by furosemide [164]. As previously explained, the NKCC2 transporter is electroneutral, but back-leak of potassium into the tubular fluid takes place through specific potassium channels in the apical membrane. This recycling of potassium creates a lumen-positive voltage across the epithelium that drives other positively charged ions, including calcium, into the peritubular space via the paracellular shunt pathway, accounting for calcium reabsorption in this part of the tubule [139].

Distal tubule

Calcium ions are actively reabsorbed in the distal convoluted tubule and collecting duct [188]. Transport in this segment varies independently of sodium reabsorption: it is probable that homeostatic changes in calcium excretion are effected here. Factors increasing calcium reabsorption include parathyroid hormone (PTH) [189], hypocalcaemia (probably by PTH-independent mechanisms as well as by promoting PTH release), metabolic alkalosis [190] and hyperphosphataemia [191]. Hypoparathyroidism, hypercalcaemia, chronic metabolic acidosis and phosphate depletion are inhibitory (i.e. they increase calcium excretion). Vitamin D has been reported to have both enhancing [192] and inhibiting [193] effects on calcium excretion; a physiologically important role for vitamin D in renal calcium excretion has not been demonstrated in humans [194]. The apparent discrepancies among these reports may be due to species differences. Calcium enters distal tubular cells across the apical membrane through nifedipine-sensitive calcium channels. The driving force appears to be the electrical polarisation of the membrane, which is strongly influenced by intracellular chloride concentration. Measures that decrease intracellular chloride (such as thiazide diuretics) cause hyperpolarisation of the membrane and enhance calcium uptake, thus decreasing its excretion [195]. This, incidentally, explains why thiazides decrease calcium excretion while increasing sodium excretion.

Renal handling of magnesium

Magnesium is processed by the kidney in a manner similar, but not identical, to calcium. The major difference is that the proximal tubule is proportionately less important and Henle's loop more important in the case of magnesium. Also, unlike calcium, overall renal magnesium handling is of the Tm-threshold type (Figure 3.6).

Glomerular filtration

Like calcium, magnesium is present in plasma in protein-bound, complexed and ionised forms. Unfilterable magnesium (Mg_{UF}) is about 80% of total plasma magnesium [196], a rather higher fraction than for calcium.

Proximal tubule

Magnesium is absorbed less avidly in the proximal tubule than sodium and calcium, so that its concentration rises along the length of the segment to a value about 1.6 times that in glomerular filtrate [197, 198]. This probably reflects a lower epithelial permeability to magnesium than to calcium, the forces driving reabsorption of the two being similar. Proximal magnesium reabsorption changes in parallel with that of sodium in response to changes in factors influencing the latter, but to a lesser extent.

Loop of Henle

Eighty per cent of the magnesium delivered into the loop is reabsorbed there [197]; this segment therefore accounts for quantitatively the most important fraction of magnesium reabsorption. To what extent active and passive (voltage-dependent) transports are responsible is not known. The marked inhibitory effect of furosemide on magnesium reabsorption [199] suggests that the same mechanism that accounts for calcium reabsorption in the loop is involved, but this has not been formally demonstrated.

Distal tubule

Only a small proportion (<5%) of filtered magnesium is reabsorbed in the distal tubule and collecting duct [200]. The mechanism responsible has not been identified. Although it is tempting to dismiss distal tubular reabsorption as unimportant because the amount involved is small, this is misleading because 5% of the filtered load represents a large quantity of magnesium in relation to dietary intake, and the final regulation of magnesium excretion is presumably effected at the most distal site capable of magnesium reabsorption, probably the distal convoluted tubule.

Renal handling of phosphate

Inorganic phosphate (P) is filtered and reabsorbed by a Tm-limited transport system (Figure 3.5). Although FE_P can be calculated using Equation 3, marked variability in TmP secondary to changes in GFR makes FE_P an imprecise way of describing tubular P reabsorption [201]. The quotient TmP/GFR defines the theoretical P threshold, i.e. the intercept on the x-axis of Figure 3.5 obtained by extending the P excretion curve and ignoring the splay. It is this quantity that is altered by changes in circulating PTH and other modulators of tubular P transport. TmP/GFR can be calculated from the equation [202]:

$$\frac{TmP}{GFR} = P_\mathrm{p} - \left(\frac{U_\mathrm{P} \times P_\mathrm{creatinine}}{U_\mathrm{creatinine}} \right) \qquad (14)$$

Segmental tubular phosphate reabsorption

The bulk of filtered P is reabsorbed in the proximal tubule, where it is responsive to influences such as changes in ECF volume that alter sodium reabsorption. Entry into the cell is via sodium–phosphate co-transporters in the apical membrane. Two families of such transporters have now been characterised in renal cortex from several species, including man. Designated as Type I and Type II transporters respectively, both are present in proximal tubular apical membranes. All relevant evidence indicates that the Type II transporter is the physiologically important regulator of P reabsorption. It is a protein of 635 amino acids, probably has 8 transmembrane-spanning domains, and has sites for protein phosphorylation which probably regulate transporter activity via protein kinase C. It transports with a stoichiometry of 3Na:1P. The gene is located on chromosome 5 (that for the Type I transporter is on chromosome 6). Expression of the gene is partly under the control of another gene on the X chromosome that either regulates transcription or codes for a humoral factor that up-regulates the activity of the transporter. This explains the X-linked transmission of familial hypophosphataemic rickets, in which Type II transporter activity has been shown to be reduced [203]. The role of the Type I transporter in the control of human phosphate transport, and its possible relevance to disease, is not yet clear. An authoritative review of the physiology and molecular biology of tubular P transport has recently been published [204].

PTH and phosphate reabsorption

PTH inhibits P reabsorption in both proximal [205] and distal [206] segments. Changes in proximal P reabsorption are paralleled by changes in sodium reabsorption, as would be expected from the nature of the transport process, whereas in the distal tubule PTH has no effect on sodium transport. PTH binds to proximal tubular cell receptors that activate the adenylate cyclase and protein kinase C pathways [207]. Acute changes in transporter activity are probably mediated by activation of protein kinase C which reduces activity of the Type II transporter, probably by phosphorylation. Chronic changes probably involve alterations in gene transcription and translation [208]. PTH release is controlled directly and indirectly by phosphate intake. Increasing P intake leads to transient hyperphosphataemia, which in turn causes hypocalcaemia. Hypocalcaemia stimulates PTH release both directly and by altering vitamin D metabolism (see below). The increased level of PTH inhibits P reabsorption, leading to phosphaturia that compensates for the increase in dietary P.

Renal metabolism of vitamin D

The active end-product of vitamin D metabolism is the hormone 1, 25-dihydroxycholecalciferol (1, 25-DHCC, 1, 25-dihydroxyvitamin D_3). It is produced from vitamin D by 25-hydroxylation, which takes place in the liver, and subsequent 1(-hydroxylation which takes place in the mitochondria of the proximal tubular cells [209, 210]. In conditions of 1, 25-DHCC repletion, 1α-hydroxylation is suppressed and the inactive metabolite 24, 25-DHCC is produced instead [211]. The kidney is thus an endocrine organ producing a hormone under negative feedback control: according to need, conversion of 25-HCC oscillated between 1α- and 24-hydroxylation. Apart from the circulating concentration of 1, 25-DHCC, other factors promoting 1α-hydroxylation include, in descending order of power, hypocalcaemia, hypophosphataemia and PTH [212]. As well as regulating the production of 1, 25-DHCC, the kidney is one of its target organs, along with intestine and bone. Localisation of the hormone to the nuclei of distal tubular cells [213] occurs and presumably mediates its renal action, which is to enhance tubular calcium reabsorption [214], reinforcing the elevation of ECF Ca and P concentrations mediated by its other major actions: stimulation of intestinal Ca and P transport and mobilisation of bone mineral. Failure of renal 1α-hydroxylation of vitamin D is one of the two main processes involved in the causation of the bone disease of chronic renal failure, the other being secondary hyperparathyroidism [215].

Concentration and dilution of urine

Tonicity of body fluids

The tonicity, or effective osmolality, of body fluids is controlled within narrow limits (291 ± 4 mosmol/kg H_2O) by regulation of water intake and excretion. Changes in ECF tonicity are sensed by osmoreceptors located in the anterior hypothalamus [216, 217]. ECF hypertonicity produces thirst, leading to increased water intake (providing the subject has access to water), and release of antidiuretic hormone (ADH), leading to a reduction in water excretion; hypotonicity has the opposite effects. Mammals in the wild state drink in response to thirst; they therefore oscillate between isotonicity, the point at which thirst disappears, and marginal hypertonicity, which stimulates further water intake. They rarely, if ever, need to excrete dilute urine but may need to excrete highly concentrated urine if water is not immediately available in response to the thirst stimulus. Civilised man, in contrast, frequently drinks in excess of biological need for social and cultural reasons and due to the availability of flavoured (and otherwise adulterated) drinks. The ability to excrete urine more dilute than ECF is therefore essential to the avoidance of dilutional hypotonicity.

The diluting segment

As previously discussed, proximal tubular fluid reabsorption is isotonic. The dissociation between water and solute reabsorption necessary for the production of urine with osmolality different from that of ECF takes place in more distal parts of the nephron. Micropuncture studies [218] showed that the fluid in the early distal convoluted tubule was hypotonic to plasma (about 100 mosmol/kg H_2O), irrespective of whether the final urine was concentrated or dilute at the time. Studies of isolated, perfused rabbit TALs [219, 220] confirmed that solute was actively reabsorbed without water in this segment. This is now known to be via the Na^+-K^+-$2Cl^-$ transporter NKCC2 (see above). The TAL and early distal convoluted tubule are therefore the obligate diluting segment. When maximally dilute urine is being produced, the late distal tubule and collecting ducts also become water impermeable in the absence of ADH, and continuing solute (NaCl) reabsorption in the late distal convoluted tubule and the collecting duct leads to the elaboration of urine of osmolality about 40 mosmol/kg H_2O. The production of concentrated urine depends on the establishment of interstitial hypertonicity in the medulla, a process that ingeniously utilises the same transporting process that is responsible for dilution, i.e. active electrolyte reabsorption in the TAL.

Countercurrent multiplication and exchange

The processes of countercurrent multiplication and exchange [221] convert the hyperosmolality of the interstitium surrounding the TAL, and resulting from NaCl reabsorption, into an axial concentration gradient maximal at the papillary tip. The elements of the countercurrent system are the loops of Henle (multipliers) and the vasa recta (exchangers) with the collecting duct being the site of final osmotic water reabsorption. The mechanism was described in principle many years ago by Kuhn and associates [222, 223], but a more detailed understanding of the process required methods of investigation not available until much later. A general description of the medullary countercurrent system is beyond the scope of this chapter; the reader is referred to an authoritative symposium published in *Federation Proceedings* in 1983 [224–229]. A recurring difficulty has been to account for the concentration of solute in the inner medullary and papillary interstitium (where the tonicity is highest) in the apparent absence of active solute reabsorption in the thin (inner medullary) segment of the ascending limb (Figure 3.2). This probably depends on passive recycling of urea through facilitated diffusion in the medulla [230, 231]. Various models have been constructed to account for the observed hypertonicity in the inner medulla without the need to postulate active solute reabsorption in the thin ascending limb [232–234] but none has been unequivocally validated to date.

The antidiuretic hormone

The human antidiuretic hormone is the nona-peptide arginine vasopressin (AVP) [235]:

Cys - Tyr - Phe - Glu - Asp - Cys - Pro - Arg - Gly - NH$_2$

with a ring structure formed by a disulphide bridge between the two cystine residues. It is synthesised in cells whose bodies lie in the supraoptic and paraventricular nuclei of the anterior hypothalamus, and released from their axonal endings in the posterior pituitary. It is released in response both to osmoreceptor stimulation [216] and carotid sinus and aortic arch baroreceptor stimulation [236]. The former is responsible for maintaining tonicity of body fluids in the normal range, whereas the latter causes renal water retention in the face of underfilling of the high-pressure compartment of the circulation due to, for example, volume depletion, vasodilatation

or left ventricular failure. Baroreceptor-mediated AVP release is not suppressible by hypotonicity, and so hyponatraemia is commonly seen in conditions associated with it [237]. A much larger proportional volume change is needed than osmolar change to initiate an AVP response (Figure 3.12). An increase of only 1–2% in plasma osmolality suffices to elicit a maximally antidiuretic plasma level (5 pg/ml), while a reduction in blood volume or pressure of about 8% is needed before a significant AVP response is seen. However, very high AVP levels are produced when hypovolaemia or hypotension become more severe than this.

Antidiuretic hormone receptors

AVP binds to specific receptors (V$_2$ receptors) on the collecting duct cells, causing activation of adenylate cyclase and conversion of ATP to cyclic AMP. This initiates a chain of intracellular events that culminate in the insertion of water channels in the apical membrane of the cell, rendering it permeable to water. The gene for the V$_2$ receptor is on the long arm of the X chromosome; mutations in it are responsible for the disease X-linked diabetes insipidus [239, 240].

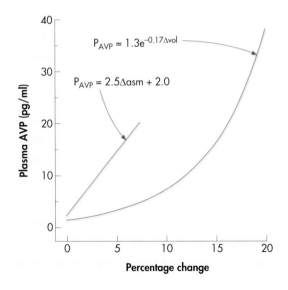

Figure 3.12 *The antidiuretic hormone response to isovolaemic increase in plasma osmolality (linear relationship) and to isotonic depletion of plasma volume (exponential relationship). The negative value of the exponent of the equation relating P$_{AVP}$ to volume arises from the fact that the volume change is in a negative direction. (Modified from Dunn* et al. *[238].)*

Aquaporins

The water channels referred to in the previous paragraph belong to a family of proteins known as *aquaporins*, of which different members are expressed in different cell types. The human collecting duct aquaporin is Aquaporin 2, and the gene that codes for it is located on chromosome 12 in the region 12q13 [241, 242]. Mutations in the gene for Aquaporin 2 cause a form of diabetes insipidus clinically indistinguishable from that caused by mutations in the V_2 receptor gene except that, as would be expected, it is inherited as an autosomal recessive condition and affects both sexes equally.

Free water clearance and reabsorption

The urinary solute excretion rate is determined by dietary and metabolic factors, but is usually in the region of 500–1500 mosmol/day for an adult on an average diet. Taking a notional value of 580 mosmol/day, and assuming a plasma osmolality of 290 mosmol/kg H_2O, it is evident that 2 litres of isotonic urine would suffice to excrete this amount of solute. Any additional water excretion will render the urine hypotonic to plasma: such additional water excretion is called free water clearance, C_{H_2O}. Osmolar clearance can be calculated using Equation 15:

$$C_{OSM} = \frac{U_{OSM} \times V}{P_{OSM}} \qquad (15)$$

When urine is isotonic, $U_{OSM} = P_{OSM}$ (by definition), and therefore $C_{OSM} = V$. When urine is hypotonic to plasma, $C_{OSM} < V$, and:

$$C_{H_2O} = V - C_{OSM} \qquad (16)$$

When urine is hypertonic, $C_{OSM} > V$ and therefore the calculated value for C_{H_2O} is negative. Reversing the sign, negative free water clearance becomes free water reabsorption, usually designated Tc_{H_2O}:

$$Tc_{H_2O} = C_{OSM} - V \qquad (17)$$

C_{H_2O} and Tc_{H_2O} define the limiting values for renal water excretion, and therefore for tolerated water ingestion. At a solute excretion rate of 580 mosmol/day, C_{OSM} is 2 litres a day.

Rearranging Equation 16:

$$V = \frac{C_{OSM} \times P_{OSM}}{U_{OSM}} \qquad (18)$$

and taking values of 40 and 1200 mosmol/kg H_2O as minimal and maximal U_{OSM} respectively, yields limiting values for V of 14.5 and 0.48 litres daily. Corresponding maximum values for C_{H_2O} and Tc_{H_2O} are 12.5 and 1.52 l/day. Thus, at any given solute excretion rate, the defence against overhydration and dilution (C_{H_2O}) is much more effective than that against dehydration and concentration (Tc_{H_2O}), a conclusion borne out by clinical experience. This huge capacity to protect the body fluids from dilution may be an evolutionary inheritance from our fish and amphibian ancestors, to whom (in fresh water) osmotic dilution is a constant threat.

References

1. Rubin MI, Bruck E, Rapoport M. Maturation of renal function in childhood: clearance studies. J Clin Invest 1949; 28: 1144–62
2. Du Bois D, Du Bois EF. A formula to estimate the approximate surface area if height and weight are known. Arch Int Med 1916; 17: 863–71
3. McCance RA, Widdowson EM. The correct physiological basis on which to compare infant and adult renal function. Lancet 1952; ii: 860–2
4. Coulthard MG, Hey EN. Weight as the best standard for glomerular filtration in the newborn. Arch Dis Child 1984; 59: 373–5
5. McCance RA. The maintenance of stability in the newly born. 1. Chemical exchange. Arch Dis Child 1959; 34: 361–70
6. Dugdale AE. Evolution and infant feeding. Lancet 1986; I: 670–3
7. Holliday, 1994.
8. Kildeberg P. Disturbances of hydrogen ion balance occurring in premature infants. II. Late metabolic acidosis. Acta Paediatr Scand 1964; 53: 517–26
9. Manz F, Kalhoff H, Remer T. Renal acid excretion in early infancy. Pediatric Nephrol 1997: in press
10. Möller E, McIntosh JF, Van Slyke DD. Studies of urea excretion. II. Relationship between urine volume and the rate of urea excretion by normal adults. J Clin Invest 1928; 6: 427–65

11. Smith, HW. The kidney. Structure and function in health and disease. Chapter 3. New York: Oxford University Press, 1951: 39–62

12. Shannon JA. The renal excretion of creatinine in man. J Clin Invest 1935; 14: 403–10

13. Arant BS, Edelmann CM Jr, Spitzer A. The congruence of creatinine and inulin clearances in children: use of the Technicon AutoAnalyzer. J Pediatr 1972; 81: 559–61

14. Calcagno PL, Rubin MI. Renal extraction of para-aminohippurate in infants and children. J Clin Invest 1963; 42: 1632–9

15. Christensen JA, Meyer DS, Bohle A. The structure of the human juxtaglomerular apparatus. A morphometric, light microscopic study on serial sections. Virchows Archiv 1975; 367: 83–92

16. Tisher CC, Bulger RE, Trump BF. Human renal ultrastructure: I. Proximal tubule of healthy individuals. Lab Invest 1966; 15: 1357–94

17. Tisher, 1968.

18. Bulger RE, Tisher CC, Meyers CH, Trump BF. Human renal ultrastructure: II. The thin limb of Henle's loop and the interstitium in healthy individuals. Lab Invest 1967; 16: 124–41

19. Beeuwkes R III, Bonventre JV. Tubular organisation and vascular-tubular relations in the dog kidney. Am J Physiol 1975; 229: 695–713

20. Kriz W. Structural organization of the renal medullary counterflow system. Fed Proc 1983; 42: 2379–85

21. Walker AM, Bott PA, Oliver J, MacDowell MC. The collection and analysis of fluid from single nephrons of the mammalian kidney. Am J Physiol 1941; 134: 580–95

22. Arakawa M. A scanning electron microscopic study of the glomerulus of normal and nephrotic rats. Lab Invest 1970; 23: 489–96

23. Arakawa M. A scanning electron microscopic study of the human glomerulus. Am J Pathol 1970; 64: 457–66

24. Jorgensen F, Bentzon MW. The ultrastructure of the normal human glomerulus. Thickness of glomerular basement membrane. Lab Invest 1968; 18: 42–8

25. Vernier RL. Electron microscopic studies of the normal basement membrane. In: Siperstein MD, Colwell AR Sr, Meyer K (eds) Small blood vessel involvement in diabetes mellitus. Publication 57, American Institute of Biological Sciences, Arlington, Virginia, 1964

26. Jorgensen F. The ultrastructure of the normal human glomerulus. Ejinar Munksgaard, Copenhagen, 1966

27. Caulfield JP, Farquar MG. Distribution of anionic sites in glomerular basement membranes: their possible role in filtration and attachment. Proc Natl Acad Sci USA 1976; 73: 1646–50

28. Kanwar YS, Farquar MG. Characterization of anionic sites in the glomerular basement membrane (GBM). Kidney Int 1978; 14: 713 (abstract)

29. Kanwar YS, Farquar MG. Anionic sites in the glomerular basement membrane. In vivo and in vitro localization in the laminae rarae by cationic probes. J Cell Biol 1979; 81: 137–53

30. Venkatachalam MA, Karnovsky MJ, Fahimi HD, Cotran RS. An ultrastructural study of glomerular permeability using catalase and peroxidase as tracer proteins. J Exp Med 1970; 132: 1153–67

31. Robson AM, Giangiacomo J, Kienstra RA, et al. Normal glomerular permeability and its modification by minimal change nephrotic syndrome. J Clin Invest 1974; 54: 1190–9

32. Brenner BM, Hostetter TH, Humes HD. Glomerular permselectivity: barrier function based on discrimination of molecular size and charge. Am J Physiol 1978; 234: F455–60

33. Groniowski J, Biczysko W, Walski M. Electron microscopic studies on the surface coat of renal podocytes in albuminuric rats. Lab Invest 1974; 30: 58–63

34. Goode NP, Shires M, Davison AM. The glomerular basement membrane charge-selectivity barrier: an oversimplified concept? Nephrol Dial Transplant 1996; 11: 1714–16

35. Starling, 1896.

36. Brenner BM, Troy JL, Daugherty TM. The dynamics of glomerular ultrafiltration in the rat. J Clin Invest 1971; 50: 1776–80

37. Deen WM, Robertson CR, Brenner BM. A model of glomerular ultrafiltration in the rat. Am J Physiol 1972; 223: 1178–83

38. Brenner BM, Troy JL, Daugherty TM, et al. Dynamics of glomerular ultrafiltration in the rat. II. Plasma flow dependence of GFR. Am J Physiol 1972; 223: 1184–90

39. Maddox DA, Deen WM, Brenner BM. Dynamics of glomerular ultrafiltration. VI. Studies in the primate. Kidney Int 1974; 5: 271–8

40. Deen WM, Troy JL, Robertson CR, Brenner BM. Dynamics of glomerular ultrafiltration in the rat. IV. Determination of the ultrafiltration coefficient. J Clin Invest 1973; 52: 11500–8

41. Navar LG, Bell PD, White RW, et al. Evaluation of the single nephron glomerular filtration coefficient in the dog. Kidney Int 1977; 12: 137–49

42. Kirkman H, Stowell RE. Renal filtration surface in the albino rat. Anat Record (Philadelphia) 1942; 82: 373–91

43. Shea SM, Morrison AB. A stereological study of the glomerular filter in the rat. Morphometry of the slit

diaphragm and basement membrane. J Cell Biol 1975; 67: 433–43

44. Landis EM. Micro-injection studies of capillary permeability. II. Relationship between capillary pressure and the rate at which fluid passes through the walls of single capillaries. Am J Physiol 1927; 82: 217–38

45. Zweifach BW, Intaglietta M. Mechanics of fluid movement across single capillaries in the rabbit. Microvascular Res 1968; 1: 83–101

46. Myers *et al*, 1975.

47. Baer PG, Navar LG, Guyton AC. Renal autoregulation, filtration rate and electrolyte excretion during vasodilatation. Am J Physiol 1970; 219: 619–25

48. Baylis C, Deen WM, Myers BD, Brenner BM. Effects of some vasodilator drugs on trancapillary fluid exchange in the renal cortex. Am J Physiol 1976; 230: 1148–58

49. Ausiello DA, Kreisberg JJ, Roy C, Karnovsky MJ. Contraction of cultured rat glomerular mesangial cells after stimulation with angiotensin II and arginine vasopressin. J Clin Invest 1980; 65: 754–60

50. Dworkin LD, Ichikawa I, Brenner BM. Hormonal modulation of glomerular function. Am J Physiol 1983; 244: F95–104

51. Robertson CR, Deen WM, Troy JL, Brenner BM. Dynamics of glomerular ultrafiltration in the rat. III. Hemodynamics and autoregulation. Am J Physiol 1972; 223: 1191–200

52. Burg MB, Orloff J. Electrical potential difference across proximal convoluted tubule. Am J Physiol 1970; 219: 1714–16

53. Gyory AZ, Brendel V, Kinne R. Effect of cardiac glycosides and sodium ethacrynate on transepithelial sodium transport in in vivo micropuncture experiments and on isolated plasma membrane Na-K-ATPase in vitro of the rat. Pflügers Arch 1972; 335: 287–96

54. Brant SR, Yun CH, Donowitz M, Tse CM. Cloning, distribution, and functional analysis of the human Na^+/H^+ exchanger isoform, NHE3. Am J Physiol 1995; 269: C198–206

55. Burg MB, Green N. Bicarbonate transport by isolated perfused rabbit proximal convoluted tubules. Am J Physiol 1977; 233: F307–14

56. Burg MB, Patlak C, Green N, Villey D. Organic solutes in fluid absorption by renal proximal convoluted tubules. Am J Physiol 1976; 231: 627–37

57. Kokko JP. Proximal tubule potential difference. Dependence on glucose, HCO_3^- and amino acids. J Clin Invest 1973; 52: 1362–7

58. Kinne R. Properties of the glucose transport system in the renal brush border membrane. In: Bronner F, Kleinzeller A (eds) Current topics in membranes and transport. New York: Academic Press, Vol 8, 1976; 209–67

59. Giebisch G, Windhager E. Electrolyte transport across tubular membranes. In: Orloff J, Berliner RW (eds) Handbook of physiology. Section 8: Renal physiology. Am Physiol Soc 1973: 315–76

60. Diamond J, Bossert W. Standing gradient osmotic flow. A mechanism for coupling of water and solute transport in epithelia. J Gen Physiol 1967; 50: 2061–83

61. Martino & Earley, 1968.

62. Spitzer A, Windhager. Effect of peritubular oncotic pressure changes on proximal tubular fluid reabsorption. Am J Physiol 1970; 218: 1188–93

63. Berry CA, Cogan MG. Influence of pertubular protein on solute absorption in the rabbit proximal tubule. J Clin Invest 1981; 68: 506–16

64. Malvin RL, Wilde WS, Sullivan LP. Localisation of nephron transport by stop-flow analysis. Am J Physiol 1958; 194: 135–42

65. Strickler JC, Thompson DD, Klose RM, Giebisch G. Micropuncture study of renal phosphate excretion in the rat. J Clin Invest 1964; 43: 1596–1607

66. Pitts RF, Alexander RS. The renal absorptive mechanism for inorganic phosphate in normal and acidotic dogs. Am J Physiol 1944; 142: 648–62

67. Segal S, Thrier SO. Renal handling of amino acids. In: Orloff J, Berliner RW (eds) Handbook of Physiology. Section 8: Renal physiology. American Physiology Society, Washington DC, 1973: 653–76

68. Ullrich KJ. Renal tubular mechanisms of organic solute transport. Kidney Int 1976; 9: 134–48

69. Bernier GM, Conrad ME. Catabolism of human microglobulin by the rat kidney. Am J Physiol 1969; 217: 1359–62

70. Waldmann TA, Strober W, Mogielnicki BP. The renal handling of low molecular weight proteins. II. Disorders of serum protein catabolism in patients with tubular proteinuria, the nephrotic syndrome, or uremia. J Clin Invest 1972; 51: 2162–74

71. Walsmann *et al*. 1972

72. Ullrich 1972

73. Park CH, Maack T. Albumin absorption and catabolism by isolated perfused proximal convoluted tubules of the rabbit. J Clin Invest 1984; 73: 767–77

74. Irish JM III, Grantham JJ. Renal handling of organic anions and cations. In: Brenner BM, Rector FC (eds). The kidney. Philadelphia: W.B. Saunders, Vol 1, Chapter 13, 1981; 619–49

75. de Wardener HE. The control of sodium excretion. In: Orloff J, Berliner RW (eds) Handbook of physiology. Section 8: Renal physiology. Chapter 21. Washington DC: Am Physiol Soc, 1973: 677–720

76. Brenner BM, Bennett CM, Berliner RW. The relationship between glomerular filtration rate and sodium reabsorption by the proximal tubule in the rat. J Clin Invest 1968; 46: 1358–74

77. Ichikawa I, Hoyer JR, Seiler MW, Brenner BM. Mechanism of glomerulotubular balance in the setting of heterogeneous glomerular injury: preservation of a close functional linkage between individual nephrons and surrounding microvasculature. J Clin Invest 1982; 69: 185–98

78. Wright FS, Briggs JP. Feedback regulation of glomerular filtration rate. Am J Physiol 1977; 233: F1–7

79. Schnermann J, Ploth DW, Hermle M. Activation of tubuloglomerular feedback by chloride transport. Pflügers Arch 1976; 362: 229–40

80. Stowe NT, Schnermann J. Renin-aldosterone mediation of tubulo-glomerular feedback control of filtration rate. Fed Proc 1974; 33: 247 (abstract)

81. Thurau K, Boylan JW. Acute renal success. The unexpected logic of oliguria in acute renal failure. Am J Med 1976; 61: 308–15

82. Brezis M, Rosen S, Silva P, Epstein FH. Selective vulnerability of the medullary thick ascending limb to anoxia in the isolated perfused rat kidney. J Clin Invest 1984; 73: 182–90

83. Strauss MB, Lamdin E, Smith WP, Bleifer DJ. Surfeit and deficit of sodium: a kinetic concept of sodium excretion. Arch Int Med 1958; 102: 527–36

84. McCance RA. Experimental sodium chloride deficiency in man. Proc Roy Soc London, Series B 1936; 119: 245–68

85. Epstein M. Cardiovascular and renal effects of head-out water immersion in man. Circulation Res 1976; 39: 619–28

86. Gillespie DS, Sandberg RL, Koike TI. Dual effect of left atrial receptors on excretion of sodium and water. Am J Physiol 1973; 225: 706–10

87. Guyton AC, Scanlon CJ, Armstrong GG. Effects of pressoreceptor reflex and Cushing's reflex on urinary output. Fed Proc 1952; 11: 61–62

88. Keeler R. Natriuresis after unilateral stimulation of carotid receptors in unanesthetized rats. Am J Physiol 1974; 226: 507–11

89. Epstein FH, Post RS, McDowell M. Effects of an arteriovenous fistula on renal hemodynamics and electrolyte excretion. J Clin Invest 1953; 32: 233–41

90. Daly JJ, Roe JW, Horrocks P. A comparison of sodium excretion following the infusion of saline into systemic and portal veins in the dog. Evidence for a hepatic role in sodium excretion. Clin Sci 1967; 33: 481–7

91. Martino JA, Earley LE. Demonstration of the role of physical factors as determinants of natriuretic response to volume expansion. J Clin Invest 1967; 23: 371–86

92. Schrier RW, McDonald KM, Marshall RA, Lauler DP. Absence of natriuretic response to acute hypotonic saline loading in dogs. Clin Sci 1968; 34: 57–72

93. Schrier RW, Fein RL, McNeil JS, Cirksena WJ. Influence of interstitial fluid volume expansion and plasma sodium concentration on the natriuretic response to volume expansion in the dog. Clin Sci 1969; 63: 371–85

94. Paintal AS. Vagal sensory receptors and their reflex effects. Physiol Rev 1973; 53: 159–227

95. Olsson K. Further evidence for the importance of cerebrospinal fluid sodium concentration in central control of fluid balance. Acta Physiol Scand 1973; 88: 183–8

96. de Wardener HE, Mills IH, Clapham WF, Hayter CJ. Studies on the efferent mechanism of the sodium diuresis which follows the administration of intravenous saline in the dog. Clin Sci 1961; 21: 249–58

97. Dirks JH, Cirksena WJ, Berliner RW. The effect of saline infusion on sodium reabsorption by the proximal tubule of the dog. J Clin Invest 1965; 44: 1160–1170

98. Lindheimer MD, Lalone RC, Levinsky NG. Evidence that an acute increase in glomerular filtration rate has little effect on sodium excretion in the dog unless extracellular volume is expanded. J Clin Invest 1967; 46: 256–65

99. Howards SS, Davis BB, Knox FG, et al. Depression of fractional sodium reabsorption by the proximal tubule of the dog without sodium diuresis. J Clin Invest 1968; 47: 1561–2

100. Sonnenberg H. Medullary collecting duct function in antidiuretic and in salt or water diuretic rats. Am J Physiol 1974; 226: 501–6

101. Sonnenberg H. Secretion of salt and water into the medullary collecting duct of Ringer-infused rats. Am J Physiol 1975; 228: 565–8

102. Shipley RE, Study RS. Factors regulating renal blood flow and urine flow following acute changes in renal artery perfusion pressure. Am J Physiol 1950; 163: 750 (abst)

103. Selkurt EE. Effect of pulse pressure and mean arterial pressure modification on renal haemodynamics and electrolyte and water excretion. Circulation 1951; 4: 541–51

104. Arendshorst WJ, Navar LG. Renal circulation and glomerular hemodynamics. In: Schrier RW, Gottschalk CW (eds) Diseases of the Kidney. Chapter 2, 5th Edition. Boston: Little, Brown & Co., 1993: 75

105. LaGrange RG, Sloop CH, Schmid HE. Selective stimulation of renal nerves in the anaesthetised dog. Circulation Res 1973; 33: 704–12

106. Slick GL, Di Bona GF, Kaloyanides GJ. Renal sympathetic nerve activity in sodium retention of acute caval constriction. Am J Physiol 1974; 226: 925–32

107. Bello-Reuss E, Colindres RE, Pastoriza-Munoz E et al. Effects of acute unilateral denervation in the rat. J Clin Invest 1975; 56: 208–17

108. Muller J, Barajas L. Electron microscopic and histochemical evidence for a tubular innervation in the renal cortex of the monkey. J Ultrastructural Res 1972; 41: 533–49

109. Moss NG. Renal function and renal afferent and efferent activity. Am J Physiol 1982; 243: F425–33

110. Laragh JH, Sealey J, Brunner HR. The control of aldosterone secretion in normal and hypertensive man: abnormal renin-aldosterone patterns in low renin hypertension. Am J Med 1972; 53: 649–63

111. August JT, Nelson DH, Thorn GW. Response of normal subjects to large amounts of aldosterone. J Clin Invest 1958; 37: 1549–55

112. Young DB, McCaa RE, Pan Y-J, Guyton AC. Effectiveness of the alsosterone-sodium and potassium feedback control system. Am J Physiol 1976; 231: 945–53

113. Young DB, Guyton AC. Steady state aldosterone dose-response relationships. Q Circulation Res 1977; 40: 138–42

114. Moyer JH, Handley CA. Norepinephrine and epinephrine effect on renal haemodynamics. Circulation 1952; 5: 91–7

115. McDonald RH Jr, Goldsberg LI, McNay JL, Tuttle EP Jr. Effect of dopamine in man: augmentation of sodium excretion, glomerular filtration rate and renal plasma flow. J Clin Invest 1964; 43: 1116–24

116. Eble JN. A proposed mechanism for the depressor effect of dopamine in the anaesthetized dog. J Pharmacol Exp Ther 1964; 145: 65–70

117. Lee MR. Dopamine and the kidney. Clin Sci 1982; 62: 439–48

118. Finlay GD, Whitsett TL, Cucinell EA, Goldberg LI. Augmentation of sodium and potassium excretion, glomerular filtration and renal plasma flow by levodopa. New Engl J Med 1971; 284: 865–70

119. Haycock GB, Al-Dahhan J, Mak RHK, Chantler C. Effect of indomethacin on clinical progress and renal function in cystinosis. Arch Dis Child 1982; 57: 934–9

120. Kaojarera S, Chennavasin P, Anderson S, Brater DC. Nephron site of effect of nonsteroidal anti-inflammatory drugs on solute excretion in humans. Am J Physiol 1983; 244: F134–9

121. Henrich WL, Berl T, McDonald KM, Anderson RJ, Schrier RW. Angiotensin II, renal nerves and prostaglandins in renal hemodynamics during hemorrhage. Am J Physiol 1978; 235: F46–51

122. Scicli AG, Gandolfi R, Carretero OA. Site of formation of kinins in the dog nephron. Am J Physiol 1978; 234: F36–40

123. McGiff JC, Terragno NA, Malik KO. Release of prostaglandin E-like substance from canine kidney by bradykinin. Circulation Res 1972; 31: 36–43

124. Atlas SA, Kleinert HD, Camargo M J, et al. Purification, sequencing and synthesis of natriuretic and vasoactive rat peptide. Nature 1984; 309: 717–19

125. Flynn TG, Davies PL. The biochemistry and molecular biology of atrial natriuretic factor. Biochem J 1985; 232: 313–21

126. Cargill RI, Lipworth BJ. Pulmonary vasorelaxant activity of atrial natriuretic peptide and brain natriuretic peptide in humans. Thorax 1995; 50:183–5

127. Amin J, Carretero OA. Mechanisms of action of atrial natriuretic factor and C-type natriuretic peptide. Hypertension 1996; 27: 684–7

128. Veldkamp PJ, Carmines PK, Inscho EW, Navar LG. Direct evaluation of the microvascular actions of ANP in juxtamedullary nephrons. Am J Physiol 1988; 254: F440–4

129. Appel RG, Wang J, Simonson MS, Dunn MJ. A mechanism by which atrial natriuretic factor mediates its glomerular action. Am J Physiol 1986; 251: F1036–42

130. Meher-Lehnert H, Taai P, Caramelo C, Schrier RW. ANP inhibits vasopressin-induced Ca^{2+} mobilization and contraction in glomerular mesangial cells. Am J Physiol 1987; 255: F763–70

131. Scavone C, Scanlon C, McKee M, Nathanson JA. Atrial natriuretic peptide modulates sodium- and potassium-activated adenosine triphosphatase through a mechanism involving cyclic GMP and cyclic

GMP-dependent protein kinase. J Pharmacol Exp Ther 1995; 272: 1036–43

132. Brenner BM, Ballerman BJ, Gunning ME, Zeidel ML. Diverse biological actions of atrial natriuretic peptide. Ann Rev Physiol 1990; 70: 665–99

133. Lohmeier TE, Mizelle HL, Reinhart GA. Role of atrial natriuretic peptide in long-term volume homeostasis. Clin Exp Pharmacol Physiol 1995; 22: 55–61

134. Manoogian C, Pandian M, Ehrlich L, et al. Plasma atrial natriuretic hormone levels in patients with the syndrome of inappropriate antidiuretic hormone secretion. J Clin Endocrinol Metab 1988; 67: 571–5

135. Goetz KL. Physiology and pathophysiology of atrial peptides. Am J Physiol 1988; 254: E1–15

136. Raine AEG, Firth JG, Ledingham JGG. Renal actions of atrial natriuretic factor. Clin Sci 76: 1–8

137. Kenyon CJ, Jardine AG. Atrial natriuretic peptide: water and electrolyte homeostasis. Baillière's Clin Endocrinol Metab 1989; 3: 431–50

138. Clerico A, Iervasi G, Iascone MR, et al. Evaluation of the endocrine function of the heart in humans: proposal for an integrated approach for the assessment of production, secretion, distribution and degradation of atrial natriuretic factor and related peptides. Int J Pharmacol Res 1995; 15: 65–86

139. Delpire E, Kaplan MR, Plotkin MD, Hebert SC. The Na-(K)-Cl cotransporter family in the human kidney: molecular identification and function(s). Nephrol Dial Transplant 1996; 11: 1967–73

140. Simon DB, Karet FE, Hamdan JM, Di Pietro A, Sanjad SA, Lifton RP. Bartter's syndrome, hypokalemic alkalosis with hypercalciuria, is caused by mutations in the Na-K-2Cl cotransporter NKCC2. Nat Genet 1966; 13: 183–8

141. Simon DB, Nelson-Williams C, Johnson Bia M. Gitelman's variant of Bartter's syndrome, inherited hypokalaemic alkalosis, is caused by mutations in the thiazide-sensitive Na-Cl cotransporter. Nat Genet 1996; 12: 24–30

142. Lemmink HH, van den Heuvel LPWJ, van Dijk HA, et al. Linkage of Gitelman syndrome to the thiazide-sensitive sodium-chloride cotransporter gene with identification of mutations in Dutch families. Pediatr Nephrol 1996; 10: 403–7

143. Gitelman HJ, Graham JB, Welt LG. A new familial disorder characterized by hypokalemia and hypomagnesemia. Trans Assoc Am Physicians 1966; 79: 221–35

144. Korbmacher C, Letz B, Ackermann A, Volk T. Sodium channels and non-selective cation channels in the cortical collecting duct. Nephrol Dial Transplant 1995; 10: 1546–50

145. Canessa CM, Schild L, Buell G et al. Amiloride-sensitive epithelial Na^+ channel is made of three homologous subunits. Nature 1994; 367: 463–7

146. Shimkets RA, Warnock DG, Bositis CM, et al. Liddle's syndrome: heritable human hypertension caused by mutations in the β subunit of the epithelial sodium channel. Cell 1994; 79: 407–14

147. Hansson JH, Nelson-Williams C, Suzuki H, et al. Hypertension caused by a truncated epithelial sodium channel α subunit: genetic heterogeneity of Liddle syndrome. Nat Genet 1996; 11: 76–82

148. Hanukoglu A. Type 1 pseudohypoaldosteronism includes two clinically and genetically distinct entities with either renal or multiple target organ defects. J Clin Endocrinol Metab 1991; 73: 936–44

149. Chang S-S, Grunder S, Hanukoglu A, et al. Mutations in the subunits of the epithelial sodium channel cause salt wasting with hyperkalaemic acidosis, pseudohypoaldosteronism type 1. Nat Genet 1996; 12: 248–53

150. Malnic G, Klose RM, Giebisch G. Micropuncture study of renal potassium secretion in the rat. Am J Physiol 1964; 206: 674–86

151. Reineck HJ, Osgood RW, Ferris TF, Stein JH. Potassium transport in the distal tubule and collecting duct of the rat. Am J Physiol 1975; 229: 1401–9

152. Reineck HJ, Osgood RW, Stein JH. Net potassium addition beyond the superficial distal tubule of the rat. Am J Physiol 1979; 235: F104–10

153. Grantham JJ, Burg MB, Orloff J. The nature of transtubular Na and K transport in isolated rabbit collecting tubules. J Clin Invest 1970; 49: 1815–26

154. MacKnight ADC. Epithelial transport of potassium. Kidney Int 1977; 11: 391–414

155. Giebisch G, Stanton B. Potassium transport in the nephron. Ann Rev Physiol 1979; 41: 241–56

156. Silva P, Hayslett JP, Epstein FH. The role of Na-K-activated adenosine triphosphatase in potassium adaptation. Stimulation of enzymatic activity by potassium loading. J Clin Invest 1973; 52: 2665–71

157. Khuri RN, Agulian SK, Kallioghlian A. Intracellular potassium in cells of the distal tubule. Pflügers Arch 1972; 335: 297–308

158. Rossier BC, Palmer LG. Mechanism of aldosterone action on sodium and potassium transport. In: Seldin

DW, Giebisch G (eds) The kidney, physiology and pathophysiology. New York: Raven Press, 1992: 1373–409

159. Feldman D, Funder J, Edelmann IS. Subcellular mechanism of the action of adrenal steroids. Am J Med 1971; 53: 545–60

160. Toussaint C, Vereerstraeten P. Effects of blood pH changes on potassium excretion in the dog. Am J Physiol 1962; 202: 768–72

161. Gennari FJ, Cohen JJ. The role of the kidney in potassium homeostasis: lessons from acid–base disturbances. Kidney Int 1975; 8: 1–5

162. Green R, Giebisch G. Some ionic requirements of proximal tubular sodium transport. I. The role of bicarbonate and chloride. Am J Physiol 1975; 229: 1205–15

163. Burg MB, Green N. Effect of mersalyl on the thick ascending limb of Henle's loop. Kidney Int 1973a; 4: 245–51

164. Burg MB, Stoner L, Cardinal J, Breen N . Furosemide effect on isolated perfused tubules. Am J Physiol 1973; 225: 119–24

165. Burg MB, Green N. Effect of ethacrynic acid on the thick ascending limb of Henle's loop. Kidney Int 1973b; 4: 301–8

166. Kunau RT Jr, Weller DR, Webb HL. Clarification of the site of action of chlorothiazide in the rat nephron. J Clin Invest 1975; 56: 401–7

167. Vander AJ, Wilde WS, Malvin RL. Stop-flow analysis of aldosterone and steroidal antagaonist, SC8109, on renal tubular transport kinetics. Proc Soc Exp Biol Med 1960; 103: 525–7

168. Lacy FB, Dobyan DC, Jamison RL. Effect of triamterene on the mammalian distal tubule in vivo. Renal Physiol 1979; 2: 36

169. Baer JE, Jones CB, Spitzer SA, Russo HF. The potassium-sparing and natriuretic activity of N-amidino-3,5-diamino-6-chloropyrazinecarboxamide hydrochloride (amiloride hydrochloride). J Pharmacol Exp Ther 1967; 157: 472–85

170. Gottschalk CW, Lassiter WE, Mylle M. Localisation of urine acidification in the mammalian kidney. Am J Physiol 1960; 198: 581–5

171. Cogan MG, Maddox DA, Lucci M S, Rector FC Jr. Control of proximal bicarbonate reabsorption in normal and acidotic rats. J Clin Invest 1979; 64: 1168–80

172. DuBose TD, Pucacco LR, Seldin DW, et al. Microelectrode determination of pH and pCO$_2$ in rat proximal tubule after benzolamide: evidence for hydrogen ion secretion. Kidney Int 1979; 15: 624–9

173. Lucci MS, Pucacco LR, DuBose TD, et al. Direct evaluation of acidification by the rat proximal tubule: the role of carbonic anhydrase. Am J Physiol 1980; 238: F372–9

174. Warnock DG, Rector FC Jr. Proton secretion by the kidney. Ann Rev Physiol 1979; 41: 197–210

175. Rodriguez-Soriano J, Boichis H, Stark H, Edelmann CM Jr. Proximal renal tubular acidosis. A defect in bicarbonate reabsorption with normal urinary acidification. Pediatric Res 1967; 1: 81–98

176. Brenes LG, Brenes JN, Hernandez MM. Familial proximal renal tubular acidosis: a distinct clinical entity. Am J Med 1977; 63: 244–52

177. Relman AS, Lennon EJ, Lemann J Jr. Endogenous production of fixed acid and the measurement of the net balance of acid in normal subjects. J Clin Invest 1961; 40: 1621–30

178. Pitts RF. The renal excretion of acid. Fed Proc 1948; 7: 418–26

179. Hutcheon RA, Kaplan BS, Drummond KS. Distal renal tubular acidosis in children with chronic hydronephrosis. J Paediatr 1976; 89: 372–6

180. Sebastian A, McSherry E, Morris RC Jr. Impaired renal conservation of sodium and chloride during sustained correction of systemic acidosis in patients with type 1, classic renal tubular acidosis. J Clin Invest 1976; 58: 454–69

181. Rodriguez-Soriano J, Vallo A, Castillo G, Oliveras R. Renal handling of water and sodium in children with proximal and distal renal tubular acidosis. Nephron 1980; 25: 193–8

182. Schwartz WB, Cohen JJ. The nature of the renal response to chronic disorders of acid–base equilibrium. Am J Med 1978; 64: 417–28

183. Harris CA, Baer PG, Chirito E, Dirks J. Composition of mammalian glomerular filtrate. Am J Physiol 1974; 227: 972–6

184. Le Grimellec C. Micropuncture study along the proximal tubule. Electrolyte reabsorption in first convolutions. Pflügers Arch 1975; 354: 133–50

185. Taylor A, Windhager EE. Possible role of cytosolic calcium and Na-Ca exchange in regulation of epithelial sodium transport. Am J Physiol 1979; 236: F505–12

186. Edwards BR, Baer PG, Sutton RAL, Dirks J. Micropuncture study of diuretic effects on sodium and calcium reabsorption in the dog nephron. J Clin Invest 1973; 52: 2418–72

187. Lassiter WE, Gottschalk CW, Mylle M. Micropuncture study of renal tubular reabsorption of calcium in normal rodents. Am J Physiol 1963; 205: 771–5

188. Constanzo LS, Windhager EE. Calcium and sodium transport by the distal convoluted tubule of the rat. Am J Physiol 1978; 235: F492–506

189. Gregor R, Lang F. Distal site of calcium reabsorption in the rat nephron. Pflügers Arch 1978; 374: 153–7

190. Sutton *et al*, 1979.

191. Coburn JW, Hartenbower DL, Massry SG. Modification of calciuretic effect of extracellular volume expansion by phosphate infusion. Am J Physiol 1971; 220: 377–83

192. Litvak J, Moldawer JP, Forbes AP, Henneman PH. Hypocalcaemic hypercalciuria during vitamin D and dihydrotachysterol therapy of hypoparathyroidism. J Clin Endocrinol Metab 1958; 18: 246–52

193. Ney R, Kelly G, Bartter FC. Actions of vitamin D independent of the parathyroid glands. Endocrinology 1968; 82: 760–6

194. Bernstein D, Kleeman CR, Maxwell MH. The effect of calcium infusions, parathyroid hormone, and vitamin D on renal clearance of calcium. Proc Soc Exp Biol Med 1963; 112: 353–5

195. Gesek FA, Friedman PA. Mechanism of calcium transport stimulated by chlorothiazide in mouse distal convoluted tubule cells. J Clin Invest 1992; 90: 429–38

196. Walser M. Divalent cations: physicochemical state in glomerular filtrate and urine and renal excretion. In: Orloff J, Berliner RW (eds) Handbook of physiology. Section 8: renal physiology. American Physiological Society, Washington DC, 1973; 555–86

197. Morel F, Roinel N, Le Grimellec C. Electron probe analysis of tubular fluid composition. Nephron 1969; 6: 350–64

198. Quamme GA, Wong NLM, Dirks J, *et al*. Magnesium handling in the dog kidney: a micropuncture study. Pflügers Arch 1978; 377: 95–99

199. Eknoyan G, Suki WN, Martinez-Maldonado M. Effect of diuretics on urinary excretion of phosphate, calcium and magnesium in thyroparathyroidectomised dogs. J Lab Clin Med 1979; 76: 257–66

200. Brunette MG, Vigneault N, Carriere S. Micropuncture study of magnesium transport along the nephron in the young rat. Am J Physiol 1974; 227: 891–6

201. Parfitt & Frame, 1975.

202. Brodehl J, Krause A, Hoyer P. Assessment of maximal tubular phosphate reabsorption: comparison of direct measurement with the nomogram of Bijvoet. Pediatr Nephrol 1988; 2: 183–9

203. Tenenhouse HS, Werner A, Biber J, Ma S, Roy S, Murer H. Renal Na–phosphate cotransport in murine X-linked hypophosphataemic rickets. J Clin Invest 1994; 93: 671–3

204. Murer H, Biber J. Molecular mechanisms in renal phosphate reabsorption. Nephrol Dial Transplant 1995; 10: 1501–4

205. Agus ZS, Gardner LB, Beck LH, Goldberg M. Effects of parathyroid hormone on renal tubular reabsorption of calcium, sodium and phosphate. Am J Physiol 1973; 224: 1143–8

206. Pastoriza-Munoz E, Colindres RE, Lassiter WE, Lechene C. Effect of parathyroid hormone on phosphate reabsorption in rat distal convolution. Am J Physiol 1978; 235: F321–30

207. Muff R, Fischer JA, Biber J, Murer H. Parathyroid hormone receptors in control of proximal tubular function. Ann Rev Physiol 1992; 54: 67–79

208. Levi M, Lötscher M, Sorribas V. Cellular mechanisms of acute and chronic adaptation of rat renal P_i transporter to alterations in dietary P_i. Am J Physiol 1994; 267: F900–8

209. Gray RW, Omdahl JL, Ghazarian JG, DeLuca HF. 25-hydroxycholecalciferol-1-hydroxylase: subcellular location and properties. J Biol Chem 1972; 247: 7528–32

210. Brunette MG, Chan M, Ferriere C, Roberts KC. Site of 1,25 dihydroxyvitamin D_3 synthesis in the kidney. Nature 1978; 276: 287–9

211. De Luca HF, Schnoes HK. Metabolism and actions of vitamin D. Ann Rev Biochem 1976; 45: 631–66

212. De Luca HF, Schnoes HK. Vitamin D: recent advances. Ann Rev Biochem 1983; 52: 411–39

213. Stumpf WE, Sar M, Reid FA, Tanaka Y, DeLuca HF. Target cells for 1, 25-dihydroxyvitamin D. Science 1979; 206: 1188–90

214. Steele TH, Engle JE, Tanaka Y, *et al*. Phosphatemic action of 1,25-dihydroxyvitamin D_3. Am J Physiol 1975; 229: 489–95

215. Mehls O, Ritz E, Kreusser W, Krempien B. Renal osteodystrophy in uraemic children. Clin Endocrinol Metab 1980; 9: 151–76

216. Verney EB. The antidiuretic hormone and the factors which determine its release. Proc R Soc London, Series B 1947; 135: 25–106

217. Sladek CD, Knigge KM. Osmotic control of vasopressin release by rat hypothalamo-neurohypophyseal

explants in organ culture. Endocrinology 1977; 101: 1834–8

218. Gottschalk CW, Mylle M. Micropuncture study of the mammalian urinary concentrating mechanism: evidence for the countercurrent hypothesis. Am J Physiol 1959; 196: 927–36

219. Burg MB, Green N. Function of thick ascending limb of Henle's loop. Am J Physiol 1973c; 224: 659–68

220. Rocha AS, Kokko JP. Sodium chloride and water transport in the medullary thick ascending limb of Henle. J Clin Invest 1973; 52: 612–23

221. Jamison RL. Countercurrent systems. In: Thurau K (ed) Kidney and urinary tract physiology. London: Butterworths, Chapter 7, 1974; 199–245

222. Kuhn W, Ryffel K. Herstellung konzentrierte Losungen aus verdunnten durch blosse Membranewirkung: ein Modellversuch zur function der Niere. Hoppe-Seylers Zeitschrift fur Physiologische Chemie 1942; 276: 145–78

223. Wirz H, Hargitay B, Kuhn W. Lokalisation des Konzentrierungsprozesses in der Niere durch direkte Kryoskopie. Helv Physiol Pharmacol Acta 1951; 9: 196–207

224. Stephenson JL. Renal concentrating mechanism: introduction. Fed Proc 1983a; 42: 2377–8

225. Stephenson JL. The renal concentrating mechanism: fundamental theroretical concepts. Fed Proc 1983a; 42: 2386–91

226. Stephenson JL, Berliner RW. The renal concentrating mechanism: summary. Fed Proc 1983; 42: 2405

227. Kriz W. Structural organization of the renal medullary counterflow system. Fed Proc 1983; 42: 2379–85

228. Jamison RL. The renal concentrating mechanism: micropuncture studies of the renal medulla. Fed Proc 1983; 42: 2392–7

229. Marsh DJ. Computer simulation of renal countercurrent systems. Fed Proc 1983; 42: 2398–404

230. Levinsky NG, Berliner RW. The role of urea in the urinary concentrating mechanism. J Clin Invest 1959; 38: 741–8

231. Bray GA, Preston AS. Effect of urea on urine concentration in the rat. J Clin Invest 1961; 40: 1952–60

232. Stephenson JL. Concentration of urine in a central core model of the renal counterflow system. Kidney Int 1972; 2: 85–94

233. Kokko JP, Rector FC. Countercurrent multiplication system without active transport in inner medulla. Kidney Int 1972; 2: 214–23

234. Bonventre JV, Lechene CP. Renal medullary concentrating process: an integrative hypothesis. Am J Physiol 1980; 239: F578–88

235. du Vigneaud V. Hormones of the posterior pituitary gland: oxytocin and vasopressin. Harvey Lectures, 1954/55 Series 50: 1–26

236. Schrier RW, Bichet DG. Osmotic and non-osmotic control of vasopressin release and the pathogenesis of impaired water excretion in adrenal, thyroid and edematous disorders. J Lab Clin Med 1981; 98: 1–15

237. Berl T, Schrier RW. Water metabolism and the hypo-osmolar syndromes. In: Brenner BM, Stein JH (eds) Sodium and water homeostasis. Chapter 1. Churchill Livingstone, New York, 1978: 1–23

238. Dunn FL, Brennan TJ, Nelson AE, Robertson GL. The role of blood osmolality and volume in regulating vasopressin secretion in the rat. J Clin Invest 1973; 52: 3212–9

239. Knoers N, van den Ouweland AM, Dreesen J et al. Nephrogenic diabetes insipidus: identification of the genetic defect. Pediatr Nephrol 1993; 7: 685–8

240. Knoers N, van den Ouweland AM, Verdijk M, Monnens LA, van Oost BA. Inheritance of mutations in the V_2 receptor gene in thirteen families with nephrogenic diabetes insipidus. Kidney Int 1994; 46: 170–6

241. Deen PMT, Weghuis DO, Sinke RJ, et al. Assignment of the human gene for the water channel of renal collecting duct Aquaporin 2 (AQP2) to chromosome 12 region q12→q13. Cytogenet Cell Genet 1994; 66: 260–2

242. Sesake S, Fushimi K, Saito H. Cloning, characterization and chromosomal mapping of human aquaporin of collecting duct. J Clin Invest 1994; 93: 1250–6

Structure and function of the upper urinary tract in health and disease

4

J. M. Fitzpatrick and P. G. Horgan

The kidneys play a major role in regulating the physico-chemical status of the extracellular fluid bathing the cells of the body. Fluid and electrolyte homeostasis is maintained by the processes of glomerular filtration, selective tubular absorption, and tubular secretion. Additionally, the kidney displays important endo-crine activity and plays a prominent role in intermedi-ate metabolism. The basic physiological functions of the kidney are reviewed in the first part of this chap-ter, after which alterations in kidney function and physiology, resulting from obstruction of the urinary tract, prolonged hypotension and drug therapy are considered.

Basic anatomy and physiology

The kidneys, which are paired organs, are situated on either side of the vertebral column and lie on the pos-terior abdominal wall. The renal nerves, vessels and the renal pelvis – formed from the funnel-like dilata-tion of the upper ureter – pass through the hilum, which is located on the medial border of each kidney (Figure 4.1). Each kidney is composed of two macro-scopically distinct regions, as revealed by bisection, comprising the outer cortex, with its characteristic granular appearance, and the inner medulla. The latter is composed of a number of renal pyramids, the apices of which project into the major and minor calyces, which in turn drain into the renal pelvis. The pelvis is considered to be the first functional section of the ureter and plays no role in the formation of urine.

The basic unit of renal function is the nephron, the fine structure of which is illustrated in Figure 4.2; this comprises the glomerulus surrounded by Bowman's capsule, which drains into the proximal tubule. The latter is connected to the distal tubule via the loop of Henle, which consists of a descending and an ascend-ing limb. Urine formation starts at the glomerulus, where filtration occurs in a process that excludes plasma proteins and blood cells from the filtrate. The composition of the filtrate is further altered as it passes through the proximal convoluted tubule, loop of Henle and distal convoluted tubule, where tubular reabsorption and secretion occur before drainage into the collecting duct. Each of the two kidneys contains in the region of one million nephrons. Based on the cortical location of their glomeruli, three distinct nephron populations have been described and classi-fied as: (1) superficial, where the glomeruli are situated within 1 mm of the capsular surface of the kidney; (2) midcortical, where the glomeruli are located deeper within the cortex; and (3) juxtamedullary, where the glomeruli are located immediately above the corti-comedullary junction. The length of the loop of Henle provides the main distinguishing feature between each type of nephron, with the loops of the juxtamedullary nephrons being long, and often reach-ing the tips of the renal papillae, as opposed to those of the superficial nephrons which are short and only reach the outer medulla.

Within each kidney, the renal artery divides to form progressively smaller branches known as interlo-bar, arcuate and interlobular arteries (see Figure 4.1). As the interlobular arteries extend towards the surface

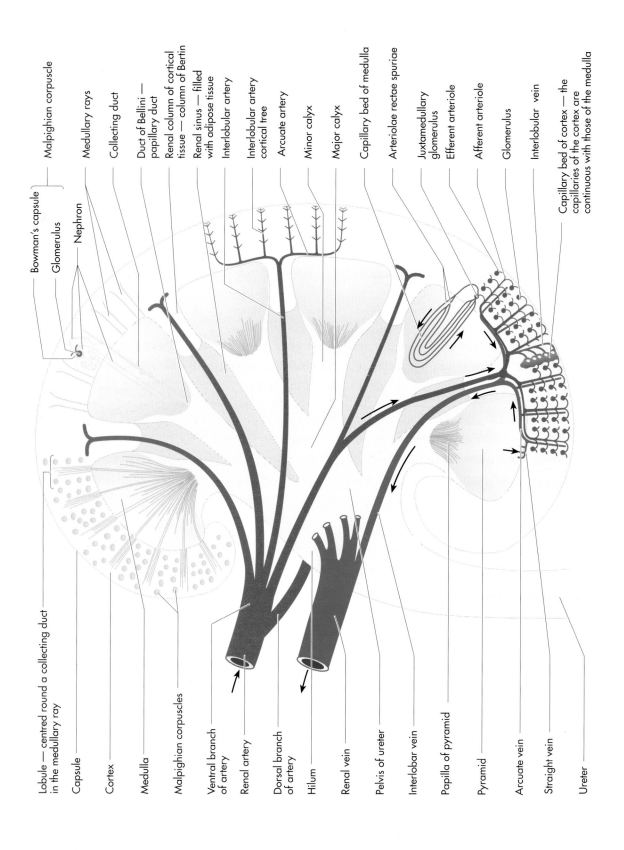

Bowman's capsule
Glomerulus
Nephron

Malpighian corpuscle

Medullary rays

Collecting duct

Duct of Bellini — papillary duct

Renal column of cortical tissue — column of Bertin

Renal sinus — filled with adipose tissue

Interlobular artery

Interlobular artery cortical tree

Arcuate artery

Minor calyx

Major calyx

Capillary bed of medulla

Arteriolae rectae spuriae

Juxtamedullary glomerulus

Efferent arteriole

Afferent arteriole

Glomerulus

Interlobular vein

Capillary bed of cortex — the capillaries of the cortex are continuous with those of the medulla

Lobule — centred round a collecting duct in the medullary ray

Capsule

Cortex

Medulla

Malpighian corpuscles

Ventral branch of artery

Renal artery

Dorsal branch of artery

Hilum

Renal vein

Pelvis of ureter

Interlobar vein

Papilla of pyramid

Pyramid

Arcuate vein

Straight vein

Ureter

Figure 4.1 *The structure and blood supply of the human kidney.*

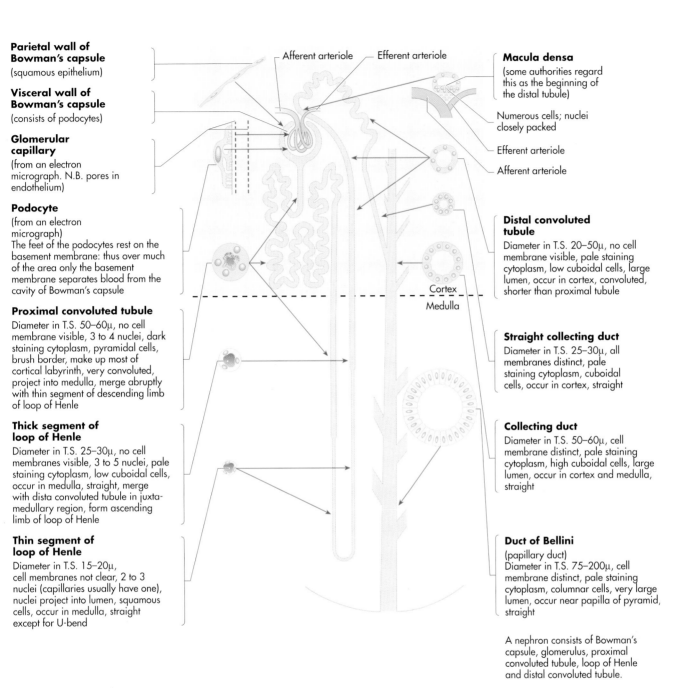

Parietal wall of Bowman's capsule
(squamous epithelium)

Visceral wall of Bowman's capsule
(consists of podocytes)

Glomerular capillary
(from an electron micrograph. N.B. pores in endothelium)

Podocyte
(from an electron micrograph)
The feet of the podocytes rest on the basement membrane: thus over much of the area only the basement membrane separates blood from the cavity of Bowman's capsule

Proximal convoluted tubule
Diameter in T.S. 50–60μ, no cell membrane visible, 3 to 4 nuclei, dark staining cytoplasm, pyramidal cells, brush border, make up most of cortical labyrinth, very convoluted, project into medulla, merge abruptly with thin segment of descending limb of loop of Henle

Thick segment of loop of Henle
Diameter in T.S. 25–30μ, no cell membranes visible, 3 to 5 nuclei, pale staining cytoplasm, low cuboidal cells, occur in medulla, straight, merge with dista convoluted tubule in juxta-medullary region, form ascending limb of loop of Henle

Thin segment of loop of Henle
Diameter in T.S. 15–20μ, cell membranes not clear, 2 to 3 nuclei (capillaries usually have one), nuclei project into lumen, squamous cells, occur in medulla, straight except for U-bend

Afferent arteriole   Efferent arteriole

Macula densa
(some authorities regard this as the beginning of the distal tubule)

Numerous cells; nuclei closely packed

Efferent arteriole

Afferent arteriole

Distal convoluted tubule
Diameter in T.S. 20–50μ, no cell membrane visible, pale staining cytoplasm, low cuboidal cells, large lumen, occur in cortex, convoluted, shorter than proximal tubule

Cortex
Medulla

Straight collecting duct
Diameter in T.S. 25–30μ, all membranes distinct, pale staining cytoplasm, cuboidal cells, occur in cortex, straight

Collecting duct
Diameter in T.S. 50–60μ, cell membrane distinct, pale staining cytoplasm, high cuboidal cells, large lumen, occur in cortex and medulla, straight

Duct of Bellini
(papillary duct)
Diameter in T.S. 75–200μ, cell membrane distinct, pale staining cytoplasm, columnar cells, very large lumen, occur near papilla of pyramid, straight

A nephron consists of Bowman's capsule, glomerulus, proximal convoluted tubule, loop of Henle and distal convoluted tubule.

Figure 4.2 *Diagram of a nephron.*

of the cortex, afferent arterioles, which supply the nephron, are given off at right angles. An efferent arteriole emerges from the glomerulus, and peritubular capillaries arising from the subdivision of this arteriole enmesh the tubules of a neighbouring nephron. Venous channels, through which blood leaves the kidney, are formed from the reunion of these capillaries.

Glomerular filtration

The complex microvascular structure forming the renal glomerulus is made up from endothelial, epithelial and mesangial elements. The glomerulus is composed of a vascular bundle of capillaries projecting into the concavity of Bowman's capsule, which forms the first part of the nephron. Bowman's space lies within the capsule and it is across the barrier between the vascular lumen and this space that the process of filtration occurs. The barrier making up Bowman's capsule is composed of three layers: capillary endothelium, basement membrane and a single-celled layer of epithelial cells (Figure 4.3).

Fenestrations of large aperture occur within the vascular endothelial layer, and a homogenous acellular network of glycoproteins and mucopolysaccharide forms the basement membrane on which lies the visceral epithelial layer of podocytes, which are distinct from the rest of Bowman's capsule. The bulk of the glomerulus is composed of mesangial and endothelial cells. Endothelial cells lining the glomerular capillaries perform an important role in the movement of macromolecules across the capillary layer. Synthesis of the basement membrane of the glomerulus involves roles played by both the endothelial and epithelial cells. Podocytes, which form the visceral wall of Bowman's capsule, consist of interdigitating foot-like processes between which filtration slits occur and through which ultrafiltrate passes into Bowman's space (see Figure 4.2). A thick layer of glycosialoproteins lines the foot processes of the podocytes and adversely affects free filtrate flow; thin diaphragms bridging the filtration slits, lying between the foot processes of the podocytes at the level of the basement membrane, further impede this flow. The mesangial cells, which have contractile properties, are predominantly located at the glomerular stalk.

Filtration of fluid from capillary lumen to capsular space is controlled by the same forces as those described by Starling in 1899 for fluid movements in other capillaries. The barrier between capillary lumen and capsular space is not permeable to colloids but is freely permeable to crystalloids. Inulin (molecular weight <6 kDa) passes freely into the nephron, whereas albumin, which is a relatively small (7 kDa), anionic molecule, is almost totally excluded. The electrolyte concentration of fluid in Bowman's space is almost identical to that of plasma but the fluid contains only small concentrations (50 mg/l or less) of albumin, approximating to 100 times less than that found in plasma. Molecules of less than 7 kDa pass unhindered across the barrier, but larger molecules are excluded by a sieving process, performed initially by the endothelial fenestrae and then by the hydrated spaces between the glycoprotein chains of the basement membrane. Macromolecules that do reach the podocytes are prevented from passing into the capsular space by the glycosialoprotein coating of the foot processes and the diaphragms bridging the filtration slits.

The three parts making up the glomerular barrier – endothelial cells of the glomerular capillary, glomerular basement membrane, and epithelial cells of Bowman's capsule – are composed of fixed polyanions; these have a tendency to repel negatively charged ions, thus preventing their permeation across the membranes. This electrical barrier represents another limiting factor, regarding protein diffusion into the capsular space, because most proteins carry a net

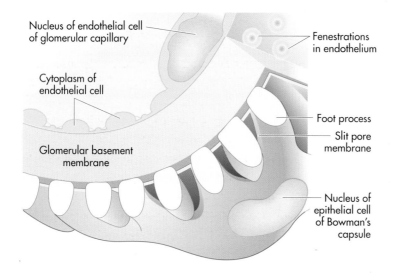

Nucleus of endothelial cell of glomerular capillary

Fenestrations in endothelium

Cytoplasm of endothelial cell

Foot process

Slit pore membrane

Glomerular basement membrane

Nucleus of epithelial cell of Bowman's capsule

Figure 4.3 *Structure of the glomerular filter. (Reproduced with permission from Blandy J. Lecture notes on urology, fourth edition. Oxford: Blackwell Scientific Publications, 1991: 37.)*

negative charge. In addition to the influence of molecule size, the shape of molecules also affects the ease, or otherwise, with which they pass across the glomerular barrier. The net filtration pressure (NFP) – defined as the net forces favouring ultrafiltration – is determined by the difference between the forces aiding filtration (transcapillary hydraulic pressure) and the difference between the forces that oppose filtration (colloid osmotic pressures), as indicated in Table 4.1 and demonstrated in the equation below:

$$NFP = (P_{GC} + O_{BC}) \; - \; (P_{BC} + O_{GC}) \qquad (1)$$

where P_{GC} = glomerular hydraulic pressure, O_{BC} = oncotic pressure of fluid in Bowman's capsule, P_{BC} = hydraulic pressure in Bowman's capsule, O_{GC} = oncotic pressure of plasma in capillary.

Because there is an insufficient quantity of protein in Bowman's space to contribute appreciably to oncotic pressure, the above equation can be amended as follows:

$$NFP = P_{GC} \; - \; P_{BC} \; - \; O_{GC} \qquad (2)$$

The evolution of experimental techniques has enabled the evaluation of nanolitre samples of fluid obtained from the glomeruli of experimental animals, using micropuncture techniques, and has provided a means of measuring pressures in individual nephrons directly. In a widely available strain of Wistar rat, possessing glomeruli on the renal cortical surface, direct measurements of glomerular capillary pressure have been successfully made and found to be 40% lower than aortic pressure.

Moving from the afferent to the efferent end of the

Table 4.1 Glomerular filtration rate

Average GFR in men = 125 ml/min per 1.732 m^2
Lower in women
Falls by 10 ml/min per decade after age 40
Increased in pregnancy
Dependent on the hydraulic pressure difference between
  glomerulus and tubule
Ultrafiltration forces
  Hydrostatic pressure (Bowman's capsule, glomerular
    capillary)
  Oncotic pressure (plasma, tubular fluid)
  Permeability and surface area of glomerular capillaries
Greater in juxtamedullary than in cortical nephrons

capillary vessel, hydraulic pressure gradually decreases due to the inherent resistance to flow along the capillary. Glomerular capillary oncotic pressure increases along the length of the capillary due to the glomerular barrier being relatively impermeable to plasma proteins, so resulting in an increased concentration of colloids as crystalloids are filtered. A combined increase in oncotic pressure and decrease in hydraulic capillary pressure can therefore result in net filtration ceasing. This phenomenon – known as filtration pressure equilibrium – may occur in humans in cases such as those following severe haemorrhage when glomerular capillary pressure is unusually low. In such circumstances, renal plasma flow is used as the major determinant of glomerular filtration rate (GFR).

Glomerular filtration rate is the rate at which filtration from the capillary into Bowman's space occurs. It is measured by determining the renal clearance of any substance freely filterable at the glomerulus but that is not secreted, metabolised or absorbed by the renal tubules. Each day, the average healthy man filters 180 l into Bowman's capsule, or 125 ml/min per 1.73 m^2 surface area (see Table 4.1). Permeability of the glomerular barrier, surface area available for filtration and the net filtration pressure all affect GFR. The permeability of glomerular vessels is far greater ($\times$ 10–100) than that of capillaries located elsewhere in the body and the process of filtration is facilitated by the large surface area resulting from the anatomical arrangement of the glomerulus.

The filtration coefficient (Kf) is defined as the product of surface area and hydraulic (water) permeability as described in the following equation:

$$GFR = Kf \; \times \; NFP \qquad (3)$$

Glomerular filtration rate is predictably affected by changes in any of the parameters in Equation 3 (Table 4.2).

Diseases of the glomerulus that reduce the available surface area for filtration alter the filtration coefficient. Hypertension, acute renal failure, obstructive uropathy, glomerulonephritis and experimental nephrotoxicity are examples of diseases that reduce available surface area in this way. Vasoactive substances have been reported to stimulate the mesangial cells of the glomerulus to reduce surface area and in

Table 4.2 Summary of influences on glomerular filtration rate

Parameters affecting GFR GFR = Kf × (P_{GC} − P_{BC} − O_{GC})		Changes to GFR
Kf	Increase	Increase
	Decrease	Decrease
P_{GC}	Afferent constriction Efferent dilatation	} Decrease
	Afferent dilatation Efferent constriction	} Increase
P_{BC}	Tubular/distal obstruction	Decrease
O_{GC}	Increase systemic oncotic Decrease pressure/plasma flow	} Decrease

so doing reducing GFR. In laboratory studies, it has been confirmed that the filtration coefficient is unaffected by changes in renal plasma flow and that it stays constant even when renal plasma flow is doubled.

Glomerular capillary hydraulic pressure is the most physiologically sensitive of the variables contributing to the net filtration pressure. Glomerular filtration rate tends to decrease in response to an increase in afferent arteriolar resistance; conversely, filtration is increased by any reduction in inflow resistance. Upstream pressure and glomerular filtration rate are increased by constriction of the efferent arteriole, whereas a reduction in GFR tends to result from efferent vasodilatation. There is a predictable relationship between the afferent arteriolar plasma protein concentration (afferent oncotic pressure) and GFR in which the latter varies inversely with afferent oncotic pressure (as net filtration pressure is decreased by increased oncotic pressure). However, experimental evidence has indicated the situation is far more complex than it would first seem. The evidence suggests that an in-vivo fall in afferent oncotic pressure goes hand in hand with a fall in the filtration coefficient; this may be due to hormonal stimulation of glomerular mesangial cells. Among the variety of hormones having this stimulatory affect are antidiuretic hormone (vasopressin), angiotensin II and parathormone.

Obstruction of the tubular system distal to the glomerulus results in an increase in the pressure within Bowman's capsule. Such obstructions (e.g.

ureteric calculi) may occur within the kidney or in other areas of the urinary tract. As a result of the obstruction, there is a damming of urine, a raised pressure in Bowman's capsule, and subsequently a reduced GFR. Various substances (as shown in Table 4.3) are used as markers of renal clearance, the measurement of which is used to determine GFR. Glomerular filtration rate approximates clearance of the chosen substance if that substance is filtered at the glomerulus but is not secreted or absorbed in other segments of the nephron. The various methods used to measure GFR, with their advantages and disadvantages, are considered in Table 4.3.

Tubular function

The tubular system consists of a monolayer of epithelial cells lying on a basement membrane and stretches from the glomerulus to the calyx. Tight junctions interconnect the cells forming the tubule, with each named segment of the tubule being composed of cells with a different structure and function. The pars convoluta forms the first part of the proximal tubule and then gives way to the straight pars recta, which forms the latter part of the proximal tubule and merges with the loop of Henle. The loop of Henle leads to the short, intraglomerular macula densa, which then merges with the distal tubule. The quanity of a substance lost to the body is determined by the amount of that substance transported by the tubules. The following equation expresses the tubular transport of substance x (T_x):

$$T_x = GFR \times P_x - U_x V \qquad (4)$$

Where P_x = plasma concentration of x, U_x = urinary concentration of x, V = volume of urine per unit time.

With net absorption, the value of T_x is positive and with net secretion its value is negative. The reabsorptive capacity of the kidneys is maximal for substances such as glucose, and their secretory capacity is maximal for substances such as para-aminohippurate.

Tubular reabsorption

Hydraulic flow facilitates the transfer of fluids and electrolytes across the glomerular barrier. Because of the absence of filtration pores, and due to the lack of any effective hydraulic pressure, little transfer of this sort occurs in the tubule. Transport mechanisms facilitating tubular reabsorption are varied, and these are summarised in Table 4.4.

Table 4.3 Glomerular filtration rate measurement and renal clearance

Concept of renal clearance
  Clearance = GFR if:
  substance freely filterable
  not absorbed, secreted, metabolised, e.g. inulin
Inulin clearance
  Accurate; complex; little clinical utility
Endogenous creatinine clearance

$$C_{cr} = \frac{U_{cr} \times V}{P_{cr}}$$

  Overestimates GFR because creatinine filtered and secreted
  Drug interference, e.g. cimetidine, trimethoprim
  Overestimation greater at lower GFR levels
Radioisotope clearance
  ^{125}I-iothalamate
  Slight overestimate of GFR
Extraction factor
  Computerised calculation of decay of injected labelled DTPA
Exogenous creatinine clearance
  Creatinine clearance measured by following loading dose of creatinine
  Mainly an experimental technique

Table 4.4 Tubular reabsorption transport mechanisms

Facilitated diffusion

Diffusion

Primary active transport (ATPase dependent)

Secondary active transport (co-transport, e.g. glucose, sodium transport)

Endocytosis

Transcellular through luminal basolateral membranes

Paracellular across tight junctions

Simple diffusion

This mechanism requires no energy expenditure, nor does it involve membrane carriers. Simple diffusion depends upon membrane lipid solubility and occurs along downhill electrochemical gradients.

Simple facilitated diffusion

This process, which involves movement along downhill electrochemical gradients, is facilitated by membrane carrier proteins. The process is subject to competitive inhibition due to its having specificity and saturability.

Secondary active transport

In this mechanism, two substances bind to a common membrane carrier; one substance moves, by simple facilitated diffusion, in a downhill direction and in doing so releases sufficient energy to carry the second substance in an uphill manner against its electrochemical gradient.

Primary active transport

The direct splitting of ATP provides the energy required for this transport mechanism. A specific membrane carrier binds the substance and transports it against an uphill gradient.

Endocytosis

This is a form of primary transport in which ATP is split to provide the energy to facilitate the process. The substance being transported (usually macromolecules) is enveloped by the plasma membrane, which invaginates and wraps itself around the substance.

Most transport, with the exception of that of the minority of substances that are transported across the intercellular tight junctions, occurs through the luminal and basolateral membranes. Therefore, in order to reach the peritubular capillaries, a substance may utilise one of two distinct transport processes. In the case of sodium, passage across the luminal membrane is by way of simple facilitated diffusion; the sodium–potassium-dependent ATPase pump provides the energy required for the active transport of sodium across the basolateral membrane. In the final step of the transport process, sodium ions migrate from the interstitial fluid, by bulk flow along with

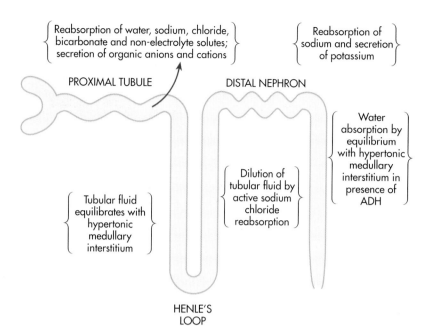

Figure 4.4 *Nephron with sites of major fluid and electrolyte transport functions. (Adapted from Webster G, Kirby K, King I et al. (eds) Reconstructive urology. Vol. 1. Boston: Blackwell Scientific Publications, 1993: 686.)*

water, into the peritubular capillaries. For all substances, this is the final step in the reabsorption process.

The greater part of sodium reabsorption (80%) takes place in the proximal tubules, 15% of reabsorption occurs in the ascending loop of Henle, and the remainder in the distal tubule by way of coupling to potassium (Figure 4.4). Reabsorption in the distal tubule is aldosterone dependent. The complex process of reabsorption in the proximal tubule is mediated by a variety of mechanisms including feedback control of the GFR by the macula densa, the putative existence of natriuretic hormone, and GFR variation with the state of the extracellular fluid. Amino acid absorption takes place by way of at least five distinct transport systems: (1) neutral, (2) dibasic, (3) dicarboxylic, (4) iminoglycine, and (5) beta. Cyclic 3'5'-AMP-mediated parathormone activity decreases phosphate reabsorption and enhances phosphate excretion. Reabsorption of chloride is a passive process linked with the active transport of sodium. The proximal tubule reabsorbs almost all filtered potassium. The process of pinocytosis facilitates the reabsorption of low molecular weight proteins.

Tubular secretion

As with the reabsorptive mechanisms, secretory processes in the tubular epithelium are categorised as being passive or active. For all substances, the first step in the secretory process involves passive simple diffusion across the peritubular capillary endothelium into the interstitial fluid. Simple diffusion through the tight junctions results in the subsequent passage of the substance in question into the tubular lumen; alternatively, subsequent passage occurs either passively or actively via the basolateral and luminal membranes, as described for reabsorption. Pre-existing electrochemical gradients are disrupted by the active carriage of substances into and out of cells, so allowing an element of back-diffusion. This back-diffusion element is variously termed a pump-leak or bidirectional transport system.

Complete removal of a substance from one compartment and into another by the transport mechanisms described above is rendered difficult by the pump-leak system, but in these terms the system is of more importance where leaky epithelia are concerned (good crystalloid permeability) than is the case with tight epithelia. As shown in Table 4.5, the tubules actively secrete a variety of substances, including cations, anions and drugs. Substances actively secreted in this way are usually of exogenous origin (e.g. drugs), slowly metabolised agents or poorly metabolised substances such as para-aminohippurate.

It should be remembered that in addition to the

Table 4.5 Substances secreted by tubules

Penicillin	Creatinine
Probenecid	Cimetidine
Trimethoprim	Procaine
Chlorothiazide	Acetylcholine
Frusemide (furosemide)	Dopamine
Hippurates	Histamine
Prostaglandins	Serotonin

described functions of the nephron, incorporating glomerular filtration, tubular reabsorption and secretion, the tubule also has its own metabolic requirements. To satisfy such requirements, the tubular cells may metabolise organic nutrients. Alternatively, the metabolites may be utilised to change the environment or composition of the urine or plasma, via the manufacture of bicarbonate and ammonia (Figure 4.5).

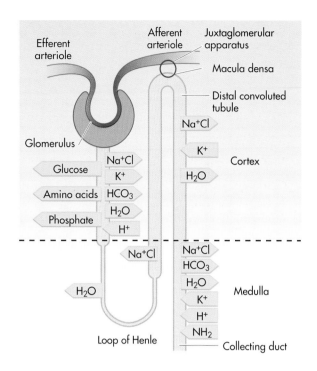

Figure 4.5 *Diagrammatic representation of the main sites for removal or addition of electrolytes and solutes from or to the tubular lumen. (Reproduced with permission from Webster G, Kirby K, King I et al. (eds) Reconstructive urology, Vol. 1. Boston: Blackwell Scientific Publications, 1991: 8.)*

Renal blood flow

The control of GFR and the regulation of the internal environment are optimised by the complex physiological mechanisms that operate within the unique organ of the kidney. Based on a total renal blood flow of 1100 ml/min, renal plasma flow is estimated to be 650 ml/min. Of this, 20% is filtered (125 ml/min) and the remainder leaves the glomerulus by way of the efferent arteriole (filtration fraction). Glomerular filtration rate is under the control of the sympathetic nervous system, autoregulation, the juxtaglomerular apparatus and prostaglandins. Internal blood flow is autoregulated by two intrarenal mechanisms: (1) the myogenic system, and (2) tubular glomerular feedback (Table 4.6).

Increased tension on the vessel smooth muscle wall, induced by afferent arteriolar blood pressure, results in reflex vasoconstriction and a subsequent increase in resistance to blood flow, together with a

Table 4.6 Renal absorption

Mechanisms
  Myogenic
  Tubuloglomerular feedback
  Metabolic
  Hormonal
  Renal sympathetic innervation

Sodium/water reabsorption
  Angiotensin II
  Aldosterone
  Atrial natriuretic factor
    28-amino-acid peptide
    Produced in atria
    Reduced sodium absorption

Renal sympathetic activity
  Rise in activity leads to sodium retention

Renin release
  Systemic baroreceptors
  Juxtaglomerular cells
  Macula densa

reduction of what would, in other circumstances, be an increased GFR. An augmented flow of water and filtered solutes through the macula densa is produced by the initial increase in GFR and this in turn activates the local release of vasoconstrictors, which raise afferent arteriolar resistance. Adenosine or angiotensin may cause these effects.

Arterial and venous baroreceptors are stimulated by decreases in systemic arterial blood pressure and volume; the consequence of such stimulation is an increase in sympathetic outflow. This, together with the release of adrenaline from the adrenal glands, constricts the afferent arterioles and in so doing reduces renal blood flow and GFR. However, in site of the overall drop in renal blood flow, the GFR is preserved due to the fact that the efferent arterioles are also constricted. The same net result may also occur as a consequence of the stimulation of the higher brain centres and peripheral chemoreceptors, which increase sympathetic drive. Recovery of total blood pressure is aided by a reduced GFR causing an increase in renal peripheral resistance and a reduction in salt and water excretion.

As shown in Table 4.6, juxtaglomerular influences are also an important regulator of blood flow.

Decreases in renal blood flow result in the release of renin, which catalyses the conversion of angiotensin to angiotensin I; the latter is then metabolised in the lungs to angiotensin II. The release of renin is achieved by: (1) internal baroreceptors located in the renin-secreting granular cells of the juxtaglomerular apparatus: these respond inversely to afferent arteriolar pressure, thus a reduction in pressure results in the induction of increased renin secretion; (2) a direct stimulatory effect of circulating adrenaline and of the sympathetic nervous system on renin secretion; (3) the fact that the concentrations of sodium and chloride ions in the macula densa cells and tubule have an inverse relationship with renin release by the granular cells, thus renin secretion is promoted by a low concentration of tubular sodium chloride and a low GFR; and (4) the influence of angiotensin II (negative feedback) on renin release. Negative feedback on renin secretion is exerted by calcium ions, potassium ions and vasopressin, otherwise known as antidiuretic hormone. The vasodilatory effects of the prostaglandins (E2 and I2) antagonise vasoconstrictor effects on the vasculature of the kidney; the synthesis and release of prostaglandins are induced by increased sympathetic drive or angiotensin II stimulation. The net effect of all the influences discussed above and summarised in Table 4.6 is to maintain a steady GFR when total renal blood flow is in a state of fluctuation.

Renal handling of sodium chloride and water

Transport of sodium from the tubular lumen into the cell occurs by facilitated downhill diffusion and from the cell into the capillary by way of the sodium chloride-dependent ATPase pump. Sodium moves on its own, by co-transport with amino acids and glucose, and by countertransport with hydrogen ions. Due to the influence of osmotic gradients, water and chloride follow passively. The above process is primarily dependent upon the permeability of membranes and tight junctions (Table 4.7).

Movement of chloride takes place in three ways: (1) along a concentration gradient produced secondary to the flow of sodium and water; (2) with the help of active sodium transport, along an electrochemical gradient from lumen to interstitial fluid; and

Table 4.7 Specialised functional segments of nephron

Proximal tubule
Reabsorption of water, sodium, chloride, bicarbonate, non-electrolyte solutes
Secretion of organic anions, cations
Thin limbs of Henle's loop
Water permeable
Tubular fluid equilibration with hypertonic medulla
Thick limbs of Henle's loop
Water impermeable
Dilution of tubular fluid by active sodium, chloride reabsorption
Distal nephron segments
Fine regulation volume, composition urine
Sodium, water reabsorption (antidiuretic hormone-dependent)
Potassium secretion

(3) by a secondary active process linked to primary active transport of sodium. The third process is the main means of chloride movement in the thick ascending loop of Henle.

Proximal tubule

The proximal tubule is the site in which the greatest proportion of sodium and water absorption (65% of that filtered) occurs. The concentration of sodium and the fluid osmolality are the same as those for plasma at the end of the proximal tubule. Reabsorption of filtered bicarbonate is driven by sodium countertransport with hydrogen ions. Reabsorption of bicarbonate couples with sodium reabsorption in the later part of the tubule. Sodium and water absorption is retarded in the presence of osmotic diuretics such as mannitol or glucose in diabetics.

Loop of Henle

The loop of Henle is the site at which a further 25% of filtered water and sodium is reabsorbed. Active sodium or chloride absorption does not occur in the thin descending or ascending limbs of the loop. Primary active sodium transport in the thick ascending limb of the loop gives rise to a tubular fluid having lower sodium concentration and osmolality relative to those of the plasma entering the distal tubule. The loop's ascending limb is impermeable to water, which is in distinct contrast to the case in the descending limb, which is highly permeable to water.

Distal tubule

In the distal tubule, the reabsorption of sodium chloride by active transport continues and, due to the tubule's low permeability to water, osmolality decreases still further. The influences of antidiuretic hormone on the luminal membrane affect water permeability in the terminal segments of the distal tubule. Antidiuretic hormone receptors located on the basolateral membrane interact with antidiuretic hormone, with the consequent activation of adenylate cyclase and the release of cyclic AMP. Prostaglandin synthesis is also induced by antidiuretic hormone and this opposes adenylate cyclase activation of intracellular cyclic AMP, so increasing luminal membrane permeability (negative feedback).

Urine concentration

The minimum obligatory water loss required to excrete wastes is 0.42 l/day and the maximum urine concentration attainable is 1400 mosmol/l. The countercurrent multiplier system located in the loop of Henle operates to achieve the concentration of urine. Although the descending limb of the loop of Henle does not actively absorb sodium chloride, it is freely permeable to water; the opposite is true for the thick ascending limb of the loop. As a result, fluid becomes progressively diluted in the ascending limb and progressively concentrated in the descending limb. At any horizontal level within the medulla there is a gradient of 200 mmol/l, whereas from the top of the medulla to the bottom of the medulla there is a variance of 300 to 700 mosmol/l. Under the influence of antidiuretic hormone, tubular fluid is progressively concentrated along this gradient as it flows along the collecting tubules.

Urea exerts an important influence in the concentration of urine. Both the outer medullary and cortical sections of the collecting tubules and the distal tubule are impermeable to urea, hence the luminal concentration of urea rises at these locations. Conversely, the permeability to urea of the inner medullary area allows diffusion of urea into the medullary interstitium, adding to the high osmolality and concentrating ability of the medulla. The loop of Henle's countercurrent multiplier function is complemented by the vasa recta's similarly looped configuration; this passively protects the osmalality gradient in the medulla. The loops of the vessel allow water to diffuse out of and sodium chloride to diffuse into the descending limb; in the ascending limb, the effects are opposite. This function is referred to as countercurrent exchange.

Renal control of extracellular volume

Plasma sodium concentration is the most important influence on extracellular volume. The difference between filtered sodium (GFR × plasma sodium) and the quantity of sodium reabsorbed is equivalent to sodium secretion. Although the main regulators of plasma sodium concentration are those factors responsible for the homeostatic control of extracellular volume, receptors that are sensitive to fluctuations in plasma sodium are located in the brain, adrenal cortex and kidney. A fall in extracellular volume is manifested by a reduced intravascular volume and pressure, the reflex restoration of which returns plasma sodium levels to normal. As already discussed, a decreased GFR results from a fall in systemic blood pressure and is corrected by autoregulation, sympathetic drive and angiotensin II, as summarised in Table 4.6. A reduction in the excretion of water and salt and the restoration of extracellular volume are the net effect.

Aldosterone

Sodium reabsorption in the distal tubule is promoted by aldosterone – a steroid hormone secreted by the zona glomerulosa of the adrenal cortex. Even though 90% of filtered sodium is absorbed proximal to the distal tubule, the role of aldosterone and its affect on the latter are important. Aldosterone exerts its action by binding to cell cytosolic receptors and moving into the nucleus, where it stimulates protein synthesis. As a result of this action, luminal membrane sodium permeability is increased, as is the activity of the sodium–potassium-dependent ATPase pump. Although aldosterone secretion is primarily controlled by angiotensin II, it is also influenced by plasma potassium and sodium concentrations as well as by endorphins, dopamine and adreno-corticotrophic hormone.

Natriuretic hormone

Natriuretic hormone, which is a 28-amino-acid peptide originating from the cardiac atrium, antagonises the sodium–potassium-dependent ATPase pump and reduces sodium reabsorption.

Interstitial hydraulic pressure

A direct relationship exists between interstitial hydraulic pressure and peritubular capillary pressure, one varying with the other. Increased back-leakage of water and sodium across tight junctions into the lumen of the tubule, with the consequent reduction in reabsorption, results from elevations in interstitial hydraulic pressure. Elevations in capillary oncotic pressure (induced by an increased filtration fraction) reduce interstitial hydraulic pressure and, by reducing back-leakage, favour the reabsorption of sodium and water.

It is thought that two distinct nephron populations with differing abilities to reabsorb sodium may exist. If this is the case, sodium excretion would be dramatically altered with the redistribution of blood to either population of nephrons. Angiotensin II and the catecholamines increase sodium reabsorption by their direct effects on the proximal tubule. Sodium reabsorption is also increased by insulin, cortisol, growth hormone and oestrogen, whereas parathormone, glucagon and progesterone all increase sodium excretion.

Antidiuretic hormone

Nerve endings located in the posterior pituitary, the cell bodies of which lie in the supra-optic and paraventricular ganglia of the hypothalamus, release antidiuretic hormone, which is an octapeptide. Decreases in atrial pressure result from a fall in systemic blood pressure which reflexly inhibits the tonic firing of baroreceptors. As a consequence, antidiuretic hormone is released from the posterior pituitary, causing vasoconstriction and so increasing peripheral resistance and restoring blood pressure. This action of antidiuretic hormone is in addition to its sodium-sparing effects in the kidney. The generation of angiotensin II also stimulates the release of the hormone. Another direct influence on antidiuretic hormone release is that of plasma osmolality, changes in which are detected by osmoreceptors located in the hypothalamus. Secretion can be altered by the thirst centre, alcohol, pain and fear.

Renal control of potassium

The flow of potassium across body cell membranes is regulated by the sodium–potassium ATPase pump. The pump is under the influence of aldosterone, adrenaline and insulin, all of which stimulate movement of potassium into cells. Potassium is freely filterable in the kidney, but less than 10% is excreted. It can either be secreted or absorbed by the tubules. Of filtered potassium, 50% is reabsorbed in the proximal tubule by the process of passive diffusion along the concentration gradient created by water absorption. Potassium is secreted along the length of the descending loop of Henle, but reabsorption occurs along the ascending limb of the loop. In the distal tubules, potassium is actively pumped through the basolateral membrane and into the tubular cells. As a result, potassium concentration is increased, with the consequent creation of a chemical gadient for flow into the lumen. Potassium-specific channels and weak pumping activity are present within the luminal membrane, thus enabling reabsorption of potassium into the cell. In response to elevations in plasma potassium, the adrenal cortex secretes aldosterone. This increases the activity of the basolateral ATPase pump, as well as increasing the number of pumps directly, with the net result being an increase in potassium secretion into the luminal fluid. The renin–angiotensin system is influenced by reductions in extracellular volume and produces the same effects by way of aldosterone secretion.

Acid–base influences on potassium secretion

Basolateral entry of potassium into tubular cells, with the consequent increase in potassium excretion, is stimulated in the presence of alkalosis. In some forms of acidosis, for the first 24 hours, the opposite effects to those just described are evident.

Renal handling of calcium

Bone, kidney and the gastrointestinal tract all play a role in controlling the homeostasis of calcium. Vitamin D exerts an influence on intestinal absorption and increases the uptake of dietary phosphate and calcium. Of the total body calcium, 99% is sequestered in bone and undergoes a constant flux of interchange with the extracellular fluid. Vitamin D facilitates the reabsorptive effects of parathormone and increases reabsorption of calcium from bone.

Plasma calcium that is unbound to protein (60%) is freely filtered at the glomerulus and thereafter is actively reabsorbed in all parts of the nephron other than the descending loop of Henle. Most of the calcium is reabsorbed proximally and is closely linked with the reabsorption of sodium. In the distal tubules, calcium absorption and sodium absorption are under the influence of parathormone and aldosterone, respectively. The total amount of calcium absorbed in the gastrointestinal tract is equivalent to the amount of calcium excreted (1–2%). Metabolic acidosis increases calcium excretion.

As plasma calcium concentration falls, parathormone is released from the parathyroid glands. The ensuing effects are threefold: (1) phosphate absorption and calcium absorption from the intestine are increased; (2) reabsorption of calcium by the tubules is increased and phosphate reabsorption reduced; and (3) bone and intestinal absorption of calcium and phosphate increases in response to the action of dihydroxycholecalciferol formed from the hydroxylation of vitamin D in the kidney. High plasma calcium concentrations stimulate the secretion of calcitonin from the parafollicular cells of the thyroid gland. Calcitonin inhibits bone reabsorption and in so doing decreases plasma calcium concentration. Intestinal absorption of calcium is depressed by cortisol and increased by growth hormone. Urinary excretion of calcium is also increased by growth hormone.

Acid–base balance

A pH range of 7.36–7.45 is maintained in the circulating blood of healthy individuals. The basic process of oxidative metabolism provides the principal supply of hydrogen ions, as shown in the equation below:

$$CO_2 + H_2O = H_2CO_3 = H^+ + HCO_3^-$$

Plasma hydrogen ion concentration is also increased by the formation of fixed acids such as sulphuric, lactic and phosphoric acid as well as by ketones. An important role is played by the kidney in acid–base balance. Extracellular (CO_2^+ and HCO_3^-) and intracellular (phosphates and proteins) mechanisms buffer acid–base changes extrarenally. The Henderson–Hasselbalch equation, reproduced below, outlines the key factors regulating hydrogen ions:

$$pH = 6.1 + \log HCO_3^- /0.03 Pa_{CO_2}$$

Therefore, the respiratory control of plasma carbon dioxide tension and the renal control of bicarbonate excretion are sufficient to achieve acid–base balance.

In situations of acidosis, maximum quantities of filtered bicarbonate are reabsorbed by the kidneys; additionally, the kidneys contribute still more bicarbonate to the plasma by secreting hydrogen ions into the tubular lumen. Filtered bicarbonate is excreted by the kidney when alkalosis prevails. Reabsorption of bicarbonate (which is freely filterable) in healthy subjects is by means of an active process. Because of the impermeability of the tubular luminal membranes to bicarbonate, relative to sodium chloride water, passive reabsorption is negligible. The absorption of bicarbonate by active means involves the secretion of hydrogen ions into the tubular fluid, where they join the filtered bicarbonate. Entry of carbon dioxide into the intracellular carbonic anhydrase pathway, with the generation of a molecule of bicarbonate to enter the plasma, is preceded by the formation of carbonic acid and its subsequent dissociation into carbon dioxide and water (Figure 4.6).

The secretion of hydrogen ions is achieved by countertransport with sodium (secondary active transport) and by the primary hydrogen ion ATPase pump located in the distal tubule. In cases of acidosis, more bicarbonate is synthesised by the nephron by tubular secretion of acid. In this circumstance, hydrogen ions bind to buffers in the lumen and are excreted; they are not, as would be the case in a healthy individual, reabsorbed as water. Ammonia and phosphates are the more important of the tubular buffers. Because phosphate undergoes 75% reabsorption, making less available for buffering, there are limitations to this form of buffering system. Ammonia is formed from the conversion of glutamine, in the tubular cell, by glutaminase and glutamic acid dehydrogenase. In circumstances of acidosis, this synthesis increases (adaptation of ammonia synthesis). Due to the lipid-soluble nature of non-ionised ammonia, it passes easily into the lumen along a concentration gradient. The binding of ammonia with secreted acid results in its conversion to ammonium, which is non-absorbable and thus easily excreted. Buffered acid is quantified in the urine as titratable acid.

Influences on tubular acid secretion

There is a directly proportional relationship between the rate of tubular acid secretion and glomerular filtration rate (by a glomerulo-tubular feedback system similar to that described for sodium). The relationship between the rate of tubular acid secretion and changes in plasma carbon dioxide tension, as detected by the tubular arteriole, is also direct. In cases of respiratory acidosis (e.g. pulmonary failure), an increased plasma carbon dioxide tension occurs which, by mass action in the tubular cell, results in tubular acid secretion, reabsorption of filtered bicarbonate, and synthesis of more bicarbonate with excretion of buffered acid. In the case of respiratory alkalosis, the opposite holds

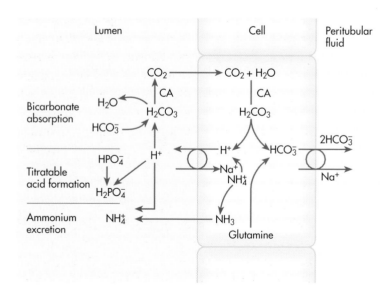

Figure 4.6 Mechanisms for the excretion of hydrogen ions. CA, carbonic anhydrase. (Reproduced with permission from Webster G, Kirby K, King I et al. (eds) Reconstructive urology, Vol. 1. Boston: Blackwell Scientific Publications, 1991: 11.)

true, there being a net excretion of filterable bicarbonate. Kidney compensation in metabolic acidosis (e.g. loss of bicarbonate or increased fixed acid production) is the same as that for respiratory acidosis; however, the stimulus is not an increased plasma carbon dioxide tension. Plasma bicarbonate increases, and the tubular cell easily reabsorbs all filtered bicarbonate; hydrogen ions are secreted for luminal buffering. This is the case even with a hydrogen ion secretion that is reduced overall (secondary to low pCO_2). The opposite situation is true in metabolic alkalosis.

The ability of the kidney to compensate for a metabolic alkalosis is reduced by salt depletion. This is due to a reflex increase in the reabsorption of sodium chloride by the tubule, with a consequent increase in hydrogen ion secretion, which then curtails the excretion of bicarbonate. By stimulating hydrogen ion secretion and sodium reabsorption, aldosterone causes the same effects as salt depletion. In the presence of potassium deficiency, this situation is compounded further. A reduction in plasma potassium concentration stimulates hydrogen ion secretion, decreases renal cell pH and worsens the alkalotic condition. Salt depletion can induce such an alkalosis in the absence of pre-existing acid–base disorders. The mineralocorticoid effects of cortisol can precipitate metabolic acidosis by the same mechanism as aldosterone.

Acute renal failure

Decreased GFR is the hallmark of acute renal failure. A reduction in renal blood flow with the diversion of the flow away from the afferent glomerular arteriole is the main cause of the reduced GFR seen in this situation. From a clinical point of view, in critically ill patients acute renal failure is manifest as a urine output of below 20 ml/hour (oliguria) (Table 4.8). Acute renal failure can be conveniently classified into three groups: (1) pre-renal, (2) renal or (3) postrenal failure (obstructive uropathy). Pre-renal failure, often progressing to acute tubular necrosis, and obstructive uropathy are the categories most often faced by urologists. Acute renal failure may also be classified by its aetiology: (1) vascular (major arteries, small vessels

Table 4.8 Biochemical changes in oliguria

	Pre-renal	Acute tubular necrosis
Plasma urea	Rises	Rises
Plasma creatinine	Rises	Rises
Urinary sodium	<20 mmol/l	>40 mmol/l
Urinary:plasma urea ratio	>10	<5
Urinary:plasma osmolality	>1.4	<1.1

or veins), (2) glomerulonephritic (post-streptococcal, systemic lupus erythematosus, antibody nephritis), (3) acute tubular necrosis, (4) interstitial nephritis (infection) and (5) obstructive uropathy.

Pre-renal azotaemia

The condition of pre-renal azotaemia, which is reversible, occurs when there is either a decrease in cardiac output (e.g. congestive cardiac failure or postmyocardial infarction) or a decrease in the effective extracellular volume (e.g. gastrointestinal obstruction, major burns or haemorrhagic shock). Three major changes in renal function are caused by the ensuing reduction in renal blood flow. The first of these changes is a reduction in salt and water excretion; the excretion of sodium is closely dependent (direct relationship) on changes in arterial blood pressure. The extrarenal hormones vasopressin (also known as antidiuretic hormone) and aldosterone also influence sodium handling by the nephron. In hypovolaemic states, the secretion of these hormones is increased. This results in further retention of sodium and water with a consequent reduction in urine flow and a decreased urinary sodium concentration (<20 mEq/l). These changes occur even before GFR is seen to decrease.

A reduction in the clearance of urea also occurs before GFR falls. Maximum tubular reabsorption of urea, with a consequent increase in plasma urea concentration, is allowed by the reduction of urine flow alluded to above. The increased plasma urea concentration may be further compounded by catabolism or absorption of partially digested blood from the gastrointestinal tract increasing urea formation. As a result, the use of plasma urea concentration as an indicator of renal function is of limited value. The deterioration in urine flow and composition is exaggerated by the time that GFR eventually falls below normal values. Urine flow is reduced in pre-renal failure and sodium; creatinine and urea are retained.

Acute tubular necrosis

The commonest cause of acute renal failure is acute tubular necrosis, which occurs following hypoxia, sepsis or exposure to nephrotoxic compounds. In the oliguric patient, an isotonic, acidic urine containing protein plus white cell and granular casts is secreted. In terms of morphology, extensive and patchy necrosis of the tubules is visible; intratubular casts are evident and there is leakage of tubular fluid.

The generation of angiotensin II and the generation of prostaglandin are two important vascular influences on the development of acute tubular necrosis. In the case of angiotensin II, vasoconstriction is induced and potassium filtration decreases. Although prostaglandin usually acts protectively via its vasodilatory effect, it also has a renin-releasing capability. In the experimental situation, glycerol-induced acute tubular necrosis is aggravated by the infusion of indomethacin – a prostaglandin synthetase inhibitor – whereas infusion of prostaglandin E2 has a protective effect.

Differentiating acute tubular necrosis from pre-renal failure

In seriously ill patients, the serial measurement of GFR is impractical, and diagnosis depends on the detection of changes in urinary and plasma osmolality and urea and creatinine levels. The latter are the most reliable as urea is often a superior indicator of catabolism than is renal function. It is seldom necessary to conduct complicated measurements involving fractional sodium excretion or free water clearance. The most useful factors in differentiating pre-renal failure from acute tubular necrosis in oliguric patients are summarised in Table 4.8.

Postrenal azotaemia

The effects of ureteric obstruction depend on whether the problem is unilateral (e.g. ureteric calculus) or bilateral (e.g. posterior urethral valves, prostatic hyperplasia). If obstruction is total, complete anuria in the affected kidney develops rapidly, but there may be no overall physiological changes. Characteristic renal changes occur as a result of partial obstruction and these are looked at further in the section on obstructive uropathy (see page 107).

Drug-induced renal disease

Disorders in renal function occurring as a result of adverse drug reactions are a common problem. Table 4.9 summarises drug-induced nephropathies, from which it can be seen that renal involvement in such adverse reactions may take the form of acute renal failure as a result of interstitial nephritis or acute tubular necrosis, transient fluid and electrolyte abnormalities, and chronic renal failure.

Acute interstitial nephritis

Often, acute interstitial nephritis is first seen as renal failure; it may be severe and oliguric. Drug-related causal agents implicated in this condition include

Table 4.9 Drug-induced nephropathies

Renal syndrome	Drugs
Acute interstitial nephritis	Methicillin, ampicillin, diuretics, non-steroidal anti-inflammatory drugs, allopurinol, phenytoin, cimetidine, sulphonamides
Acute tubular necrosis	Aminoglycosides, cisplatin, tetracycline, methoxyflurane, amphotericin B, cephalosporins, contrast agents used in radiology
Chronic renal failure	Analgesics: phenacetin, aspirin, acetaminophen, non-steroidal anti-inflammatory drugs (especially in combination); cyclosporin

beta-lactam antibiotics, diuretics, cimetidine, non-steroidal anti-inflammatory drugs, and allopurinol. The symptoms with which patients present are acute renal failure, joint pains, rash and pyrexia. Pathognomonic to acute interstitial nephritis is urinary eosinophilia, but pyuria, haematuria and proteinuria are often encountered. Renal biopsy is diagnostic of the condition. Gallium renal scanning reveals an increased uptake in acute interstitial nephritis but uptake is normal in acute tubular necrosis.

Acute tubular necrosis

Acute tubular necrosis implies direct toxicity to the epithelial cells of renal tubules. The aminoglycosides are especially recognised for their nephrotoxicity and their reputation in this respect is well earned. Of the aminoglycosides, gentamicin possesses the greatest potential for causing renal damage; it is followed by tobramycin, amikacin and then netilmicin. Serious harm occurs in less than 10% of patients. Initially, lysosomal and brush border enzymes are detectable in the urine; this is followed by proteinuria and impaired tubular function. The aminoglycosides exert their deleterious effects with regard to nephrotoxicity by altering phospholipids within the lysosomes of tubular cells and by causing cell necrosis. Intracellular binding of aminoglycosides may be limited by the administration of calcium supplements, which on this basis may be useful therapeutically. The use of cephalosporin antibiotics has been associated with renal toxicity and this has especially been the case with the use of cephaloridine. Synergism with aminoglycoside toxicity is possible. Non-oliguric renal failure due to vasoconstriction is induced by amphotericin B; this leads ultimately to tubular acidosis, concentrating defects, and loss of potassium. Avoidance of volume depletion during administration of this agent minimises these adverse effects.

Acute tubular necrosis with calcium and potassium wasting is induced by cisplatin and carboplatin; these are platinum-containing anticancer agents. These risks can be reduced by prehydration.

Paracetamol induces liver toxicity and acute tubular necrosis, but the clinical picture is usually dominated by the former. In a small proportion of patients, the ionic and more recently developed non-ionic contrast agents used in radiographic investigations cause acute tubular necrosis. However, the risk is estimated to be less than 10%. Aetiological factors associated with acute tubular necrosis include diabetes, liver failure, multiple myeloma (particularly with dehydration), volume depletion, renal insufficiency, heart failure, old age, and volume of contrast infused.

Chronic renal failure

Analgesic nephropathy is prone to develop in patients taking analgesics over extended periods of time. Renal insufficiency, sterile pyuria and impaired ability to concentrate are indicative of the condition. Induction of chronic recurrent papillary necrosis by medullary ischaemia and toxic metabolite injury result in the symptoms described above. Sloughed papillae are detectable in the urine; they may cause ureteral obstruction. Loss of vasodilatory prostaglandins with subsequent ischaemic damage results from the inhibition of renal prostaglandin synthetase by aspirin and non-steroidal anti-inflammatory drugs. Changes resulting from ischaemic damage can be imaged using ultrasound (small kidney and thinned cortex) or intravenous urography (ring sign). Progression to end-stage disease in some of these patients will make them candidates for transplantation. Patients with chronic renal failure also have an increased risk of developing transitional cell carcinomas of the upper urinary tract.

Obstructive uropathy

Obstruction of the urinary tract has diverse effects on renal function. Where the obstruction is gradual, which is often the case, the situation is reflected clinically by the development of chronic renal insufficiency. Acute renal failure accompanied by severe acidosis and hyperkalaemia occurs as a result of sudden and complete bilateral obstruction. Preservation of kidney function by preventing damage to the nephron, especially secondary to infection, is the main aim of investigation and treatment. Atrophy is one of the pathological signs associated with the obstructed kidney and, within seven days of obstruction, such atrophy commences in the distal nephron.

By day 14, atrophy can be seen to have spread to the cortical regions of the kidney, with eventual glomerular damage. Marked changes in renal blood flow and glomerular filtration rate are associated with obstructive uropathy. The distal nephron forms the major site of injury, the consequence of which manifests as an inability to concentrate urine; additionally, alterations in hydrogen ion secretion lead to acidosis. Hypertension and systemic electrolyte disorders may be consequences of alterations in tubular handling of electrolytes. The degree of completeness of urinary obstruction (obstruction may be unilateral or bilateral) and its duration determine its effects on renal function.

Sodium and water excretion

Where ureteric obstruction is unilateral, the absolute quantity of sodium excreted by the postreleased kidney is equivalent to that excreted by the contralateral, unobstructed kidney. This is in spite of the fact that in the obstructed kidney GFR is reduced overall to 10–20% of normal. Following relief of unilateral ureteral obstruction, postobstructive diuresis does not occur unless the contralateral kidney is missing or severely damaged.

After the release of bilateral ureteric obstruction, the situation is somewhat different, with dramatic increases in the absolute quantity of water and sodium in the excreted urine. A reduction in absolute and fractional sodium excretion, as a result of an increase in the tubular reabsorption of water and sodium, is associated with the increased ureteric, and hence intratubular, pressure that occurs in obstruction. Therefore, in itself, increased tubular pressure is not natriuretic and the postobstructive diuresis observed following chronic bilateral ureteric obstruction results from other factors. The period of anuria prior to the removal of the ureteric obstruction is important in the genesis of diuresis that occurs following the relief of urinary obstruction.

Single-nephron GFR falls following the release of ureteric obstruction. Although reabsorption is decreased or unchanged in bilateral obstruction, this is not the case in unilateral obstruction, in which reabsorption in the proximal distal tubules is increased. In all types of obstruction, reabsorption in juxtaglomerular proximal tubules is decreased. The ability of the thick ascending limb of the loop of Henle to reabsorb salt is inhibited in both unilateral and bilateral obstruction. The volume of fluid delivered to the distal tubules increases following the release of bilateral obstruction; in unilateral obstruction, the increase is relatively less. In unilateral obstruction, reabsorption increases in the distal tubules, whereas in bilateral obstruction it decreases.

In obstruction, a certain amount of reabsorption of the continuing, albeit reduced, volume of glomerular filtrate may be allowed by the opening up of pyelovenous and pyelolymphatic pathways. Ruptures have been identified in the pelvipapillary fornices; pelvicalyceal permeability is altered and there is leakage of urine into the systemic circulation. Additionally, leakage may occur into the interstitial spaces; systemic absorption may occur via the renal lymphatics and damaged capillaries. Renal lymph volume is approximately that of renal flow; in ureteral obstruction, renal lymph volume increases. Pyelocanicular and pyelosinus back-flow occurs in low-pressure obstruction. With higher pressures, there is urine flow into the venous and lymphatic systems.

Renal blood flow

A transient increase in renal blood flow occurs in complete ureteric obstruction (unilateral or bilateral) as a result of changes in preglomerular vascular resistance. The release of vasoactive hormones by the kidney contributes to these changes. A fall in renal blood flow to preobstruction levels follows its initial rise; preobstruction levels are reached within about four hours. Blood flow continues to fall for more than 24 hours, after which it stabilises at a lower level. At eight weeks following complete unilateral ureteric obstruction, the estimated renal blood flow is 12% below normal values.

In the canine experimental model, permanent focal arteriolar damage occurs after partial ureteric obstruction. These findings lend support to the view that postobstructive renal failure results from vascular injury. Renal blood flow and its intrarenal distribution normalise following the release of bilateral obstruction. In unilateral obstruction, blood flow following the removal of the obstruction remains low and is shunted primarily to the outer cortex of the kidney. This blood flow pattern contributes to the raised fractional reabsorption of salt and water by the proximal and distal tubules of the nephrons located in the outer cortex of the kidney.

Inhibition of the cyclo-oxygenase pathway reverses renal blood flow and renin secretion effects, implying that prostaglandins play a regulatory role. Renal blood flow is unaffected by adrenergic blockade. Increases in blood flow are also influenced by histamine, the involvement of which can be abrogated by H_1-receptor blockade. After the initial four hours of obstruction, increasing levels of thromboxane A_2 may mediate the vasoconstriction and reduced blood flow alluded to above. Atrial natriuretic protein may also be involved in the changes in renal blood flow that occur in obstruction.

Glomerular filtration rate

In ureteric obstruction, GFR falls but filtration does not cease completely. A fall in GFR is induced by a decrease in renal blood flow and an increase in intratubular pressure. Additionally, the ultrafiltration coefficient decreases, possibly due to renin release, thus reducing GFR further. Both in unilateral and in bilateral obstruction, there is an estimated fourfold to fivefold reduction of filtration rate. Release of the obstruction results in return of the GFR to about 50% of pre-obstruction levels.

Postobstructive diuresis

Raised volumes of filtrate arrive at the distal tubules and collecting ducts during partial ureteric obstruction and after the release of bilateral ureteric obstruction. Additionally, polyuria and increased urinary sodium result from the kidney's decreased ability to concentrate urine. Changes in renal blood flow patterns and increased fractional reabsorption by cortical nephrons, following the release of chronic unilateral ureteric obstruction, may reduce salt and water excretion.

Although these changes are not apparent in bilateral obstruction, a fivefold increase in salt and water excretion occurs in spite of a GFR that has been reduced by 80%. The accumulation of natriuretic factors during anuria may be contributory to postrelease

diuresis. A possible candidate is urea as it is known to have an osmotic diuretic effect. Postobstructive diuresis has been observed in humans in spite of normal plasma urea levels, suggesting that other natriuretic factors in addition to urea must be involved (Table 4.10).

Studies have demonstrated that the deterioration in function is greater and the time to recovery longer as the period of time over which the obstruction is present increases. The potential for a postrelease diuresis increases as the osmotic load from retained fluids and solutes increases and as the GFR increases. That is, the higher the GFR or osmotic load, the greater the potential for a postrelease diuresis.

During the recovery period, large volumes of electrolytes (particularly sodium) and water are lost. In extreme cases, the patient may become hypotensive. Systemic acidosis or hyperkalaemia may be induced by defects in urine acidification and potassium excretion. Hypomagnesaemia due to magnesium loss has also been reported.

Recovery of renal function

The kidneys' ability to recover functionally after the release of bilateral and unilateral ureteric obstruction is dependent upon two factors: (1) the severity of the renal injury, and (2) the presence of absence of infection. Renal deterioration is accelerated by supervening infection. The immediate intervention of a urologist is warranted in cases of infection to effect renal

Table 4.10 Postobstructive diuresis

Loss of salt, water after release
Bilateral ureteric obstruction or unilateral obstruction with contralateral nephrectomy/poor function
Associated with azotaemia
Causes
Elevated plasma urea
Atrial natriuretic factor
Damage to intrinsic reabsorptive distal tubular mechanisms
Treatment
Cautious replacement of fluids, electrolytes
Monitor serum electrolytes

drainage and establish aggressive antimicrobial therapy.

A shift from aerobic to anaerobic renal metabolism is a consequence of ureteral obstruction. The utilisation of fatty acids and alpha-ketoglutarate deteriorate significantly, and eventually there is a loss of renal gluconeogenesis. These changes are marked and possibly irreversible by six weeks postobstruction.

Due directly to an increase in renin secretion, acute ureteral obstruction may lead to hypertension. In chronic hydronephrosis, hypertension is secondary to expansion of extracellular fluid by sodium and water retention; it is independent of renin secretion.

Functional assessment of obstructive uropathy

Urinalysis may reveal macroscopic or microscopic haematuria in patients who have ureteric or renal calculi. Urinary infection secondary to stasis is signified by bacteriuria.

Polycythaemia may present as a consequence of urinary obstruction; this probably results from erythropoietin release. Depending on the degree of uraemia, haemoglobin levels may be decreased or normal. The diagnosis of infection is supported by a polymorphonuclear leucocytosis. Blood urea concentration rises disproportionately to creatinine levels in postrenal obstruction due to an increased reabsorption of urea in the obstructed tubules. The blood urea : creatinine ratio is not uncommonly above 15. Plasma phosphate and calcium levels fall in longstanding ureteric obstruction.

Opaque calculi may be revealed by plain films of the abdomen and an estimate of renal size may also be made from such plain films. Renal calculi are often difficult to identify in spite of the fact that over 95% are radiopaque. In view of this, the usefulness of plain radiographs is limited. Glomerular filtration alone is responsible for the excretion of contrast media such as Renografin, Hypaque and Miokon. A delay in the opacification of the parenchyma, by contrast in the tubules (nephrogram phase), and a decrease in kidney size occur in acute hydronephrosis. Where there is supervening infection and pyonephrosis develops, the intravenous urogram may show non-function or poor visualisation.

Obstructing ureteric calculi are demonstrated by retrograde catheterisation. Where obstructing ureteric calculi are present, renal pelvic drainage and a cessation of the deterioration of renal function may be accomplished by the placement of an indwelling stent. The presence of an obstructed urinary tract can be confirmed using renal ultrasound. Thinning of the renal cortex and hydronephrosis are easily visualised.

Useful information regarding retroperitoneal causes of obstruction or the presence of tumours can be obtained using magnetic resonance imaging and computerised tomography techniques. In some patients, the performance of antegrade perfusion pressure measurements (Whitaker test), by way of an indwelling nephrostomy tube, can provide additional information regarding the obstruction. The prolonged passage time of non-reabsorbable radiolabelled agents enables increased rates of salt and water reabsorption from obstructed tubules to be monitored directly. Using this technique, the individual contribution to overall renal function of the nephrons in each of the kidneys can be measured.

Conclusions

Glomerular filtration, selective tubular reabsorption, tubular secretion and tubular metabolism are the four fundamental renal functions maintaining the physiological balance of the body. Multiple extrarenal controls that fine-tune urine production are superimposed on this intrinsic regulatory function. These extrarenal controls include the cardiovascular regulatory systems, the parathyroid glands, the pituitary glands and the adrenal medulla and cortex. Renal failure is the end result of many disease states and is accompanied by a rise in serum creatinine and urea concentrations, acidosis, anuria and hyperkalaemia. It is the clinician's responsibility to recognise and treat these disorders at a stage at which they can be reversed (prerenal failure); progression to established tubular necrosis must be prevented. The task of preventing such progression is made more difficult by the widespread employment of potentially nephrotoxic drugs.

A condition increasingly seen by urologists is that

of renal obstruction; this reflects the ageing population. The effects of partial versus complete obstruction or unilateral versus bilateral obstruction are now predictable and reproducible. Rapid deterioration of renal function can result from superinfection in the obstructed renal tract. The development of post-obstructive diuresis is predictable, so enabling the initiation of appropriate therapeutic intervention.

Further knowledge on renal function is accrued every year and an understanding of renal function is required for the management of renal disease. The urologist should be aware of the most recent advances in the understanding of renal function both in health and disease.

Further reading

Berry CA. Heterogeneity of tubular transport processes in the nephron. Ann Rev Physiol 1982; 44: 181

Brenner BM, Humes HD. Mechanics of glomerular ultra-filtration. N Engl J Med 1977; 297: 148

Gottshalk CW, Lassiter WE. Micropuncture methodology. In: Orloff J, Berliner RW (eds) Handbook of renal physiology. Washington DC: American Physiological Society, 1973: 129

Kassirer JP. Clinical evaluation of kidney function: glomerular function. N Engl J Med 1971; 285: 385

Kincaid-Smith P. Analgesic abuse and the kidney. Kidney Int 1980; 17: 250

Kokko JP, Rector FC Jr. Countercurrent multiplication system without active transport in inner medulla. Kidney Int 1972; 2: 214

Laragh JH. Atrial natriuretic hormone, the renin–aldosterone axis and blood pressure–electrolyte hemostasis. N Engl J Med 1985; 313: 1330

Leahy AI, Ryan PC, McEntee GM, Nelson AC, Fitzpatrick JM. Renal injury and recovery in partial ureteric obstruction. J Urol 1989; 147(7): 199

Levey AS. Measurement of renal function in chronic renal disease. Kidney Int 1990; 38: 167

McDougal WS. Pathophysiology of glomerular dysfunction following ureteral obstruction. Dialogues in Pediatr Urol 1990; 13(6): 7

Porter GA, Bennett WM. Nephrotoxic acute renal failure due to common drugs. Am J Physiol 1981; 241: F1

Vaughan ED Jr, Gillenwater JY. Diagnosis, characteristics and management of postobstructive diuresis. J Urol 1973; 109: 286

Upper urinary tract obstruction

5

L. S. Young, N. J. Hegarty and J. M. Fitzpatrick

Introduction

Ureteric obstruction causes pressure and blood flow changes that damage the kidney and interfere with its functions of excretion and homeostasis. Obstructive uropathy occurs as a result of numerous disease processes. Early recognition and treatment are important in preserving renal function. A greater understanding of the pathophysiological changes as well as a review of current strategies help us to define diagnostic and therapeutic instruments for optimal management of this disease.

Aetiology

Ureteric obstruction can arise from disease of the ureter, the retroperitoneum or the abdomen or as ureteric involvement in systemic disease. Obstruction can be acute or chronic, partial or complete, constant or intermittent.

Congenital causes of obstruction (Table 5.1)

Intraluminal
Absence or atresia of the ureter is associated with severe renal dysplasia. Bilateral involvement results in Potter's syndrome and is incompatible with life. Persistence of fetal folds is frequently seen in premature infants, but generally resolves with growth. Congenital strictures occur most commonly in the area of the vesico-ureteric junction and may be the result of scarring following reflux in the fetus. They present in a

Table 5.1 Congenital upper tract obstruction

Intraluminal	Extraluminal
PUJ obstruction	Ureterocoele
Ureteric atresia	Ectopic
Ureteric valve	Orthotopic
Ureteric folds	Bladder diverticulum
Congenital stricture	Vascular
Vesico-ureteric reflux	Retrocaval ureter
Primary mega-ureter	Retroiliac ureter
	Lower pole renal vessels
	Persistent umbilical artery
	?Gonadal vessels

similar manner to primary mega-ureter. Primary mega-ureter classically refers to functional obstruction of the distal ureter, but differentiation from stenotic obstruction can be difficult. The term has been more broadly applied to describe other forms of ureteric enlargement, which are classified as obstructed mega-ureter, reflux mega-ureter and non-reflux–non-obstructed mega-ureter.

Extraluminal
Ureterocoele and bladder diverticula can cause obstruction of the distal ureter or bladder outflow. Retrocaval ureter usually causes incomplete obstruction. Treatment by dismembered pyeloplasty bringing the ureter anterior to the inferior vena cava is usually possible if obstruction is significant. Occasionally, when there is extensive renal atrophy, nephrectomy is performed. Gonadal vessels often create an indent on the ureter on intravenous pyelography, but are unlikely to cause obstruction.

Acquired causes of obstruction (Table 5.2)

Intraluminal

Ureteric calculi are the commonest intraluminal obstruction. Obstruction secondary to transitional cell carcinoma or benign polyp is more gradual in onset. Clot from haemorrhage can also cause acute obstruction, but more sinister causes of haematuria need to be ruled out. Sloughed papillae can also present acutely. Their soft consistency allows them to be readily removed ureteroscopically. Obstruction with metallic stents is associated with epithelial hyperplasia, ingrowth of tumour, the creation of an adynamic ureteric segment or kinking of the ureter (see below).

Extraluminal

Dilatation in pregnancy is most commonly due to hormonal dilatory effects, but compression by the gravid uterus can occur. Aneurysmal disease of the aorta or iliac vessels can cause ureteric obstruction. Insertion of a nephrostomy tube greatly increases the risk of graft infection, and other means of relieving obstruction should initially be considered. Primary retroperitoneal tumours or direct or lymphatic spread from pelvic tumours can involve the ureters unilaterally or bilaterally. Idiopathic retroperitoneal fibrosis typically involves the middle portion of the ureter, and obstruction can also result from the extension of intra-abdominal inflammatory processes.

Table 5.2 Acquired upper tract obstruction

Intraluminal	Extraluminal
Calculus	Malignancy
Stricture	Pelvic: prostate, colorectal,
Urothelial tumour	ovarian, uterine, cervical
Blood clot	Retroperitoneal: lymphoma,
Sloughed papilla	sarcoma, mesothelioma,
Benign polyp	secondary
Fungal ball	Gastrointestinal
Foreign body (stent)	Pancreatitis, appendicitis,
	diverticulitis, Crohn's disease
	Vascular
	Abdominal aortic aneurysm,
	iliac artery aneurysm
	Pregnancy
	Gynaecological
	Fibroids, endometriosis
	Retroperitoneal fibrosis
	Idiopathic, secondary

Renal function

Glomerular function is altered following obstructive uropathy, depending on the severity and duration of the obstruction and whether the obstruction is unilateral or bilateral. The glomerular filtration rate of single nephrons is determined by the glomerular blood flow rate, the net ultrafiltration pressure and the ultrafiltration coefficient. Whole kidney glomerular filtration rate is determined by the proportion of glomeruli actually receiving blood flow and filtering as well as by the filtration rate of functional glomeruli.

There is a triphasic relationship between ipsilateral blood flow and ureteral pressure. The initial response is an increase in renal blood flow and ureteral pressure, suggesting preglomerular vasodilatation. The initial vasodilatation is transient and lasts for up to 90 minutes. The second phase of the response occurs between 90 minutes and five hours, when renal blood flow is decreased and ureteral pressure continues to rise. During the third and chronic stage (5–18 hours), both renal blood flow and ureteral pressure decrease. Measurement of ureteral and regional blood flow under pathophysiological conditions has proved difficult using conventional methods. Advances in imaging and analytical technology, however, enables study of flow in precisely defined anatomical locations [1, 2].

Acute ureteric obstruction

Acute unilateral obstruction

Pressure changes (Table 5.3)

Following obstruction, the hydrostatic pressure of fluid proximal to the obstruction is elevated. Increasing proximal tubular pressure occurring due to obstruction, together with raised tubular and capsular hydrostatic pressures result in a lowering of net effective filtration pressure.

Ureteral pressure increases to between 50 and 70 mmHg within a few minutes of obstruction [3].

Table 5.3 Triphasic pressure – blood flow response in the obstructed kidney following the onset of unilateral ureteric obstruction

	Time	Collecting system pressure	Renal blood flow
Phase I	0–90 mins	⇑	⇑
Phase II	90 mins–4 hrs	⇔ (Remains elevated)	⇓ (To below control)
Phase III	4–18 hrs	⇓ (To resting)	⇓ (Continued decrease)

This raised pressure can be further elevated during diuresis [4].

Glomerular filtration rate and blood flow

In the first two to three hours following the onset of obstruction, the lack of antegrade urine flow results in striking increases in proximal tubule hydraulic pressure. This pressure increase transmitted back to the Bowman's space would be expected to decrease the glomerular filtration rate [5–7]; however, increases in the glomerular capillary pressure (PCG) during the early phase of obstruction results in a relative preservation of glomerular filtration rate [7]. A greater reduction is seen, however, during osmotic diuresis. Dilatation of the afferent arteriole resulting in reduced arteriolar resistance (RA) is responsible for the increase in PCG. Alterations in afferent arteriolar tone are thought to result from intrarenal mechanisms, as the hyperaemic response is observed in denervated as well as in isolated perfused kidneys [8, 9]. Neither catecholamines nor electrical stimulation reduce the increase in renal blood flow following obstruction [10]. Furthermore, increased pressure has also been demonstrated in individual nephrons when antegrade urine flow is retarded by the placement of wax blocks in the tubules [11].

There are several potential mechanisms responsible for afferent vasodilatation, including regulation by the macula densa, direct myogenic reflex, and increases in vasodilating hormones. Reduced urine flow passing the macula densa due to obstruction may induce the tubuloglomerular feedback mechanism, resulting in reduced arteriolar resistance and thereby increasing arteriolar blood flow and glomerular pressure [11]. Raised interstitial pressure resulting from obstruction reduces the transmural gradient in the afferent arteriolar wall, leading to reduced contractility of the smooth muscle cells of the vascular wall.

Vascular mediators are also known to modulate early rises in blood flow following obstruction. Prostaglandin synthesis inhibition has been shown to prevent early renal vasodilatation during unilateral obstruction [11]. Nitric oxide has also been demonstrated to be important in these renal haemodynamic changes [12]. During acute obstruction, the increase in blood flow and ureteral pressure abrogated by prostaglandin synthesis inhibition has been shown to be completely restored by the exogenous infusion of L-arginine. Nitric oxide production stimulated by ureteric obstruction is therefore capable of superseding the prostaglandin system in sustaining high renal blood flow and ureteral pressure [13].

Acute ureteric obstruction is associated with an increased secretion of angiotensin II. There is now substantial evidence to indicate that all of the components necessary for the local formation of angiotensin II exist in the kidney, and that they may operate, wholly or in part, independently of the circulating renin–angiotensin system [14]. It has been suggested that, in ureteric obstruction, a compensatory increase in renal blood flow to the contralateral kidney may be inhibited in part by an enhanced secretion of angiotensin II in the ipsilateral kidney [15].

Acute bilateral obstruction

The early haemodynamic response is absent or markedly attenuated during bilateral obstruction.

Studies of ureteral obstruction in the denervated kidney suggest a possible mechanism for this difference. Francisco *et al.* demonstrated that obstruction increased nerve trafficking to the contralateral kidney [16]. When either the obstructed or the non-obstructed kidney was denervated, the contralateral vasoconstrictor response to obstruction was abolished. This study suggests that, in bilateral obstruction, increased renal nerve activity may counteract the early vasodilatory effects of obstruction [16].

Chronic ureteric obstruction

Chronic unilateral obstruction

Pressure changes

Ureteral pressure decreases within 24 hours to about 50% [17]. Over the next six to eight weeks, ureteral pressure continues to decline despite the persistence of obstruction. Initially, proximal tubular pressure remains elevated, but declines to 30% of control values 24 hours following obstruction. Intratubular pressures are also decreased. Collapsed tubules are seen within the outer cortex, and glomerular pressure is reduced as a consequence of afferent arteriole constriction.

Glomerular filtration rate and blood flow

After three hours of unilateral obstruction, renal blood flow declines. On examination of regional blood flow, unperfused and underperfused areas of the cortex are evident. In the ipsilateral kidney, there is a shunting of flow from the outer to the inner cortical zone. A similar, if somewhat less marked, shunting of blood flow from outer to inner cortex is seen in the contralateral kidney [18]. A major reason for reduced whole kidney glomerular filtration rate is therefore the lack of perfusion of many of the glomeruli. Glomerular filtration rate of the single nephron is also decreased due to markedly reduced PCG owing to afferent vasoconstriction. These changes have been demonstrated in the individual nephron blocked with oil, indicating that the late vasoconstrictive response, like the early hyperaemic phase, is due to intrarenal blood flow [19, 20].

Both renal vasoconstrictive hormonal systems – the renin–angiotensin and the prostaglandin–throm-

boxane systems – have increased activity during ureteral obstruction. Inhibition of angiotensin II during chronic ureteral obstruction in rats results in significant preservation of both renal mass and function. Captopril, the angiotensin-converting enzyme inhibitor, has been shown to ameliorate the decline in renal blood flow and glomerular filtration rate observed in both unilateral and bilateral obstruction [21]. Though captopril can also act by increasing the levels of kinins, it is not via this pathway, but rather by reducing the generation of angiotensin II, that captopril reduces RA [22]. Angiotensin II has also been implicated as a mediator of mesangial cell contractility, thereby reducing the ultrafiltration coefficient in the chronically obstructed kidney [23].

Thromboxane A2 has also been implicated as a vasoconstrictor in chronic ureteric obstruction [23–25]. Inhibition of thromboxane A2 using both imidizol and the more specific, potent inhibitors UR-37248 and UK-38485 has been shown to reduce vasoconstriction and improve renal blood flow and glomerular filtration rate [26–28]. Thromboxane A2 may be responsible for altered vessel geometry following obstruction. Vessel elongation and decreased diameter account in part for increased vascular resistance.

The origin of thromboxane A2 remains undetermined. Inflammatory cells, predominantly macrophages and suppressor T cells that infiltrate the cortex and medulla following obstruction, may generate thromboxanes as well as other vasoconstrictors [29]. Schreiner *et al.* have demonstrated that irradiation of obstructed kidneys, markedly reducing the extent of cellular infiltration, results in a significant reduction in urinary thromboxane B2, increased glomerular filtration rate and renal blood flow, and an improvement of sodium and water excretion [30]. Obstruction therefore stimulates infiltration of inflammatory mononuclear cells that generate vasoconstrictors, among which is thromboxane A, contributing to an increase in RA in the obstructed kidney. Platelet activating factor has also been shown to release thromboxane B2 and prostaglandin E2, a potent inflammatory mediator; it is synthesised by mesangial cells of the glomerulus and by medullary interstitial cells [31]. Polymorphonuclear leucocytes infiltrating the kidney during disease processes [32], including obstruction, also synthesise platelet activating factor [33].

Thromboxane A2 generation by isolated glomeruli from obstructed kidneys has been demonstrated by some but not all investigators [29, 34, 35]. Thromboxane from this source may mediate changes in the ultrafiltration coefficient, but it is unlikely to play a major role in alterations in RA as the afferent arteriole is upstream from the glomerulus [36].

Renal vasodilatation during the early phase of obstruction may augment renal vascular production of endothelin-1, a potent vasoconstrictor, thereby contributing to the subsequent decline in renal blood flow. Increased renal release of endothelin-1 in chronic obstruction in dogs has been demonstrated, and the renal vasoconstriction that persists after the relief of obstruction is reversed by the calcium channel blocker verapamil, resulting in a marked increase in renal blood flow and in glomerular filtration rate [37]. Further studies may elucidate whether calcium channel blockers could offer long-term therapeutic benefits in the treatment of obstruction.

There are a number of vasodilatory factors that may ameliorate the vasoconstrictive effects of obstruction, including atrial natriuretic peptide, arachidonic derivatives such as prostaglandin E2, and nitric oxide. Atrial natriuretic peptide increases renal blood flow and glomerular filtration rate, through vasodilatation of the afferent arteriole, constriction of the efferent arteriole and increasing the ultrafiltration coefficient. Atrial natriuretic peptide also reduces renin release by the macula densa, thereby reducing circulating angiotensin II [38]. Prostaglandin E2, and nitric oxide may also ameliorate chronic obstructive constriction.

Chronic bilateral obstruction
As with the acute phase of ureteric obstruction, there are distinct differences in the haemodynamic responses of the obstructed kidney in the presence of unilateral and bilateral obstruction. There is a reduction in vasoconstriction observed in bilateral obstruction that is likely to be mediated by extrarenal pathways and influenced to some extent by inter-renal communication. It has been demonstrated that during 24 hours' obstruction, glomerular filtration rate was preserved somewhat if the contralateral kidney was either obstructed or removed [39]. Several factors have been identified as possible mediators, including the nervous system. The accumulation of urea, atrial natriuretic peptide, urodilatin and other natriuretic substances also tends to ameliorate the effects of obstructive vasoconstriction on the glomerular filtration rate in bilateral obstruction. Atrial natriuretic peptide levels increase in bilateral but not in unilateral obstruction, and is a major factor in the reduction of the vasoconstrictive effect of obstruction [38, 40]. Atrial natriuretic peptide is stimulated by volume expansion resulting from obstruction. It is this increase in atrial natriuretic peptide release as well as a reduction in its degradation that contribute to the known increase in plasma atrial natriuretic peptide levels in animals and patients with bilateral ureteric obstruction.

The interplay between intrarenal and extrarenal factors results in dramatic decreases in glomerular filtration rate during and immediately following chronic ureteric obstruction. Decreased glomerular filtration rate resulting from a decrease in the number of functioning glomeruli is caused by a reduction and redistribution of renal blood flow. Reductions in the glomerular filtration rate of single nephrons are brought about by increased RA and increased ultrafiltration coefficient. Augmented angiotensin II activity and release of thromboxane A2, in part by inflammatory cells, contribute to these perfusion defects. In bilateral obstruction, retention of natriuretic substances and increases in plasma levels of atrial natriuretic peptide offset the vasoconstrictive influences to some degree.

Pathophysiology

Pathology

In the first few weeks following ureteric obstruction, the renal pelvis dilates. There is an increase in mean kidney weight owing to oedema, despite renal atrophy. After several weeks, atrophy of the kidney is greater than intrarenal oedema, and the weight decreases. The kidney becomes dark in appearance due to discrete areas of ischaemia, red blood cell swelling and necrosis.

Thickening of glomerular basement membrane and obliteration of filtration slits occur as early as 30 hours following ureteric obstruction [41]. During the first few days, there is dilatation of the proximal and distal tubules. By two weeks, atrophy and necrosis of the epithelial cells of the tubules can be observed. By four weeks following obstruction, the medulla is reduced to half its normal mass, the cortex is also significantly reduced, with the parenchymal strip consisting primarily of connective tissue and small, irregular glomeruli [42].

Obstruction has been noted to damage the polar regions of the kidney initially [43]. The openings of Bellini's ducts into the papilla have been shown to be more dilated and gaping than in the midportion, which may account for the earlier and greater transmission of back pressure to the polar tubules.

Proliferation of medullary interstitial cells, which are thought to secrete prostaglandins, has been observed during the first week of obstruction [44]. In experimental animals, proliferation of interstitial fibroblasts and infiltration of macrophages and T lymphocytes have been demonstrated. These infiltrating cells are thought to be responsible for the increased release of thromboxane A2 and prostaglandin E2. The influx of inflammatory cells begins at four hours and peaks at 12 hours [45]. Using histochemical techniques, the loss of the normal high alkaline phosphatase content of the proximal tubules has been shown five days following following total obstruction in rats [46].

A fundamental aspect of the pathogenesis of chronic ureteric obstruction is the complex changes in the renal cell phenotype and the loss of tissue mass, reflecting an imbalance between cell proliferation and cell death in the obstructed kidney. These changes may potentially represent an important avenue through which many pathogenic factors of obstruction proceed, yet the cellular process in various compartments of the kidney with obstruction remains poorly understood. Truong et al. employed an in-situ end-labelling technique and several antibodies with specificity for proliferating cells to study the frequency of cell apoptosis and cell proliferation in rat kidneys with ureteric obstruction [47]. Their data suggested that tubular cell apoptosis may be pathologi-

cally related to the tubular atrophy and renal tissue loss characteristic of chronic obstruction, and that proliferation and apoptosis of interstitial cells may play a role in the observed interstitial cell damage in this model.

Increased cell proliferation following long-term ureteric obstruction is evidenced by significant increases in proliferating cell nuclear antigen-positive nuclei during obstruction. During renal injury and recovery, numerous growth factors and cell cycle-related genes are expressed. p53 is associated with cell proliferation, DNA repair, maintaining DNA integrity and regulation of apoptosis. In addition, p53 expression regulates inductive processes that increase the levels of two other proteins that also control cell replication, wild-type p53 activated fragment 1 (p21) and growth-arrested DNA damage 45 (GADD45). During chronic obstruction, p53 and p21 genes, but not GADD45, have been shown to be activated [48]. Inhibition of the angiotensin system reduces p53 and p21 expression; this is thought to be due, at least in part, to an inhibition of interstitial cell proliferation.

Ricardo et al. delineated the time course of the intercellular adhesion molecule, ICAM-1, and the vascular adhesion molecule, VCAM-1, mRNA and protein expression following obstruction [49]. Adhesion molecules are thought to play a role in macrophage recruitment following the mechanical disturbance following obstruction. ICAM-1 has been demonstrated to be important in the initiation of macrophage recruitment into the renal cortex of the obstructed kidney. Angiotensin II has been implicated in the induction of fibrosis following ureteric obstruction.

Transforming growth factor (TGF-β1) is a potential mediator of tubulointerstitial fibrosis in the rat following obstruction. Decorin is a protein composed of a core protein and a chondroitin sulphate side-chain, and is capable of inactivating TGF-β1. Elevations of decorin mRNA and protein have been reported in the cortex of the ipsilateral, but not the contralateral, kidney in parallel with active TGF-β1, following ureteric obstruction [50]. TGF-β1 has also been implicated in the development of kidney pathology following fetal obstruction [51].

Tubular injury in unilateral ureteric obstruction

has been associated with rapid gene activation in both the obstructed and the contralateral kidney. Increased activity in the testosterone-repressed prostate message (*TRPM-2*) gene, which is associated with apoptosis, has been demonstrated [42]. Examination of the nucleotide sequence of this gene reveals that it is equivalent to clusterin, a dimeric glycoprotein. Clusterin gene products have been detected in the collecting ducts and distal tubules following 24 hours of unilateral obstruction and are linked with loss of renal function. Obstruction is also thought to cause reverse filtration of the Tamm–Horsfall protein across the Bowman's capsule [52]. The protein is present only in the urinary tract, and approximately 50 mg per day is synthesised in the ascending limb of the loop of Henle and the distal convoluted tubules. Detection of Tamm–Horsfall protein within Bowman's space and increased activity of clusterin may prove to be important clinical markers in the detection of obstructive injury.

The lymphatic system

Obstruction of the ureter is followed by dilatation of the efferent renal lymphatics (Figure 5.1). Renal lymphatic drainage is through both hilar and capsular lymphatics. Normal lymph flow is similar to that of urine output; however, during obstruction this flow is increased [53], which is thought to be as a result of raised intrarenal venous pressure [54].

The preservation of renal function following obstruction is due to pyelolymphatic backflow. Reabsorption of renal pelvis urine into the lymphatics allows replacement glomerular filtration to occur, and penetration of urine into the interstitial spaces induces liberation of histamine, with the resultant increase in capillary permeability. Ligation of the lymphatics in the presence of obstruction produces severe renal damage, with necrosis and destruction seen in several days instead of several months [55].

Tubular function (Table 5.4)

Tubular reabsorption of sodium

Excretion by the postobstructed kidney has been found to be normal or mildly elevated. Given that the glomerular filtration rate is significantly reduced, the excretion of normal urine volume implicates an increase in free sodium excretion. It has been shown that, between the loop of Henle and the beginning of the papillary collecting duct, there is diminished net reabsorption of salt and water [56]. There is a striking impairment of volume reabsorption in the proximal

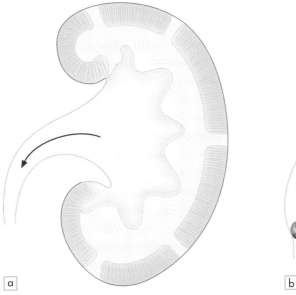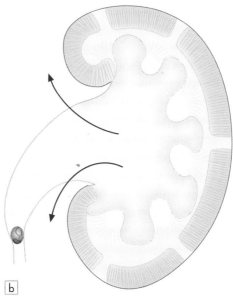

Figure 5.1 *Dilation of perirenal lymphatics allows urine output to be maintained, while lowering collecting system pressure in the obstructed kidney. (a) Anterograde flow of urine in unobstructed kidney; (b) obstructed kidney with dilated collecting system and pyelolymphatic backflow of urine.*

Table 5.4 Effects of ureteric obstruction on tubular function

	Sodium reabsorption	Potassium excretion	Urine acidification and concentration
Unilateral	⇓	⇓	⇓
Bilateral	⇓	⇑	⇓⇓

straight tubule, the medullary thick ascending limb, the cortical collecting duct and the inner medullary collecting duct. Despite the lack of major ultrastructural damage, the cellular mechanisms of active transport are impaired in obstructive nephropathy [57, 58]. Both unilateral obstruction and bilateral obstruction result in an identical decrease in function, implicating tubule cell injury rather than the continuous action of natriuretic substances as the cause of defective active transport.

There is a selective down-regulation of transporter activity and levels of expression of transporter proteins after 24 hours of obstruction. There would also appear to be a down-regulation of the metabolic machinery in response to a decrease in active transport. The disruption of urine flow, increased interstitial pressure, alterations in blood flow to the tubules and the generation of natriuretic substances in the kidney may all be avenues by which obstruction down-regulates transporter activity. Intrarenal hormones have also been implicated in these processes. As mentioned previously, obstruction markedly increases medullary levels of prostaglandin E2, which are thought to inhibit sodium reabsorbtion by reducing Na^+, K^+-ATPase [59–61].

Excretion of potassium

In unilateral obstruction, potassium excretion is reduced approximately in proportion to the fall in the glomerular filtration rate [62]. Following bilateral obstruction, however, potassium excretion is markedly increased, in parallel with the increase in sodium excretion. Studies have shown that proximal potassium reabsoption is normal, but that additional potassium is added to the urine in the collecting duct, due to increased distal delivery of sodium and volume post-obstruction [63].

Urine concentration and acidification

Urine osmolarity following obstruction approaches that of plasma, denoting a reduced capacity to concentrate and dilute the urine. This defect results from a reduction in the ability of the medullary thick ascending limb to remove solute without water from the urine and a failure of the collecting duct to increase water permeability in response to antidiuretic hormone and cyclic adenosine monophosphate [64, 65].

Obstruction also results in a significant impairment of urine acidification, though release of obstruction is not accompanied by bicarbonaturia, indicating a relative preservation of proximal tubule biacarbonate reabsorption. There is, however, a reduced ability to lower urine pH in response to acid loading, suggesting a defect in the ability of the distal nephron to acidify the urine after relief of the obstruction [66, 67]. In addition to defects in distal nephron acid transport, reduced ammoniagenesis in the proximal tubule has also been shown to contribute to reduced acid excretion in obstruction. A reduced capacity to generate ammonia from glutamine at several steps along the pathway, including decreased glutamine uptake and oxidation, reduced generation of glucose and ammonia and reduced oxygen consumption, has been demonstrated [68, 69].

Investigation and treatment

Location of the obstruction dictates the most appropriate choice of treatment. The degree of obstruction, the presence of infection and the premorbid renal function determine the urgency for intervention. Advances in understanding of physiological processes allow the development of novel investigative and therapeutic tools. The search for an accurate, non-invasive means for the detection of ureteric obstruction has focused attention on the renal resistive index [70–72] The renal resistive index has been developed as an adjunct to ultrasound to aid in the differentiation of obstructive from non-obstructive upper tract dilatation. It is defined as:

$$\text{Renal resistive index} = \frac{(\text{peak systolic velocity} - \text{lowest diastolic velocity})}{\text{peak systolic velocity}}$$

using Doppler ultrasonography to measure the velocity of renal artery blood flow. It appears to be of particular use in patients with complete obstruction and is less sensitive in those with partial obstruction [71]. As the resistive index is dependent on blood flow measurement, the series of blood flow changes occurring in early ureteric obstruction and following the administration of non-steroidal anti-inflammatory drugs or other analgesics will lead to inaccurate readings.

The Whitaker test is regarded by many as the gold standard for the diagnosis of obstruction. Percutaneous needle puncture of the renal pelvis allows direct measurement of intrapelvic pressure. Its invasive nature, however, generally limits its use to cases in which the results of other modalities are inconclusive, though it can be readily used in patients with a nephrostomy already in place.

All methods used to treat ureteric obstruction have inherent effects on renal physiology. Open renal surgery can result in nephron loss and impaired renal function. Bivalve, anatrophic intersegmental and serial radial nephrotomies lead to parenchymal distortion and up to 50% decrease in renal function. The extended sinus approach (development of the plane between the renal parenchyma and pelvis) is associated with little tissue or functional loss [73]. Similarly, percutaneous nephrostomy causes no detectable alteration in function [74]. Stone transit is dependent on hydrostatic pressure and ureteric motility. Nephrostomy insertion lessens the hydrostatic pressure but does not interfere with peristalsis, facilitating stone propulsion. Double J ureteric stents are associated with ureteric dilatation, diminished peristalsis and impaired stone passage [75]. Metal stents, used in the treatment of strictures in advanced malignancy, interfere with peristalsis in the portion of ureter they occupy, and it remains to be determined what ureteric length can be stented while still allowing peristalsis

[76]. Insertion in the distal ureter can lead to vesicoureteric reflux if the stent occupies the ureteral orifice, or kinking with resultant obstruction if placed just promimal to the intramural ureter [77].

Agents that have a relaxant effect on ureteric smooth muscle, such as phentolamine, glucagon and theophylline, may relieve renal colic and facilitate stone passage. Opiates have central analgesic action, but also affect ureteric motility. In-vitro studies have shown morphine to cause sustained ureteric spasm, whereas pethidine causes initial spasm, followed by relaxation, implicating it as a more suitable agent for the treatment of ureteric colic [78]. Similarly, non-steroidal anti-inflammatory drugs have a relaxant effect on the ureter in vitro [78], but also have a profound effect on renal blood flow, as discussed earlier.

Recovery of function after the relief of obstruction

The ability of the kidney to regain its functioning capacity depends to a large extent not only on the duration and the severity of the obstruction, but also on the presence or absence of a viable contralateral kidney. In an animal model of partial ureteric obstruction, relief of obstruction after four weeks did not restore the renal circulation to its preoperative profile [79]. In the same model, relief of obstruction did lead to significant improvement in glomerular filtration [80]. This difference may occur as a consequence of a divergence in the distribution pattern of renal blood flow and glomerular filtration following ureteric obstruction. The distribution of blood flow and glomerular filtration are significantly different following the release of complete obstruction, with perfusion being more markedly decreased in the outer cortex and filtration being most significantly impaired in the inner cortex [81, 82]. Thus, the relief of obstruction may lead to an improvement in filtration without restoration of intrarenal blood flow to its preoperative profile. Animals obstructed for one, two or three weeks have permanently decreased renal function, to approximately half, one-third and one-sixth of normal, respectively. If the angiotensin-converting enzyme inhibitor, captopril, is administered during the obstructive period, there is a decrease in loss of renal function to only 40% of control at one week, 50% at two weeks and 50% at three weeks. Bilateral obstruction or contralateral nephrectomy ameliorates the haemodynamic effect of obstruction [83]. This is likely to be due to the accumulation of solutes, urea and other vasodilatory substances such as atrial natriuretic peptide when the contralateral kidney is absent.

Conclusions

The response of the kidney to ureteric obstruction depends not only on the severity and duration of the obstruction, but also on the pre-existing renal function. There are defined changes that occur at both the vascular and cellular level. Understanding of these factors continues to evolve slowly, enabling the development of investigative and therapeutic tools for early diagnosis, treatment and prevention of renal injury associated with ureteric obstruction.

References

1. Mooney EF, Geraghty JG, O'Connell M, *et al*. Radiotracer measurement of ureteric blood flow. J Urol 1994; 152: 1022–4

2. Geraghty JG, Nsubuga M, Angerson W, *et al*. A study of regional distribution of renal blood flow using quantitative autoradiography. Am J Physiol 1992; 263: F958–62

3. Backlund L, Nordgren L. Pressure variations in the upper urinary tract and kidney at total ureteric occlusion. Acta Soc Med Ups 1966; 71: 285–301

4. Vaughan ED Jr, Shenasky JH, Gillenwater JY. Mechanism of acute haemodynamic response to ureteral occlusion. Invest Urol 1971; 9: 109–18

5. Canton AD, Stanziale R, Corradi A, Andreucci VE, Mignole L. Effects of acute ureteral obstruction on glomerular haemodynamics in rat kidney. Kidney Int 1977; 12: 403–11

6. Ichikawa I. Evidence for altered glomerular haemodynamics during acute nephron obstruction. Am J Physiol 1982; 242: F580–5

7. Gaudio KM, Siegel NJ, Hayslett JP, Kashgarian M. Renal perfusion and intratubular pressure during ureteral occlusion in the rat. Am J Physiol 1980; 238: F205–9

8. Navar LG, Baer PG. Renal autoregulatory and glomerular filtration responses to graduated ureteral obstruction. Nephron 1970; 7: 301–16

9. Schramm LP, Carlson DE. Inhibition of renal vasoconstriction by elevated ureteral pressure. Am J Physiol 1975; 228: 1126–33

10. Wright FS, Briggs JP. Feedback control of glomerular blood flow, pressure and filtration rate. Physiol Rev 1979; 59: 958–1006

11. Allen JT, Vaughan ED, Gillenwater JY. The effect of indomethacin on renal blood flow and ureteral pressure in unilateral ureteral obstruction in awake dogs. Invest Urol 1978; 15: 324–7

12. Lanzone J, Gulmi F, Chou S, Moopan U, Kim H. Renal haemodynamics in acute unilateral ureteral obstruction: contribution of endothelium-derived relaxing factor. J Urol 1995; 153: 2055–9

13. Shulsinger D, Gulmi F, Chou S-Y, Mooppan U, Kim H. Activation of the endothelium-derived relaxing factor system in acute unilateral ureteral obstruction. Abstract. J Urol 1997; 157: 1951

14. Ichikawa I, Harris RC. Angiotensin actions in the kidney: renewed insight into the old hormone. Kidney Int 1991; 40: 583–96

15. Frokiaer J, Djurhuus J, Neilsen M, Pedersen E. Renal haemodynamic response to ureteral obstruction during converting enzyme inhibition. Urol Res 1996; 24: 217–27

16. Francisco LL, Hoversten LG, DiBona GF. Renal nerves in the compensatory adaptation to ureteral occlusion. Am J Physiol 1980; 238: F229–34

17. Vaughan ED Jr, Sweet RE, Gillenwater JY. Mechanism of acute haemodynamic response to ureteral occlusion. Invest Urol 1971; 9: 109–18

18. Grace PA, Gillen P, Dowsett DJ, Fitzpatrick JM. Partial unilateral ureteric obstruction alters regional renal blood flow. World J Urol 1990; 8: 170–4

19. Harris RH, Yarger WE. Renal function after release of unilateral ureteral obstruction in rats. Am J Physiol 1974; 227: 806–15

20. Yarger WE, Griffith LD. Intrarenal haemodynamics following chronic unilateral ureteral obstruction in dogs. Am J Physiol 1974; 227: 816–26

21. Wahlberg J, Stenberg A, Wilson DR, Persson AE. Tubuloglomerular feedback and interstitial pressure in obstructive nephropathy. Kidney Int 1984; 26: 294–301

22. Yarger WE, Schocken DD, Harris RH. Obstructive nephropathy in the rat: possible roles for the renin–angiotensin system, prostaglandins and thromboxanes in postobstructive renal function. J Clin Invest 1980; 65: 400–12

23. Ichikawa I, Purkerson ML, Yates J, Klahr S. Dietary

protein intake conditions the degree of renal vasoconstriction in acute renal failure caused by ureteral obstruction. Am J Physiol 1985; 249: F54–61

24. Morrison AR, Benabe JE. Prostaglandins in vascular tone in experimental obstructive nephropathy. Kidney Int 1981; 19: 786–90

25. Sheehan SJ, Moran KT, Dowsett DJ, Fitzpatrick JM. Renal haemodynmics and prostaglandin synthesis in partial unilateral ureteric obstruction. Urol Res 1994; 22: 279–85

26. Purkerson ML, Klahr S. Prior inhibition of vasoconstrictors normalises GFR in postobstructed kidneys. Kidney Int 1989; 35: 1305–14

27. Loo MH, Egan D, Vaughan ED, Marion D, Felsen D, Weisman S. The effect of the thromboxane A$_2$ synthesis inhibitor OKY-046 on renal function in rabbits following release of unilateral ureteral obstruction. J Urol 1987; 137: 571–6

28. Klotman PE, Smith SR, Volpp BD, Coffman TM, Yarger WE. Thromboxane synthetase inhibition improves function of hydronephrotic rat kidneys. Am J Physiol 1986; 250: F282–7

29. Schlondorff D, Folkert VW. Prostaglandin synthesis in glomeruli from rats with unilateral ureteral obstruction. Adv Prostaglandin Thromboxane Res 1980; 7: 1177–9

30. Schreiner GF, Harris KPG, Purkerson ML, Klahr S. Immunological aspects of acute ureteral obstruction: immune cell infiltrate in the kidney. Kidney Int 1988; 34: 487–93

31. Weisman SM, Freund RM, Felsen D, Vaughan ED Jr. Differential effect of platelet activating factor (PAF) receptor antagonists on peptide and PAF-stimulated prostaglandin release in unilateral ureteral obstruction. Biochem Pharmacol 1988; 37: 2927–32

32. Bouchier Hayes DM, Young LS, Fitzpatrick JM. Role of the activated neutrophil and nitric oxide in ureteric obstruction. Surg Forum 1997; 83: 778–80

33. Schlondorff D, Neuwirth R. Platelet-activating factor and the kidney. Am J Physiol 1986; 251: F1–11

34. Yanagisawa H, Morrissey J, Morrison AR, Klahr S. Eicosanoid production by isolated glomeruli of rats with unilateral ureteral ligation. Kidney Int 1990; 37: 1528–35

35. Folkert VW, Schlondorff S. Altered prostaglandin synthesis by glomeruli from rats with unilateral ureteral ligation. Am J Physiol 1981; 241: F289–99

36. Curhan GC, Zeidel ML. Urinary tract obstruction. In: Brenner BM and Rector FC (eds) The kidney. Philadelphia: WB Saunders, 1996: 1936–58

37. Khan S, Gulmi F, Chou S-Y, Moopan U, Kim H. Contribution of endothelin-1 to renal vasoconstriction in unilateral ureteral obstruction: reversal by verapamil. J Urol 1997; 157: 1957

38. Brenner BM, Ballermann BJ, Gunning ME, Zeidel ML. The diverse actions of atrial natriuretic factors in rat urine. Physiol Rev 1990; 70: 665–99

39. Harris RH, Yarger WE. The pathogenesis of postobstructive diuresis: the role of circulating natriuretic and diuretic factors, including urea. J Clin Invest 1975; 56: 880–7

40. Purkerson ML, Blaine EH, Stokes TJ, Klahr S. Role of atrial peptide in natriuresis and diuresis that follow relief of obstruction. Am J Physiol 1989; 256: F583–9

41. McDougal WS. Pathophysiology of glomerular dysfunction following ureteral obstruction. Diagnosis Pediatr Urol 1990; 13: 7–12

42. Gillenwater JY. The pathophysiology of urinary tract obstruction. In: Walsh PC, Retik AB, Stamey TA, Vaughan ED. (eds) Campbell's urology, 6th ed. Vol. 2. Philadelphia: WB Saunders, 1992: 499–532

43. Ransley PG, Risdon RA. Renal papillae and intrarenal reflux in the dog. Lancet 1974; 2: 1114

44. Sheehan HL, Davis JC. Experimental hydronephrosis. Arch Pathol 1959; 68: 185–93

45. Klahr S. Immunologic aspects of urinary tract obstruction. Dialogues Pediatr Urol 1990; 13(6): 3–9

46. Wilmer HA. The disappearance of phosphatase from the hydronephrotic kidney. J Exp Med 1943; 78: 225–30

47. Truong L, Petrusevska G, Yang G, et al. Cell apoptosis and proliferation in experimental chronic obstructive uropathy. Kidney Int 1996; 50: 200–7

48. Morrissey J, Ishidoya S, McCraken R, Klahr S. Control of p53 and p21 (WAF1) expression during unilateral ureteral obstruction. Kidney Int 1996; 57: S84–92

49. Ricardo SD, Levinson ME, DeJoseph MR, Diamond JR. Expression of adhesion molecules in rat renal cortex during experimental hydronephrosis. Kidney Int 1996; 50: 2001–10

50. Diamond JR, Levinson M, Kreisberg R, Ricardo D. Increased expression of decorin in experimental hydronephrosis. Kidney Int 1997; 51: 1133–9

51. Medjebeur A, Bussieres L, Gasser B, Gimonet V, Laborde K. Experimental bilateral urinary obstruction in foetal sheep: transforming growth factor β1 expression. Am J Physiol 1997; 273: F372–9

52. Dziukas LJ, Sterzel RB, Hodson CJ, Hoyer JR. Renal localisation of Tamm–Horsfall protein in unilateral

obstructive uropathy in rats. Lab Invest 1982; 47: 185–93

53. Sugarman J, Friedman M, Barret E, Addis T. The distribution, flow, protein and urea content of renal lymph. Am J Physiol 1942; 138: 108–17

54. Naber, KG, Madsen PO. Renal function in chronic hydronephrosis with and without infection and the role of lymphatics: an experimental study in dogs. Urol Res 1974; 2: 1–9

55. Rusznyak I, Foldi M, Szabo G. Lymphatics and lymph circulation. London: Pergamon Press, 1960

56. Sonnenberg H, Wilson DR. The role of the medullary collecting ducts in postobstructive diuresis. J Clin Invest 1976; 57: 1564–74

57. Hanley MJ, Davidson K. Isolated nephron segments from the rabbit models of obstructive nephropathy. J Clin Invest 1982; 69: 165–74

58. Campbell HT, Bello-Reuss E, Klahr S. Hydraulic water permeability and transepithelial voltage in the isolated perfused rabbit cortical collecting tubule following acute unilateral obstruction. J Clin Invest 1985; 75: 219–25

59. Lear S, Silva P, Kelley VE, Epstein FH. Prostaglandin E2 inhibits oxygen consumption in rabbit medullary thick ascending limb. Am J Physiol 1990; 258: F1372–8

60. Jabs K, Zeidel ML, Silva P. Prostaglandin E2 inhibits Na/K-ATPase in rabbit inner medullary collecting duct cells. Am J Physiol 1989; 257: F424–30

61. Stokes JB, Kokko JP. Inhibition of sodium transport by prostaglandin E2 across isolated perfused rabbit collecting tubule. J Clin Invest 1977; 59: 1099–104

62. Buerkert J, Martin D, Head M. Effect of acute ureteral obstruction on terminal collecting duct function in the weanling rat. Am J Physiol 1979; 236: F260–7

63. Buerkert J, Head M, Klar S. Effect of acute bilateral ureteral obstruction on deep nephron and terminal collecting duct function in the young rat. J Clin Invest 1977; 59: 1055–65

64. Zeidel ML, Strange K, Emma F, Harris HW Jr. Mechanisms and regulation of water transport in the kidney. Semin Nephrol 1993; 13: 155–67

65. Harris HW Jr, Strange K, Zeidel ML. Current understanding of the cellular biology and molecular structure of the antidiuretic hormone-stimulated water transport pathway. J Clin Invest 1991; 88: 1–8

66. Ribeiro C, Suki WN. Acidification in the medullary collecting duct following ureteral obstruction. Kidney Int 1986; 29: 1167–71

67. Laski ME, Kurtzman NA. Site of the acidification defect in the perfused postobstructed collecting tubule.

Miner Electrolyte Metab 1989; 15: 195–200

68. Blondin J, Purkerson ML, Rolf D, Schoolwerth AC, Klahr S. Renal function and metabolism after relief of unilateral ureteral obstruction. Proc Soc Exp Biol Med 1975; 150: 71–6

69. Klahr S, Schwab SJ, Stokes TJ. Metabolic adaptations of the nephron in renal disease. Kidney Int 1986; 29: 80–9

70. Shokeir A, Provoost A, Nijman R. Resistive index in obstructive uropathy. Br J Urol 1997; 80: 195–200

71. Cole T, Brock J, Pope J, Schrum F. Evaluation of renal resistive index, maximum velocity, and mean arterial flow velocity in a hydronephrotic partially obstructed pig model. Invest Radiol 1997; 32: 154–60

72. Shokeir A, Nijman R. Partial uretral obstruction: role of renal resistive index in stages of obstruction and release. Urology 1997; 49: 528–35

73. Fitzpatrick JM, Sleight MW, Braack A, Marberger M, Wickham JEA. Intrarenal access: effects on renal function and morphology. Br J Urol 1980; 52: 409–14

74. Horgan PG, Sarazen AA, Lennon GM, Fitzpatrick JM. The effect of stones on renal and ureteric physiology. World J Urol 1993; 11: 7–12

75. Lennon GM, Thornhill JA, Grainger R, McDermott TED, Butler MR. Double pigtail ureteric stent versus percutaneous nephrostomy: effects on stone transit and ureteric motility. Eur Urol 1997; 31: 24–9

76. Young LS, Hegarty NJ, Fitzpatrick JM. Obstructive uropathy. Curr Opin Urol 1998; 8/2: 119–24

77. Lugmayr HF, Pauer W. Wallstents for the treatment of extrinsic malignant ureteral obstruction: midterm results. Radiology 1996; 198: 105–8

78. Lennon GM, Bourke J, Ryan PC, Fitzpatrick JM. Pharmacological options for the treatment of acute ureteric colic. Br J Urol 1993; 71: 401–7

79. Leahy AH, Ryan PC, McEntee GM, Nelson AC, Fitzpatrick JM. Renal injury and recovery in partial ureteric obstruction. J Urol 1989; 142: 199–203

80. Harris RH, Yarger WE. Renal function after the release of unilateral ureteral obstruction in rats. Am J Physiol 1974; 227: 806–15

81. Yarger WE, Giffith LD. Intrarenal haemodynamics following chronic unilateral ureteral obstruction in the dog. Am J Physiol 1974; 227: 816–26

82. McDougal WS. Pharmacologic preservation of renal mass and function in obstructive uropathy. J Urol 1982; 28: 418–21

83. Prevoost AP, Molenaar JC. Renal function during and after a temporary complete unilateral ureter obstruction in rats. Invest Urol 1981; 18: 242–6

Interactive obstructive uropathy: observations and conclusions from studies on humans

6

N. J. R. George

It has been known for many years that dysfunctional abnormalities of the lower urinary tract may affect the performance of the upper urinary tract in several respects. Typical examples of such bladder dysfunction include those associated with benign prostatic hypertrophy and the changes that are observed after neurological damage to the spinal cord – the neuropathic bladder. It is recognised that the renal damage caused by such interaction between the lower and upper tract may be severe, silent and progressive, leading to terminal renal failure if the abnormalities are not recognised and corrected.

In this chapter, the basis of our physiological understanding of the mechanisms involved in the interactive urinary tract dysfunctional states is explored. Animal studies of such abnormalities have been few and far between, partially because of the difficulties with complex animal experimentation and partly because natural models of lower/upper tract dysfunction do not exist. This account therefore deals with neurologically normal human subjects found to have a particular form of bladder dysfunction (high-pressure chronic retention), which is particularly appropriate to demonstrate the physiological changes that occur synchronously within lower and upper tract. Naturally, all subjects gave informed consent for the procedures, which, being undertaken without any form of anaesthesia, benefited additionally from the ability of the patient to speak and comment throughout on the test procedures. Before describing the observations and discussing the conclusions of these studies, it is pertinent first to review the historical perspective relating to interactive dysfunction; such an appreciation explains previous misunderstandings and lays a more secure foundation for a rational understanding of the interactive disorder.

Historical perspective

In the 1840s, dissections by Guthrie in England and Civiale in France identified a number of abnormalities in the region of the bladder neck (Figure 6.1). Clearly visible in many cases were large lateral lobes of the prostate, with a bladder showing trabeculation and sacculation. However, in a number of cases, there was equivalent detrusor hypertrophy, trabeculation etc., but little to be seen in the way of prostatic hypertrophy, a thickened median bar at the bladder neck being the only possible source of obstruction (Figure 6.1b). A short while later, again in Paris at the Necker Hospital, Professor Guyon described a third type of dysfunctional bladder, which was essentially thin walled yet still associated with typical 'prostatic' symptoms. Guyon called this entity 'prostatisme vesicale'. At the time, the relationship between these three apparently discrete forms of bladder dysfunction was far from clear, and the situation was not assisted by the very high prevalence of lower urinary tract stones and infection (urgency, frequency, incontinence) in both middle-aged and older men.

However a hypothesis was formed, which, in the subsequent 70–100 years, became known as 'the three-stage theory of prostatism' (Figure 6.2). In this theory, the bladder first becomes trabeculated and hypertrophied because of outflow tract obstruction,

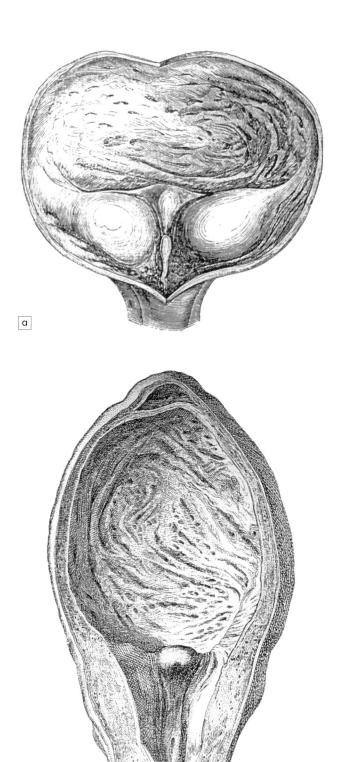

a

b

Figure 6.1 *Drawings of original dissections by early investigators.*

usually as a result of an easily palpable and enlarged prostate. As obstruction develops, sacculation and diverticulum formation take place and, with 'increased pressure', the ureters and subsequently the upper tracts dilate, leading to hydronephrosis and eventual renal failure. In the third phase of the classically described course of events, the bladder becomes decompensated – flaccid, large and overdistended. Overflow incontinence was said to occur.

'The three-stage theory of prostatism' was widely accepted in the latter part of the nineteenth century and first half of the twentieth century, and typical accounts are to be found in urological texts published as late as the 1980s. Examination of the theory, however, revealed inconsistencies that it was impossible to explain on a rational basis. In particular, it was not clear why a detrusor muscle which in stage two had developed hypertrophy, trabeculation and sacculation should suddenly give way into a thin-walled, atonic bag associated with overflow incontinence and upper tract hydronephrosis.

In fact, an explanation of this dilemma had been offered by some careful observational studies undertaken after the Second World War. In 1948, Badenoch studied 26 patients with bladder neck obstruction (similar to that in Figure 6.1b) whose mean age was 43, 16 of the patients being under 50 years. He noted no prostatic enlargement whatsoever in these cases, but made the highly significant observation that 25 of the 26 cases had diverticulum formation and bilateral hydroureter, with hydronephrosis in the majority. In 1951, Wallace complemented this study. He looked at the association between lateral lobe enlargement, median lobe enlargement, normal and dilated upper tracts. He found that 89% of cases with large prostatic lateral lobes had no upper tract dilatation, but that 72% of patients with bladder neck hypertrophy alone demonstrated clear hydronephrosis with hydroureter. These studies showed clearly that whereas upper tract dilatation was indeed related to obstruction, this relatively rarely involved the expected prostatic hypertrophy but was much more strongly correlated with pure bladder neck obstruction. These and other studies eventually led to the conclusion that the unifying 'three-stage theory of prostatism' was unlikely to be correct and that individual or discrete disorders of the

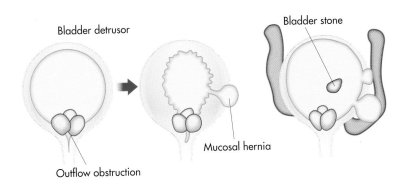

Bladder detrusor

Outflow obstruction

Mucosal hernia

Bladder stone

Figure 6.2 *The classically described 'three stage' theory of prostatism.*

lower urinary tract (i.e. bladder neck obstruction, primary atonic/thin-walled bladder) offered a more plausible explanation for the observed clinical symptom complexes. The particular group of patients with upper tract dilatation associated with bladder neck hypertrophy originally described and clarified by Badenoch was subsequently investigated in greater detail, and the advent of sophisticated urodynamic measuring equipment enabled precise recordings of this dysfunctional state – subsequently named high-pressure chronic retention – to be made for the first time. Simultaneous advances in uroradiology and nephrostomy placement, in particular, finally allowed for the possibility of sophisticated simultaneous urodynamic and radiological studies of both the upper and lower urinary tracts. This chapter therefore describes and illustrates the physiological interactive changes in both the lower and upper tracts, using records obtained by the author and colleagues from such studies on patients with uncomplicated (sterile urine) high-pressure chronic retention.

The micturition cycle

It is important to consider the bladder in terms of the micturition cycle. Traditionally, the words 'obstruction' and 'blockage' have been associated with difficulty in passing urine, and the idea of blockage has somehow become extended to the upper tracts – rather as in the 'three-stage theory of prostatism'. However, a moment's consideration of the micturition cycle (Figure 6.3) shows that the bladder spends very little time indeed on micturition and the vast percentage of its functional existence is spent in storage

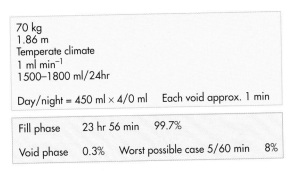

70 kg
1.86 m
Temperate climate
1 ml min^{-1}
1500–1800 ml/24hr

Day/night = 450 ml × 4/0 ml   Each void approx. 1 min

Fill phase	23 hr 56 min	99.7%	
Void phase	0.3%	Worst possible case 5/60 min	8%

Figure 6.3 *Volumes and events during the micturition cycle.*

mode. A normal, 70-kg adult will micturate four times in 24 hours, passing approximately 1500 ml of urine. Assuming that each micturition takes approximately one minute to complete, it is clear that the bladder is contracting for only 0.3% of 24 hours; more emphatically, the bladder is in storage phase for 23 hours 56 minutes of the day. Even in a case severe enough to spend five minutes micturating every hour, the bladder still spends 92% of its time in the filling phase.

These simple calculations show that if there is to be any effect of the lower tract on the upper tract, any abnormality thought to be responsible must act chiefly during the filling phase. An abnormality during the micturition phase – however severe – would not have sufficient time to act and lead to permanent change in the ureters or renal pelvis. Thus, the state of the bladder during filling is of critical importance to a concept of interactive urinary tract dysfunction and, in this respect, the mechanical and physical properties of the bladder wall (bladder compliance) require detailed consideration.

The bladder wall in high-pressure retention

The bladder wall in patients with high-pressure chronic retention is characteristically thick, with massive detrusor hypertrophy. Endoscopically, bars of trabecular muscle stand out, often described as a cathedral-roof appearance (Figure 6.4). Histological examination and analysis of sections taken from such trabecular bars (Figure 6.5) show degeneration of the smooth muscle bundles into collagen, as illustrated using the Masson trichrome stain. It is not difficult to imagine that the course of the ureter to the vesico-ureteric junction through the wall of such a bladder may well become obstructed. The normal co-apting process of ureteric peristalsis may be lost (Figure 6.6, *top*) and, indeed, obstruction at the vesico-ureteric junction may become worse as the bladder empties (Figure 6.6, *bottom left*). The situation is well illustrated by occasional whole mounts of such bladders (Figure 6.7). Massive trabeculation and hypertrophy may well cause intramural obstruction to the ureter, seen in the figure with a wire probe emerging from the ureteric orifice.

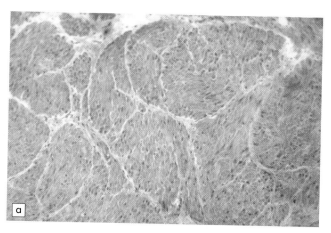

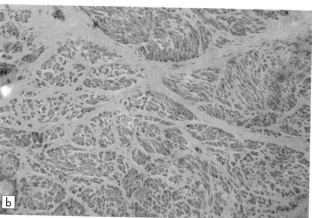

Figure 6.5 Histological appearances of detrusor muscle in high-pressure chronic retention. Muscle hypertrophy (a) may degenerate (b) with collagen infiltration (green stain).

The effect of bladder wall hypertrophy

As might be expected, the increase in detrusor muscle mass together with the collagen infiltration illustrated above fundamentally alter the urodynamic characteristics of the bladder as a storage organ. Furthermore, in high-pressure chronic retention, an intrinsic detrusor pressure remains within the bladder after micturition has been completed, and accurate recording of this intrinsic 'end void' pressure is critical with regard to the analysis of associated renal dysfunction. It is not known at the present time (and it is extremely difficult to determine by experimental means) whether the upper tract dilatation develops as a result of the bladder wall hypertrophy illustrated in Figure 6.6 or as a result of the intrinsic detrusor post-void pressure remaining within the bladder after micturition. This is

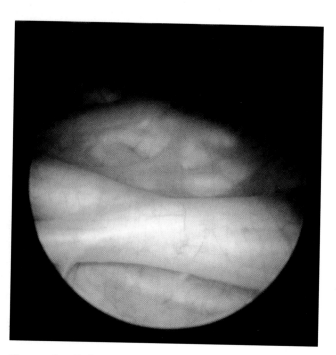

Figure 6.4 Endoscopic appearance in high-pressure chronic retention.

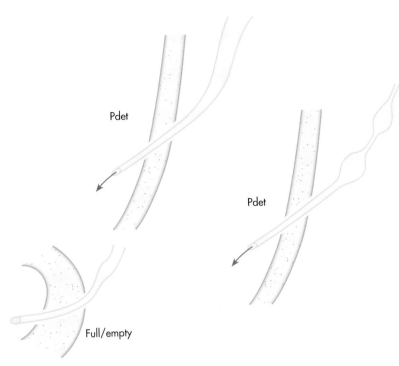

Pdet

Pdet

Full/empty

Figure 6.6 *Ureteric passage through thickened detrusor wall. Right, normal; centre, loss of peristalsis; left, increasing wall thickness after micturition.*

perhaps a slightly academic point as, regardless of whether pressure precedes hypertrophy or vice versa, the end result – progressive upper tract dilatation – remains the same.

Measurement of end void pressure

As noted above, the accurate recording of end void pressure is an important measurement, which correlates with renal dysfunction. Figure 6.8 illustrates such a measurement taking place. The typical patient with high-pressure retention (painless, protuberant bladder) micturates in an entirely normal fashion in private and without any Valsalva manoeuvre (artificial pushing). Following the void, the patient lies on the table and, under local anaesthetic, a small needle is placed suprapubically through the abdominal and bladder walls. Fluid rises up the tube as illustrated, clearly demonstrating the end void intrinsic detrusor pressure remaining within the bladder; this can easily be measured with reference to the pubic bone as is standard practice, and is responsible for the 'high-pressure' name applied to this form of chronic retention.

This simple procedure is important because it exactly mimics the patient's natural state. On occasion,

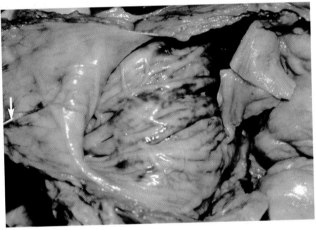

Figure 6.7 *Whole mount bladder from case of high-pressure retention. Note the wire in the ureteric orifice (arrow).*

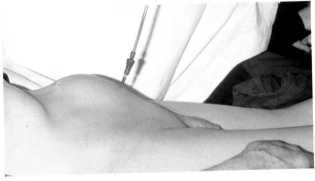

Figure 6.8 *Direct measurements of intrinsic detrusor post void pressure by suprapubic puncture.*

investigators have attempted to obtain such measures following urodynamic investigation of the bladder during which the organ has almost invariably been artificially filled at supranormal rates. Such abnormal filling rates significantly disrupt the normal working of high-pressure bladders, and false recordings are invariably obtained. The measurement of end void pressure as described above is the simplest and the best method of obtaining the critical pressure that relates to renal dysfunction.

Summary of the urodynamic data relating to bladders with high-pressure retention

Figure 6.9 illustrates the important concept of the 'pressure cycle' that occurs within the bladder of patients with high-pressure chronic retention. Following micturition (end void point), the pressure within the bladder rises as filling takes place from the upper tracts. Eventually, the end fill pressure is reached, at which point the patient is experiencing the normal desire to void. A detrusor contraction takes place (over and above the intrinsic pressure within the bladder) and urine is expelled in the usual fashion. At the end of micturition, the pressure returns once again to the end void point, thus completing the pressure 'loop'.

It can thus be seen that, in the state of high-pressure chronic retention, the bladder fills and empties in cyclical fashion at an abnormally raised

pressure *throughout the 24 hours*. Micturition may occur with apparent normality but at no time are the upper tracts able freely to empty into the bladder storage organ. Thus, it might be predicted that within the upper tracts a similar cycle might be observed – reduced pressure when urine was able to drain easily into the bladder but rising pressure as the bladder filled and passage of urine distally through the vesico-ureteric junction became more difficult. This hypothesis is tested by the experiment described below.

The patient with high-pressure retention never drains the bladder below the end void point unless urine is removed artificially. If a catheter is placed in the bladder and urine is withdrawn (dashed line in Figure 6.9), pressure will drop towards zero and, of course, the suprapubic mass will disappear. As already noted, measurements taken under these circumstances are highly misleading and do not give useful prognostic information regarding renal function.

Summary of filling phase abnormalities

The broad categories of filling phase abnormality that may be seen in the human bladder are noted in Figure 6.10. Normal patients with normal inflow phases have a pressure rise to the physiological bladder capacity (approximately 500 ml) of less than 5 cmH$_2$O. Such patients never develop upper tract dilatation; these are the majority with 'simple' bladder outflow obstruction. Cases of poor compliance are those in whom the bladder pressure rises during filling. This can be easily

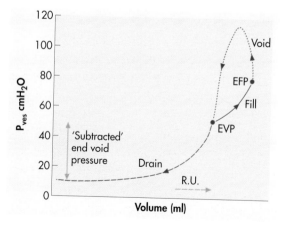

Figure 6.9 *Pressure–volume relationship in high pressure chronic retention. EFP, end fill pressure; EVP, end void pressure; RU, residual urine.*

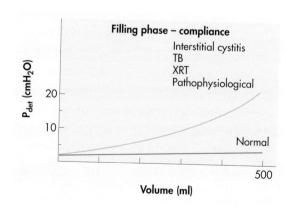

Figure 6.10 *Types of abnormal bladder compliance.*

understood when the bladder wall has been replaced by fibrous tissue such as occurs in interstitial cystitis, tuberculosis or after radiation therapy. In high-pressure retention, the reduced compliance during filling is related to a pathophysiological abnormality of smooth muscle – detrusor hypertrophy and associated collagen formation, as illustrated earlier. It is important to note that the depiction of poor compliance as illustrated in Figure 6.10 is related to abnormal (urodynamic) filling of an initially empty bladder during the test. By contrast, the abnormal pressure relationships seen in Figure 6.9 are purely the result of *natural* filling and voiding characteristics.

The reason for the development of the high-pressure, obstructed characteristic remains unknown. Undoubtedly, this detrusor reaction to obstruction may occur with any form of distal urethral lesion such as a dense phimosis, urethral stricture or, in children, urethral valves. Obstruction that involves typical prostate hypertrophy rarely seems to lead to the high-pressure type of change (as noted above in the historical series). This may be related to the irritation caused by prostatic obstruction, such detrusor instability perhaps protecting against the development of painless retention.

The radiological assessment of high-pressure bladders

Reflux cystograms (Figure 6.11) show, as might be expected, a trabeculated, sacculated picture entirely consistent with the cystoscopic appearance. It might also be expected that reflux would not be seen when one considers the oblique path of the ureter through the massively hypertrophied bladder wall (Figure 6.7). Naturally, for the purpose of these human studies into interactive dysfunction, all patients received cystograms to exclude the possibility of reflux that would be expected to lead to unrelated and entirely different changes within the upper tracts. In the patients studied, urine was always sterile and reflux never present.

Intravenous urography demonstrates the typical picture of well-preserved renal parenchyma with general distension of the collecting system from the calyces to the vesico-ureteric junction (Figure 6.12).

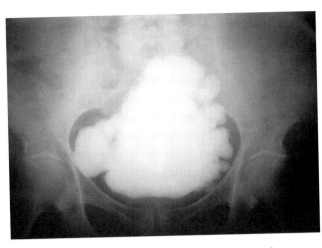

Figure 6.11 *Reflux cystogram in high-pressure retention demonstrating competent vesico-ureteric junction.*

Figure 6.12a illustrates particularly well the typical 'snake's head' appearance of high-pressure retention at the lower end of the left ureter – a near-certain sign of raised intravesical pressure and a warning, if not otherwise suspected, that renal function might subsequently be at risk. Such appearances present a relatively easy target for a skilled nephrostomist, and the placement of a nephrostomy at last allows the synchronous measurement of upper and lower urinary tract pressures to be contemplated.

Interactive pressure recordings in patients with high-pressure chronic retention and hydroureter/hydronephrosis

Following careful screening to exclude default conditions such as prostate cancer or urinary tract infection, consenting patients underwent the investigation protocol as illustrated in Figure 6.13. A nephrostomy tube was placed in the renal pelvis (via the renal substance to avoid leakage) and connected to standard Whitaker pump/measurement apparatus. A suprapubic pressure line was inserted and finally a urethral catheter allowed bladder volume to be increased or decreased at will. The patient was made warm and comfortable on the investigation table as the studies took an extended period of time. Patients rarely experienced any discomfort during the tests and commonly fell asleep during measurements.

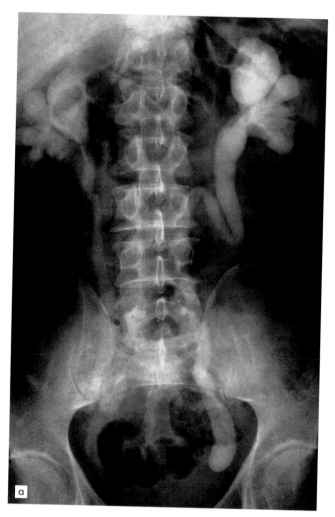
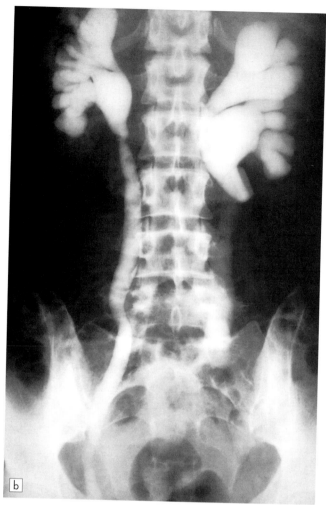

Figure 6.12 (a, b) *Radiological aspects of high-pressure retention.*

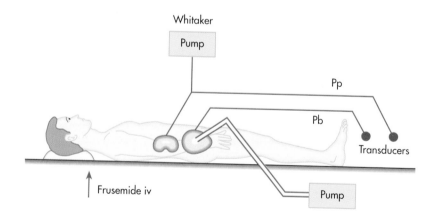

Figure 6.13 *Experimental protocol for bladder and renal pressure measurement.*

States of hydration

Three differing states of hydration were identified. Baseline hydration determined that the patient was comfortable – enough water had been drunk to satisfy thirst. Water drinking determined that the patient was asked to drink 1–1.5 litres of water fairly rapidly, a load well in excess of what he would normally ingest. A third level of fluid loading was attained by the administration of frusemide 0.5 mg/kg intravenously. These three forms of hydration were used to 'front end load' the urinary tract, i.e. to present differing diuretic loads to the drainage system of the urinary tract.

In addition to fluid loads presented to the kidney, it was possible to vary the rate with which the fluid passed through the vesico-ureteric junction. This was performed by filling and emptying the bladder through the urethral catheter, the resultant pressure being recorded by the suprapubic pressure line. As will be evident from Figure 6.9, such artificial filling and emptying of the bladder results in marked swings of intrinsic detrusor pressure, which may be expected to affect vesico-ureteric transport.

Experimental observations

The results of these experiments are illustrated in the following figures. During prolonged baseline recordings (Figure 6.14) in which the patient was resting comfortably and simply hydrated, there was no identifiable correlation or connection between bladder and pelvic pressure measurements. Occasional pelvic pressure waves were seen, as were occasional detrusor contractions (unstable waves), but these bore no temporal relationship to each other. Subsequently (Figure 6.15), the bladder was filled at a rate of 60 ml per minute and the effect on the bladder and pelvic pressures was noted. As expected from the pressure/ volume characteristic of high-pressure bladders, the bladder pressure rose rapidly but at the same time the pelvic pressure was also seen to rise, albeit much more slowly. When 100 ml of water was removed from the bladder (Figure 6.16), the bladder pressure dropped

rapidly, as again would be expected, but pelvic pressure also dropped following the slow initial rise, demonstrating that the artificial 'cycling' of bladder pressure (see above) had induced a form of artificial 'cycling' of the upper tract pressure.

The cycling linkage continued but was more precisely interlinked when oral water loading increased the perfusion pressure at the proximal end of the urinary tract (Figure 6.17). Natural diuresis and subsequent bladder drainage (100 ml) produced sharp

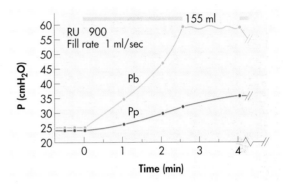

Figure 6.15 Subsequent pressure variations.

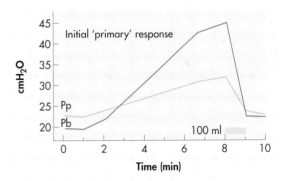

Figure 6.16 Effect of bladder pressure variation.

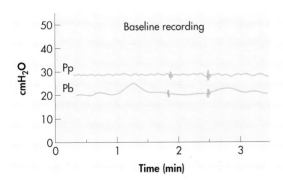

Figure 6.14 Baseline recordings of renal pelvic (P_p) and bladder (P_b) pressures.

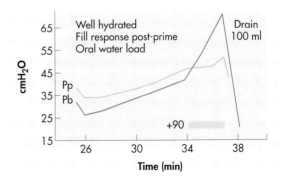

Figure 6.17 Further pressure variations with water loading and an additional 90 ml in the bladder.

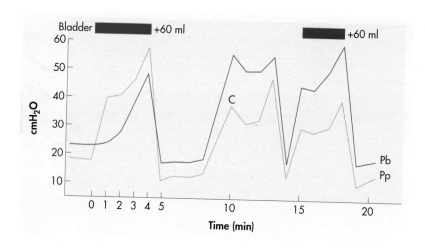

Figure 6.18 Co-ordinated pressure movements within bladder and renal pelvis. Drainage volumes not shown. C, possible time of ureteric 'creep'.

swings in bladder and pelvic pressure measurements although, as might be expected, bladder pressure swings were more acute than those seen in the renal pelvis.

Subsequently, under maximal 'front end loading' caused by frusemide IV, bladder pressure cycling via the urethral catheter led to similar sharp swings of pressure being recorded from the renal pelvis (Figure 6.18). Occasionally, small reductions in pelvic pressure were observed; these were thought to represent periods of ureteric 'creep', during which time smooth muscle of the upper urinary tract dilated marginally, thus reducing the pressure and accommodating a greater volume. This is the mechanism – also detected in the bladder – thought experimentally to account for the development of hydroureter and hydronephrosis over the long term (Figure 6.19).

The interactive pressure experiments are summarised in Figure 6.20. During baseline periods, bladder and renal pressures are dissociated and variation of bladder pressure, in particular, has no effect on upper tract distension. However, prolonged increase of bladder pressure (unlikely to be tolerated by the patient) or increased fluid loading/diuretic therapy (a reasonably common occurrence) might well 'prime' the upper tracts, and thereafter pressures within the pelvis may mimic precisely pressures within the bladder. It is very important to appreciate that this synchronous pressure state occurs in the *absence* of vesico-ureteric reflux. The pressure measured within the pelvis is not a reflection of bladder pressure 'passing backwards' up the ureter; it is a pressure required

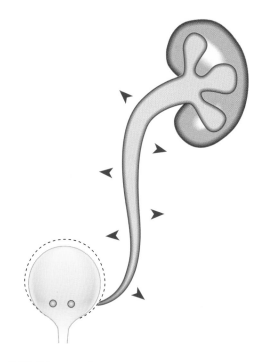

Figure 6.19 Schematic diagram of ureteric 'creep' – gradual dilatation under stress.

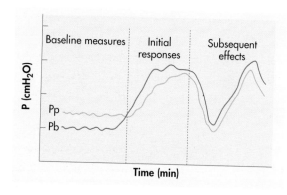

Figure 6.20 Summary of interactive pressure–volume effects.

to be exerted by the upper tract if perfusion through the vesico-ureteric junction is to occur.

It is proposed, therefore, that these experiments give some insight into the development of hydronephrosis in the simple, uncomplicated (uninfected) case of high-pressure retention. It is now possible to consider what might be the consequences of such changes for renal function. Using the same experimental model, both renographic and biochemical aspects of renal function may be examined, and the technique and results of these studies are briefly described.

Excretory function measured by gamma camera renography

It has already been noted that the lack of co-apting peristaltic waves would be likely fundamentally to affect drainage function from the upper urinary tract. The ureter, previously divided into segments, becomes an open column of fluid as hydronephrosis supervenes, and such an open column is capable of exerting forces very dissimilar to those acting in the normal state. It might be hypothesised, for example, that such an open hydroureter would, under certain critical circumstances, exert pressures on the vesico-ureteric junction in the vertical position that would not be present in the horizontal position. Clearly, in this respect, the pressure on the other side of the vesico-ureteric junction (i.e. within the bladder) would be critical, but there might be defined circumstances in which significant differences in drainage from the upper tracts would be seen when the patient was in the erect rather than in the horizontal position.

Such circumstances, can in fact, be identified and one such patient is illustrated in Figures 6.21–6.23. The intravenous pyelogram of this 41-year-old man is not at first glance overtly hydronephrotic, but an open hydroureter can be seen on both sides, most marked on the left, and the typical 'snake's head' at the lower end of the ureter (typical of high-pressure retention) can be seen. The relatively small but high-pressure bladder fails to opacify. Iodine-123 gamma camera renography was performed in the erect and supine positions under identical circumstances a few days

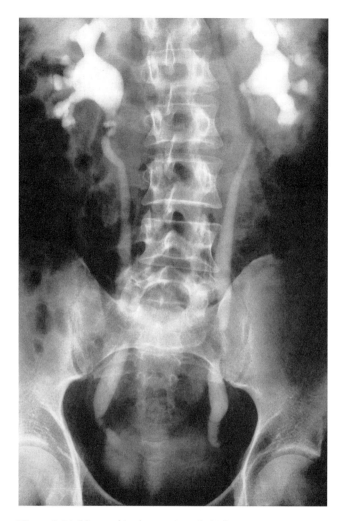

Figure 6.21 *Urographic changes in early high-pressure retention.*

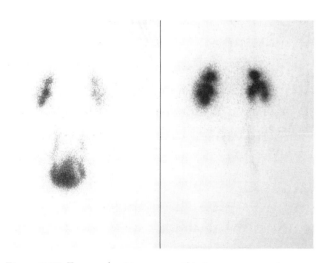

Figure 6.22 *Erect and supine renographic images.*

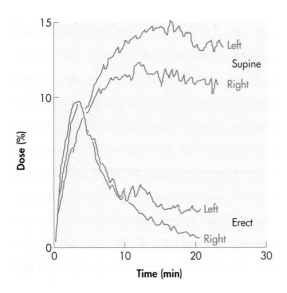

Figure 6.23 *Erect and supine renographic curves.*

apart. Figure 6.22 shows accumulated frames between 10 and 15 minutes. The panel showing the erect study clearly demonstrates upper tract drainage, particularly from the left, and bladder filling, whilst the panel relating to the supine study shows near-total stasis within the renal pelvis and calyces and no image whatsoever of the bladder. Graphical analysis (Figure 6.23) shows equally good uptake for either test but little excretion in the supine position as compared to near-normal excretion (renal area of interest demonstrated) in the erect position. This simple study in a young man with early, high-pressure retention demonstrates conclusively that drainage through the vesico-ureteric junction can be affected by postural conditions; loss of the normal co-apting mechanism might well be responsible for the observations.

The gravitational theory of drainage

This gravitational theory of the open hydroureter may be tested using the human high-pressure retention model (Figure 6.24). In these studies, men with sterile high-pressure retention have a suprapubic line and catheter inserted under local anaesthetic. Thus, the volume and therefore the pressure within the bladder may be varied at will whilst the patient is seated or lying in front of a gamma camera.

The results of various studies are depicted in Figures 6.25–6.28. In the first experiment, a man underwent ^{123}I gamma camera renography in the sitting position. He was comfortably hydrated but had been asked not to void prior to the examination. It was thus envisaged that his bladder pressure would be relatively advanced up the pressure–volume curve illustrated in Figure 6.9. An injection of the isotope

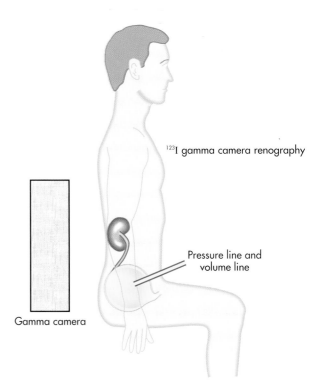

Figure 6.24 *Experimental protocol for drainage experiments.*

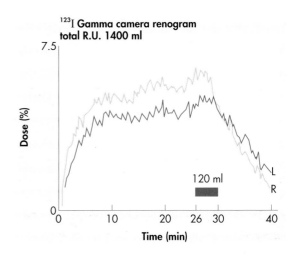

Figure 6.25 *Effect of bladder drainage.*

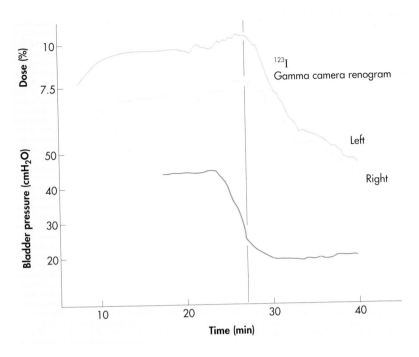

Figure 6.26 Bladder pressure and renal drainage compared.

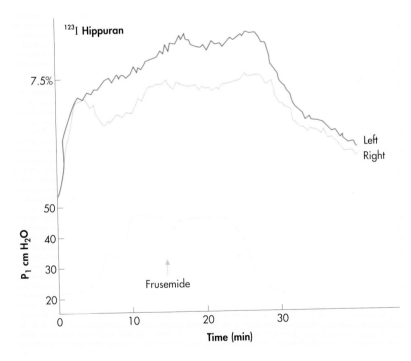

Figure 6.27 Lack of frusemide effect until bladder drained. See text for details.

was given and the curves elaborated are shown. At 25 minutes, 120 ml of urine was withdrawn through the suprapubic catheter and the effect on the renal clearance of the isotope was observed. The acute reduction in intravesical volume, and thus pressure, allowed vesico-ureteric transport to take place, urine from the previously obstructed kidney passing rapidly onwards and down the hydroureter. In Figure 6.26, the same experiment is repeated but the intravesical pressure is recorded on the same time base as the renogram curves. Under these conditions, little isotope escapes the renal substance until the reduction of the bladder volume once again causes a sharp drop of bladder pressure, following which rapid reduction in isotope counts from the kidney takes place. These experiments demonstrate an important hydrodynamic aspect of high-pressure retention. A vertical line drawn at the moment net isotope counts begin to reduce bisects the intravesical pressure recording at approximately 25 cmH$_2$O. Thus, when the intravesical pressure is above this level, little or no drainage occurs from the upper tract. As the pressure falls through 25 cmH$_2$O, rapid drainage starts to commence, suggesting that the figure of 25 cmH$_2$O is particularly important for the maintenance of upper tract function.

The robust and resilient nature of the lower tract changes is illustrated in Figure 6.27. In these experiments bladder pressure was recorded as before during gamma camera renography. However, to stimulate the upper tract to the maximum – and thus, if possible, to force perfusion into the bladder – an injection of frusemide was given 15 minutes after the isotope injection. As can be seen, despite this 'front end loading', the renographic counts do not diminish and the renographic curves do not deflect until once again bladder pressure has been significantly reduced by removing fluid from within. Lower tract intrinsic pressure and dynamics appear to dominate renal function, and such an effect may still be seen in relatively advanced obstructive renal failure (Figure 6.28). In this case, relatively poor uptake during gamma camera renography signifies relatively high serum creatinine, but on draining the bladder there is still an effect seen in the erect position that is not identified if the renography is carried out supine.

In conclusion, therefore, it is possible to advance an hypothesis in high-pressure chronic retention to account for the variation seen in upper and lower tract pressures. It is postulated that an open hydroureter (approximate length in the adult 25 cm, Figure 6.29) may maintain profusion through the vesico-ureteric junction as long as the cyclic intrinsic detrusor pressure remains under 25 cmH$_2$O for the majority of the cycle. If the intrinsic detrusor pressure rises to more than 25 cmH$_2$O for the majority of the filling phase, ureteric stasis should supervene and obstructed renal failure should follow. This hypothesis was explored in the original paper describing high-pressure retention in which a graph of intrinsic detrusor pressure against serum creatinine (Figure 6.30) appeared to show that

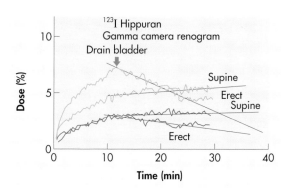

Figure 6.28 *Bladder effect in advanced renal failure.*

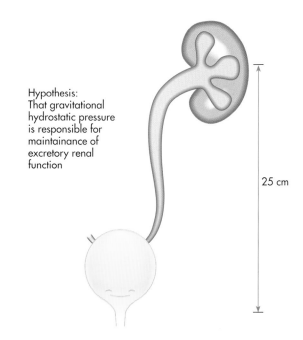

Figure 6.29 *Hypothesis for gravitational theory in open hydroureter.*

above 25 cmH$_2$O there was indeed a steep rise in creatinine, as would be expected from the experimental evidence. Although there were few patients with significantly raised creatinine levels in this series, results from other workers have tended to support the importance of the 25–30 cmH$_2$O pressure range with respect to the maintenance of renal profusion and function. Similar figures also guide those who reconstruct the bladder, who should ensure that either tonic or phasic reservoir contraction waves do not reach this critical pressure limit for significant periods of the 24 hours.

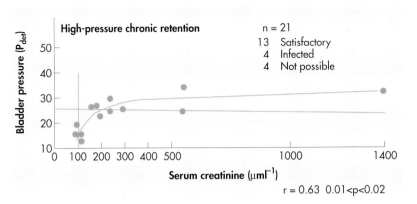

Figure 6.30 *Intrinsic detrusor pressure related to serum creatinine.*

Biochemical studies before and after the relief of obstruction

This subject has been extensively studied in the literature and in the author's own department during the last few years by Jones and co-workers. An understanding of the abnormalities of tubular function that may occur under such circumstances is important for the practising urologist, who not infrequently has to manage a patient with postobstructive diuresis on the urology ward. Absolute excretory volumes (Figure 6.31) and electrolyte excretion (Figure 6.32) are maximal within 24 hours and usually stabilise by 14 days. Synchronous studies of glomerular filtration rate estimated by various techniques (Figure 6.33) illustrate that most of the early improvement is related to tubular recovery, although a late glomerular recovery phase can be identified. Precisely similar urodynamic, renographic and biochemical changes may

be seen in children as well as in adults: infants and children with urethral valves have a syndrome nearly identical to high-pressure retention (the valve bladder) and, in those cases that are not associated with reflux, similar patterns of obstructive renal failure take place. Unfortunately, the destructive nature of the severe obstruction on the detrusor muscle frequently leads to marked collagen infiltration and fibrotic damage, with resultant very poor compliance. By contrast, in the adult, long-term studies, from the author's own unit and others, suggest that the majority of cases recover well, as regards both bladder and renal function.

The observations recorded above have, of course, been made in a particular group of patients with a particular form of bladder dysfunction. It might be argued that patients with neurogenic bladder dysfunction – acknowledged to be chiefly at risk because of obstructive renal problems – could not be linked urodynamically or therapeutically with the high-pressure retention group. There is no doubt that neurogenic

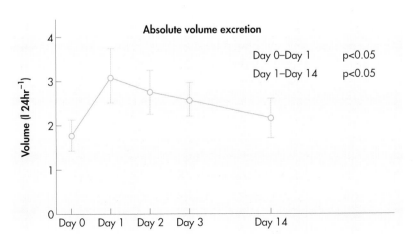

Figure 6.31 *Volume excretion before and after relief of obstruction. Day 0: prior to relief of obstruction by bladder catheterisation.*

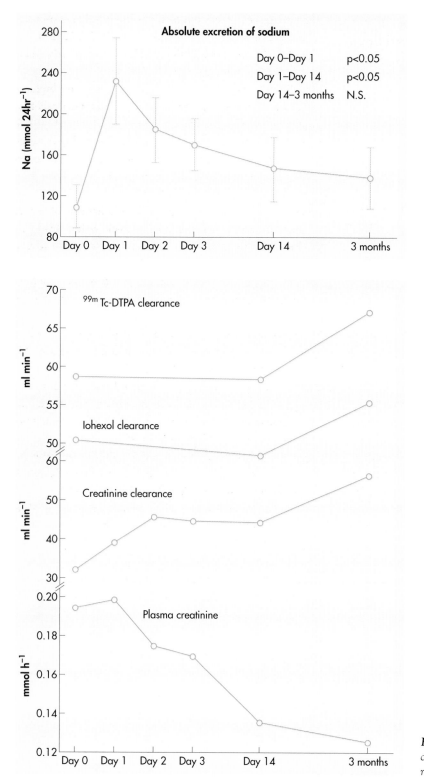

Figure 6.32 Sodium excretion before and after release of obstruction. Day 0: as in Figure 6.31.

Figure 6.33 Summary of glomerular and tubular changes in obstructive uropathy before and after the release of obstruction. Day 0: as in Figure 6.31.

bladders may demonstrate a profile of much more aggressive hyper-reflexic contractions than that seen in high-pressure retention cases (although, in the latter, moderate instability may be seen on ambulatory stud-ies), and it is possible that the hyper-reflexic contrac-tions themselves may be responsible for the obstruc-tive renal failure. Nevertheless, there are enough signs in common (clinical, radiological, renographic and biochemical) to consider that the conditions may be associated, at least in part; the therapeutic and reconstructive lessons learned in one group may well be applicable to the other.

Further reading

Badenoch AW. Congenital obstruction of the bladder neck. Ann RCS 1949; 4: 295–307

George NJR, Feneley RC, Roberts JBM. Identification of the poor risk patient with 'prostatism' and detrusor failure. Br J Urol 1986; 58: 290–5

George NJR, O'Reilly PH, Barnard RJ, et al. High pressure chronic retention. Br Med J 1983; 286: 1780–3

George NJR, O'Reilly PH, Barnard RJ, et al. Practical management of patients with dilated upper tracts and chronic retention of urine. Br J Urol 1984; 56: 9–12

Ghose RR. Prolonged recovery of renal function after prostatectomy for prostatic outflow obstruction. Br Med J 1990; 300: 1376–7

Holden D, George NJR, Rickards D, et al. Renal pelvic pressures in human chronic obstructive uropathy. Br J Urol 1984; 56 565–70

Jones DA, Atherton JC, O'Reilly PH, et al. Assessment of the nephron segments involved in post-obstructive diuresis in man, using lithium clearance. Br J Urol 1989; 64: 559–63

Jones DA, George NJR, O'Reilly PH, et al. Reversible hypertension associated with unrecognised high pressure chronic retention of urine. Lancet 1987; 11: 1052–4

Jones DA, George NJR, O'Reilly PH. Post-obstructive renal function. Semin Urol 1987; 5: 176–90

Jones DA, George NJR, O'Reilly PH, et al. The biphasic nature of renal functional recovery following relief of chronic obstructive uropathy. Br J Urol 1988; 61: 192–7

Jones DA, Gilpin SA, Holden D, et al. Relationship between bladder morphology and long-term outcome of treatment in patients with high pressure chronic retention of urine. Br J Urol 1991; 67: 265–85

Jones DA, Holden D, George NJR. Mechanism of upper tract dilatation in patients with thick walled bladders, chronic retention of urine and associated hydroureteronephrosis. J Urol 1988; 140: 326–9

Jones DA, Lupton EW, George NJR. Effect of bladder filling on upper tract urodynamics in man. Br J Urol 1990; 65: 492–6

Sacks SH, Aparicio SAJR, Bevan A, et al. Late renal failure due to prostatic outflow obstruction: a preventable disease. Br Med J 1989; 298: 156–9

Styles RA, Neal DE, Griffiths CJ, et al. Long term monitoring of bladder pressure in chronic retention of urine: the relationship between detrusor activity and upper tract dilatation. J Urol 1988; 140: 330–4

Styles RA, Neal DE, Ramsden PD. Chronic retention of urine. The relationship between upper tract dilatation and bladder pressure. Br J Urol 1986; 58: 647–51

Wallace DM. The bladder neck in urinary obstruction. Proc R Soc Med 1951; 44: 434–7

N. J. R. George

Introduction

The infectious process encompasses a highly complex series of events that surrounds the relationship between the host and parasite as the former attempts to defend itself against the offensive properties of the latter. Virulence factors available to the micro-organism will be combated by a wide range of specific and non-specific defence mechanisms, and the result of this encounter – 'the microbiological battle ground' – will determine whether or not infectious disease is established.

Conventionally, accounts of infection of the urinary tract concentrate on the response of the urothelium to bacterial invasion. However, a continuing and perhaps increasing tendency to open surgery in certain groups of patients determines that a basic understanding of the broader concepts of the infectious process is likely to be advantageous for the practising urological surgeon. Therefore, in this account of urinary tract infection, before dealing with specific issues relating to organisms and the urothelium, a general description is given of the host–parasite relationship as it applies to the urogenital system both in health and disease. Some important fundamental definitions are noted in Table 7.1. Such general microbiological points may be considered under the following headings:

Colonising micro-organisms in health.
General defence mechanisms.
General modifying factors.
Properties of commensal organisms.

Table 7.1 Essential definitions of basic microbiological terms

Term	Definition
Pathogenicity	Ability to cause disease
Opportunistic infection	Weakened defences predispose to infection, often by non-pathogens
Virulence	Degree of pathogenicity

Colonising micro-organisms in health

Table 7.2 lists common colonising micro-organisms by site in healthy humans. The widespread presence of Staphylococci and Streptococci on the skin and surrounding the lower genitourinary tract will be appreciated, as will the occurrence of Candida and Lactobacilli within vaginal flora. The colon contains enormous numbers of bacteria – up to 10^{11} organisms/g. The majority of these organisms are obligate anaerobes, although aerobic and facultative anaerobic organisms such as Enterobacteriaceae and *Enterococcus* spp. are present in significant numbers (approximately 10^8/g of colonic contents), these species being the most common source of uropathogens.

The normally balanced environment of the bowel flora is significantly affected by antimicrobial agents. Antibiotic therapy results in normally sensitive *Escherichia coli* strains as well as anaerobic species being replaced by more resistant strains and organisms such as *Pseudomonas aeruginosa* [1]. Cessation of broad-spectrum therapy allows recolonisation by resident

Table 7.2 Organisms by site in health (normal flora). Commensal organisms which exist in symbiotic relationship with the host protecting against uropathogens

Skin

Staphylococci (*Staph. aureus* and *Staph. epidermidis*)
Corynebacterium spp.
Candida spp.

Lower genitourinary tract

Staphylococci
Streptococci
Anaerobic cocci
Corynebacterium spp.
Lactobacilli (vagina)

Large intestine

Anaerobes
Bacteroides spp.
Clostridium spp.
Fusobacterium spp.
Aerobes/facultative anaerobes
Escherichia coli
Klebsiella spp.
Streptococci – Enterococci (*Strep. faecalis*)
Yeasts

flora, but slower growing anaerobic organisms may initially be displaced by faster growing Enterobacteriaceae. Thus, injudicious broad-spectrum therapy may increase the size of the colonic reservoir from which uropathogens are normally drawn [2] – as noted above, these organisms usually account for only 0.1% of total colonic flora. The presence of a large volume of potential uropathogens may clearly be an ascending threat to the lower urinary tract, particularly in the presence of any abnormality such as outflow tract obstruction or congenital anomalies.

General defence mechanisms

Non-specific host defence mechanisms are outlined in Table 7.3. General resistance to invasion may be described in terms of events at the surface of the host, events at a deeper level and mechanisms that depend on cellular function.

The role of commensal flora is further explored below. The mechanical integrity of skin and mucous membranes may clearly be breached in a number of ways. Breakdown of lipids into fatty acids (approximate pH 5–6) by skin flora constitutes a mildly hostile environment for pathogens. Lysozyme, found in every mucosal secretion, splits the muramic acid linkage in cell walls of Gram-positive organisms in particular. The iron-binding properties of lactoferrin disrupt the normal metabolism of the micro-organism. Immunoglobulin A (IgA) secretion may prevent the attachment of organisms to host cells.

Penetration of the initial line of defence leads to more substantial but non-specific reactions such as the acute phase response and the inflammatory response. Humoral and cellular components such as protease inhibitors and adherence proteins are delivered to the site and the classical inflammatory reaction supervenes. Activation of the complement cascade by the alternative pathway may lead to bacterial lysis as well as to enhancement of phagocytosis. The anti-adherence properties of the glycoprotein fibronectin may prevent the attachment of pathogenic organisms. Increased phagocytosis by various cells, including neutrophil polymorphs, mononuclear phagocytes and natural killer cells, is stimulated by a complex series of events that may vary according to the nature of the microbiological challenge.

General modifying factors

A number of generalised factors may affect the standard host defence mechanisms. Patients at the extremes of life are vulnerable to infections. Postmenopausal hormonal changes in the lower urinary tract are of particular interest to urologists

Poor nutrition or overt malnutrition, particularly in the elderly, may weaken defences in a number of ways relating to protein synthesis and vitamin deficiency. Generalised disorders such as diabetes mellitus, alcoholism and renal failure may markedly increase susceptibility to disease, as will overwhelming infection and certain types of drug therapy, as well as the general debility related to advanced malignancy. Pathological conditions that further expose the individual to the risk of infection, such as stone disease or obstruction, are considered below.

Properties of commensal organisms

Commensal organisms have an important role to play in the protection of the host by resisting the growth of

Table 7.3 General non-specific (constitutive) host defence mechanisms. These are conveniently described in terms of the degree to which the organism penetrates the surface. General factors that may compromise or modify these defences are noted

Surface	Compromised	Subsurface	Compromised	Cellular	Compromised
Commensal Flora	Antibiotics	Lysozyme	Drugs Corticosteroids Immunosuppression Infections	Phagocytosis Polymorpho-nuclear Mononuclear	Alcoholism
Mechanical Integrity Acidity	Surgery Cannulae	Lactoferrin Acute phase response			Advanced cancer Renal disease Liver disease HIV
Secretions Lysozyme Lactoferrin IgA		Inflammatory response			
Flow Peristalsis Irritation	Surgery Obstruction	Complement Fibronectin			

more pathogenic organisms. The mechanisms by which they attain this objective are listed in Table 7.4. Competition for a limited supply of nutrients acts to restrict the growth of pathogens, whilst the ability of the commensal organisms to occupy certain cell surface receptors (tropism) limits the adherence possibilities for the invader. Bacterial products known as bacteriocins may be toxic to other organisms, often of the same species. As noted above, fatty acid production from sebum and lipids results in a hostile microenvironment. Low-level but continued stimulation of

Table 7.4 Mechanisms of protection by commensal flora. See text for details

Competition for nutrients	(interference)
Competition for receptors	(tropism)
Bacteriocin production	
Fatty acid production	
Stimulation of immune system	
Stimulation of natural antibodies	

the immune system as well as the stimulation of cross-reacting 'natural' antibodies (such antibodies are raised to organisms that the host has not encountered because of antigenic cross-reaction with organisms that have been experienced) further enhance resistance to pathogenic bacteria. Apart from antibiotic therapy, the normal commensal flora may be significantly affected by general factors such as diet, hygiene habits and underlying disease.

The described general mechanisms are, under the normal circumstances of health, remarkably effective at excluding pathogenic invasion. For a more complete account of the highly complex processes involved, the reader is referred to standard bacteriological texts. The remainder of this chapter addresses first specific microbiological aspects of urinary tract infection in humans, followed by a clinical account of the more important forms of inflammatory disease.

Host defence mechanisms: lower urinary tract

Apart from the broad concepts outlined above, the lower urinary tract has a number of specific defence mechanisms that allow it to counter the threat posed by the reservoir of potential pathogens located chiefly in the lower bowel and on the perineal skin. Naturally, the anatomy of the male and, in particular, the length of the urethra determine that ascending infection is extremely uncommon when compared with the female. Nevertheless, the lower urogenital tract, whilst clearly offering a bacteriological threat to the female urothelium, does offer some defence mechanisms against ascending infection by pathogenic bacteria.

Commensal organisms

An outline of the advantages of commensal flora has been given above. During the reproductive years, circulating oestrogens effect the vaginal epithelium, which stores increased amounts of glycogen within the cells (Figure 7.1). The glycogen is metabolised by *Lactobacillus acidophilus* into lactic acid, and the resultant drop in pH produces an unfavourable microenvironment for the majority of pathogenic bacteria attempting to ascend into the bladder. Disruption of this vaginal flora by vaginitis or other infection leads to a rise in pH and loss of the natural defence barrier. Lactobacilli (which, together with other Gram-positive rods are collectively known as Döderlein's bacilli) are one of the main causes of milk going sour and, indeed, are the active organisms in 'live' yoghurt, which for this reason is frequently advocated by health magazines as a topical application that can prevent recurrent lower urinary tract infection without the need for antibiotic therapy. Naturally, such protection

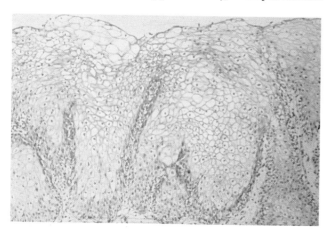

Figure 7.1 Vaginal epithelial cells stuffed with glycogen. Produced in response to oestrogens, the glycogen is broken down by Lactobacillus acidophillus, *thus increasing local vaginal acidity.*

is not available either before or after the menopause, one fact that possibly explains the increased incidence of ascending lower urinary tract infection in elderly women, whose introital skin is often thin and atrophic due to lack of circulating oestrogens.

Urine

Urine, normally a good culture medium, may, under some circumstances, be inhibitory or even bactericidal against some uropathogens. Low urinary pH levels, in particular, as well as raised blood urea and high osmolality are inhibitory for some organisms [3].

Genital skin

Although strictly unrelated to the urothelium, penetration of the natural barrier afforded by genital skin can have serious consequences for the patient (Figure 7.2). Any perforation of penile skin may be followed by infection, but this is particularly the case when the patient is diabetic, and such patients are commonly exposed to increased risk during the self-administration of vasoactive substances for erectile dysfunction.

Urine flow

Urine flow from the kidney by ureteric peristalsis and from the bladder by periodic detrusor contraction constitutes the main defence mechanism of the urinary tract against ascending infection [4]. Loss of competence at the vesicoureteric junction for any reason may lead, under certain circumstances, to significant renal damage; additionally, reflux prevents efficient bladder emptying, thus compromising the flushing mechanism of micturition, which is similarly impeded by any form of lower urinary tract obstruction.

Bladder surface mucin

In a series of experiments on rabbit bladders, Parsons *et al.* proposed that a bladder surface mucin layer consisting of a glycosaminoglycan was secreted by transitional cells and acted as an 'anti-adherence factor' by inhibiting bacterial attachment to bladder mucosa, thereby facilitating the removal of bacteria by the voiding process. These workers demonstrated that removal of the glycosaminoglycan layer by acid markedly increased adhesion to the urothelium (Figure 7.3) and, furthermore, instillation of heparin (a synthetic glycosaminoglycan) into bladders previously denuded of their glycosaminoglycan layer by acid resulted in restoration of the antimucosal adherence properties. Pretreatment of the bacteria with heparin had no effect on adherence, and the authors concluded that the surface mucin provided a protective barrier for the urothelium, thus preventing bacterial adherence to the uroepithelial cells. Subsequently, the bacteria trapped in the glycosaminoglycan layer are expelled by urination [5–7].

Tamm–Horsfall protein

Tamm–Horsfall protein is secreted by the cells of the ascending loop of Henle and is the most common mucoprotein of renal origin in urine. Also known as

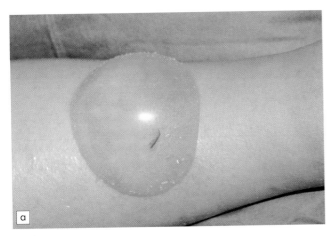

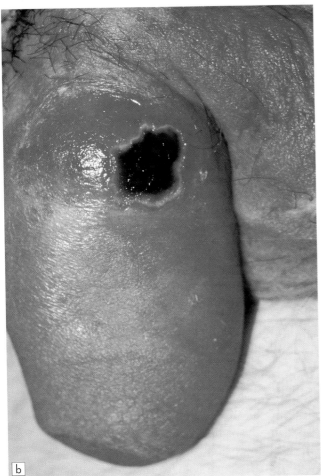

Figure 7.2 The importance of skin epithelial integrity. (a) Large blister on forearm: no infection within perfect sub-blister culture medium due to integrity of ultrathin residual epithelial covering. (b) Puncture site of intracavernosal therapy in a diabetic: despite full precautions, serious widespread inflammation has taken place.

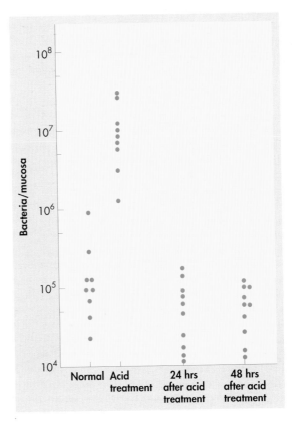

Figure 7.3 Effect of bladder surface mucin. Binding of ^{14}C-labelled E. coli to normal bladder mucosa and acid-treated mucosa. Acid treatment removes the mucin layer and bacterial adhesion to the bladder mucosa increases significantly. Twenty-four hours after acid treatment, the mucin layer has recovered sufficiently to prevent epithelial attachment. (From Parsons CL et al. Rabbit bladder. Urology 1977; 9: 48–52.)

uromucoid, Tamm–Horsfall protein was originally noted to react with influenza virus [8], but subsequently it was established that it was capable of binding strongly to E. coli expressing type 1 mannose-sensitive fimbriae [9], probably because of mannose-containing side-chains within the mucoprotein. Following entrapment, it is proposed that the uromucoid–coliform complex is mechanically cleared from the urinary tract by urination.

Local immune response

The role of immunity in the defence of the urinary tract remains poorly understood. Although considerable humoral and cellular response may be observed in upper urinary tract infection, serum production of urinary antibody is characteristically difficult to detect in bladder infection, perhaps reflecting the relative superficiality of the infection.

Virulence mechanisms

Virulence mechanisms are those properties of the parasite that enable it first to colonise and subsequently to flourish within the host. Such mechanisms may be directed against external agents administered in order to eradicate the organism or against the host itself, including natural host defences that have developed over time to counter the invading micro-organism. (Table 7.5)

Virulence against external agents: antimicrobial resistance

Before the Second World War, there were few agents with reliable antimicrobial properties, and the virulence capability of organisms was almost entirely directed against the natural properties of the host. Following the discovery and clinical usage of penicillin, organisms rapidly developed systems for evasion of the toxic effects of antibiotics, and the consequent emergence of resistant strains today constitutes a significant threat, particularly for certain groups of the population such as hospital in-patients. Staphylococcus aureus, once almost entirely penicillin sensitive, is now approximately 90% resistant to the agent. Neisseria gonorrhoeae remained penicillin sensitive for many years, but the acquisition of β-lactamase activity has resulted in high levels of penicillin resistance. Hospital-based doctors will be well aware of the extremely serious threat posed by methicillin-resistant Staph. aureus (MRSA) infections, which may spread rapidly throughout whole wards and effectively be untreatable. These examples underscore the extreme flexibility and adaptability of the invading micro-organism, which, through evolutionary processes, has managed to match and subsequently often overcome the best efforts of scientific antibiotic endeavour.

Types of resistance

Organisms may acquire antimicrobial resistance by two basic mechanisms. Intrinsic resistance implies that the organism may naturally resist antibiotics, by the production of natural enzymes such as β-lactamases, or because the usual antibiotic target within the cell is lacking, or by the presence of an impenetrable cell wall. Acquired resistance develops as a result of the evolution of new or altered genetic material, which may occur either through mutations or gene transfer. Such mutations and transfers result in a number of well-described mechanisms by which the organism may evade the action of the antibiotic.

Enzyme inactivation

β-lactamase production is the most important resistance mechanism of the penicillins and cephalosporins. The enzyme hydrolyses the β-lactam bond in the antibiotic structure, which renders it inactive. β-lactamase production is commonly found in Staph. aureus, N. gonorrhoeae and Enterobacteriaceae.

Altered permeability

Various alterations in receptor activity and transport mechanisms may prevent access of the antibiotic to the micro-organism. Aminoglycosides and tetracyclines

Table 7.5 General classification of virulence mechanisms

Against external agents	Antimicrobial resistance
Against the host	Toxin production General mechanisms Adherence mechanisms

are actively taken up into organisms, and resistance may occur either by inactivation of the transport mechanism or by development of additional systems allowing increased expulsion of the drug from the cell.

Alteration of binding site

Antibiotics may bind to specific targets within the cell. Genetic variation may alter or delete the antibiotic target, thus leading to resistance to the drug. The sites of action of the more commonly used antibiotics are summarised in Table 7.6. The complex nature of antimicrobial resistance determines that a detailed account is beyond the scope of this text and for a comprehensive overview the reader is referred to definitive studies of resistance mechanisms [10].

Virulence against the host itself

Toxin production

Toxins are proteins that are able to harm the cells or tissues of the host. Many organisms elaborate toxins, which may either assist with the process of local invasion or be themselves responsible for the characteristics of disease. Important examples of such virulent toxins are those that produce the clinical manifestations of diphtheria, tetanus and botulism.

A number of organisms, including *E. coli*, exhibit haemolysin activity that may damage erythrocytes in a variety of ways, including phospholipase C activity (cell membrane damage) and osmotic lysis. *E. coli* strains commonly associated with urinary tract infection (01, 02, 04, 06, 07, 016, 018, 075) frequently elaborate haemolysins, and such strains may be disproportionately promoted from the colonic reservoir [11, 12]. Despite the strong association of such strains with the ability to cause ascending urinary tract infection, the precise mechanism of enhanced virulence remains unknown.

General mechanisms

Apart from toxin production, there are numerous general mechanisms that facilitate the organism in its attempt to enter and multiply within the host:

penetration,
antihumoral activity,
evasion of phagocytosis,
competition for nutrients.

Penetration

In general, organisms are unable to penetrate the intact epithelium of the host unless prior damage (see Figure 7.2b) has taken place. However, certain parasites may do so, the best example in the urinary tract being the cercariae of *Schistosoma haematobium*, which are able to penetrate unbroken skin for a few hours after being shed by the intermediate snail host (Figure 7.4).

Table 7.6 Target sites of common antimicrobial drugs. It is convenient to consider the action of the antibiotic as it relates to bacterial cell structure – cell wall, cytoplasmic membrane, ribosomal function and nucleic acid synthesis

Drug	Target/mechanism
β-lactam (penicillin, cephalosporin)	Cell wall: disruption of peptidoglycan X-linkage
Aminoglycosides	Ribosomal interference: misreading mRNA
Erythromycin	Translocation interference
Tetracyclines	RNA-binding interference
Trimethoprim	Nucleic acid interference: dihydrofolate reductase inhibition
Fluoroquinolones (ciprofloxacin)	Inhibit DNA gyrase

Antihumoral activity

As noted above, antibodies such as secretory IgA may be active against organisms before mucosal invasion occurs. Organisms such as *N. gonorrhoeae* and *Proteus mirabilis* elaborate anti-IgA proteases that inactivate this defence mechanism. A further antihumoral virulence factor is exhibited by certain isolates of *N. gonorrhoeae* that are able to resist the lytic effects of complement. Such strains are thus able to multiply and enter the host bloodstream, whereas those isolates that lack this virulence factor are unable to invade and remain localised on the surface of the genital tract [13]. Resistance to the bactericidal effect of serum/complement has been linked to the integrity of the lipopolysaccharide cell wall (O antigen). Additionally, loss of capsular polysaccharide (K antigen) has been associated with lack of resistance to complement-mediated lysis [14].

Evasion of phagocytosis

A number of bacteria have developed mechanisms for resisting phagocytic attack by the host. Variation in surface antigens and the properties of some polysaccharide capsules may constitute a successful defence mechanism by preventing interaction between the phagocytic cell and the invading organism [13].

Competition for nutrients

To be successful, any invading micro-organism will require an adequate supply of nutrients. Free iron, in particular, is required for metabolism and multiplication of *E. coli*, iron uptake being facilitated by the siderophore aerobactin. The ability to produce aerobactin thus confers an advantage on strains invading the urinary tract, and an association has been observed between aerobactin production and the expression of P fimbriae (see below) in patients with symptomatic urinary tract infection [15].

Adherence mechanisms

The adherence of a cell to another structure is an extremely important biological characteristic that can be observed widely throughout nature. Early reports of this phenomenon [16] were slightly misleading as the particular mechanisms of attachment were not fully understood at that time. General observations of bac-

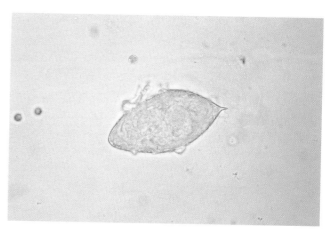

Figure 7.4 Schistosoma haematobium. *The spike-like projection at the end of the egg identifies the organism compared to the projections of* Schistosoma mansoni, *which are located in the equatorial region. The cercariae are uniquely able to perforate intact human skin. (Photomicrograph courtesy of Dr Alan Curry, UHSM.)*

teria and algae adhering to inert plastic or rocks in streams were brought together with other observations of various bacteria adhering in vivo to a number of epithelial surfaces. It is now possible to distinguish the individual mechanisms by which adhesion takes place in each of these specialised circumstances (Table 7.7). Although fimbriae are of overriding importance in urinary tract infection, it is helpful briefly to describe and contrast other methods of adhesion. Adherence is defined as the initial interaction of a micro-organism with the host. An adhesin is a microbiological molecule that leads to bacterial adhesion to cells or tissues. Adhesins predominantly react with specific receptors on the host cell surface, although non-specific adhesion (by surface charge etc.) may occur.

Types of adhesins

Afimbrial adhesins consist of polymers, polysaccharides, lipoteichoic acid and other proteins associated with the cell wall of the organism. Collectively, these

Table 7.7 Recognised adhesion mechanisms. See text for details

Afimbrial adhesins
Adherence pedestals
Fimbriae

are known as a 'glycocalix' and together they serve to attach the organism to the target cell. The classical studies into glycocalix formation involved *Streptococcus mutans*, an organism that colonises human teeth, leading to decay. Enzymatic activity at the cell surface degrades sucrose, providing fructose for ongoing nutrition, but also polymerises glucose into polysaccharide chains used to construct the glycocalix. Thus, the organism attaches itself to its target at the same time as protecting itself against attack and concentrating its nutrients by wrapping itself within the glycocalix – also known as a 'biofilm' [17].

Helicobacter pylori provides a typical example of an organism that attaches via small cellular projections known as adherence pedestals. This organism, with its unmistakable flagella (approximately three times the size of fimbriae, see below), attaches to cells within the gastric epithelium, leading to ulceration and perhaps gastric carcinoma (Figure 7.5a). Presumably, the flagella drives the organism downwards into the mucosa, following which, adhesion to the target cells take place (Figure 7.5b).

Fimbriae (also known as pili) are important virulence structures that mediate attachment to host tissues and are particularly important in the pathogenesis of *E. coli* urinary tract infection. A typical organism may have 100–500 appendages, each approximately 5–10 nm in diameter and 2 μm in length (Figure 7.6). Isolates of *E. coli* may produce a number of antigenically distinct fimbriae, although some strains produce no fimbriae at all.

Functional and structural definition of fimbriae

Various methods, such as electron microscopy and erythrocyte agglutination, have been used to characterise the different types of fimbriae. Type I fimbriae cause haemagglutination of guinea-pig erythrocytes, this reaction being inhibited by the presence of mannose; hence, these adhesins are commonly known as mannose-sensitive pili. Such fimbriae are to be found on most *E. coli* isolates and the precise role of the adhesin (see below) has yet to be defined. Mannose-sensitive pili may facilitate general attachment to epithelial cells of the lower genitourinary tract and are certainly responsible for attachment to uromucoid [9] and to urinary catheters [18].

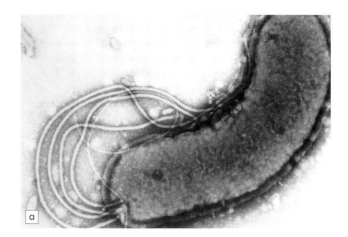

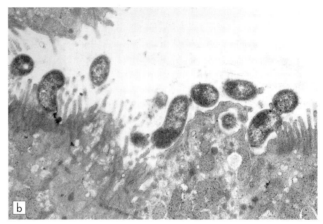

Figure 7.5 Helicobacter pylori. *(a) The flagellae of the organism are easily identified (significantly larger than fimbriae). (b) The flagellae are used to propel the organism into gastric mucosa, where adhesins provide attachment. (Photomicrographs courtesy of Dr Alan Curry, UHSM.)*

P fimbriae, so called as they specifically adhere to uroepithelial cells and P blood group antigens on human erythrocytes, are also known as mannose-resistant pili as addition of the sugar does not inhibit the haemagglutination reaction. P fimbriae are particularly important in diseases of the urinary tract, and the clinical significance is discussed below. Some strains of organisms may express both type I and type P pili and such expression may vary according to the conditions of growth, a factor that may complicate attempts to identify virulence factors by in-vitro bacteriological studies. Variation in pilus expression is known as phase variation [19].

In addition to the above fimbrial types, there are a number of adhesins, including S, type 1c, G, M and X, which have been identified to date. These adherence

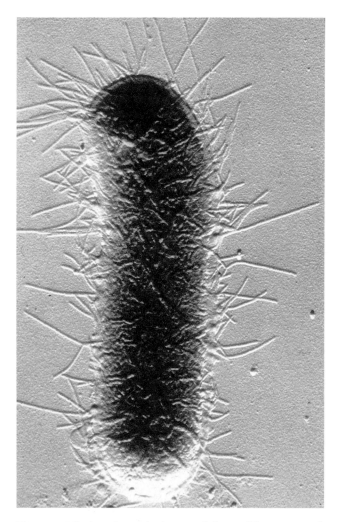

Figure 7.6 Escherichia coli *showing fimbriae. (Photomicrograph courtesy of Dr Pauline Handley, University of Manchester.)*

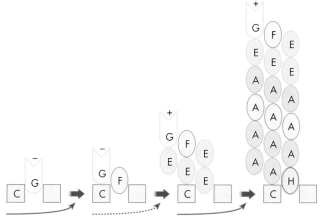

Figure 7.7 *Pilus assembly and structure. The P pilus is constructed and assembled on a platform of PapC protein. The adhesion characteristics are chiefly determined by the terminal PapG protein, which must be some distance from the platform before it is able to function (− = no adhesion; + = able to adhere). The PapA subunits are formed in a helical fashion into the stem of the pilus, the entire structure being approximately 1000 subunits long. (Data from Lindberg et al. [20].)*

mechanisms may be associated with some strains of uropathogenic *E. coli*, although a full description is outside the scope of this text.

Structure and ultrastructure of P fimbriae

Advances in molecular biology have enabled the structure of P fimbriae to be elucidated (Figure 7.7). The Pap pili (*p*ili *a*ssociated with *p*yelonephritis) essentially consist of four proteins, PapA, PapE, PapF and PapG, constructed and assembled on a platform of PapC protein. PapG is chiefly responsible for binding to the receptor, whilst protein PapA constitutes the bulk of the 'stem' of the pilus, approximately 1000 subunits being arranged in a helical fashion between the surface of the organism and the active tip proteins [20]. Experimental observations suggest that

the adhesion characteristics are maintained by the GFE tip proteins, even in the absence of the helical structure PapA stem subunits. It has been suggested that the reason for the seemingly dispensable fibre structure is that this length places the adhesin outside the lipopolysaccharide cell surface structure of *E. coli* (see below), thus maintaining the integrity of the individual virulence mechanisms [20].

Recent advances in the understanding of receptor structure for the G tip protein are leading to significant advances in knowledge concerning the mechanisms of urinary tract infection. Table 7.8 annotates the globoseries glycolipid isoreceptor types, each of which contains the disaccharide α-GAL-1-4-β-GAL (known colloquially as GAL-GAL), and their association with disease. Different positioning of the disaccharide within the molecule in each of the isoreceptors determines the adherence capability of the G tip proteins. Organisms with class I tip proteins do not adhere and do not cause disease in humans due to the absence of the globo-isoreceptor. Those with class II are strongly associated with pyelonephritis, whilst class III adhesins are commonly found in patients with cystitis [21]. Thus, the structure of the globo isoreceptor determines the outcome between invading organism and host: patients with infections from

Table 7.8 Globoseries glycolipid isoreceptor types and their association with disease. The essential chemical structure of the receptor has been emphasised by bold underlined text. For further details concerning the site of the disaccharide GAL-GAL core receptor, see reference 21. Globo A is similar but not identical to the Forssman antigen and has been investigated as part of comparative receptor studies [23, 24]

Pilus G tip protein epitope class	Glycolipid isoreceptor	Agglutinate red cells from	Disease association
I	Globo<u>tria</u>osylceramide	Rabbit	Not in human
II	Globo<u>tetra</u>osylceramide (globoside)	Human Pig	Pyelonephritis
III	Globo<u>penta</u>osylceramide (Forssman antigen)	Goat Sheep ?Human	Cystitis

coliforms expressing class II adhesins are unlikely to suffer from cystitis, globoside being the major isoreceptor in the human kidney [22]. Similarly, the association of class III adhesin with cystitis suggests a predominance of Forssman receptors on the urothelium of the lower urinary tract. Further studies of receptor expression by means of differential blood group analysis [23] have demonstrated that minor differences in receptor core structure profoundly affect disease patterns and emphasise the importance of precise 'fitness' if bacteria are to persist and multiply within the lower urinary tract [24]. Nevertheless, despite these studies of adhesin/receptor interactions, the importance of non-specific mechanisms such as electrostatic and hydrophobic attractive forces should not be overlooked [22].

Clinical relevance of fimbrinated status

Long before the mechanisms of adherence were fully understood, observational studies had indicated a connection between macroscopically observed bacterial adherence and the severity of urinary tract infection. This phenomenon was first reported in the *Lancet* in 1976 by Catharina Svanborg Edén and colleagues from the Department of Immunology in Göteborg, Sweden, a department that has continued at the forefront of adherence research. Uroepithelial cells from freshly voided morning urine samples were added to bacterial cells and the mixture incubated during rotation for 60 minutes. Adherent bacteria (Figure 7.8) were counted under direct light microscopy. The

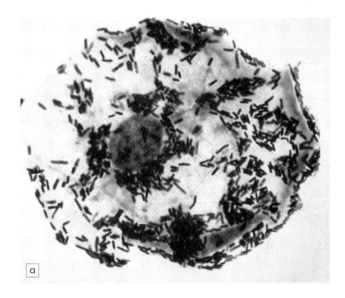

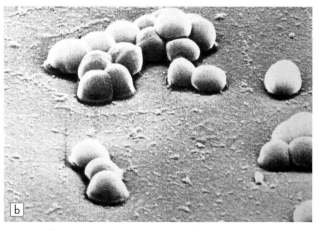

Figure 7.8 *Examples of bacterial adherence. (a) Adherence of* Escherichia coli *to epithelial cell. (b) Adhesion of colonies to the surface of a urinary catheter. Such adhesion is thought to be mediated by type 1 fimbriae [18].*

results (Figure 7.9) demonstrated convincingly that pyelonephritic strains were more adherent than strains from other disorders of the lower urinary tract [25]. This effect was negated when the organisms were incubated with antibodies against the strain tested. These observations were extended by Fowler and Stamey, who studied adherence to vaginal cells from controls and from women susceptible to lower urinary tract infection (Figure 7.10). Significant adherence was demonstrated, suggesting the possibility that general cellular characteristics might be involved in the adherence process [26]. This concept was taken further by Schaeffer and co-workers, who confirmed the findings on vaginal cells and then showed that the same phenomenon could be observed on buccal cells (Figure 7.11). These observations clearly indicated that there might be a widespread alteration in the surface characteristics of mucosal epithelial cells in particular susceptible individuals [27].

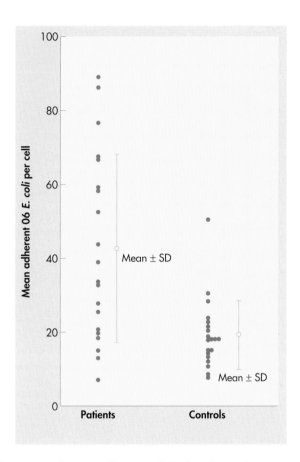

Figure 7.10 *In-vitro adherence of* Escherichia coli *to vaginal epithelial cells in patients susceptible to recurrent urinary tract infection compared to controls. (Data from Fowler and Stamey [26].)*

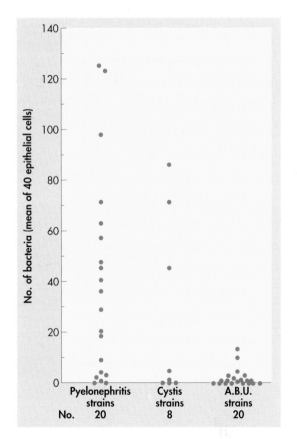

Figure 7.9 Escherichia coli *adhering to 40 healthy, human, urinary tract epithelial cells. Organisms from patients with asymptomatic bacteriuria adhered minimally when compared to those from cases of pyelonephritis. (Data from Svanborg Edén et al. [25].)*

Previously, Sellwood and co-workers at the Veterinary Agricultural Research Council had noted that the administration of *E. coli* strains expressing K-88 surface antigen caused neonatal diarrhoea in some piglets but not in others. This phenomenon was observed to be due to K-88 adherence to intestinal cell brush borders in piglets that developed diarrhoea, whereas those that remained well did not show this phenomenon [28, 29]. Subsequently, it was found that 'adhesive' and 'non-adhesive' piglets inherited these intestinal cellular characteristics in a simple Mendelian manner and these findings have since been acknowledged as the first report of a genetic basis for resistance to enteric disease [30]. Schaeffer, quoting this work, noted that it might explain in part why some patients' resistance to infectious disease could correlate with their blood groups [31].

The subsequent ability to identify P fimbrinated varieties of *E. coli* allowed further investigation into

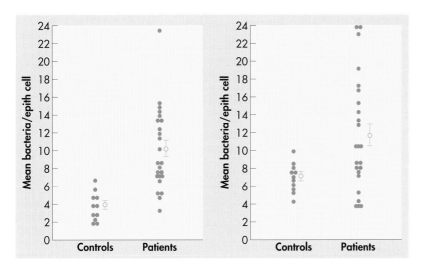

Figure 7.11 In-vitro adherence of Escherichia coli to vaginal cells (left) and buccal cells (right) from patients with recurrent urinary tract infections as compared to controls. (Data from Schaeffer et al. [27].)

the mechanisms of urinary tract infection. Källenius et al. [32] examined 97 children with urinary tract infection and compared them with 82 healthy controls. P fimbrinated forms were found in 33/35 (94%) of urinary strains causing acute pyelonephritis but in only 19% of patients with cystitis and in 14% of cases with asymptomatic bacteriuria (Table 7.9). By contrast, only 7% of faecal isolates from healthy controls carried such fimbriae. Further evidence of the importance of P fimbrination was observed by Johnson and co-workers [33], who investigated host conditions that might be associated with increased frequency of P fimbriae or other virulence factors. These studies clearly showed that, whilst P fimbrinated forms remained relatively common in the presence of anatomical urinary tract abnormality or after instrumentation, the fimbrinated form was absolutely essential if infection was to occur when none of these predisposing abnormalities was present. Summarising, coliform strains with a variety of characteristics are capable of causing upper urinary tract infection in the presence of (i.e. with the help of) obstruction or other abnormalities; however, for infection to supervene in a completely normal upper urinary tract, the presence of the P-fimbrinated form of E. coli is near essential.

By contrast, debate continues as to the influence of the various fimbrinated forms in lower urinary tract infection. Type I fimbriae are found in a majority of Enterobacteriaceae, on both non-pathogenic as well as pathogenic E. coli. As noted above, such mannose-sensitive fimbriae adhere powerfully to urinary slime [9], although the advantage conferred by such adherence remains obscure. Other established host targets of mannose-sensitive pili include vaginal cells and vaginal mucus as well as the surface of foreign bodies such as catheters (see Figure 7.8b). Recent studies of

Table 7.9 Study by Källenius et al. [32] of 97 children with urinary tract infection (UTI) compared to 82 healthy controls

Collection place and time	Febrile, symptomatic UTI (clinical pyelonephritis)	Afebrile, symptomatic UTI (cystitis)	Afebrile, asymptomatic UTI (ABU)	Controls (faeces)
Stockholm area:				
Jan–Nov 1979	11/12	—	—	1/30*
Jan 1979–Dec 1980	16/17[†]	4/19	4/35	5/40**
Malmö area:				
March–Dec 1980	6/6	1/7	1/1	0/12**
Total	33/55 (p < 0.001)[§]	5/26 (p = 0.17)	5/36 (p = 0.43)	6/82

*Adults. One colony per specimen examined; [†]Collecting period Dec 1979–Dec 1980; **Children. Six colonies per specimen examined; [§]Significance level compared with faecal controls.

cystitis in young schoolgirls [34], chosen (by age) to exclude the effect of sexual intercourse, observed that the clones of organisms responsible for the infection were P fimbrinated, whereas these forms were not usually found on the perineum – where clones exhibiting type I fimbriae and other virulence factors predominated. These observations, when summarised, indicate that type I fimbriae are commonly to be found in the faecal reservoir as well as in the periurethral zone and may well facilitate the initial move towards the lower urinary tract. Thereafter, however, the evidence suggests that P-fimbrinated forms determine the course of disease. Strains exhibiting class II G tip protein are likely to cause upper urinary tract infection and pyelonephritis; strains exhibiting class III G tip protein (ab initio or by phase variation) are able to bind to the Forssman receptor and initiate significant lower urinary tract infection.

Therapeutic implications

The observations noted above might assist the treatment of affected individuals in a number of ways. Variation in adhesion potential might identify at-risk groups. Fimbriae would appear to be a rational target for antimicrobial therapy and vaccine development. In the veterinary piglets experiment referred to above, effective vaccines based initially on the K-88 antigen were developed and successfully prevented neonatal diarrhoea in the susceptible groups. Immunisation with purified P fimbriae has been attempted in a number of animal models, with variable success. As might be expected, phase variation and other types of antigen variability might be expected to cause problems in this type of therapeutic approach.

Virulence factors in other uropathogens

Not surprisingly, studies of other species involved in urinary tract infection have demonstrated the presence of adherence mechanisms. *Proteus mirabilis* and *Klebsiella* spp. have been found to express fimbriae in animal experiments [35, 36]. *Staph. saprophyticus* is acknowledged as being able to adhere avidly to uroepithelial cells, probably by non-specific adherence mechanisms.

Summary of virulence factors in urinary tract infections

It is appropriate to bring together those factors that are thought to be important with respect to the virulence of Gram-negative bacteria in general and *E. coli* in particular (Figure 7.12; Table 7.10).

The antigenic structure of the bacterial surface is classically described in terms of three classes of antigens. O antigens represent the polysaccharide sidechains of the lipopolysaccharide structure found in all Gram-negative bacteria. The polysaccharide is anchored to the outer membrane by lipid A (see Figure

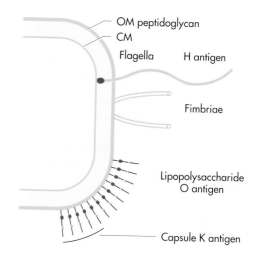

Figure 7.12 *Schematic diagram of cell wall Gram-negative bacteria and associated structures. CM = cytoplasmic membrane; OM = outer membrane. Note differential size of flagella and fimbriae. Lipid A (see text) is on the innermost aspect of the lipopolysaccharide O antigen next to the outer membrane (see also Figure 7.20).*

Table 7.10 Virulence factors associated with *E. coli*

Specific O serotypes
K capsular antigen
Adherence mechanisms
Resistance to serum bactericidal activity
Haemolysin production
Aerobactin production
Colicin V

7.20), the agent thought to be responsible for endotoxic shock, as described below. O antigens are heat stable and, classically, certain serogroups (01, 02, 04, 06, 07, 016, 018 and 075) are responsible for urinary infections, such strains being responsible for up to 80% of cases of pyelonephritis. Modern theory suggests that the O antigen is not itself specifically responsible for pathogenicity but rather the identified serogroupings represent clones of organisms with a selection or panel of various virulence properties that enable successful colonisation of the urinary tract. Other serogroupings, and hence other combinations of virulence factors, may enable successful colonisation of other areas such as the gastrointestinal tract. K capsular antigen is partially heat stable and may on occasion partially obscure the O antigen (Figure 7.12). K capsular polysaccharide antigen has been strongly associated with pyelonephritis for many years, both in adults [37] and in children [38]. Seventy per cent of strains from children with pyelonephritis were associated with K1, K2, K3, K12 and K13 antigens, of which K1 is acknowledged to be the most frequently associated strain with pyelonephritic disease. Interestingly, K1 strains have also been associated with 80% of E. coli strains causing neonatal meningitis [38].

Adherence mechanisms have been fully described above, and the relationship between type 1 fimbriae, P fimbriae and the ability to cause urinary tract infection has been noted. Typically, E. coli may be killed by serum bactericidal activity relating to both the classical and alternative pathways of complement. Cell wall lipopolysaccharide (O antigen) is thought to provide a degree of resistance against complement-mediated digestion and, recently, Leying and associates have suggested that the K1 polysaccharide antigen may also confer significant levels of serum resistance to the organism [14]. The advantages conferred on those organisms expressing haemolysin and aerobactin have been noted above. Colicin V is another virulence factor that has selectively been found to be present in isolates from urine but not in isolates from the faecal reservoir. Colicin V is assumed to interfere with host defence mechanisms [11, 12].

Organisms responsible for urinary tract infection

The great majority of urinary tract infections are caused by single bacterial species and, amongst these, E. coli is by far the most common, accounting for approximately 85% of general or community-based infections at the present time. Previous studies (Table 7.11) have emphasised the differences between general practice and hospital practice, where E. coli accounts for only approximately 50% of the isolates. Proteus, Klebsiella, Enterococci and Pseudomonas are all more frequently isolated from hospital patients, especially if an indwelling catheter is present [39, 40]. Remaining organisms include Enterobacter, Citrobacter and Serratia; fungal infections are rarely encountered outside hospital practice.

The presence of abnormalities in the urinary tract, as may be found in congenital abnormality or obstruction, often leads to infection by non-coliform organisms such as Proteus and Klebsiella and, additionally, under these circumstances, mixed infections are frequently encountered. Naturally, obstruction related to stone formation is often associated with P. mirabilis. Staph. saprophyticus has been identified, particularly in the USA, as a cause of acute cystitis in young sexually active females [41]. Anaerobic organisms are rarely pathogens in the urinary tract. Maskell and co-workers supported the concept that slow-growing, carbon dioxide-dependent Gram-positive bacteria might be responsible for the 'urethral syndrome' [42], although these suggestions that 'fastidious' organisms could be responsible for the symptom complex were strongly denied by other workers [43]. Apart from Lactobacilli, Gardinerella vaginalis and Ureaplasma urealyticum are not infrequently isolated, but their role in infection of the lower urinary tract remains unproven.

Routes of infection
Organisms may enter the urinary tract via the ascending route, the haematogenous route or the lymphatic route.

Ascending route
The difference in the incidence of lower urinary tract infection between men and women strongly suggests

Table 7.11 Organisms causing urinary tract infection in community and hospital practice. Although the proportions of organisms have remained relatively similar, it is accepted that in the 1990s approximately 80–85% of community urinary tract infection is related to *Escherichia coli*. The comparable figure for hospital-based infections has remained steady, at approximately 50%

	General practice		Hospital practice	
	1976[1]	1971[2]	1971[2]	1978[2]
E. coli	72	78.5	55.4	50.7
Proteus mirabilis	9	9.2	11.4	10.6
Staphylococci	6	5.1	3.3	2.7
Strep. faecalis	3.3	2.3	4.0	4.3
Klebsiella spp.	2.7	2.3	16.8	21.6
Pseudomonas	–	–	2.7	2.8
Remainder	7.0	2.6	6.4	7.3

[1] Ref. 39.
[2] Ref. 40.

that the ascending urethral route is the most common pathway for infection and, in the female, organisms have been isolated from the bladder after both urethral massage [44] and sexual intercourse [45]. One insertion of a urinary catheter into the bladder has been observed to result in lower urinary tract infection in 1–2% of patients [46]. It is widely agreed that the presence of a urethral catheter for more than 36–48 hours almost invariably results in bladder bacteriuria. Recent studies suggest that spermicidal agents encourage the colonisation of the introital region with uropathogenic bacteria [47]. The relationship between the introital flora and lower urinary tract infection is further considered below.

The question of ascent into the upper tract from the bladder in the absence of reflux appears problematical. Presumably, various virulence factors must aid progression through the vesicoureteric junction; perhaps mucosal oedema caused by local inflammation disrupts the valvular mechanisms and allows passage of organisms, which then successfully colonise the upper tracts by means of the appropriate fimbrinated structures. Diuresis and loss of the usual co-apting ureteral mechanisms have also been suggested as mechanisms whereby organisms may gain entry into the upper tract.

Haematogenous route

Blood-borne infection of the kidney is a well described though uncommon mechanism of renal infection in individuals who are otherwise normal. Staphylococcal spread from dental abscesses may occur, and these and other organisms may originate from sites such as diseased heart valves. Haematogenous spread of *Candida albicans* has been observed in experimental circumstances, although this fungus is not usually observed unless a chronic indwelling catheter is present. Interestingly, if one ureter is tied and bacteria are introduced into the bladder during experimentation on animals, infection supervenes in the non-obstructed kidney but not on the hydronephrotic side [48]. This convincingly demonstrates the overriding importance of the ascending route and the relative resistance to haematological spread, even in the presence of severe obstruction – conditions under which it is acknowledged that haematogenous infection should easily supervene.

Lymphatic route

Theoretically, infection could spread via the lymphatics into various parts of the urinary tract, but in practice there is little clinical evidence for such a mode of infection. Occasional experimental reports have failed to provide evidence that the lymphatic route is other than of academic interest.

Clinical aspects of urinary tract infection

The significance of 'significance'

Historically, there have always been difficulties in distinguishing between true bacteriuria – defined as actual residence of bacteria within the urinary tract – and contamination – defined as the adventitious entry of bacteria into the urine during the collection of the specimen. This problem was most notably tackled in the mid-1950s by Edward H. Kass from Boston, who performed a number of studies on women with various disorders of the lower urinary tract in both the normal and pregnant states. In his most important study, the urine of female patients attending outpatient clinics was studied, specimens being obtained by catheterisation and cultured promptly thereafter [49]. Kass found (Figure 7.13) that the patients could broadly be divided into two groups. In the first group were patients with bacterial counts between 0 and 100 000 per ml of urine and, of these, only approximately 15% had a past history of urinary tract infection, instrumentation or catheterisation of the urinary

tract. Kass noted that the bacteria obtained in this group were usually the common saprophytes of the urinary tract and his contention that these were contaminated specimens was further supported by the fact that second samples obtained from the same group usually demonstrated dissimilar organisms and counts.

By contrast, in the second group, with more than 100 000 bacteria per ml, 55% had a past history of urinary tract infections and repeat sampling in these patients revealed similar high counts, both specimens yielding commonly accepted pathogens of the urinary tract. These simple yet ground-breaking observations define the level of 'bacterial significance' widely used to this day: 10^5 organisms or colony-forming units (CFU) per ml from midstream urine.

For a quarter of a century, the scientific distinction between patients with contaminants and patients with true infection was broadly welcomed. Gradually, however, it became clear that there were a significant number of women with dysuria and frequent urination whose midstream urines did not contain 'significant' bacteriuria and to these women the label 'acute urethral syndrome' was applied. In an important study, Stamm and co-workers investigated 59 women with the 'acute urethral syndrome' from whom bladder urine was obtained by either suprapubic aspiration or clean urethral catheterisation. Forty-two patients had abnormal pyuria and 37 of these were infected with coliforms, *Staph. saprophyticus* or *Chlamydia trachomatis*. Patients without pyuria had little demonstrable infection. Stamm concluded that the classic

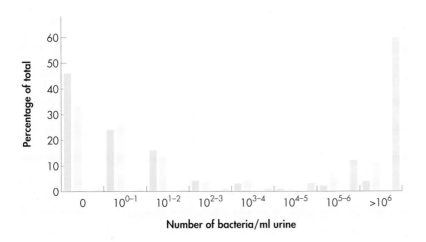

Figure 7.13 Bacterial counts in the urine of various population groups. Kass noted that most of the patients with low counts did not have a history of urinary tract infection and, in these cases, reculture frequently demonstrated different organisms. However, patients with >10^5 organisms frequently had pure cultures associated with significant clinical infections (pyelonephritis). ■ *'Asymptomatic' women in medical OPD (335).* *'Asymptomatic' diabetic women (89).* *'Asymptomatic' women with cystocele (92).* ■ *Patients with diagnosis of pyelonephritis (74). (Data from Kass [49].)*

Kass criteria of $>10^5$/ml was an insensitive diagnostic criterion when applied to symptomatic lower urinary tract infection in this group of relatively young, sexually active women [50].

This and other similar studies [51] provoked a flurry of editorial comment [52, 53]. Doubt was cast over the suggestion that 10^2 organisms per ml could reliably discriminate between patients with infected and uninfected lower urinary tracts. Additionally, it was noted that many midstream urine cultures were mixed – ignoring conventional wisdom that true pathogens are usually found in pure culture. Nevertheless, it was acknowledged that most of Stamm's bacteriuric patients ($>10^2$, $<10^5$) had pyuria, suggesting that this was indeed a true infection [52]. Stamm himself made further comment and reviewed the situation in 1984 [53]. He pointed out that the essence of Kass's original work (often forgotten) concerned patients with pyelonephritis, not women with acute frequency/dysuria lower tract symptoms. He made a plea for closer communication between clinicians and laboratory so as to obtain better information from the more flexible approach to quantitative bacteriological sampling. There is little doubt that urologists should be aware that 'no significant growth' may mean different things according to definitions in different bacteriological laboratories. It is the responsibility of each clinician to determine whether such a report refers to 10^5 CFU/ml or 10^2 CFU/ml; as usual, optimum results only arise from close co-operation between clinicians and the laboratory service.

The introital question

Another major microbiological debate concerns the means whereby pathogenic organisms pass from the (presumed) faecal reservoir to the lower urinary tract. In particular, the importance of organisms that colonise the vaginal introitus and periurethral region has been discussed at great length and the debate continues to the present day.

There seems little doubt that E. coli – pathogenic or otherwise – may obtain a foothold in the introital area and in this respect it has been noted above that mannose-sensitive type 1 pili adhere powerfully to vaginal epithelial cells [27], vaginal mucous [54] and uromucoid [9]. It has additionally been emphasised that type 1 fimbriae are to be found on non-pathogenic as well as on pathogenic Enterobacteriaceae.

Three essential questions may be asked. (i) Do women at risk from urinary tract infections carry pathogenic organisms in the introital and periurethral area? (ii) If so, are these organisms responsible for the symptomatic bladder or pyelonephritic infection? (iii) In such cases, what is the state of the introital and periurethral area between overt symptomatic clinical infections?

A number of workers support the concept that abnormal periurethral flora is to be found in women with recurrent infections. Hinman's group [55] studied 43 patients and found that the flora contained a higher percentage of pathogenic micro-organisms than that of female subjects without urological disease. In a general practice study from London, Grüneberg observed that the infecting strain of E. coli was isolated from rectal, vaginal and periurethral flora in nearly all cases. Furthermore, he noted that chemotherapy eradicated the organism from the urine but not necessarily from the introital/urethral area [56]. Stamey studied cultures from 20 premenopausal controls compared to cultures from nine women with recurrent urinary infections [57]. He observed that not only was introital colonisation significantly higher in the patients but, additionally, Enterobacteriaceae persist after the infectious episode, and he postulated that the introital mucosa in women with infection was biologically different from the same area in women who never suffer from lower urinary tract infection. This postulate was supported some years later by Pfau and Sacks [58], who had previously shown that the predominant bacterial flora of the introital and periurethral area consisted of Lactobacilli and Staphylococci, Gram-negative bacteria being infrequent and transitory. These workers found E. coli to be the predominant micro-organism recovered from 68% of introital, 60% of vaginal and 42% of urethral cultures. Despite these apparently conclusive results by American researchers, a number of British workers failed to confirm the findings [59–62]. Nevertheless, although an absolute association between periurethral flora and lower urinary tract infection could not be demonstrated, it was acknowledged that the presence of E. coli in the introital area might constitute a 'permissive factor' for the subsequent development of overt infection [59]. Similarly, O'Grady and co-workers could find no difference in the carriage rate between normal women and women with symptoms suggestive of urinary tract infection, although again these workers acknowledged that introital bacteria were more commonly recovered in patients when symptomatic (34%) than when symptom free (19%) [60]. In a further development, Brumfitt observed that women with recurrent urinary infections were susceptible to perineal and periurethral colonisation with Gram-negative bacteria, but they noted that the infection need not be with the colonising enterobacteria [61]. Kunin attempted to reconcile these positions [58 – editorial comment] by suggesting that most workers could agree that infections were indeed preceded by colonisation of the periurethral area with Gram-negative bacteria but he considered that the evidence for colonisation of this area between infections was less convincing. It may be argued that the presence or absence of organisms is not as critical as the ability of any organisms that may be present – i.e. the virulence mechanism carried on those organisms – to ascend and invade the lower urinary tract. In summary, colonisation is important but the critical factor relates to the presence or absence of essential virulence mechanisms.

Urinary tract infection: variation by age and sex

It is appropriate at this point to review the changes that may occur in the urinary tract of either sex as a result of invasion by micro-organisms. Table 7.12 records the prevalence of bacteriuria by age in either sex as determined by studies in the literature. It is immediately apparent that bacteriuria is more common in females at all times of life, with the single exception of babies under three months old, in which group boys are more than twice as likely as girls to have clinical infection.

Infants

In the first month of life, there is a virtually identical incidence of urinary tract infection in girls compared to boys [63]. Interestingly, in babies under three months old, the infection rate in boys depends on whether circumcision has been performed. For those who have had the operation, the incidence of infection is significantly less than that of girls of the same age. For uncircumcised infants, however, the risk is considerably greater and it is clear that the presence of the foreskin is linked to an increased incidence of lower urinary tract infection. These observations were made in a remarkable study of 422 328 children born to members of the American services over a ten-year

Table 7.12 Prevalence of bacteriuria by age (%). The identified groups of patients are fully discussed in the text

	Age (years)									
	<½	<3/12	<5	School age	Young men	Non-pregnant females	Pregnant females	Pregnant females previous bacteriuria	65–70	>80
Male	0.075	Circumcised 0.07 Non-circumcised 0.77	0.5	0.03	<0.1	–	–	–	2–3	>20
Female	0.077	0.3	4.5	1.2	–	1.3	4–7	35	20	>20
Reference	63	63	67	68, 69, 70, 71, 72	–	73	72, 74, 75	70, 71	76	76

period. Precision military record keeping allowed the results of circumcision to be accurately documented (Figure 7.14). A surprising 80% of the male population underwent circumcision but the 20% who did not suffered 70% of the male urinary tract infections [63]. The authors later proved their point by noting that a subsequent decline in the circumcision rate was associated with an increased incidence of male infant infection [64].

Preschool children

Urinary tract infection is important in children of this age group as renal development is usually considered to be most at risk at this time. Both symptomatic and asymptomatic infections are more common in girls, although the line between the two is difficult to draw – careful history taking in children with so-called 'asymptomatic bacteriuria' often reveal symptoms strongly suggestive of urinary tract infection [65]. From the first year onwards, infections become increasingly uncommon in male infants and, indeed, the presence of such an infection may indicate significant pathology or other abnormality of the urinary tract. Infections in girls may be troublesome and, as noted above, permanent damage relating to the reflux of infected urine may occur by mechanisms such as those described by Ransley [66]. It is difficult to avoid the conclusion that bacteriuria is a very important finding in this group of children [67].

Bacteriuria in schoolchildren

As can be seen from Table 7.12, the problem of bacteriuria in schoolchildren relates almost entirely to girls. There is an impressive body of evidence concerning the nature and outcome of such infections. In Charlottesville, Virginia, an area with a stable local population, Kunin prospectively studied the characteristics and natural history of urinary tract infection in schoolgirls between 1959 and 1968. It was observed that bacteriuria was common in schoolgirls and symptoms were often absent; recurrences frequently occurred [68]. Approximately one-third of girls had symptoms of the infection at the time of detection. In the UK, Meadow and co-workers reported broadly similar findings in Birmingham schoolchildren. Infection in male schoolchildren was essentially undetectable, but 1% of girls had significant asymptomatic bacteriuria [69]. In another important prospective study, the Cardiff/Oxford Bacteriuria Study Group followed 208 girls from 5 to 12 years of age who had been identified as suffering from bacteriuria. The girls were followed for four years and the authors noted that treatment had little effect on the emergence of symptoms, the clearance of vesicoureteric reflux, renal growth or the progression of renal scars. These observations seemed to suggest that renal damage had occurred before five years of age, as noted above [70].

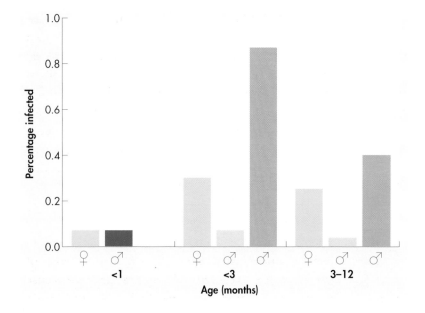

Figure 7.14 Urinary tract infection in infants under the age of one year. The incidence of infection is approximately similar for both sexes under one month, but thereafter girls have more infections than boys unless the boys have not been circumcised. ■ Circumcised; ■ uncircumcised. (Data from Wiswell and Roscelli [63].)

The effect of bacteriuria on subsequent pregnancy
Both Kunin's group and the Oxford/Cardiff group continued to follow their young ladies as they grew up and eventually became pregnant. These irreplaceable studies have emphasised the importance of vigilance with respect to young bacteriuric schoolgirls.

Gillenwater reported the American results in 1979. Sixty schoolgirls with bacteriuria and 38 matched controls had been followed for periods up to 18 years. Renal scars and/or caliectasis were observed to occur only in the bacteriuric group, but renal function and blood pressure were not affected. The study group had ten times as many bacteriuric episodes as did controls, and infections were particularly common during subsequent pregnancy. Most interestingly, seven children of the bacteriuric mothers but none of the controls themselves showed urinary tract infections [71].

The Oxford/Cardiff group studied 52 pregnancies in 34 women who had been found to have bacteriuria in childhood. At the first antenatal visit, the prevalence of bacteriuria in the study group was significantly greater (35%) than that in the control group (5%). During pregnancy, pyelonephritis developed in 10% of the study group and in 4% of controls. The data suggested that previously bacteriuric women known to have renal scars were at increased risk from hypertension and pre-eclampsia of pregnancy, findings that have not been universally accepted. No comment was made about the children resulting from these pregnancies and their susceptibility or otherwise to urinary tract infection [72].

In summary, therefore, these observations show that asymptomatic bacteriuria in schoolgirls persists over long periods of time. Subsequently, such young ladies are at greater risk of infections during pregnancy and, if renal damage has occurred in earlier life, the pregnancy may perhaps be complicated by hypertension or pre-eclampsia. The children of such women appear to inherit an ongoing susceptibility to bacteriuria and infection.

Young non-pregnant females
It is generally accepted that the prevalence of bacteriuria in this group is approximately 1% per decade. To investigate the assumption that this was largely inter-course related, Kunin's group compared the prevalence of significant bacteriuria in nuns and married women. It was found, as expected, that celibacy was associated with a lower frequency of infection, but young nuns still had a higher frequency of urinary infection than young males. Kunin commentated later that it was not clear from this study whether there was a subpopulation of women who were inherently susceptible to urinary infection that was not the result of sexual intercourse [73].

Bacteriuria during pregnancy
There is general agreement that between 4% and 7% of pregnant women have bacteriuria [74, 75] and, of these, between 20% and 40% will develop symptomatic infection later in the pregnancy, usually in the third trimester. Bacteriuria in the lower urinary tract more commonly leads to pyelonephritis in pregnant rather than in non-pregnant women, presumably because of the various changes that occur in the upper tracts as a result of the pregnancy. The prevalence of bacteriuria during pregnancy rises with parity, sexual activity, age, diabetes mellitus and the presence of the sickle cell trait. It has already been mentioned that pregnant women who were bacteriuric as schoolgirls carry a significantly greater risk of urinary tract infection during pregnancy [70, 71].

Urinary tract infection in young adult men
As previously emphasised, urinary tract infection in otherwise healthy adult men is very uncommon. Presumably, the large difference in prevalence between men and women is related to the length of the urethra and the difficulties which face uropathogens attempting to reach the urethral meatus from the faecal reservoir. The antibacterial nature of prostatic fluid is noted below. Presumably, most infections that occur arise due to sexual intercourse with an infected female partner or, in the case of homosexuality, direct contamination from the faecal reservoir.

Older patients
The higher incidence of urinary tract infection in female patients that operates throughout most of life begins to reverse in old age. Presumably because of prostatic obstruction, residual urine and other

problems in the lower urinary tract of older men, the incidence of bacteriuria rises steeply to significant levels, particularly after the age of 70 (Table 7.12). It has been observed that the place of residence has an important influence on the presence or otherwise of bacteriuria. Older men living at home have a lower incidence of bacteriuria than those living in nursing home accommodation, where the prevalence in both sexes is approximately 20%. Figures for those resident in hospital in-patient facilities are even higher [76].

Uncomplicated cystitis in females

Approximately 20% of women experience an episode of simple cystitis during their lifetime. Most of these episodes settle rapidly, but 2% or 3% suffer from repeat infections. In a Danish study, non-pregnant women between the ages of 16 and 65 years were referred to the medical out-patient clinic where a placebo study of patients with acute symptomatic lower urinary tract infection was undertaken. Fifty-three female patients were given placebo and were followed for more than 12 months following the initial infection; 43 of these (81%) spontaneously cleared their urine within five months [77]. Unfortunately, nearly half these patients became re-infected within a year, and similar observations were found in the antibiotic-treated group. The author concluded that host defence and eradication mechanisms could be very effective, but to keep the recurrence of bacteriuria to a minimum, it would be necessary to recheck urine samples for at least six months after the initial elimination of bacteriuria.

Typically, uncomplicated lower urinary tract infection is caused by E. coli in 80% of domicillary cases. Staph. saprophyticus may be implicated in up to 5% of cases, this organism being particularly noted in the literature from North America. The causes of the 'acute urethral syndrome' as reported by Stamm et al. have already been noted [50]. It seems reasonable that a pure growth of organisms at concentrations between 10^2 and 10^5 accompanied by pyuria should be accepted as a case of true cystitis. The case of bladder urine with mixed organisms and equivocal pyuria is much more debatable; this may perhaps be better described as equivocal cystitis, in contradistinction to the true urethral syndrome described below, in which the symptoms of urethral irritation are accompanied by neither organisms nor pyuria – the female equivalent of 'prostatodynia'.

The urethral syndrome

A critical definition of the female urethral syndrome refers to the symptoms of frequency and dysuria in the absence of bacteriuria and pyuria in both initial (voided bladder I, VB1) and midstream (VB2) urine when analysis is made on several separate occasions. This definition assumes that such female patients have been thoroughly screened to exclude vesical motor dysfunction (bladder instability) as well as systemic and local (e.g. trauma, tumour, irradiation injury) disease [78].

A number of workers have stressed the importance of pyuria in patients with such urethral symptomatology. O'Grady and co-workers [79] proposed that pyuria was significant even when tests failed to identify bacteriuria. In their studies, if cultures were performed over extended periods of time, bacteria were eventually identified and thus this patient group was designated as being 'between infections' [79]. Chlamydia trochomatis was identified in 10 of 16 patients with pyuria but in only 1 of 16 patients without white cells in the urine [50]. The controversy surrounding more fastidious carbon dioxide-dependent organisms – chiefly Lactobacilli – has also been noted [42]. In summary, although considerable effort may be required, the presence of pyuria may often give a clue as to the true bacteriological cause of the frequency dysuria syndrome. Those who have neither bacteriuria nor pyuria constitute the essential core of those who are said to suffer from the true 'urethral syndrome'.

Pyelonephritis

The clinical, radiographic and therapeutic aspects of acute and chronic pyelonephritis are outwith the remit of this chapter. The important virulence factors that enable colonisation of the upper tract have been noted, as have those factors in childhood that later predispose to pyelonephritis of pregnancy. It is generally agreed that uncomplicated pyelonephritis in adults – as opposed to infants under five years – rarely leads to permanent and progressive renal damage with scarring. Renal function usually remains stable.

Stones and infection

Most urinary infections are caused by *E. coli*, but a substantial minority – around 10% – may be due to *Proteus mirabilis*, which is also found in the normal faecal flora. Most patients with simple *Proteus* infections do not form stones, but stone formation is a risk, one that is particularly high when stones are already present. Urease-producing bacteria, of which *Proteus* is the most notable species, may split urea into ammonia and carbon dioxide, with alkalisation of the urine and precipitation of crystals of magnesium, ammonia and calcium phosphate 'triple phosphate', leading to stone formation. Such struvite stones may grow rapidly in infected urine and a vicious circle ensues whereby the organisms themselves are trapped within the stone, safe from the action of antibiotics and the natural host defence mechanisms. Urine cultures at these times may show pyuria but, misleadingly, no bacterial growth. Thus, removal of the stone is an essential part of the treatment of patients with *Proteus* and other urea-splitting urinary tract infections.

Infections of the male genital tract

Prostatitis

Until relatively recently, considerable confusion surrounded the symptom complex of men thought to have 'prostatitis'. In no small part, this was related to problems of terminology: various authorities were describing aspects of prostatitis in the literature but calling these symptom complexes by different names such as 'pelvic floor tension myalgia'. As a result, no-one was very sure exactly who was investigating which group of patients.

This situation was clarified by Drach *et al.*, who suggested a classification in a letter to the *Journal of Urology* [80] that has since become accepted by most workers in the field. The categories are:

1. acute bacterial prostatitis,
2. chronic bacterial prostatitis,
3. non-bacterial prostatitis,
4. prostatodynia.

These four conditions have many symptoms in common but they are also distinguished by specific clinical and microbiological features. Successful treatment in each group depends on meticulous attention to diagnostic detail, without which failure is inevitable.

Organisms responsible for acute bacterial and chronic bacterial prostatitis are generally similar and resemble those organisms responsible for lower urinary tract infection. The majority are grown in pure culture; most often, *E. coli* is isolated, whereas institutionalised patients may harbour more virulent organisms such as *Pseudomonas* or *Streptococcus faecalis*. It has been suggested that the (rare) episodes of cystitis that occur in young men are all secondary to infection of the prostatic ducts.

Aetiological factors thought to be important in acute or chronic bacterial prostatitis include ascending urethral infection and reflux of infected urine into ejaculatory and prostatic ducts. Blacklock [81] noted that patients with chronic bacterial prostatitis frequently had the same pathogens as those identified in the vaginal cultures of their sexual partners. Kirby and co-workers injected carbon particles into the bladders of men about to undergo transurethral resection and found the particles within the prostate on later histological examination, thus proving that significant intraprostatic reflux had taken place [82].

Localisation of infection

It is evident that with a unified genitourinary tract emerging at the urethral meatus, specimens obtained therefrom may relate to urethral, prostatic or bladder infections. To overcome this difficulty, specific techniques have been developed for the localisation of infection [83]. A possible scheme for carrying out such studies is illustrated in Figure 7.15. The localisation tests are not difficult, but require attention to detail and a state of preparedness – failure to attend to such detail usually results in negative findings and a disappointed tertiary referral.

Following arrival in the clinic, the patient passes a VB1 specimen (10 ml – voided bladder 1). This is a 'washout' specimen and relates to urethral disease. After the passage of a further 100–200 ml, the patient collects a standard specimen of midstream urine (VB2 – voided bladder 2). Following this, the prostate is massaged in the usual fashion and prostatic secretion is collected for analysis, as described below. Subsequently, the next voided 10 ml is collected for further

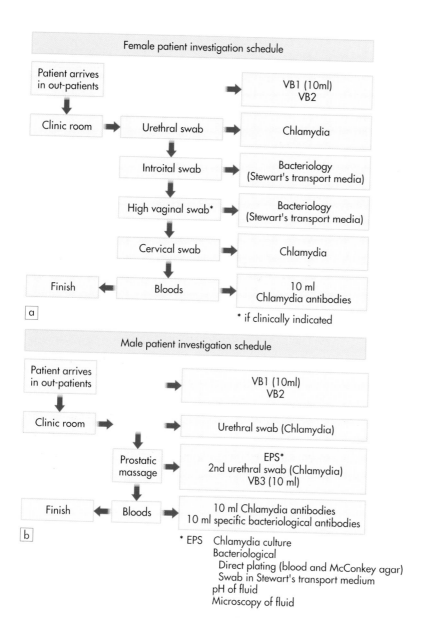

Figure 7.15 *Possible investigation schedules for (a) female and (b) male patients with possible urogenital infection. The tests are time intensive and require meticulous planning (see text for details).*

examination (VB3 – voided bladder 3) and, within this specimen, organisms of prostatic origin may be cultured. Thus, by comparison of specimens obtained from urethral urine, bladder urine and post-massage urine, it is generally possible to localise the source of the patient's infection.

Examination of prostatic fluid

Examination of material obtained after prostatic massage is an important step in the diagnosis of genital infection. In general, cases of prostatic inflammation are found to have more than 15 white cells per high-powered field when such microscopy is performed;

as noted above, it is important to check that urethral and bladder specimens do not have similar levels of pyuria. A number of biochemical examinations may be made of expressed prostatic fluid (Figure 7.16). The pH of the fluid, normally around 6.5, becomes alkaline as a result of decreased levels of citric acid [84]. Zinc levels also reduce significantly [85], this element having previously been known as prostatic antibacterial factor (PAF) due to its potent bactericidal action on most bacteria capable of causing urinary tract infection. It is not clear, however, whether these changes are the cause or the result of bacterial infection of the prostate gland.

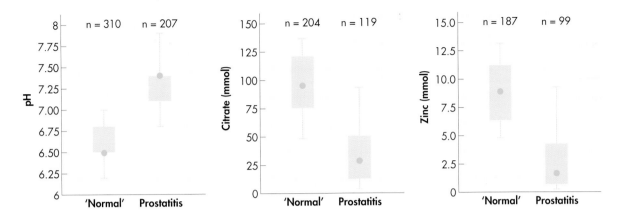

Figure 7.16 *Differences in expressed prostatic secretion (EPS) composition between 'normal' samples and men with prostatitis. Circles, median values; boxes, central 50% of samples. Error bars 10th/90th percentile. All differences significant (P < 0.001). Infection causes a rise in pH but a decrease in citrate and zinc concentrations. (See text for details.) (Data from Kavanagh et al. [85].)*

Non-bacterial prostatitis

The cause of non-bacterial prostatitis is essentially unknown. Meticulous investigations may reveal pyuria but no positive cultures may be obtained by the selective methodology described above. It is not clear whether the symptom complex – which is similar to chronic bacterial prostatitis – is related to infectious disease by an unidentified pathogen or is a non-infectious inflammatory process (Figure 7.17). A num-

ber of causes of non-bacterial prostatitis have been discussed in the literature, including previous antibiotic therapy, viral infection (herpes), *Ureaplasma urealyticum*, chemical inflammatory processes and autoimmune disease. The role of *Chlamydia trochomatis* is controversial. Mardh studied 53 patients with non-bacterial prostatitis and found only one positive chlamydial isolate [86], and most other investigators have been similarly unsuccessful in identifying this

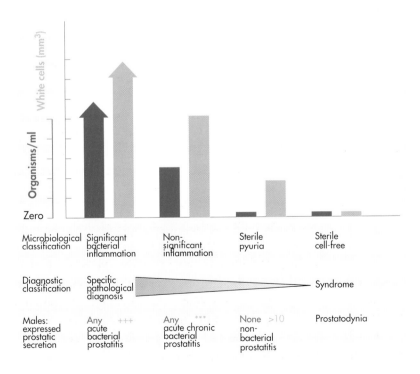

Figure 7.17 *The spectrum of microbiological activity in expressed prostatic secretion. Anticipated levels of both organisms and white cells in the four conditions classified by Drach et al. [80] are illustrated. The major clinical problems relate to patients with non-bacterial prostatitis and prostatodynia.*

organism in prostatic fluid or even in prostatic aspirates obtained by direct transrectal ultrasound-guided needle puncture of the gland [87]. Nevertheless, identification of this agent as the causative organism of epididymitis in younger men (Figure 7.18) raises questions as to how the infection reaches the epididymis [88]. In this study, a tender, swollen epididymis was associated with chlamydial infection in 19 of 23 patients (83%) aged between 15 and 25 years, and these findings were consolidated by the observation that 9 of 12 consorts were also positive for this infection. Presumably, these observations are reconciled by assuming that the organism may pass from urethra to epididymis but the biological environment within the prostate ducts themselves is hostile to this agent.

Antibiotic penetration in prostatitis
The specific physicochemical characteristics of the prostate and prostatic fluid govern the penetration of antibiotics into the organ. To penetrate the lipid membrane of the prostatic epithelium, a drug must be lipid soluble and, furthermore, the acid–base characteristic of the drug will determine the concentration of the antibiotic in the fluid. Experiments on normal dog prostates (secretion pH 6.4) demonstrate that only bases are able to penetrate successfully into prostatic fluid. However, as noted above, during infection of the human prostate, pH becomes more alkaline and the dissociation gradient may reverse. Nevertheless,

fat-soluble bases such as erythromycin and trimethoprim are effective in acute or chronic bacterial prostatitis despite experimental evidence that suggests that concentration of the drug should deteriorate as the pH of the expressed prostatic fluid becomes more alkaline.

Tuberculosis

Genitourinary tuberculosis is an important infection of the urinary tract. Although the incidence of the disease has declined in Western Europe and North America, it remains highly prevalent elsewhere, particularly in Africa and South East Asia. Despite classical teaching that the disease affects groups with poor health and inadequate nutrition, new cases are constantly identified amongst apparently healthy sections of the population. Although outside the remit of this chapter, the urologist will be aware that the infection has to be considered in the differential diagnosis of those patients with persistent sterile pyuria.

Bacteraemia and septic shock

Septic shock is a relatively common and extremely serious complication of infection, usually of Gram-negative origin. In urological practice, the complication is most often encountered in the management of stones, usually complex in nature and located in the upper tract. Septicaemic shock, however, may occur after apparently simple and uncomplicated instrumentation of the urinary tract.

Figure 7.19 illustrates organisms isolated from blood cultures and the surgical procedures involved, taken from a typically busy stone service. The endotoxin that is thought to trigger the septic cascade lies between the outer membrane and the core oligosaccharide that makes up the O serotype antigen common to Gram-negative bacteria (Figure 7.20; see also Figure 7.12). Known as lipid A, this lipopolysaccharide may trigger the release of large amounts of cytokines such as tumour necrosis factor and interleukins, which participate in the classically described cascade illustrated in Figure 7.21. A full description of the sepsis syndrome is beyond the scope of this chapter, but urologists will be aware of the urgent need to maintain adequate tissue profusion by volume replacement at the same time as instituting

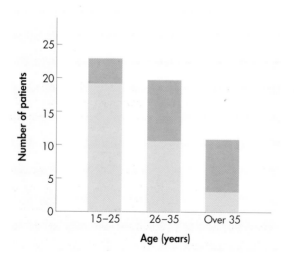

Figure 7.18 *Age distribution of patients with epididymitis according to recovered organism.* ■ *Negative for* C. trachomatis; ■ *Positive for* C. trachomatis. *(Data from Grant et al. [88].)*

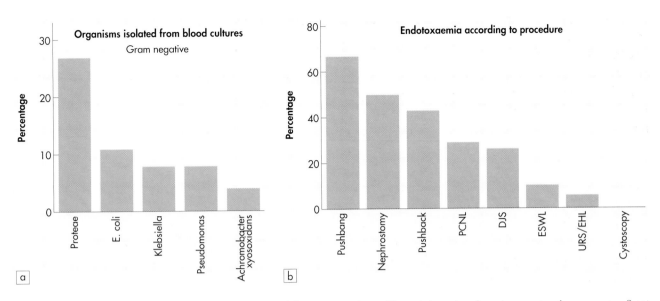

Figure 7.19 *Organisms (a) recovered from blood cultures following procedures (b) carried out in a busy interventional stone centre. Septic shock unfortunately occurs in a significant number of these cases.*

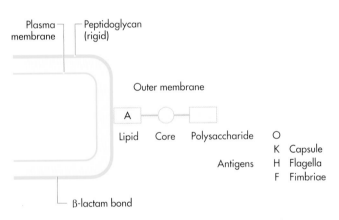

Figure 7.20 *Detailed structure of the O polysaccharide antigen associated with Escherichia coli. Lipid adjacent to the outer membrane (lipid A) is thought to be responsible for the manifestations of endotoxic shock.*

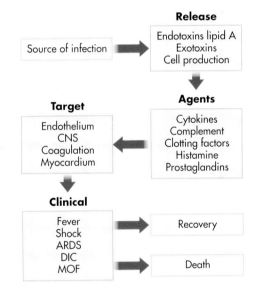

Figure 7.21 *The classical cascade described in endotoxic septicaemic shock. ARDS, adult respiratory distress syndrome; DIC, disseminated intravascular coagulation; MOF, multiple organ failure.*

appropriate antimicrobial therapy, as judged by repeated blood cultures if necessary.

Papilloma viruses and cancer

Human papilloma viruses (HPV) are DNA-containing viruses that stimulate rapid cell division. External genital warts (Figure 7.22) are most frequently caused by HPV types 6 and 11. Other HPV types (mainly 16 and 18) are frequently present in the anogenital region and have been associated with the development of high-grade, premalignant cervical lesions – cervical intraepithelial neoplasia (CIN) III – as well as anogenital cancer, principally of the anus and vulva. DNA sequences from such HPVs are detectable in the majority of cervical and anal tumours; PCR studies of apparently normal cervical smears showed increased levels of sequences from 'high-risk virus types' and subsequent colposcopy confirmed the presence of underlying high-grade CIN III [89]. Not all women infected with high-risk HPV types develop cancer, and the reason for this discrepancy remains unclear at the present time.

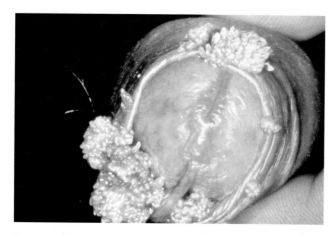

Figure 7.22 *Exophytic papilloma virus, usually caused by type 6 or type 11 infection.*

Localisation studies in the urinary tract

It is pertinent to summarise the various localisation studies that may be employed to identify the site of infection of any particular organism. Such studies, when efficiently and accurately performed, can be of great help to the urologist attempting to identify the source of organisms within the urinary tract.

Studies on prostatic fluid described by Meares and Stamey [83] have already been noted. Stamey has also been responsible for refining localisation studies designed to determine the source of bacteriuria emanating from the upper urinary tract. Essentially, this test involves ureteric catheterisation of the appropriate unit in question after meticulous steps to eradicate bacteria from the bladder that would otherwise contaminate the ureteric sample. Such techniques have been equally useful when attempting to determine the source of cells with abnormal cytological features. Earlier methods for differentiating kidney from bladder infections (Fairley bladder washout test) have fallen into disuse, although such studies can, on occasion, be clinically helpful.

Summary of definitions

Adherence
Initial interaction of micro-organism with host.

Adhesin
Microbiological molecule that leads to adhesion to cells or tissues.

Bacteriuria
The residence of bacteria within the urinary tract.

Contamination
Adventitious entry of bacteria during urine collection.

Fitness
The ability of bacteria to establish and maintain a population in a specific ecological habit.

GAL-GAL
The essential core of the disaccharide receptor for P fimbriae.

Pathogenicity
The ability to cause disease.

Phase variation
Variation of virulence antigens, often to protect the organism.

Tropism
The restriction of commensals and pathogens to certain host tissues and cell types.

Virulence
The degree of pathogenicity.

References

1. Lincoln K, Lidin-Janson G, Winberg J. Resistant urinary infections resulting from changes in resistance pattern of faecal flora induced by sulphonamide and hospital envirnoment. Br Med J 1970; 3: 305–9
2. Finegold SM, Mathisen GE, George WL. Changes in human intestinal flora related to administration of antimicrobial agents. In: Hentges DJ (ed) Human intestinal micro flora in health and disease. New York: Academic Press, 1983; 355–446
3. Kaye D. Antibacterial activity of human urine. J Clin Invest 1968; 47: 2374–90
4. Cox CE, Hinman F Jr. Experiments with induced bacteriuria, vesical emptying and bacterial growth on a mechanism of bladder defence to infection. J Urol 1961; 86: 739–48
5. Parsons CL, Greenspan C, Mulholland SG. The primary antibacterial defence mechanism of the bladder. Invest Urol 1975; 13: 72–6
6. Parsons LC, Shrom SH, Hanno PM, Mulholland SG. Bladder surface mucin – examination of possible mechanisms for its antibacterial effect. Invest Urol 1978; 60: 196–200

7. Parsons CL, Mulholland SG, Anwar H. Antibacterial activity of bladder surface mucin duplication by exogenous glycosaminoglycan (heparin). Infect Immun 1979; 24: 552–7

8. Tamm I, Horsfall FL. A mucoprotein derived from human urine which reacts with influenza, mumps and Newcastle disease viruses. J Exp Med 1952; 95: 71–97

9. Ørskov I, Ferencz A, Ørskov F. Tamm–Horsfall protein or uro-mucoid is the normal urinary slime that traps type I fimbrinated Escherichia coli. Lancet 1980; 1: 887

10. Mayer KH, Opal SM, Mederios AA. Mechanisms of antibiotic resistance. In: Mandell GL, Benett JE, Dolin R (eds). Principles and practice of infectious diseases. Churchill Livingstone, 1995: 212–24

11. Cooke EM, Ewins SP. Properties of strains of Escherichia coli isolated from a variety of sources. J Med Microbiol 1975; 8: 107–11

12. Minshew BH, Jorgenson J, Swanstrum M. Some characteristics of E. coli strains isolated from extra-intestinal infections of humans. J Infect Dis 1978; 137: 648–54

13. Mayer TF. Pathogenic Neisseriae – a model of bacterial virulence and genetic flexibility. Int J Microbiol 1990; 274: 135–54

14. Leying H, Suerbaum S, Kroll H-P, Stahl D, Opferkuch W. The capsular polysaccharide is a major determinant of serum resistance in K-1 positive blood culture isolates of Escherichia coli. Infect Immun 1990; 58: 222–7

15. Jacobson SH, Hammarlind M, Lidefeldt KJ, Österberg E, Tullus K, Brauner A. Incidence of areobactin-positive Escherichia coli strains in patients with symptomatic urinary tract infection. Eur J Clin Microbiol Infect Dis 1988; 7: 630–4

16. Costerton JW, Geesey GG, Cheng K-J. How bacteria stick. Sci Am 1978; 238: 86–95

17. Gibbons RJ, van-Houte J. Bacterial adherence in oral microbial ecology. Ann Rev Microbiol 1975; 29: 19–41

18. Mobley HLT, Chippendale GR, Tenney JH, Hull RA, Warren JW. Expression of type I fimbriae may be required for persistence of Escherichia coli in the catheterised urinary tract. J Clin Microbiol 1987; 25: 2253–7

19. Eisenstein BI. Phase variation of type I fimbriae in Escherichia coli is under transcriptional control. Science 1981; 214: 337–9

20. Lindberg F, Lund B, Johansson L, Normark S. Localisation of the receptor-binding protein adhesin at the tip of the bacterial pilus. Nature 1987; 328: 84–7

21. Roberts JA. Tropism in bacterial infections: urinary tract infections. J Urol 1996; 156: 1552–9

22. Roberts JA, Kaack MB, Baskin G, Marklund B-I, Normark S. Epitotes of the P-fimbrial adhesin of E. coli cause different urinary tract infections. J Urol 1997; 158: 1610–13

23. Senior D, Baker N, Cedergren B, et al. Globo-A – a new receptor specificity for attaching Escherichia coli. FEBS Letters 1988; 237: 123–7

24. Lindstedt R, Larson G, Falk P, Jodal U, Leffler H, Svanborg C. The receptor repertoire defines the host range for attaching Escherichia coli strains that recognise Globo-A. Infect Immun 1991; 59: 1086–92

25. Svanborg Edén C, Hanson LÅ, Jodal U, Lindberg U, Åkerlund AS. Variable adherence to normal human urinary tract epithelial cells of Escherichia coli strains associated with various forms of urinary tract infection. Lancet 1976; 2: 490–2

26. Fowler JE, Stamey TA. Studies of introital colonisation in women with recurrent urinary tract infections – role of bacterial adherence. J Urol 1977; 117: 472–6

27. Schaeffer AJ, Jones JM, Dunn JK. Association of in vitro Escherichia coli adherence to vaginal and buccal epithelial cells with susceptibility of women to recurrent urinary tract infections. N Engl J Med 1981; 304: 1062–6

28. Sellwood R, Gibbons RA, Jones GW, Rutter JM. A possible basis for the breeding of pigs relatively resistant to neonatal diarrhoea. Vet Rec 1975; 95: 574

29. Sellwood R, Gibbons RA, Jones GW, Rutter JM. Adhesion of enteropathogenic Escherichia coli to pig intestinal brush borders: the existence of two pig phenotypes. J Med Microbiol 1975; 8: 405–11

30. Rutter JM, Burrows MR, Sellwood R, Gibbons RA. A genetic basis for resistance to enteric disease caused by E. coli. Nature 1975; 257: 135–6

31. Buckwalter JA, Naifeh GS, Auer JE. Rheumatic fever and the blood groups. Br Med J 1962; 2: 1023–7

32. Källenius G, Möllby R, Svenson SB, et al. Occurrence of P-fimbrinated Escherichia coli in urinary tract infections. Lancet 1981; 2: 1369–72

33. Johnson JR, Roberts PL, Stamm WE. P-fimbriae and other virulence factors in Escherichia coli urosepsis: association with patients' characteristics. J Infect Dis 1987; 156: 225–8

34. Schlager TA, Whittam TS, Hendley JO, et al. Comparison of expression of virulence factors by Escherichia coli causing cystitis and E. coli colonising the peri-urethra of healthy girls. J Infect Dis 1995; 172: 772–8

35. Silverblatt FS. Host–parasite interaction in the rat renal pelvis: a possible role of pili in the pathogenesis of pyelonephritis. J Exp Med 1974; 140: 1696–9

36. Fader RC, Davis CP. Effect of pilation on *Klebsiella pneumoniae* infection in rat bladders. Infect Immun 1980; 30: 554–61

37. Glynn AA, Brumfitt W, Howard CJ. K antigens of *Escherichia coli* and renal involvment in urinary tract infections. Lancet 1971; 1: 514–16

38. Kaijser B, Hanson LA, Jodal U, Lidin-Janson G, Robins JB. Frequency of *E. coli* K antigens in urinary tract infections in children. Lancet 1977; 2: 663–4

39. Crump J, Pead L, Maskell R. Urinary infections in general practice. Lancet 1976; 1: 1184

40. Grüneberg RN. Antibiotic sensitivities of urinary pathogens, 1971–1978. J Clin Pathol 1980; 33: 853–6

41. Jordan PA, Iravani A, Richard GA. Urinary tract infection caused by *Staphylococcus saprophyticus*. J Infect Dis 1980; 142: 510–15

42. Maskell R, Pead L, Allen J. The puzzle of 'urethral syndrome': a possible answer? Lancet 1979; 1: 1058–9

43. Brumfitt W, Hamilton-Miller JMT, Ludlam H, Gooding A. Lactobacilli do not cause frequency and dysuria syndrome. Lancet 1981; 2: 393–4

44. Bran JL, Levison ME, Kaye D. Entrance of bacteria into the female urinary bladder. N Engl J Med 1972; 286: 626–9

45. Buckley RM, McGuckin M, MacGregor RR. Urine bacterial counts following sexual intercourse. N Engl J Med 1978; 298: 321–4

46. Hinman F Jr. Mechanisms for the entry of bacteria and the establishment of urinary infection in female children. J Urol 1966; 96: 546–50

47. Hooton TM, Hillier S, Johnson C. *Escherichia coli* bacteriuria and contraceptive method. JAMA 1991; 265: 64–9

48. Vivaldi E, Cotran R, Zangwill DP. Ascending infection as a mechanism in pathogenesis of experimental non-obstructive pyelonephritis. Proc Soc Exp Biol Med 1959; 102: 242–7

49. Kass EH. Bacteriuria and the diagnosis of infections of the urinary tract. AMA Arch Int Med 1957; 100: 709–14

50. Stamm WE, Wagner KF, Amsell R, *et al.* Causes of the acute urethral syndrome in women. N Engl J Med 1980; 303: 409–15

51. Stamm WE, Counts GW, Running KR, Fihn S, Turck M, Holmes KK. Diagnosis of coliform infection in acutely dysuric women. N Engl J Med 1982; 307: 463–8

52. Editorial. Can Kasstigation beat the truth out of the urethral syndrome? Lancet 1982; 2: 694–5

53. Editorial. Stamm WE. Quantitative urine cultures revisited. Eur J Clin Microbiol 1984; 3: 279–81

54. Venegas MF, Navas EL, Gaffney RA, Duncan JL, Anderson BE, Schaeffer AJ. Binding of type I pilated *Escherichia coli* to vaginal mucous. Infect Immun 1995; 63: 416–21

55. Cox CE, Lacy SS, Hinman F Jr. The urethra and its relationship to urinary tract infection. II. The urethral flora of the female with recurrent urinary infection. J Urol 1968; 99: 632–8

56. Grüneberg RN. Relationship of infecting urinary organism to the faecal flora in patients with symptomatic urinary infection. Lancet 1969; 2: 766–8

57. Stamey TA, Sexton CC. The role of vaginal colonisation with enterobacteriaceae in recurrent urinary infections. J Urol 1975; 113: 214–17

58. Pfau A, Sacks T. The bacterial flora of the vaginal vestibule, urethra and vagina in premenopausal women with recurrent urinary tract infections. J Urol 1981; 126: 630–4

59. Marsh FP, Murray M, Panchamia P. The relationship between bacterial cultures of the vaginal introitus and urinary infection. Br J Urol 1972; 44: 368–75

60. O'Grady FW, Richards B, McSherry MA, O'Farrell SM, Cattell WR. Introital enterobacteria, urinary infection and the urethral syndrome. Lancet 1970; 2: 1208–10

61. Brumfitt W, Grogan RA, Hamilton-Miller JMT. Periurethral enterobacterial carriage preceding urinary infection. Lancet 1987; 1: 824–6

62. Cattell WR, McSherry MA, Northeast A, Powell E, Brooks HJL, O'Grady F. Periurethral enterobacterial carriage in the pathogenesis of recurrent urinary infection. Br Med J 1974; 4: 136–9

63. Wiswell TE, Roscelli JD. Corroborative evidence for the decreased incidence of urinary tract infections in circumcised male infants. Paediatrics 1986; 78: 96–9

64. Wiswell TE, Enzenauer RW, Holton ME, Cornish JD, Hankins CT. Declining frequency of circumcision: implications for changes in the absolute incidence and male to female sex ratio of urinary tract infections in early infancy. Paediatrics 1987; 79: 338–42

65. Feld L, Greenfield S, Ogra P. Urinary tract infections in infants and children. Paediatric Rev 1989; 11: 71–7

66. Ransley PG, Risdon RA. The pathogenesis of reflux nephropathy. Contrib Nephrol 1979; 16: 90–8

67. Siegel S, Siegel B, Sokoloff B. Urinary infection in infants and preschool children. Am J Dis Child 1980; 134: 369–72

68. Kunin CM. A ten-year study of bacteriuria in school girls: final report of bacteriologic, urologic, and epidemiologic findings. J Infect Dis 1970; 122: 382–93

69. Meadow RS, White RHR, Johnston NM. Prevalence of symptomless urinary tract disease in Birmingham schoolchildren. I. Pyuria and bacteriuria. Br Med J 1969; 3: 81–4

70. Cardiff/Oxford Bacteriuria Study Group. Sequelae of covert bacteriuria in school girls. A four-year follow-up study. Lancet 1978; 1: 889–94

71. Gillenwater JY, Harrison RB, Kunin CM. Natural history of bacteriuria in school girls. N Engl J Med 1979; 301: 396–9

72. Sacks SH, Verrier Jones K, Roberts R, Asscher AW, Ledingham JGG. The effect of symptomless bacteriuria in childhood on subsequent pregnancy. Lancet 1987; 2: 991–4

73. Kunin CM. Sexual intercourse and urinary infections. New Engl J Med 1978; 298: 336–7

74. Norden CW, Kass EH. Bacteriuria of pregnancy: a critical appraisal. Ann Rev Med 1968; 19: 431–7

75. Kass EH. Bacteriuria and pyelonephritis of pregnancy. AMA Arch Int Med 1960; 105: 194–8

76. Brocklehurst JC, Dillane JB, Griffiths L. The prevalence and symptomatology of urinary infection in an aged population. Gerontol Clin 1968; 10: 242–53

77. Mabeck CE. Treatment of uncomplicated urinary tract infection in non-pregnant women. Postgrad Med J 1972; 48: 69–75

78. George NJR. Urethral syndrome – clinical features. In: George NJR, Gosling JA (eds) Sensory disorders of the bladder and urethra. Springer Verlag, 1986: 91–102

79. O'Grady FW, Charlton CAC, Fry IK, McSherry A, Catell WR. Natural history of intractable 'cystitis' in women referred to a special clinic. In: Brumfitt W, Ascher AW (eds) Urinary tract infection. Oxford: Oxford University Press, 1973: 81–91

80. Drach GW, Fair WR, Meares EM, Stamey TA. Classification of benign diseases associated with prostatic pain: prostatitis or prostatodynia? J Urol 1978; 120: 226

81. Blacklock NJ. Anatomical factors in prostatitis. Br J Urol 1974; 46: 47–50

82. Kirby RS, Lowe D, Bultitude MI. Intraprostatic urinary reflux: an aetiological factor in abacterial prostatitis. Br J Urol 1982; 54: 729–31

83. Meares EM Jr, Stamey TA. Bacteriologic localisation patterns in bacterial prostatitis and urethritis. Invest Urol 1968; 5: 492–518

84. Blacklock NJ, Beavis JP. Response of prostatic fluid pH in inflammation. Br J Urol 1974; 46: 537–42

85. Kavanagh JP, Darby C, Costello CB. Differences in expressed prostatic secretion composition (EPS) between 'normal' samples and from men with prostatitis. Int J Androl 1982; 5: 487–96

86. Mardh PH, Ripa KT, Colleen S, Treharne JD, Darouga RS. Role of *Chlamydia trochomatis* in non-acute prostatitis. Br J Vener Dis 1978; 54: 330–4

87. Doble A, Thomas BJ, Walker MM. The role of *Chlamydia trochomatis* in chronic abacterial prostatitis: a study using ultrasound-guided biopsy. J Urol 1989; 141: 332–5

88. Grant JBF, Costello CB, Sequeira PJL, Blacklock NJ. The role of *Chlamydia trochomatis* in epididymitis. Br J Urol 1987; 60: 355–9

89. Cuziack J, Szarewski A, Terry G. Human papilloma virus testing in primary cervical screening. Lancet 1995; 345: 1533–6

The scientific basis of calcium oxalate stone formation

8

R. L. Ryall

The given

Background

Since the beginning of recorded history, human beings have grappled with the consequences of unwanted precipitation of insoluble salts from body fluids, especially within the urinary tract. Bladder stones were a scourge to the ancient Egyptians, and were so commonplace in early Greek societies that even the great Hippocrates himself, who recognised and described their symptoms, considered the disease of sufficient import to justify its specific mention in his famous Oath. These days, however, bladder stones are relatively rare, occurring endemically in children in underdeveloped or developing regions of the world where nutrition is based largely on grain, and where dairy products and protein are scarce [1]. But we in the West are not rid of the problem; throughout this century, a decline in the incidence of bladder calculi has been gradually matched by a corresponding increase in the occurrence of kidney stones [2], until now, when the incidence of renal stones has completely eclipsed that of the disease it effectively replaced. And its price is high. Six years ago, a list of the cost of medical consultations and hospitalisation for kidney and urological diseases in the USA in 1986 ranked urolithiasis as the fourth most expensive condition, superseded only by urinary tract infection, chronic renal failure and benign prostatic hyperplasia [3]. By 1993, urolithiasis was estimated to cost the American public a staggering $1.7 billion per annum. Indirect costs, such as loss of productivity, accounted for a hefty portion of this figure, because the victims

of stone disease generally include those falling within the most financially productive age groups [4], and are predominantly men, who typically earn higher salaries than women.

Yet, we have tended to become rather blasé about kidney stones. They are rarely fatal; in fact, they have come to be regarded almost as a medical nuisance rather than a serious problem, their consequences having been overshadowed by those of other urological diseases and, to some extent, trivialised by the advent of percutaneous and extracorporeal shock wave lithotripsy. What once involved major surgical intervention, significant morbidity and weeks off work is now complacently regarded as requiring only a slick trip to a day surgery unit and a few thousand uncomfortable blasts of shock waves, a misconception that has not escaped the attention of the popular tabloid press (Figure 8.1)! It is hardly any wonder that society at large, and the medical profession in particular, have come to regard stone blasting as a simple, non-invasive cure-all, and so to overlook the fact that urolithiasis is still a monumental, worldwide problem that continues to exact an enormous medical and economic price from modern communities and their individual members. Extracorporeal shock wave lithotripsy does not cure stones. It merely removes, with misleadingly apparent ease, an unfortunate by-product of an underlying metabolic abnormality, and in so doing it has left an insidious legacy: it has effectively smothered the performance of basic stone research aimed at identifying means of preventing the disease. When the author performed a cursory electronic analysis of the international urolithiasis

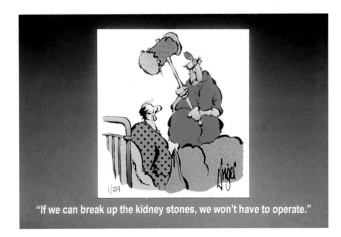

Figure 8.1 A sign of the times – the prevailing attitude to kidney stone management. ('Copyright of Herman': Universal Press Syndicate.)

literature published during 1995, she found that papers dealing with lithotripsy and the surgical management of stones outnumbered those devoted to the basic science of stone formation – by at least three to one. Perhaps of even greater concern is that a disproportionately high number of those publications were concerned with the occurrence and sequelae of significant problems caused by the procedure itself: extracorporeal shock wave lithotripsy is not the panacea it was expected to be. It is therefore becoming increasingly apparent that treatment of stones, even by this method, is no substitute for their prevention, and that there is an urgent need to prevent stones using strategies or medical treatments based on sound, basic principles. This will come only by directing attention once more to the scientific foundations of urolithiasis, and in this chapter that is what the author will attempt to do.

Composition

Kidney stones are a painful and unwelcome manifestation of biomineralisation – the formation of inorganic salts by living organisms, a natural process that, under normal conditions, is an absolute prerequisite for life and health in human beings and throughout the animal and plant kingdoms. However, unlike their salubrious counterparts, such as bones, shells and teeth, renal stones are pathological structures exhibiting features typical of uncontrolled biomineralisation [5]. Thus, their composition is dictated by environ-

mental factors rather than by cellular processes that have evolved to control the deposition of mineral for specific functional purposes. The minerals of stones, therefore, reflect the ionic composition of human urine and, not unexpectedly therefore, consist of salts combining various urinary ions in their most insoluble forms. Two large, long-term studies, one in the USA [6] and the other in Japan [7], provided data on the mineral composition of thousands of human stones, and despite the fact that they were performed 30 years apart, their results are surprisingly consistent. Calcium oxalate, either alone or mixed in varying proportions with calcium phosphate, is the principal mineral of most calculi, comprising approximately 80% of all human uroliths [6, 7]. Of the remainder, struvite stones account for between 6% and 14%. Composed of magnesium ammonium phosphate, these have a well-established aetiology, resulting from infection of urine by bacteria that cleave urea to ammonia and raise the urinary pH, thereby causing precipitation of the salt. Uric acid stones are the next most common (6–10%), followed by cystine (1–2%) and pure calcium phosphate (0–1.5%) [6, 7]. Because of their overwhelming preponderance, unless otherwise stated, this chapter reviews what is known, or is presumed, to influence the formation of calcium oxalate stones.

The apparent

Epidemiology

Although renal colic enjoys the dubious distinction of being, anecdotally at least, the worst imaginable pain, surprisingly perhaps, kidney stones often remain undetected for years. This silence, combined with the fact that some stoic stalwarts simply grit their teeth, pass their stones and never present to a hospital, means that the true incidence of stones is difficult to assess: data are usually derived from hospital discharge summaries, which tend to underestimate the true incidence of the disease [1]. Nonetheless, there seems to be general agreement among urolithiasists that, at least in the Western world, approximately one-tenth of all men can expect to suffer at least one stone episode during their lifetime [8]. Recurrences are common, two prospective studies having shown that up to 50% of stone formers will suffer at least one further episode [9, 10]. Women succumb to the disease much less frequently, forming stones one-half to one-third as often as men, although, not unexpectedly, they are more prone to infection-related stones. However, gender is just one of a variety of factors that have come to be associated with stone disease. No single factor causes stones: literally centuries of observation have provided sufficient empirical evidence to suggest that age, race, heredity, geography, local water supply, climate, hygiene, occupation and diet (Figure 8.2) are associated with urolithiasis, although data have often been conflicting and sometimes tenuous. The picture is also clouded somewhat by the fact that some of these factors are interdependent. Geography, water and climate cannot be regarded as independent variables; neither can race and heredity; nor can race and diet. Obviously, these various factors embrace an enormously wide range of influences affecting stone formation, but because the brief here is to present the scientific basis of stone formation, these will not be discussed further in any detail. Instead, interested readers are referred to an excellent article on calcium oxalate stone epidemiology by Milliner [1]. This discussion focuses on the factors shown in Figure 8.2, each of which, directly or indirectly and to varying degrees, affects one or both of just two basic phenomena that are essential events in stone pathogenesis. These are the nucleation of insoluble crystals and their subsequent retention within the kidney. From this point, this chapter is concerned specifically with what is known about these two events as they relate to calcium oxalate stones.

The likely

Physicochemical processes in stone formation

The published literature devoted to research on stone formation, like that of virtually any other subject of medical research, fairly bristles with inconsistencies, contradictions, assumptions and gigantic leaps of faith. However, there is at least one truism of which we can be absolutely confident: stones cannot form if crystals do not precipitate in the renal collecting system. For crystal nucleation to occur, the urine must be supersaturated with calcium oxalate, although as we shall see, other factors may also influence the likelihood of precipitation. However, supersaturation is a more complex term than might first seem apparent, and is illustrated simply in Figure 8.3 using calcium oxalate as a model. If an inorganic salt is added to water, some of it will dissolve. With calcium oxalate, only tiny quantities will dissolve because it is very insoluble. As long as dissolution continues, the solution is said to be undersaturated and spontaneous precipitation of crystals from solution cannot occur. If we continue to add calcium oxalate crystals, we will reach a point where no more will dissolve, because the rate of entry of calcium and oxalate ions into solution is matched by deposition of the same ions on to the surfaces of the added crystals. The solution is now *saturated* with calcium oxalate; the product of the ionic concentrations of calcium and oxalate at this point is known as the *thermodynamic solubility product*. However, it is possible to increase the concentration of dissolved calcium oxalate further. If we take a solution containing calcium ions, such as calcium chloride, and slowly add another solution containing oxalate ions, we will obtain a solution of calcium oxalate that is *supersaturated*. Spontaneous precipitation of calcium oxalate from this solution will not occur, but if

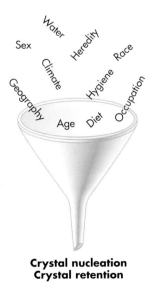

Crystal nucleation
Crystal retention

Figure 8.2 Epidemiological factors contributing to crystal nucleation and retention, two processes essential to stone formation.

we add crystals of calcium oxalate, deposition of ions will occur upon their surfaces and they will grow; they will also aggregate under these conditions. It is also possible actively to induce calcium oxalate nucleation and growth in a supersaturated solution by adding foreign matter, to produce what is known as *heterogeneous nucleation*. If we now proceed to increase the concentration of calcium oxalate, we will reach a point known as the *formation product*, at which spontaneous precipitation, or *homogeneous nucleation*, of calcium oxalate crystals will occur. The region between the solubility product and the formation product is known as the *metastable zone*, and once precipitation occurs, the solution is said to have exceeded its *metastable limit*.

Using both computational and empirical techniques, it has been shown that, under daily conditions, the urine of both stone formers and healthy subjects is supersaturated with calcium oxalate, and this is reflected in the fact that all of us, from time to time, pass crystals of calcium oxalate in our urine [11–15]. Nonetheless, the degree of supersaturation in patients does tend to be higher than that in healthy controls [16–18], although the distinction between the two groups is by no means clear cut. How, then, can we identify individuals at risk of urolithiasis? Is there some urinary feature of stone formers that sets them apart from their more fortunate fellows and enables us to predict whether precipitation is likely to occur?

Factors affecting urinary saturation with calcium oxalate

It is intuitively obvious that a number of urinary parameters must exert some influence on the degree of saturation with calcium oxalate, and thereby on the likelihood that the first essential step in stone formation, crystal nucleation, will occur. However, while some of these parameters are self-evident, the contribution of others may not be so immediately apparent. The urinary outputs of calcium and oxalate are obviously significant determinants of urinary saturation with calcium oxalate, although it is recognised that oxalate is significantly more influential than calcium [19, 20]. This stems principally from the presence of oxalate in urine at a concentration approximately one-tenth that of calcium, so that small rises in its urinary levels have far more profound effects than equivalent molar increases in calcium concentration. Precisely because it is urinary concentrations, rather than actual quantities, that will dictate whether or not the precipitation of calcium oxalate occurs, the urinary volume will also be influential: the more dilute the urine, the less probable is the occurrence of crystal nucleation. Even Hippocrates apparently recognised the significance of crystalline 'sand' in the urinary tract and the importance of diuretics for urinary stones [21] (Figure 8.4), although we can but ponder the question of whether or not he was cognizant of the scientific basis for such treatment. Calcium oxalate is more soluble under acidic conditions and decreases with increasing alkalinity; thus, the prevailing urinary pH will also contribute to the likelihood of its precipitation. Perhaps surprisingly, the urinary urate concentration is also a recognised contributor to calcium oxalate stone formation, as shall be seen later, by virtue of its demonstrated ability, at high concentrations, to cause the precipitation of calcium oxalate in urine [22]. Other urinary components that can affect the likelihood of crystal nucleation are magnesium, which binds to oxalate, thereby rendering it unavailable for complexation with calcium, and citrate, which can achieve a

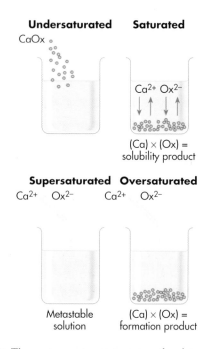

Figure 8.3 The various saturation states of calcium oxalate in solution. See text for details.

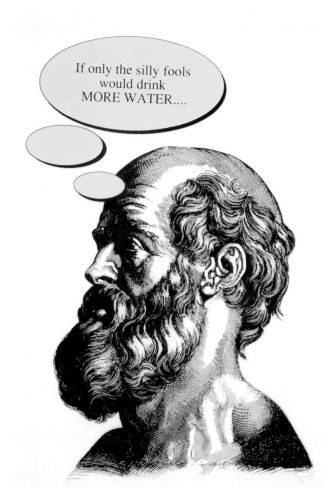

Figure 8.4 *Hippocrates' approach to the treatment of urinary stones. Little has changed in 2000 years!*

similar but converse result by chelating calcium ions. Citrate has also been reported to inhibit calcium oxalate crystal growth and aggregation, a property that is discussed in the section dealing with theories of stone formation.

It is apparent then that the first sine qua non of stone formation – namely, crystal nucleation – is influenced by several urinary constituents. We may reasonably assume, then, that derangements in one or more of these constituents may explain the occurrence of stones in affected individuals; and there is no doubt that abnormalities often occur. However, it is not possible here to review comprehensively the vast literature devoted to comparisons of the urinary excretion of calcium, oxalate, uric acid, magnesium or citrate in stone formers and healthy subjects.

Nonetheless, there is little doubt that hypercalciuria, hyperoxaluria, hypocitraturia and hyperuricosuria have frequently borne the burden of guilt for stone disease. But, with the possible exception of hypocitraturia, the evidence by no means consistently supports their damnation.

Hypercalciuria

No other urinary parameter has been so frequently measured or repeatedly blamed for the occurrence of calcium stones. Since 1939, when Flocks [23] reported that the excretion of calcium was generally higher in stone formers, much has been published on hypercalciuria. It is not the intention here to review the vast literature on the subject: a recent review on the aetiology and treatment of stones [24] deals with the matter in some depth. Nonetheless, mention should be made of the fact that consensus has not been reached regarding the true relationship between urinary calcium excretion and urolithiasis. Despite the fact that countless studies have compared the urinary calcium output between stone patients and healthy controls, the number of published papers reporting that calcium excretion is abnormally raised in stone formers is matched by others declaring that the two groups do not differ, and that renal calcium excretion therefore does not exert much influence in determining an individual's predilection to stones.

Furthermore, even where significant differences do exist, the overlap between the control and patient groups is invariably large and, for all practical purposes, renders the finding of questionable clinical value. This highlights one of the major problems associated with attempting to classify patients on the basis of any metabolic parameter: significant differences demonstrated by statistical analysis do not automatically translate to clinical usefulness. Moreover, specific mention must be made of the fact that the measurement of calcium excretion as a diagnostic or prognostic index of stone formation is pointless unless it is related to an appropriate reference range based on contemporary data from a matched cohort in the same geographical location. Yet, even today, people persist in labelling stone patients as 'hypercalciuric', either without providing the basis for that categorisation or by comparing these patients with ranges whose sources are not provided or which were derived years before in remote geographical areas. This occurs despite the well-known association between calcium excretion and diet. Added to this problem is the well-recognised phenomenon of day-to-day variation in urinary calcium excretion [25], a fact that seriously undermines the worth of a single measurement of calcium excretion as a diagnostic indicator of stone disease, and which has led to a general consensus that it is necessary to take the average of a number of determinations in order to obtain a valid classification of abnormalities. It has been shown that up to six consecutive estimations of calcium excretion may be required in order to categorise a subject, unambiguously, as normocalciuric or hypercalciuric [25]. To confuse the issue further, a large, prospective epidemiological study involving a cohort of more than 45 000 men [26] concluded that a high dietary calcium intake actually decreases the risk of kidney stones. This vindicates the recommendation [20] that a high-calcium diet be used to reduce stone recurrences in patients with mild hyperoxaluria, based on the premise that calcium in the gut binds 'free' dietary oxalate available for absorption in the lower intestine, thereby preventing its excretion in the urine. For a more lengthy discussion of the polemic surrounding the issue of hypercalciuria, readers are referred to a review detailing the opposing findings and the problems associated with attempting to categorise patients on the basis of single 24-hour urinary calcium determination [27]. It is also noteworthy that such considerations apply equally to other commonly measured urinary parameters. Obviously, the issue of hypercalciuria in stone pathogenesis is a vexed one; what about other urinary abnormalities?

Hyperoxaluria

The same controversy surrounding the role of hypercalciuria in stone disease is to be found with other urinary factors known to affect the degree of urinary saturation with calcium oxalate as definitive causes of stone formation. As stated above, oxalate concentration is significantly more influential than calcium in determining the degree of urinary saturation with respect to calcium oxalate. Nonetheless, except in individuals afflicted with primary hyperoxaluria,

which is a rare genetic condition [28], a raised urinary oxalate concentration or excretion is not invariably associated with urolithiasis. Thus, though a number of studies have reported that the daily excretion of oxalate is abnormally elevated in stone formers [e.g. 29–34], others would protest that this is not so [e.g. 35–39]. This dissension is further inflamed by the notorious technical difficulties of measuring urinary oxalate and the fact that only in the last ten years or so has it been possible to guarantee that measured values do not include a contribution from urinary ascorbate, which would have been spontaneously converted to oxalate in all but one [34] of the studies cited above.

It is apparent, then, that though both calcium and oxalate excretion undoubtedly influence the degree of saturation of urine with calcium oxalate, we cannot say just how important this influence is in determining whether or not the precipitation of calcium oxalate will actually occur. What of the other factors?

Hyperuricosuria

Unfortunately, the urinary excretion of urate is influenced by such a wide range of factors, including individuals' physical characteristics and gender, genetic make-up and dietary habits, that it is extraordinarily difficult to define a true upper limit of normal urate excretion [40]. It is probably not surprising, then, that if one carefully reviews the literary evidence that urate exerts a marked influence on a person's tendency to form calcium oxalate stones, its predictive value is even more tenuous than that of either calcium or oxalate [25, 41]. Despite this, 'hyperuricosuria' and calcium oxalate stones have long been supposed bedfellows, and this has given rise to the recognition of a subgroup of stone disease known as 'hyperuricosuric calcium oxalate urolithiasis' [42]. The notion is based on a number of empirical observations (most of which are poorly documented) suggesting that a raised urate excretion is common in calcium oxalate stone formers. Although this would appear to be supported by studies suggesting that allopurinol reduces stone recurrences in hyperuricosuric patients [43, 44], only one study has been sufficiently rigorous to demonstrate unequivocally that allopurinol slightly, but nonetheless significantly, reduces the rate of calcium oxalate stone recurrences in patients exhibiting a raised daily excretion of urate [45]. This, more than any other single observation, has ensured that, at least for the time being, urate metabolism and calcium oxalate stones will continue to be linked. Perhaps in the future a carefully controlled study will be performed, in which subjects are matched for race and geographical location (to take account of genetic and dietary influences) and height, weight and sex (all known to affect urinary urate excretion), which demonstrates unequivocally that a raised daily urate excretion encourages calcium oxalate stone disease. Also, maybe future scientific experimentation will identify the mechanism by which urate exerts its putative influence on calcium oxalate stone disease (see below). Whatever the outcome, it is clear from clinical comparative studies that even if the urinary urate concentration *does* affect the likelihood of precipitation of calcium oxalate in urine under physiological conditions, its influence is certainly not predominant: hyperuricosuria is simply not a consistent, unambiguous finding in patients with calcium oxalate urolithiasis [25, 41].

Hypocitraturia

The fact that citrate is a normal component of human urine did not escape the attention of early stone workers, who recognised that its ability to chelate calcium ions might reduce the possibility of precipitation of calcium salts in the urinary tract. It is more than 60 years since Boothby and Adams reported that urinary citrate excretion is abnormally reduced in stone formers [46], a finding that has since been corroborated by a number of workers [47–49]. However, the excretion of citrate is no different from that of the urinary parameters mentioned above, in that at least one study found no difference between patients and controls [50], while yet another pointed out that, in hypocitraturic patients who had multiple estimations performed, approximately 70% fell into the normal range on at least one occasion [51]. Nonetheless, it is now accepted that between 19% and 63% of patients with nephrolithiasis demonstrate abnormally low citrate excretion [49], and citrate supplementation has become a common form of therapy for calcium stone disease.

Other factors

In addition to those factors discussed above, the urinary pH, the prevailing magnesium concentration, and the volume of the daily urine output can all influence the degree of supersaturation with calcium oxalate and, thereby, its potential to precipitate in urine. However, at the present time, the extents of the respective influences of these factors on the chemistry of the urinary ionic soup remain unknown, because none has been unequivocally demonstrated to distinguish consistently between stone formers and healthy subjects [25]. In itself, this is hardly surprising in view of the variety of factors known to influence urinary supersaturation with calcium oxalate, but it is also a pity because the very fact that crystals precipitate from urine would provide the simplest explanation for the occurrence of stones. The problem is, as stated above, that all of us ordinarily pass calcium oxalate crystals in our urine. Crystalluria, therefore, seems to be a normal event, insofar as it occurs routinely; but it does not always proceed automatically to stone formation. Why? We may begin to answer this question by considering an observation made more than 20 years ago and upon which, uncharacteristically, there is general agreement. In marked contrast to healthy subjects, who typically pass small individual crystals, recurrent stone formers tend to excrete greater masses of crystals clustered into large aggregates [14, 15], which must increase the likelihood of crystal retention within the renal collecting system. Any theory of stone formation must take this into account.

The possible

Simple logic allows us to identify easily a number of factors that could influence the likelihood of newly formed crystals becoming lodged within the renal collecting ducts. These include factors such as the physical structure of the renal collecting system and crystal density; calcium oxalate, for instance, has a density of 2.2 g/ml, which can cause crystals to settle when the urine flow rate is insufficient to keep them in suspension. Such a mechanism explains the common association between urolithiasis and medullary sponge kidney (Figure 8.5), a genetic disease in which the terminal renal collecting ducts are dilated; this reduces the rate of urine flow and causes the deposition of a calcium oxalate sediment that often leads to stone formation in affected individuals. However, simple sedimentation cannot be used to explain the occurrence of stones in most instances; medullary sponge kidney is a rare condition. It is necessary, therefore, to invoke other mechanisms by which crystals can become trapped within the kidney. These include crystal adhesion, log-jamming, or enlargement caused by crystal growth or clustering, and can be grouped under two major headings, usually referred to as fixed-particle and free-particle stone formation. Using computational methods, renal tubular dimensions, urine transit times and published experimental data, Finlayson and Reid [52] calculated that free-particle stone formation is not feasible and that stone disease can begin only by physical sticking of crystals within the kidney. However, a similar approach using updated data later showed that free-particle disease is, indeed, possible because aggregation of free crystals can produce particles large enough to be retained in the kidney during the short transit time of urine through the collecting system [53] (Figure 8.6). Perhaps not surprisingly, there is experimental evidence lending support to both mechanisms.

Fixed-particle stone formation

Though the notion that fixation of crystalline particles is an essential step in the formation of calculi can trace its origins back to early work performed by Randall in the 1930s [54], findings related to epithelial injury and its potential role in crystal adhesion are relatively recent and are not discussed here in detail; the subject has been recently reviewed by Hackett and Shevock [54]. Based largely on work performed by Khan and colleagues, using a rat model of urolith formation [55–57], and on studies using cultured kidney cells [58, 59], Hackett and Shevock [54] and Khan [60] concluded that cellular injury plays a key role in stone formation. Such injury can be caused by high urinary oxalate concentrations, which cause exposure and release of macromolecules, which can then induce the deposition of calcium salts. This is followed by the formation of an encrustation platform, which, in the presence of continuing supersaturation, results in

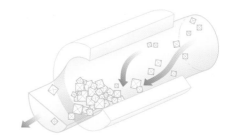

Figure 8.5 *Calcium oxalate crystal sludge formation in a dilated renal tubule in medullary sponge kidney.*

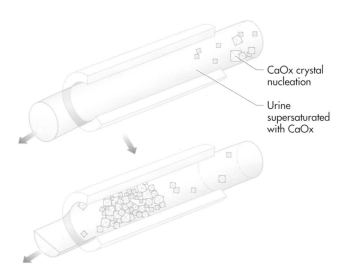

CaOx crystal nucleation

Urine supersaturated with CaOx

Figure 8.6 *Calcium oxalate crystal nucleation in supersaturated urine flowing through a kidney tubule. Crystal growth alone is insufficient to produce crystals large enough to be retained in the tubule in the several minutes urine takes to traverse the collecting system. However, aggregation can result in the formation of particles sufficiently large to occlude the tubular lumen.*

further nucleation of calcium oxalate and stone disease, following retention and stone growth. Alternatively, calcium oxalate crystals nucleated from supersaturated urine can themselves cause epithelial cell damage, which results in endocytosis of the crystals, succeeded by stone attachment and growth, and subsequent stone disease. There is, undoubtedly, compelling evidence that such mechanisms contribute to stone formation. Nonetheless, other factors almost certainly contribute to the initial formation of crystals and their potential to cause cellular trauma by enlargement, and these are considered in several theories of stone formation. Although these are grouped under the heading of free-particle stone disease, many of their elements are perfectly consistent with those of a fixed-particle mechanism of stone formation.

Free-particle stone formation

The epitaxy theory

Stones composed of a single, pure salt are rare; most consist of a mixture of compounds, notably calcium oxalate, calcium phosphate and uric acid in various proportions. In an attempt to explain the formation of mixed stones, Modlin [61] invoked the phenomenon of epitaxy. Although, as we shall see, the process can involve the association of calcium oxalate with calcium phosphate and uric acid and its salts, it has most often been cited to explain the apparent relationship between urate and calcium oxalate stones.

Epitaxy describes the process by which crystalline material of one salt is laid down upon the surface of another, chemically distinct, crystal, and depends upon the occurrence of close lattice fits between the two crystal structures. Such fits have been demonstrated to exist between calcium oxalate monohydrate and dihydrate, uric acid, monosodium urate, brushite, apatite and struvite [62]. Epitaxial nucleation of calcium oxalate by monosodium urate is depicted in Figure 8.7, which shows urine supersaturated with both monosodium urate and calcium oxalate. Crystals of urate precipitate first, thereby providing a surface for the epitaxial deposition of calcium oxalate. It has been demonstrated experimentally that crystals of sodium urate [63, 64], uric acid [65], hydroxyapatite [66] and brushite [67] can provoke nucleation of calcium oxalate from inorganic solutions. However, this property has not been shown to be retained in urine, or when seed crystals are associated with urinary macromolecules. Thus, seed crystals of pure sodium urate and uric acid have no appreciable effect on calcium oxalate crystallisation in undiluted human urine [68], nor do seed crystals of brushite or hydroxyapatite that have been generated from human urine, and which therefore contain urinary macromolecules [69]. Also, pure crystals of sodium urate and uric acid that have been pre-incubated with urinary macromolecules do not promote calcium oxalate precipitation, even in inorganic solutions [68]. Although these findings certainly diminish the possible role of epitaxy as a

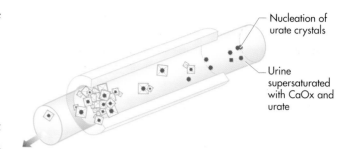

Figure 8.7 *The epitaxy theory of stone formation, showing the heterogeneous nucleation of calcium oxalate crystals by red crystals of urate, and the epitaxial deposition of calcium oxalate upon urate crystals.*

significant event in stone formation, its importance, particularly with regard to urate, is reduced even further by the fact that crystals of sodium urate or uric acid are rarely found in human urine [70] and that hyperuricosuria is not consistently demonstrable in stone formers, as discussed above.

Nonetheless, the clinical impression, so often reported, that calcium stone disease seems to be associated with high levels of urate excretion, coupled with allopurinol's success in slightly reducing the rate of calcium oxalate stone recurrence [45], would suggest that urinary urate does play some role in calcium oxalate crystal nucleation. However, it is possible that this may not depend upon its presence in a solid crystalline form. It has been known for many years that high concentrations of urate, *in solution*, can induce the spontaneous precipitation of calcium oxalate from urine, an observation that has been attributed to the phenomenon of 'salting out' [22, 71], and which explains the earlier, but poorly documented, report of Mayer and her colleagues [72] that urate affects the solubility of calcium oxalate. Moreover, high urate concentrations cause the formation of large crystalline aggregates of calcium oxalate in urine [71], a property that would encourage the retention of crystals, and thereby stone formation, within the kidney.

Whatever the basis for the assumed connection between urate metabolism and calcium stones, an accumulating body of experimental evidence would suggest that it cannot be ascribed to an epitaxial relationship between uric acid or its salts and calcium oxalate. Nor, would it seem, can epitaxy account for the frequent occurrence in stones of calcium phosphate with calcium oxalate. Although recent studies using artificial inorganic solutions designed to mimic ionic concentrations in the renal collecting system were interpreted to suggest that calcium phosphate can induce calcium oxalate crystal nucleation in the collecting duct or in urine [73], it must be remembered that the confounding effect of urinary macromolecules was not taken into account. As will be seen, macromolecules are present both within and upon the surface of calcium oxalate and calcium phosphate crystals precipitated from urine, and these interfere with the epitaxial induction of calcium oxalate nucleation by both urate [68] and calcium phosphate salts [69]. Nonetheless, although urine is typically supersaturated with respect to calcium oxalate, saturation levels are usually insufficient to allow the spontaneous precipitation of the salt. It has therefore come to be generally accepted that precipitation of calcium oxalate in the urinary tract is heterogeneous. Heterogeneous nucleation describes the process by which precipitation of a crystalline salt is brought about by a foreign agent. Anyone who has studied organic chemistry will be familiar with the oft-repeated instruction to scratch the side of a glass vessel containing a solution of an organic compound in order to expedite its precipitation by providing a focus of small particles to act as crystal 'seeds'. The most important feature of heterogeneous nucleation is that it permits crystal precipitation to occur at lower levels of supersaturation than would be required for spontaneous (homogeneous) nucleation. In stone formation, seeds could include bacteria, cellular debris, erythrocytes or urinary macromolecules, all of which have reportedly been found in stones [74], and the presence of which is regarded as evidence supporting the matrix theory of stone formation.

The matrix theory

To this point, we have been preoccupied principally with the inorganic mineral component of kidney stones. However, as discussed previously, renal calculi can be regarded as examples of uncontrolled biomineralisation, which shares a number of features with its healthy counterparts in nature. One of these counterparts is the invariable association of the mineral con-

stituent with organic material known as the matrix. Figures 8.8 and 8.9 illustrate the matrix theory of stone formation. Macromolecules, which are a normal component of all urine, are depicted as worm-like structures that act as centres for the heterogeneous nucleation of calcium oxalate from urine supersaturated with this salt. The macromolecules promote calcium oxalate crystal formation and also act as bridges binding the individual crystals together into large aggregates, which may then have further crystals deposited upon them. The theory could certainly explain the presence in stones of organic molecules and could also provide a plausible rationale for the tendency of stone formers to excrete an increased mass of large crystal aggregates. But there is, at the present time, insufficient experimental evidence to deduce that urinary macromolecules actually begin

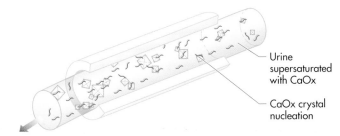

Figure 8.8 *The matrix theory of stone formation. Urinary macromolecules (represented as 'worms') induce the nucleation of calcium oxalate crystals and then act as bridges binding the crystals into aggregated structures.*

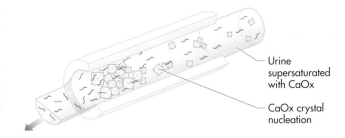

Figure 8.9 *Matrix deposition during kidney stone formation. Macromolecules in the supersaturated urine bind to the surfaces of newly formed calcium oxalate crystals and become entrapped inside the crystals as further solute ions are deposited. Such macromolecules include those normally occurring in urine (depicted as smooth, green 'worms'), and others (represented in red) arising from trauma caused by abrasion of the epithelial surface by the crystals themselves or small stones. These can also become incorporated into the stone between existing crystals, and also within individual crystals as a result of further solute deposition or crystal nucleation.*

the crystallisation events leading to stone formation and, therefore, that alterations in their structure or excretion distinguish stone formers from healthy controls.

Matrix is interlaced throughout the entire structure of all stones [75, 76], occupying disproportionately more space than would be suggested by its contribution of several per cent to the total dry weight [77]. Although its very presence suggests that it may fulfil some function in stone formation, intense investigation by Boyce and his collaborators in the 1950s and, more recently, by a number of investigators, has yielded little information about the identity of matrix macromolecules and even less about their effects on calcium oxalate crystallisation. Yet, this information is vital, for without knowing what they are, it is impossible to say what they do. There are, nonetheless, limited data from earlier studies. Boyce [78] reported that matrix consisted of 64% protein, 9.6% non-amino sugars, 5% hexosamine as glucosamine, 10% bound water, and the balance, inorganic ash; but there is good reason to be sceptical about these figures. Matrix is obstinately insoluble and the figures reported by Boyce described only the 25% of matrix that was soluble in EDTA. Also, other factors have conspired to frustrate attempts to identify its components, including the alteration of its component macromolecules caused by ageing and the crystallisation process itself [76], as well as the recognition that matrix macromolecules can derive from two physiological sources (see Figure 8.8). Macromolecules normally present in urine can become embedded inside the crystals comprising the stone, whereas others, not ordinarily present, can be released into the urine as a result of cellular trauma caused by the crystals or developing stone, and also become incorporated into the growing calculus [78, 79]. This makes it impossible to distinguish those that may have played a role in the stone's formation and those that are products of it. Nonetheless, the development of modern biotechnology has enabled us to identify specifically at least 19 individual proteins present in stones, and two of the six or so glycosaminoglycans present in urine.

Proteins shown to be in stones include human serum albumin and α- and γ-globulins [80], Tamm–Horsfall glycoprotein [81], nephrocalcin [82], α1-microglobulin [83], haemoglobin and neutrophil elastase [84], α1-antitrypsin [85], protectin [86], superoxide dismutase [87], β2-microglobulin, α1-acid glycoprotein, apolipoprotein A1, retinol-binding protein, and renal lithostathine [88], urinary prothrombin fragment 1 [89] and inter-α-trypsin inhibitor [90]. To date, the only glycosaminoglycans that have been shown to be present in stones are heparan sulphate and, to a lesser extent, hyaluronic acid [91–93]. This is despite the fact that they account for only a relatively small proportion of urinary glycosaminoglycans, the majority of which is chondroitin sulphate. However, it is one thing to know which macromolecules are in stones; it is entirely another to know why they are there and what influence they may have wrought during stone formation. The problem is compounded by our inability to distinguish between those that are potentially the cause of the stone, and those that are an effect – a dilemma overcome to some extent by analysis of the proteins and glycosaminoglycans present in calcium oxalate crystals freshly precipitated from human urine, and potentially involved in the crucial initial crystal nucleation-phase of stone formation [79, 83, 94]. Such studies have demonstrated clearly that the involvement of macromolecules in calcium oxalate crystal formation in urine is highly selective, with only a handful of the hundreds of urinary proteins and only one glycosaminoglycan (heparan sulphate) being detectable in the crystals. This suggests that perhaps the majority of proteins shown to be present in stones are simply passive adsorbents and played no active role in the stone's formation, a possibility reinforced by a lack of evidence that urinary macromolecules from stone formers differ from those of normal subjects by being able actively to induce calcium oxalate crystallisation in urine.

Thus, it is apparent at the present time that although the matrix theory of stone formation has never been proved, equally it has never been disproved. However, further extensive investigation must be undertaken in order to discover the true role of stone matrix components in stone pathogenesis because, as we are about to see, the presence of macromolecules in crystals and stones can just as easily be explained by their being inhibitors of crystallisation as by their promoting the process.

The inhibitor theory

It has long been known that urine can prevent calcification: any builder can testify that cement containing urine will not set! Urine can also inhibit physiological calcification, an observation noted by Howard and Thomas in 1958 [95] when they reported that urine from healthy subjects prevented the calcification of rachitic rat cartilage, while that from stone formers did not. This observation formed the basis of what has since come to be known as the inhibitor theory of stone formation, whose tenet is that urine normally contains substances that prevent the nucleation of insoluble crystals. Should nucleation occur, the same substances inhibit the further growth or aggregation of those crystals, thereby reducing the likelihood of their retention within the kidney. The corollary is that stone formers are susceptible to urolithiasis because their urines lack or are deficient in these inhibitors, or because the inhibitors are in some way defective, and this raises the attractive prospect, at least in theory, of being able to prevent stone recurrences by restoring the inhibitory deficit.

The principles of the inhibitor theory are shown in Figure 8.10. Naturally occurring inhibitors are depicted as worm-like structures. Once crystals have precipitated from the supersaturated urine, the inhibitor molecules bind to their surfaces and interdict the subsequent deposition of new solute ions and the clustering of the crystals into large aggregates. Although it is conceivable that high concentrations of inhibitors could completely prevent crystal growth and aggregation, in the face of overwhelming saturation their effect would be simply to retard these

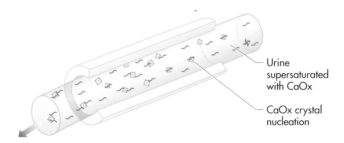

Urine supersaturated with CaOx

CaOx crystal nucleation

Figure 8.10 *The inhibitor theory of stone formation. Inhibitory substances present in urine (here represented as green 'worms') bind to the surface of newly formed calcium oxalate crystals, thereby preventing or retarding their subsequent growth or aggregation into larger crystal clusters.*

processes. Under these circumstances, inhibitors bound to the crystalline surfaces would become buried inside the growing structure as fresh calcium oxalate is deposited. Thus, although the presence of macromolecules in stones and crystals can be explained by their promotion of crystallisation, it can also result from their incompletely inhibiting the process.

The possible involvment of urinary inhibitors as modulators of stone formation is well supported by the fact that urine contains both high and low molecular weight compounds that have been shown, in various crystallisation systems, to inhibit the nucleation, growth or aggregation of calcium oxalate crystals. This is achieved either by binding to the crystal surface, as shown in Figure 8.9, or by chelating calcium or oxalate ions and thereby reducing the probablity of calcium oxalate precipitation. Naturally occurring, low molecular weight compounds in urine that have inhibitory properties are citrate, pyrophosphate and magnesium [14, 96]. As discussed above, a decreased concentration of urinary citrate is a relatively frequent finding in stone formers [47–49], and citrate supplementation is being increasingly used prophylactically for preventing stone recurrences.

Amongst the high molecular weight group can be found glycosaminoglycans [96, 97] and an ever-increasing list of proteins. Tamm–Horsfall mucoprotein can inhibit calcium oxalate crystallisation in inorganic media [98, 99], and crystal aggregation in undiluted, ultrafiltered human urine [100], but, paradoxically, promotes the deposition of both calcium oxalate [101, 102] and calcium phosphate [103] in concentrated urine. Another protein that has attracted attention for many years is nephrocalcin [82], which inhibits calcium oxalate deposition in synthetic solutions and changes in whose primary structure have been reported to account for the reduced inhibitory activity of the protein in stone formers [104]. Osteopontin, a bone protein excreted in urine, has also been implicated as an inhibitor of stone formation by virtue of its ability to inhibit calcium oxalate deposition, again, in synthetic inorganic solutions [105], a property shared with inter-α-trypsin inhibitor [106, 107], fragments of which are present in human urine. Altered molecular characteristics of inter-α-trypsin inhibitor, like those of nephrocalcin, are presumed to explain its reduced inhibitory potency in stone formers [108].

However, it is all too easy to make the gigantic leap from the demonstration of an inhibitory effect in an inorganic solution to the supposition that this is retained in urine, to the assumption that this equates to a role in stone formation. This is simply not the case. There is no doubt that much of what we know about stones has been garnered from experimental evidence obtained in synthetic, aqueous solutions, but with few exceptions, most of what we know about the inhibitory activity of urinary inhibitors tells us nothing about any likely effects they may exert on stone pathogenesis. Therefore, at the present time, it is impossible to state with certainty that the proteins mentioned actually fulfil some function under physiological conditions. However, there is one urinary protein whose effects have been tested in both inorganic media and urine. Urinary prothrombin fragment 1 is the principal protein included into calcium oxalate crystals freshly precipitated from human urine [109], is present in renal stones [89] and is a potent inhibitor of both calcium oxalate crystal growth and aggregation in undiluted, ultrafiltered urine [110]. Nonetheless, there is still no conclusive evidence that this inhibitory effect directs the course of urolithiasis. The same can be said for the urinary glycosaminoglycan heparan sulphate, which is selectively incorporated into calcium oxalate urinary crystals [92, 111] at the expense of more abundant urinary glycosaminoglycans, and which has been shown to inhibit calcium oxalate crystal aggregation in urine [97].

On the basis of the foregoing discussion, it will come as no surprise to learn that studies comparing the inhibitory effects of urine from stone formers and healthy subjects have yielded conflicting data. A number of investigators have reported that stone formers have reduced inhibitory activity [14, 112–114], but these studies are counterbalanced by others unable to confirm the observation [115–119]. These contradictory findings are almost certainly attributable to differences in patient selection and methodology, but, most importantly, to the fact that almost all tested the effects of diluted urine (usually 1% by volume) in an inorganic reaction medium. Thus, like the other theo-

ries of stone formation, the inhibitor hypothesis, though supported by a body of experimental findings, cannot be regarded as unequivocally proved. Further evidence must still be obtained before it will be possible to state with certainty that any one inhibitor, or clutch of inhibitors, can be held to account for the occurrence of stones, and even then, the effects of promotory inorganic ions such as calcium, oxalate and urate must take their share of the responsibility.

Summary

This astronaut's view of the scientific foundations of urolithiasis has, by necessity, omitted mention of most of the libraries of papers devoted to the experimental elucidation of epidemiological, genetic, metabolic and physicochemical factors leading to stone formation. It probably appears puzzling to anyone not actually involved in stone research that a disease that would at first seem to be easily explicable by recourse to simple chemical and physical principles has managed to elude our understanding, literally for centuries. But there is no need for guilt. Stone disease does not result from a single cause, and for that reason has proved extraordinarily difficult to study. As shown in Figure 8.2, it represents the end-product of multiple factors, all of which will vary in their degree of influence at any one time in a person's life. Only by painstakingly teasing out each of these factors and studying their interactions will it be possible to design therapy for preventing stone recurrences based on sound, scientific rationale.

Acknowledgement

The author would like to thank Dennis Jones for his artistic expertise.

References

1. Milliner DS. Epidemiology of calcium oxalate urolithiasis in Man. In: Khan SR (ed) Calcium oxalate in biological systems. Boca Raton: CRC Press, 1995: 169–88

2. Anderson DA. Environmental factors in the aetiology of urolithiasis. In: Cifuentes-Dellate L, Rapado A, Hogkinson A (eds) Urinary calculi. Basel: Karger, 1972: 130–44

3. Window on the 21st Century, National Kidney and Urologic Diseases Advisory Board 1990 Long-Range Plan. US Department of Health and Human Services, 1990

4. Clark JY, Thompson IM, Optenberg SA. Economic impact of urolithiasis in the US. J Urol 1995; 154: 2020–4

5. Lowenstam HA, Weiner S. On biomineralization. New York: Oxford University Press, 1989

6. Prien EL. Crystallographic analysis of urinary calculi. A 23-year survey study. J Urol 1963; 89: 917–24

7. Yoshida O, Okada Y. Epidemiology of urolithiasis in Japan: a chronological and geographical study. Urol Int 1990; 45: 104–11

8. Sierakowski R, Finlayson B, Landes RR, Finlayson CD, Sierakowski N. The frequency of urolithiasis in hospital discharge diagnoses in the United States. Invest Urol 1978; 15: 438–41

9. Ljunghal S, Danielson BG. A prospective study of renal stone recurrences. Br J Urol 1984; 56: 122–4

10. Ettinger B. Recurrence of nephrolithiasis. A six-year prospective study. Am J Med 1979; 67: 245–8

11. Robertson WG, Peacock M, Nordin BEC. Calcium crystalluria in recurrent renal-stone formers. Lancet 1969; 2: 21–4

12. Elliot JS, Rabinowitz IN. Calcium oxalate crystalluria: crystal size in urine. J Urol 1980; 123: 324–7

13. Werness PG, Bergert JH, Smith LH. Crystalluria. J Crystal Growth 1981; 53: 166–81

14. Robertson WG, Peacock M. Calcium oxalate crystalluria and inhibitors of crystallization in recurrent renal stone-formers. Clin Sci 1972; 43: 499–506

15. Hallson PC, Rose GA. Crystalluria in normal subjects and in stone formers with and without thiazide and cellulose phosphate treatment. Br J Urol 1976; 48: 515–24

16. Robertson WG, Peacock M, Nordin BEC. Activity products in stone-forming and non-stone-forming urine. Clin Sci 1968; 34: 579–94

17. Kok DJ, Papapoulos SE. Physicochemical considerations in the development and prevention of calcium oxalate urolithiases. Bone Min Metab 1993; 20: 1–15

18. Marangella M, Daniele PG, Ronzani M, Sonega S, Linari F. Urine saturation with calcium salts in normal subjects and idiopathic calcium stone formers estimated by an improved computer model system. Urol Res 1985; 13: 189–93

19. Finlayson B. Symposium on renal lithiasis. Renal lithiasis in review. Urol Clin N Am 1974; 1: 181–212

20. Robertson WG, Hughes H. Importance of mild hyperoxaluria in the pathogenesis of urolithiasis – new evidence from studies in the Arabian peninsula. Scan Micros 1993; 7: 391–402

21. Murphy L. The history of urology. Springfield, IL: Charles C Thomas, 1972

22. Grover PK, Ryall R, Marshall VR. Effect of urate on calcium oxalate crystallization in human urine: evidence for a promotory role of hyperuricosuria in urolithiasis. Clin Sci 1990; 79: 9–15

23. Flocks R. Calcium and phosphorus excretion in the urine of patients with renal or ureteral calculi. J Am Med Assoc 1939; 113: 1466–71

24. Pak CY. Etiology and treatment of urolithiasis. Am J Kidney Dis 1991; 18: 624–37

25. Ryall RL, Marshall VR. Investigation and management of idiopathic urolithiasis. In: Wickham JEA, Buck AC (eds) Renal tract stone. Metabolic basis and clinical practice. Edinburgh: Churchill Livingstone, 1990: 307–31

26. Curhan GC, Willett WC, Rimm EB, Stampfer MJ. A prospective study of dietary calcium and other nutrients and the risk of symptomatic kidney stones. N Engl J Med 1993; 328: 833–8

27. Ryall RL. The formation and investigation of urinary calculi. Clin Biochem Rev 1989; 10: 149–57

28. Danpure CJ, Rumsby G. Enzymology and molecular genetics of primary hyperoxaluria type 1. Consequences for clinical management. In: Khan SR (ed) Calcium oxalate in biological systems. Boca Raton: CRC Press, 1995: 189–206

29. Hodgkinson A. Relations between oxalic acid, calcium, magnesium and creatinine excretion in normal men and male patients with calcium oxalate kidney stones. Clin Sci Mol Med 1974; 46: 357–67

30. Robertson WG, Peacock M, Heyburn PJ, Marshall DH, Clark PB. Risk factors in calcium stone disease of the urinary tract. Br J Urol 1978; 50: 449–54

31. Cohanim M, Yendt ER. Reduction of urine oxalate during long-term thiazide therapy in patients with calcium urolithiasis. Invest Urol 1980; 18: 170–3

32. Baggio B, Gambaro G, Favaro S, Borsatti A. Prevalence of hyperoxaluria in idiopathic calcium oxalate kidney stone disease. Nephron 1983; 35: 11–14

33. Larking P, Lovell-Smith CJ, Hocken AG. Urine oxalate levels in a New Zealand reference population and renal stone formers. N Z Med J 1983; 96: 606–7

34. Cowley DM, McWhinney BC, Brown JM, Chalmers AH. Chemical factors important to calcium nephrolithiasis: evidence for impaired hydroxycarboxylic acid absorption causing hyperoxaluria. Clin Chem 1987; 33: 243–7

35. Tiselius H-G. Excretion of 4-pyridoxic acid and oxalic acid in patients with urinary calculi. Invest Urol 1977; 15: 5–8

36. Butz M, Kohlbecker G. Oxalate urolithiasis: significance of serum and urinary oxalate. Urol Int 1980; 35: 303–8

37. Galosy R, Clarke L, Ward DL, Pak CYC. Renal oxalate excretion in calcium urolithiasis. J Urol 1980; 123: 320–3

38. Ryall RL, Marshall VR. The value of the 24-hour urine analysis in the assessment of stone-formers attending a general hospital out-patient clinic. Br J Urol 1983; 55: 1–5

39. Schwille PO, Hanisch E, Scholz D. Postprandial hyperoxaluria and intestinal oxalate absorption in idiopathic renal stone disease. J Urol 1984; 132: 650–5

40. Emmerson BT. How can one define urate overproduction in man? Adv Exp Med Biol 1986; 195: 287–9

41. Ryall RL, Grover PK, Marshall VR. Urate and calcium stones – picking up a drop of mercury with one's fingers? Am J Kidney Dis 1991; 17: 426–30

42. Coe FL. Hyperuricosuric calcium oxalate nephrolithiasis. Kidney Int 1978; 13: 418–26

43. Coe FL, Raisen L. Allopurinol treatment of uric acid disorders in calcium stone formers. Lancet 1973; 1: 129–31

44. Simth MJV. Placebo versus allopurinol for renal calculi. J Urol 1977; 117: 690–2

45. Ettinger B, Tang A, Citron JT, Livermore B, Williams T. Randomized trial of allopurinol in the prevention of calcium oxalate calculi. New Engl J Med 1986; 315: 1386–9

46. Welshman SG, McGeown MG. Urinary citrate excretion in stone-formers and normal controls. Br J Urol 1976; 48: 7–11

47. Pak CYC. Citrate and renal calculi. Min Electrolyte Metab 1987; 13: 257–66

48. Menon M, Mahle CJ. Urinary citrate excretion in patients with renal calculi. J Urol 1983; 129: 1158–60

49. Pak CYC. Citrate and renal calculi: an update. Min Electrolyte Metab 1994; 20: 371–7

50. Parks JH, Coe FL. Urine citrate and calcium in calcium nephrolithiasis. Adv Exp Med Biol 1986; 208: 445–9

51. Hosking DH, Wilson JWL, Liedtke RR, Smith LH, Wilson DM. Urinary citrate excretion in normal persons and patients with idiopathic calcium urolithiasis. J Lab Clin Med 1985; 106: 682–9

52. Finlayson B, Reid F. The expectation of free and fixed particles in urinary stone disease. Invest Urol 1978; 15: 442–8

53. Kok DJ, Khan SR. Calcium oxalate nephrolithiasis, a free or fixed particle disease? J Urol 1994; 46: 847–54

54. Hackett RL, Shevock PN. The role of crystal-cell attachment and retention in stone disease: In: Khan SR (ed) Calcium oxalate in biological systems. Boca Raton: CRC Press, 1995: 323–42

55. Khan S, Hackett R. Retention of calcium oxalate crystals in renal tubules. Scan Microsc 1991; 5: 707–12

56. Khan SR, Finlayson B, Hackett RL. Experimental calcium oxalate nephrolithiasis in the rat – role of the renal papilla. Am J Pathol 1982; 107: 59–69

57. Khan SR, Hackett RL. Acute hyperoxaluria, renal injury and calcium oxalate urolithiasis. J Urol 1992; 147: 226–30

58. Lieske JC, Walsh RM, Toback FG. Calcium oxalate monohydrate crystals are endocytosed by renal epithelial cells and induce proliferation. Am J Physiol 1992; 31: F622–30

59. Lieske JC, Toback FG. Regulation of renal epithelial cell endocytosis of calcium oxalate monohydrate crystals. Am J Physiol 1993; 264: F800–7

60. Khan SR. Calcium oxalate crystal interaction with renal tubular epithelium, mechanisms of crystal ahdesion and its impact on stone formation. Urol Res 1995; 23: 71–9

61. Modlin M. The aetiology of renal stones: a new concept arising from studies on a stone-free population. Ann R Coll Surg Engl 1967; 40: 155–78

62. Lonsdale K. Epitaxy as a growth factor in urinary calculi and gallstones. Nature 1968; 217: 56–8

63. Coe FL, Lawton RL, Goldstein RB. Sodium urate accelerates precipitation of calcium oxalate in vitro. Proc Soc Exp Biol Med 1975; 149: 926–9

64. Pak CYC, Arnold LH. Heterogeneous nucleation of calcium oxalate by seeds of monosodium urate. Proc Soc Exp Biol Med 1975; 149: 930–2

65. Meyer JL, Bergert JH, Smith LH. The epitaxially induced crystal growth of calcium oxalate by crystalline uric acid. Invest Urol 1976; 14: 115–9

66. Meyer JL, Bergert GH, Smith LH. Epitaxial relationships in urolithiasis: the calcium oxalate monohydrate–hydroxyapatite system. Clin Sci Mol Med 1975; 49: 369–74

67. Meyer JL, Bergert JH, Smith LH. Epitaxial relationships in urolithiasis. The brushite–whewellite system. Clin Sci Mol Med 1977; 52: 143–8

68. Grover PK, Ryall RL. The effect of urinary macromolecules on the ability of seed crystals or uric acid, sodium urate and calcium oxalate to induce precipitation of calcium oxalate in vitro. In: Pak CYC, Resnick MI, Preminger GM (eds) Urolithiasis 1996. Dallas: Millet the Printer, Inc., 1996: 273–4

69. Kim S, Grover PK, Ryall RL. The effect of seed crystals of brushite and hydroxyapatite on calcium oxalate crystallization in undiluted human urine. In: Pak CYC, Resnick MI, Preminger GM (eds) Urolithiasis 1996. Dallas: Millet the Printer, Inc., 1996: 269–70

70. Hallson PC, Rose GA, Sulaiman S. Urate does not influence the formation of calcium oxalate crystals in whole human urine at pH 5.3. Clin Sci 1982; 62: 421–5

71. Grover PK, Ryall RL, Marshall VR. Dissolved urate promotes calcium oxalate crystallization: epitaxy is not the cause. Clin Sci 1993; 85: 1–5

72. Mayer GG, Chase T, Farvar B, et al. Metabolic studies on the formation of calcium oxalate stones, with special emphasis on vitamin B6 and uric acid metabolism. Bull NY Acad Med 1968; 44: 28–44

73. Tiselius H-G, Højgaard I, Fornander A-M, Nilsson M-A. Is calcium phosphate the natural promoter of calcium oxalate crystallization? In: Pak CYC, Resnick MI, Preminger GM (eds) Urolithiasis 1996. Dallas: Millet the Printer, Inc., 1996: 238–9

74. Ryall RL, Stapleton AMF. Urinary macromolecules in calcium oxalate stone and crystal matrix: good, bad, or indifferent? In: Khan SR (ed) Calcium oxalate in biological systems. Boca Raton: CRC Press, 1995: 265–90

75. Khan SR, Hackett RL. Role of organic matrix in urinary stone formation: an ultrastructural study of crystal matrix interface of calcium oxalate monohydrate stones. J Urol 1993; 150: 239–45

76. Warpehoski MA, Buscemi PJ, Osborn DC, Finlayson B, Goldberg EP. Distribution of organic matrix in calcium oxalate renal calculi. Calcified Tissue Int 1981; 33: 211–22

77. Boyce WH, Garvey FK. The amount and nature of the organic matrix in urinary calculi: a review. J Urol 1956; 76: 213–27

78. Boyce WH. Organic matrix of human urinary concretions. Am J Med 1968; 45: 673–83

79. Doyle IR, Ryall RL, Marshall VR. Inclusion of proteins into calcium oxalate crystals precipitated from human urine: a highly selective phenomenon. Clin Chem 1991; 37: 1589–94

80. Boyce W, King J, Fielden M. Total nondialyzable solids (TNDS) in human urine. XIII: Immunological detection of a component peculiar to renal calculous matrix and to urine of calculous patients. J Clin Invest 1962; 41: 1180–9

81. Melick RA, Quelch KJ, Rhodes M. The demonstration of sialic acid in kidney stone matrix. Clin Sci 1980; 59: 401–4

82. Nakagawa Y, Ahmed M, Hall SL, Deganello S, Coe FL. Isolation from human calcium oxalate renal stones of nephrocalcin, a glycoprotein inhibitor of calcium oxalate crystal growth. Evidence that nephrocalcin from patients with calcium oxalate nephrolithiasis is deficient in gamma-carboxyglutamic acid. J Clin Invest 1987; 79: 1782–87

83. Morse RM, Resnick MI. A new approach to the study of urinary macromolecules as a participant in calcium oxalate crystallization. J Urol 1988; 139: 869–73

84. Petersen TE, Thogersen I, Petersen SE. Identification of hemoglobin and two serine proteases in acid extracts of calcium containing kidney stones. J Urol 1989; 142: 176–80

85. Umekawa T, Kohri K, Amasaki N, et al. Sequencing of a urinary stone protein, identical to α-1-antitrypsin, which lacks 22 amino acids. Biochem Biophys Res Comm 1993; 193: 1049–53

86. Binette JP, Binette MB. A cationic protein from a urate–calcium oxalate stone: isolation and purification of a shared protein. Scan Microsc 1993; 7: 1107–10

87. Binette JP, Binette MB. Sequencing of proteins extracted from stones. Scan Microsc 1994; 8: 233–9

88. Dussol B, Geider S, Lilova A, et al. Analysis of the soluble matrix of five morphologically different kidney stones. Urol Res 1995; 23: 45–51

89. Stapleton AMF, Dawson CJ, Grover PK, et al. Further evidence linking urolithiasis and blood coagulation: urinary prothrombin fragment 1 is present in stone matrix. Kidney Int 1996; 49: 880–8

90. Dawson CJ, Grover PK, Ryall RL. Inter-α-trypsin inhibitor in urine, calcium oxalate crystals and calcium stones. In: Pak CYC, Resnick MI, Preminger GM (eds) Urolithiasis 1996. Dallas: Millet the Printer, Inc., 1996: 275–6

91. Nishio S, Abe Y, Wakatsuki A, et al. Matrix glycosaminoglycan in urinary stones. J Urol 1985; 134: 503–5

92. Yamaguchi S, Yoshioka T, Utsunomiya M, et al. Heparan sulfate in the stone matrix and its inhibitory effect on calcium oxalate crystallization. Urol Res 1993; 21: 187–92

93. Roberts SD, Resnick MI. Glycosaminoglycans content of stone matrix. J Urol 1986; 135: 1078–83

94. Iwata H, Kamei O, Abe Y, et al. The organic matrix of urinary uric acid crystals. J Urol 1988; 139: 607–10

95. Howard JC, Thomas WC. Some observations on rachitic rat cartilage of probable significance in the etiology of renal calculi. Trans Am Clin Climatol Assoc 1958; 70: 94–102

96. Ryall RL, Harnett RM, Marshall VR. The effect of urine, pyrophosphate, citrate, magnesium and glycosaminoglycans on the growth and aggregation of calcium oxalate crystals in vitro. Clin Chim Acta 1981; 112: 349–56

97. Suzuki K, Ryall RL. The effect of heparan sulphate on the crystallization of calcium oxalate in undiluted, ultrafiltered human urine. Br J Urol 1996; 78: 15–21

98. Hess B. Tamm–Horsfall glycoprotein – inhibitor or promotor of calcium oxalate monohydrate crystallization processes? Urol Res 1992; 20: 83–6

99. Hess B. The role of Tamm–Horsfall glycoprotein and nephrocalcin in calcium oxalate monohydrate crystallization processes. Scan Microsc 1991; 5: 689–95

100. Ryall RL, Harnett RM, Hibberd CM, Edyvane KA, Marshall VR. Effects of chondroitin sulphate, human serum albumin and Tamm–Horsfall mucoprotein on calcium oxalate crystallization in undiluted human urine. Urol Res 1991; 19: 181–8

101. Hallson PC, Rose GA. Uromucoids and urinary stone formation. Lancet 1979; 1: 1000–2

102. Grover PK, Ryall RL, Marshall VR. Does Tamm–Horsfall mucoprotein inhibit or promote calcium oxalate crystallisation in human urine? Clin Chim Acta 1990; 190: 223–38

103. Rose GA, Sulaiman S. Tamm–Horsfall mucoprotein promotes calcium phosphate crystal formation in whole urine: quantitative studies. J Urol 1982; 127: 177–9

104. Nakagawa Y, Parks JH, Kezdy FJ, Coe FL. Molecular abnormality of urinary glycoprotein crystal growth inhibitor in calcium nephrolithiasis. Trans Am Physiol Assoc 1985; 98: 281–9

105. Shiraga H, Min W, VanDusen WJ, et al. Inhibition of calcium oxalate crystal growth in vitro by uropontin: another member of the aspartic acid-rich protein superfamily. Proc Nat Acad Sci USA 1992; 89: 426–30

106. Sørensen S, Hansen K, Bak S, Justesen SJ. An unidentified macromolecular inhibitory constituent of cal-cium oxalate growth in human urine. Urol Res 1990; 18: 373–9

107. Atmani F, Lacour B, Strecker G, Parvy P, Drueke T, Daudon M. Molecular characteristics of uronic-acid-rich protein, a strong inhibitor of calcium oxalate crystallization in vitro. Biochem Biophys Res Comm 1993; 191: 1158–65

108. Atmani F, Lacour B, Jungers P, Drueke T, Daudon M. Reduced inhibitory activity of uronic-acid-rich protein in urine of stone formers. Urol Res 1994; 22: 257–60

109. Stapleton AMF, Simpson RJ, Ryall RL. Crystal matrix protein is related to human prothrombin. Biochem Biophys Res Comm 1993; 195: 1199–203

110. Ryall RL, Grover PK, Stapleton AMF, et al. The urinary F1 activation peptide of human prothrombin is a potent inhibitor of calcium oxalate crystallization in undiluted human urine in vitro. Clin Sci 1995; 89: 533–41

111. Suzuki K, Mayne K, Doyle IR, Ryall RL. Urinary glycosaminoglycans are selectively included into calcium oxalate crystals precipitated from whole human urine. Scan Microsc 1994; 8: 523–30

112. Dent CE, Sutor DJ. Presence or absence of inhibitor of calcium-oxalate crystal growth in urine of normals and of stone formers. Lancet 1971; 2: 775–8

113. Sarig S, Garti N, Azoury R, Wax Y, Perlberg S. A method for discrimination between calcium oxalate kidney stone formers and normals. J Urol 1982; 128: 645–9

114. Springmann KE, Drach GW, Gottung B, Randolph AD. Effects of human urine on aggregation of calcium oxalate crystals. J Urol 1986; 135: 69–71

115. Baumann JM. The role of inhibitors and other factors in the pathogenesis of recurrent calcium-containing renal stones. Clin Sci Mol Med 1977; 53: 141–8

116. Crassweller PO, Oreopoulos DG, Toguri A, Husdan H, Wilson DR, Rapoport A. Studies in inhibitors of calcification and levels of urine saturation with calcium salts in recurrent stone patients. J Urol 1978; 120: 6–10

117. Oreopoulos DG, Walker D, Akriotis DJ, et al. Excretion of inhibitors of calcification in urine. Part I. Findings in control subjects and patients with renal stones. J Can Med Assoc 1975; 112: 827–31

118. Pylypchuk G, Ehrig U, Wilson DR. Idiopathic calcium nephrolithiasis. 1. Differences in urine crystalloids, urine saturation with brushite and urine

inhibitors of calcification between persons with and persons without recurrent kidney stone formation. J Can Med Assoc 1979; 120: 658–65

119. Ryall RL, Marshall VR. The relationship between urinary inhibitory activity and endogenous concentrations of glycosaminoglycans and uric acid; comparison of urines from stone-formers and normal subjects. Clin Chim Acta 1984; 141: 197–204

Acute renal failure

9

G. H. Neild

Clinical overview

Epidemiology

Acute renal insufficiency is a sudden decline in renal function. There are no standard definitions. This chapter discusses life-threatening acute renal failure when the renal function falls towards zero. In the UK, about 50 people per million population develop acute renal failure requiring dialysis each year. Acute renal failure complicates about 5% of admissions to hospital and 30% of admissions to intensive care.

Aetiology

By far the most common causes of acute renal failure today are seen on the intensive care unit and are related to sepsis, trauma and surgery. The kidney fails, often with one or more other organs. In this setting, the kidney switches off, but if a kidney biopsy is taken, the tissue appears to be virtually normal, the kidney failure is (potentially) reversible and this is referred to as acute tubular necrosis.

In such cases, there is usually little or no doubt about the antecedent factors – although the actual cause of acute tubular necrosis is usually multifactorial, such as a combination of hypotension, sepsis and nephrotoxic drugs.

Differential diagnosis of acute renal failure
There are three levels or categories at which kidney failure may occur (see Table 9.1):

1. there is interruption of adequate blood flow (or perfusion) of the kidney;

Table 9.1 Differential diagnosis of acute renal failure

1. Prerenal failure	Inadequate blood flow to kidney
2. Renal (parenchymal) disease	Intrinsic injury to the kidney
3. Postrenal failure	Obstruction of the urine outflow

2. there is something wrong with the kidney itself;
3. there is obstruction of the ouflow of urine from the kidneys.

The different causes of acute renal failure are shown in Table 9.2.

Presentation

The clinical symptoms are usually dominated by those of the underlying pathology (Table 9.2). The symptoms of severe renal failure (uraemia) are not specific (see Chapter 10).

The classic (but not obligatory) feature of acute renal failure is reduction of the urine volume (oliguria), defined as a urine volume of less than 400 ml per day. This will often be associated with fluid retention leading to oedema. Clinical situations in which acute tubular necrosis occurs are shown in Table 9.3.

Investigations

When sick patients are admitted, there is a range of routine tests that is done (Table 9.4). This range will

Table 9.2 Aetiology of acute renal failure

Prerenal

Physiological
- Shock (hypovolaemia)
    Primary underfilling of circulating blood volume due to loss of blood, colloid or crystalloid
    Primary dilatation of peripheral circulation (loss of peripheral resistance) due to septicaemia, anaphylaxis
- Heart failure (cardiogenic shock)
- Changes in glomerulo-haemodynamics
    Hepatorenal syndrome
    Septicaemia
    Angiotensin-converting enzyme inhibitors, non-steroidal anti-inflammatory drugs

Pathological
- Renal artery thrombosis or embolus
- Dissection of aorta
- Renal artery trauma
- Cholesterol emboli

Renal

- Acute tubular necrosis
- Acute glomerulonephritis
- Acute interstitial nephritis
- Acute tubular obstruction
    Pigments (myoglobin, haemoglobin)
    Crystals
    Myeloma
- Acute infection (pyelonephritis)
- Occlusion of renal microcirculation (haemolytic uraemic syndrome)

Postrenal

- Involvement of both ureters
    Stones, papillae (intrinsic)
    Retroperitoneal fibrosis (extrinsic)
    Glands, aorta
- Bladder
    Tumour
    Prostate
    Bladder neck obstruction

be extended depending on the known diagnosis or the likely differential diagnoses.

Biochemistry

The fact that somebody has renal failure is established by the blood tests showing high values of urea and creatinine. With renal failure, whether it is acute or chronic, a number of other biochemical tests are abnormal, but these do not usually help distinguish between acute and chronic renal failure. Generally, with renal failure, the plasma potassium, phosphate and urate are raised and the calcium is reduced.

Haematology

With any patient, a full blood count (FBC) would be done and the blood clotting times checked (the prothrombin time, the activated partial thromboplastin time (APTT) or kaolin clotting time (KCT) and the thrombin time). The presence of prolonged clotting times and thrombocytopenia indicates disseminated intravascular coagulation, which is usually secondary to septicaemia.

Serology

The presence of antibodies may help to establish the cause of an autoimmune disease (e.g. antinuclear, or

Table 9.3 Clinical situations in which acute tubular necrosis occurs

Prerenal leading to ischaemic renal failure	Hypovolaemia
	Cardiac failure
	Neural (sympathetic overactivity), e.g. aortic dissection
	Septicaemia
	Cyclosporin toxicity
	Vasoactive drugs, e.g. non-steroidal anti-inflammatory drugs, angiotensin-converting enzyme inhibitors
	Renal artery occlusion, e.g. aortic surgery
Renal	Nephrotoxins, e.g. gentamicin, amphotericin, cisplatinum
	Toxin, e.g. paraquat, radio-contrast
	Toxicity, e.g. pancreatitis, multiple organ failure
	Sepsis, including pneumonia
	Idiopathic/unknown
	Myeloma
	Haemoglobinuria, myoglobinuria
Outflow obstruction	Renal colic etc.

Table 9.4 Investigations for acute renal failure

Blood tests
Biochemistry
  Blood
  Urine
Haematology
  Full blood count
  Coagulation screen
Serology (antibody tests)

Urine tests
Dipstick urine
Microscope urine
Quantify electrolytes and protein
Culture urine (midstream urine, MSU)

Bacteriology
Culture urine (MSU)
Culture blood (blood cultures)

Imaging
Radiology
Nuclear medicine

Renal biopsy

antineutrophil cytoplasm) or may be necessary in diagnosing an infectious disease.

Urine test
It is mandatory that urine is tested on admission for blood and protein. A urine sample must also be sent to the laboratory to be microscoped (looking for red cells, white cells and protein casts, and bacteria) and cultured.

Often, in acute renal failure, a spot sample of urine will be sent to the laboratory to measure the sodium, potassium and urea concentration in the urine. Pre-renal failure is characterised by urine sodium <10 mmol and a urine/plasma urea ratio >20.

Radiology and nuclear medicine
The essential information required concerning the cause of renal failure is anatomical information regarding the shape and size of the kidneys and their texture. This can all be obtained with ultrasound. The minimum information reported should be the size and shape of each kidney and whether its texture shows evidence of increased fibrosis, reported as increased echogenicity. In certain circumstances, specialist X-rays or isotope scans will be performed.

Renal biopsy
In many instances, it is clear that the injury is to the kidney itself, but the different tests will not, for example, discriminate between different types of glomerular disease. Only a renal biopsy can determine the precise diagnosis. Renal biopsies are important not only for the diagnosis but for establishing which treatment would be best and the prognosis, i.e. the likely response to the treatment.

Complications of acute renal failure

Fluid overload
This can commonly occur either before the patient is seen by the doctor or after the patient is treated with intravenous fluids. The patient will often complain of increasing breathlessness, and physical examination will show signs of fluid overload (peripheral oedema, raised jugular venous pressure or central venous

pressure, gallop rhythm) and pulmonary oedema. A chest X-ray is often necessary to confirm that there is pulmonary oedema. If the kidneys are still working, then they may be able to pass more urine after treatment with diuretics; otherwise, dialysis may be necessary to remove the fluid.

Hyperkalaemia

This is a recognised medical emergency. The patient will generally not have any specific symptoms, but an electrocardiogram will show a typical appearance of hyperkalaemia. If the potassium is not lowered, the patient may have a cardiac arrest. There are a number of strategies involving intravenous drugs to lower the potassium in the short term, but once renal failure is established, the potassium will only be controlled by dialysis.

Hypertension

The hypertension may be due to general fluid retention and/or it may be generated by the kidney. The high blood pressure may improve when fluid is removed. In addition to this, blood pressure-lowering drugs are often given. It is very important that the blood pressure should not be lowered too quickly from very high levels, particularly for patients presenting with very severe hypertension (malignant hypertension), who may suffer serious consequences. It is well known for vessels to thrombose, resulting in strokes; thrombosis of arteries to the spinal cord can result in paraplegia.

Bleeding tendency

Patients with severe renal failure have an increased likelihood of bleeding, which may occur even though their platelet count and clotting are normal. This is because the platelets, for reasons that are not clearly understood, do not adhere normally to the endothelium and arrest bleeding. In addition, sick patients may have either a low platelet count or abnormal clotting, which may be other causes of an increased bleeding tendency.

Patients are at increased risk of gastrointestinal haemorrhage, particularly from the stomach, which can be prevented by a number of therapeutic measures to reduce the acidity inside the stomach.

Infection

Patients may present with infection. Also, uraemic patients have a slightly suppressed immune system, rendering them more susceptible to infection and to severe infection.

Treatment

General conservative measures

A patient must first be resuscitated in the appropriate way. This may mean giving, or sometimes removing, fluid. All efforts should be made to re-establish a good circulatory state in the patient, which means a good cardiac output and a warm and well-perfused periphery. Patients who are anaemic may need a blood transfusion; others may be managed with intravenous saline or dextrose solutions. Attention should be paid to the blood potassium and to establishing the urine output. It is often much easier to catheterise a sick patient so that the urine output can be monitored on an hourly basis.

Specific treatment of underlying disease

This refers back to the aetiology of the renal failure. If it is established, for example, that the patient has obstruction to the ureters, then it is usually appropriate to drain the kidneys with a percutaneous nephrostomy. If the obstruction is at the level of the bladder neck or below, then simple bladder catheterisation may be sufficient.

Clearly, if the underlying problem is an infection, this should be appropriately diagnosed and treated. In some cases, the intrinsic disease to the kidney will only become clear after the biopsy, and it may require specific treatment with powerful immunosuppressive drugs.

Dialysis

There are three absolute indications for dialysis:

1. fluid overload that is resistant to diuretic therapy;
2. increasing hyperkalaemia;
3. severe uraemia and acidosis.

Generally, patients with acute renal failure will be treated with haemodialysis rather than peritoneal dialysis. However, there are times when peritoneal dialysis may be indicated or haemodialysis may be unavailable.

Prognosis

In acute renal failure, the prognosis depends on the number of organs, in addition to the kidneys, that are failing. If the kidney is the single affected organ and the patient is otherwise well, survival is in excess of 80%. Patients with more than one organ failing are likely to be managed on the intensive care unit. For such patients, the outlook is very poor. With one other organ failing (e.g. the lungs requiring ventilation), there is a 45% chance of survival. With two other organs failing (e.g. needing ventilation and cardiac support), the mortality is in excess of 80%. With three or more other organs failing, the mortality is in excess of 90%.

Those who have just renal involvement and ischaemic damage to their kidney resulting in acute tubular necrosis can expect to make an almost complete recovery, with renal function returning eventually to normal. At follow-up, they may have mild evidence of residual injury, such as small amounts of protein in the urine, but do not develop chronic renal failure.

Pathogenesis of acute tubular necrosis

Introduction

The pathogenesis of acute tubular necrosis is complex. The normal kidney filters 120 ml of ultrafiltrate from plasma per minute, or 173 litres per day. Clearly, the kidney has to have not only the normal ability to reabsorb 99% of this tubular fluid, but also multiple and complex mechanisms to protect the circulation if tubular function is compromised. Not only are there often multiple insults causing acute tubular necrosis, but there are also multiple mechanisms contributing to the final result of no urine. In attempting to unravel these mechanisms, there are three factors to consider:

1. the kidney does not function (glomerular filtration rate <5 ml/min);
2. the injury is potentially reversible;
3. the renal histology shows only (minor) tubular changes.

Two considerations underlie research into the pathogenesis of acute tubular necrosis.

1. Can strategies be developed to prevent it?
2. Can strategies be developed to accelerate its recovery?

Pathogenesis is best considered with reference to these two considerations. Firstly, what mechanisms lead to the glomerular filtration rate falling to zero? Secondly, what mechanisms maintain the glomerular filtration rate at zero even after the blood supply is returned to near normal?

There are a number of clinical situations in which acute tubular necrosis occurs (see Table 9.3). This section discusses the mechanisms initiated by these clinical insults. The key components in the pathogenesis are shown in Figure 9.1. In reality, there is rarely a

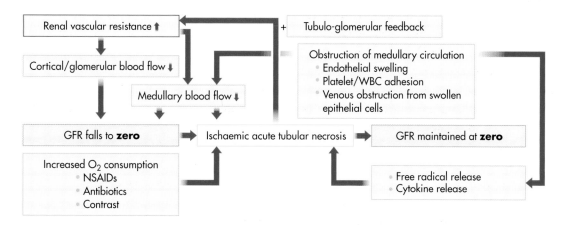

Figure 9.1 Pathogenesis of acute tubular necrosis.

single cause, but a number of events that summate and this is typified by the patient on the intensive care unit. This review only attempts to summarise the facts and present the current consensus views.

One major clue to the pathogenesis is provided by our clinical experience: in almost all experimental models of acute renal failure and in humans, volume loading with saline and the establishment of a natriuresis will prevent or minimise acute tubular necrosis. Conversely, volume contraction will increase the risk of acute tubular necrosis. If we could understand the mechanisms activated by this simple manoeuvre, then we would have real insight into the pathogenesis.

Renal anatomy and physiology relevant to acute tubular necrosis

Anatomy

The kidneys (less than 0.5% of the body mass) have one of the highest blood flow rates per unit tissue mass in the body and receive approximately 20% of the cardiac output. This is to filter the blood – only a small percentage is required to supply oxygen for metabolism. Renal blood flow, per gram of tissue, declines progressively from the outer to the inner cortex. Glomerular density shows a similar gradient and this ensures that the outer cortical glomeruli contribute most to total glomerular filtration rate.

The medullary blood supply is derived from the efferent arterioles of the inner cortical glomeruli. These arterioles branch and descend into the descending vasa rectae, which themselves descend in vascular bundles and at intervals leave to supply the adjacent peritubular capillary plexus. In the region of the thick ascending limb, the plexus is very dense.

The loops of Henle have two origins. There are short loops that descend from glomeruli in the outer cortex and they are located furthest from the vascular bundles and are most susceptible to ischaemia. Long loops, from inner cortical glomeruli, are located close to the bundles.

The capillary plexus drains upwards via the ascending vasa rectae, which empty into the arcuate veins at the corticomedullary junction. Both descending and ascending vasa rectae are resistance vessels, which reg-

ulate medullary blood flow. Ascending vessels have very thin walls and are potentially susceptible to compression by swollen tubules.

Flow in the outer cortex is approximately sixfold greater than in outer medulla and 20-fold greater than in inner medulla. Autoregulation also occurs in the medulla. The limited blood supply to the medulla prevents washout of the gradients of solute formed by the loops of Henle, which are important for normal urine concentration.

Oxygen tension

In the kidney there are gradients of oxygen availability [1]. Medullary partial pressure of oxygen (pO_2) is 10–20 mmHg and much lower than cortical pO_2 (about 50 mmHg). The corticomedullary gradient of pO_2 is maintained by the countercurrent diffusion of oxygen between arterial and venous branches of the vasa rectae, thus reducing the oxygen supply to the deeper medulla. The ambient pO_2 in the renal medulla is low, but demand for oxygen is also low because medullary tubular metabolism is mainly by anaerobic glycolysis.

Glomerular filtration

The rate of glomerular ultrafiltration depends not only on the hydrostatic pressure within the capillary but also on the total capillary surface area available for filtration. Reduction in glomerular capillary surface area due to mesangial contraction is an attractive theoretical concept and might play a role in the maintenance of reduced glomerular filtration rate. Although vasoconstrictors, such as angiotensin and endothelin, do cause mesangial cell contraction in vitro, there is no direct evidence that this does happen in vivo [2].

Vasomotor tone in the kidney is regulated by a complex series of dilator and constrictor mediators. Some are likely to be more important than others, but we no longer have the naivety to believe that one (such as endothelin) is the principal mediator. What is clear, and verified in experimental models, is that if there is afferent constriction and reciprocal efferent dilatation, then glomerular plasma flow may be normal, and yet the net hydrostatic pressure is too low to permit ultrafiltration and urine is therefore not formed.

Events that lead to a fall in glomerular filtration rate to zero

The renal tubules of healthy kidneys reabsorb over 7 litres of ultrafiltrate per hour. Failure, even partial, of tubular reabsorption would be disastrous, and so highly effective feedback mechanisms have developed to reduce or switch off glomerular filtration.

Shutdown in cortical blood flow (pre-renal failure)

When the circulation is threatened, as in hypovolaemia, the kidney reduces glomerular filtration ('pre-renal failure'). There is a great reduction in cortical blood flow, *but* at all costs medullary flow is maintained. This is partly achieved by the two circulations being independently regulated.

Heterogeneity

The immediate increase in renal vascular resistance in response to hypoperfusion, whether due to hypovolaemia or heart failure, is partly the result of massive sympathetic activity with secondary activation of the renin–angiotensin system. Although renal blood flow is decreased, glomerular filtration rate is initially preserved by a disproportionate rise in efferent tone, which is mediated in particular by angiotensin. Moreover, the increased tone in the afferent vessels is offset by vasodilatory prostaglandins and nitric oxide; for these reasons, the use of angiotensin-converting enzyme inhibitors or inhibitors of cyclo-oxgenase (e.g. non-steroidal anti-inflammatory drugs) can cause a precipitous decline in glomerular filtration rate.

A very attractive hypothesis proposes that the independent regulation of the cortical and medullary blood supplies is in part achieved by the differential action of adenosine, itself a product of ischaemia. In conditions of ischaemia in other organs, adenosine is a vasodilator and is cytoprotective. In the kidney it is a potent vasoconstrictor of the cortical circulation (via A1 receptors), but a vasodilator in the medulla (via A2 receptors) [3].

Loss of autoregulation

Following the induction of acute tubular necrosis, there is loss of endothelium-dependent vasodilatation within the kidney, which contributes to the loss of autoregulation. This may have two consequences: firstly, there will be loss of the compensatory vasodilatation following ischaemic injury, and secondly, the kidney will not be protected from any subsequent falls in perfusion pressure.

Tubulo-glomerular feedback

Glomerular haemodynamics are locally regulated by the tubulo-glomerular feedback mechanism. Early in the course of ischaemic injury to the thick ascending limb, there is loss of chloride reabsorption and activation of this feedback mechanism at the macula densa, which in turn leads to afferent arteriolar constriction and a decrease in glomerular filtration rate [4]. Adenosine is a potent enhancer of tubulo-glomerular feedback and acts in synergism with other vasoactive agents such as angiotensin to produce renal vasoconstriction. This effect is more pronounced in salt-restricted than in salt-loaded rats.

Vasoactive mediators

In addition to adenosine, there are many potent vasoactive mediators, both endogenous and exogenous, that are important. Moreover, loss of vasodilators (such as nitric oxide) will exacerbate vasoconstriction. It would be premature to single out a principal mediator, but endothelin would seem an obvious candidate as a key factor [5].

What is intriguing, and still unexplained, is the reduction in glomerular filtration rate seen in the hepatorenal syndrome (and some other situations). Although the glomerular filtration rate can be virtually zero, the kidney mimics pre-renal failure i.e. the urine is concentrated and there is avid retention of sodium, implying that the tubular (medullary) blood supply is still intact. The kidney is resistant to volume expansion. This glomerular haemodynamic state can only be achieved by afferent constriction with reciprocal efferent dilatation. No pharmaceutical intervention is yet capable of reversing this situation. Similarly, no pharmaceutical intervention will reverse cyclosporin nephrotoxicity.

Shutdown in medullary blood flow (leading to acute tubular necrosis)

Hypovolaemia

When the renal circulation is initially compromised, medullary blood flow is maintained, but beyond a certain point the medullary flow becomes inadequate to maintain oxygenation of the medullary tubules.

Sepsis and cytokine activation

In the past decade there has been an enormous increase in our understanding of the physiology of septicaemia [6]. Endotoxin (lipopolysaccharide) triggers the release of a series of cytokines and vasoactive mediators. Septic shock is associated with a fall in peripheral vascular resistance and mean arterial blood pressure. This is initially associated with a rise in cardiac output. However, venous pooling occurs, causing a fall in cardiac preload and cardiac output. This reduction in cardiac output is exacerbated by myocardial depressant factors that are generated. In the kidney, independently of these systemic effects, there is a rise in renal vascular resistance, and a fall in renal blood flow and glomerular filtration rate. These changes are due to the mediators released, which include tumour necrosis factor, interleukin-1, platelet-activating factor, thromboxane, leukotriene, and endothelin. Lipopolysaccharide itself has no direct effect on the renal circulation [6].

In septicaemia, renal haemodynamics can be altered so that, as in the hepatorenal syndrome, the glomerular filtration rate may be reduced with volume-resistant oliguria and yet there is still avid retention of sodium. More commonly, critically ill patients with septicaemia or multiple organ failure have a progressive fall in glomerular filtration rate with gradually increasing oliguria, although they may initially have non-oliguric renal failure. No pharmacological intervention significantly alters this course of events (except treatment and resolution of the underlying problem). The final sequence of events that lead to tubular ischaemia and acute tubular necrosis are still unknown.

Vascular obstruction

In experimental models of acute tubular necrosis, focal and segmental necrosis of the media in resistance arterioles is found. This is probably a consequence of the initial severe vasospasm, but may contribute to the continuing reduction in blood flow. Endothelial swelling is patchy and transient [7], except in the corticomedullary area where it is consistent and persists.

The lumens of capillaries are occluded not only by swollen endothelial cells but also by platelets and leucocytes adhering to sites of endothelial injury and thus contributing to the mechanical obstruction. Following ischaemic injury, free radical production by damaged endothelium and activated adherent neutrophils will inactivate endothelium-derived nitric oxide, thus further promoting the cycle of vasoconstriction and leucocyte adhesion. Endothelial injury will also lead to loss of endothelial tight junctions, an increase in vascular permeability, and interstitial oedema. Nevertheless, there is a rationale for giving drugs (such as prostacyclin, nitric oxide-donors) that may dilate the microcirculation and prevent leucocyte adhesion and platelet aggregation.

Although endothelial cell injury is likely to trigger thrombosis and the generation of fibrin, it is very difficult to find morphological evidence of this due to the great fibrinolytic capacity of endothelium, and fibrin may only be found when the fibrinolytic pathways are overwhelmed.

Venous obstruction

In post-mortem specimens, the dark zone at the outer medulla seen in acute tubular necrosis is due to intense vascular congestion of the ascending vasa rectae. Obstruction of the venous return from the medulla is thought to be an important factor contributing to tubular ischaemia [8]. The medullary circulation is drained by the very thin-walled ascending vasa rectae. Following ischaemic injury to medullary tubules, there is cell swelling and interstitial oedema and these swollen tubules will obstruct the ascending vessels. Sufficient cell swelling to contribute to 'no reflow' does not occur until anoxia has persisted for 30–40 minutes. Thus, a vicious circle is set up, with increasing venous obstruction increasing tubular ischaemia.

Tubular obstruction

The role of tubular obstruction in the maintenance of oliguria has provoked much debate for many years. Tubular obstruction plays a major role in some experimental models, but there is less evidence in humans. However, as described in the previous section, cell swelling is thought to play an important role in venous obstruction of the medullary circulation.

There are secondary causes of acute renal failure in which tubular obstruction is relevant. These include myeloma, crystalluria, haemoglobinuria and myoglobinuria. Although the pathogenesis of acute renal failure in, for example, myoglobinuria is complex and multifactorial, it seems sensible from a clinical point of view to minimise the risk of cast obstruction. Thus, establishing a diuresis and alkalinising the urine are logical strategies [9].

Reperfusion injury and no reflow phenomenon

In acute tubular necrosis following ischaemia and reperfusion, the mechanism of continued reduction in renal blood flow that occurs after correction of systemic pressure and volume – the so-called 'no reflow' phenomenon – is poorly understood.

There are a number of factors that contribute to it. Both the interruption and subsequent restoration of blood flow (reperfusion) cause tissue injury in any organ, although the consequences vary greatly. The impact is greatest in the heart, and cardiological science has been increasingly successful at developing interventions to protect the myocardium. Ischaemia and reperfusion in the kidney contribute not only to the renal dysfunction after periods of hypoperfusion, but to the non-immunological damage that complicates cadaveric renal transplantation and revascularisation surgery. One must be cautious about overextrapolating from the heart and central nervous system to the kidney because, in the former, interruption of flow is often complete and associated with infarction.

Leucocytes and activation of adhesion molecules

Trapping and adhesion of leucocytes in the microcirculation play a key role in ischaemic injury, and activated neutrophils can release reactive oxygen species and a variety of enzymes including proteases, elastase and myeloperoxidase. Neutrophils will adhere to endothelium when adhesion molecules on endothelial cells (such as ICAM-1) are activated, e.g. by reperfusion injury or sepsis.

In models of myocardial and intestinal ischaemia, depletion of neutrophils, blockade of neutrophil adhesion and inhibition of complement all reduce tissue injury [10, 11]. Recent powerful support for their relevance in acute renal failure comes from blocking adhesion molecules. Monoclonal antibodies against ICAM-1 protect against experimental ischaemia, even when given two hours after the insult [12], and mice deficient in ICAM-1 are protected against acute renal failure [10]. It is therefore of potential relevance that both adenosine and nitric oxide can down-regulate adhesion molecules.

Free radicals

Reperfusion with oxygenated blood is associated with free-radical generation, leading to lipid peroxidation, polysaccharide depolymerisation and deoxyribonucleotide degradation. Damaged endothelial cells not only now fail to generate vasodilators, but also release vasoconstrictors and swell, which leads to an increase in vascular permeability. These local events will also lead to progressive trapping of leucocytes, which in turn contribute to the no reflow phenomenon.

Reactive oxygen species contribute to tissue injury in models of myocardial and renal ischaemia. Although, in renal ischaemia, the use of different combinations of xanthine oxidase inhibitors, superoxide dismutase, catalase and glutathione can in general protect, the results have been disappointing. This probably reflects the difficulty in delivering exogenous antioxidants to target tissues.

Events that maintain glomerular filtration rate at zero

Ischaemic injury to tubules

Extensive research in rodent models of acute tubular necrosis have identified the thick ascending limb as the most vulnerable site for ischaemic injury. In humans, it is not certain if this part of the tubule is necessarily the most vulnerable. Histological and microdissection studies of tubules suggest a more diffuse injury (although, even by electron microscopy, changes are often inconspicuous, with little evidence of tubular necrosis).

The discussion that follows relates to work on rodent models. For the reasons given above, one must be cautious about overextrapolating the potential of protective strategies defined in these models.

Structural changes

Following ischaemic injury, a consequence of morphological changes occurs to the proximal tubule. First, 'blebs' appear on the apical surface and the brush-border is lost. Cells lose their polarity (with relocation of Na^+/K^+-ATPase from the basolateral to the apical membrane) and the integrity of their tight junctions, with integrins redistributed to the apical membrane. These changes are a consequence of alteration in the cytoskeleton and microtubule assembly. Cells (both dead and alive) exfoliate into the lumen, which may lead to an increase in intratubular pressure and exacerbate any back-leak of ultrafiltrate that is occurring through the destructive tubules into the interstitium [13].

Tubular energetics

The principal determinant of medullary oxygen consumption is the rate of active reabsorption in the thick ascending limb. Morphological injury to the thick ascending limb (in rats) can be greatly reduced by inhibiting active transport by these cells. Frusemide, which blocks chloride reabsorption, reduces the injury, and ouabain, which eliminates active transport (by inhibiting Na^+/K^+-ATPase), prevents the lesion entirely. The lesion can also be prevented by abolishing glomerular filtration (achieved by raising glomerular oncotic pressure with albumin) [1]. In contrast, increasing the work load makes the injury worse. This can be achieved acutely by fluid depletion or adding amphotericin, an ionophore that increases sodium reabsorption and thus the activity of the sodium/potassium pump and oxygen demand.

Another important way in which hypovolaemia, causing oliguria, may predispose to acute tubular necrosis is by permitting high concentrations of potential toxins (such as radiocontrast, gentamicin) to be present in the ascending tubule [1].

To cope with this potentially unstable, and hypoxic, environment in the medulla, a number of cytoprotective systems has evolved. Vasodilatory prostaglandins, nitric oxide and adenosine are all cytoprotective by inhibiting transport mechanisms (principally for sodium and chloride) and reducing tubular work. Cytochrome P-450-dependent arachidonate metabolites and platelet-activating factor also inhibit transport, and intracellular acidosis is another powerful cytoprotective force.

Biochemical events during acute ischaemic cell injury

Cortical renal tubular epithelia are strictly aerobic and are particularly susceptible to damage during periods of respiratory arrest. There have been few attempts to study biochemical events in models of acute tubular necrosis. In a study of cellular hypoxia, the ability of the rat kidney to recover and continue to pass urine following 30 minutes of ischaemia from haemorrhage was related to the magnitude and duration of the renal adenosine triphosphate (ATP) deficit (as measured in vivo by ^{32}P-NMR) [14].

There is currently much interest in in vitro models of the cell biology of acute tubular necrosis, as there are some surprising and exciting ways in which injury may be prevented. The most remarkable is glycine cytoprotection. In models of 60-minute hypoxia, re-oxygenation results in 80% cell death, which is prevented by co-incubation of cells with glycine [15]. Glycine is also cytoprotective against cell ischaemia induced by inhibitors of oxidative phosphorylation and glycolysis. The cells maintain structure and recover full metabolic function and ATP content after the removal of the inhibitors [15, 16]. The protective effect of glycine occurs at a stage beyond calcium dysregulation and ATP preservation [16].

Cellular injury is associated with an increase in intracellular calcium. The influx of calcium exacerbates the medullary hypoxia and the injury, and thus the therapeutic potential for calcium channel antagonists to protect against acute tubular necrosis [17].

Summary and therapeutic implications

Until recently, most experimental models of acute tubular necrosis involved a single massive insult, which bore little relation to the onset of acute tubular necrosis in humans. More recently, models have been developed that combine multiple insults, although individually they have no effect. These are based on inhibiting the multiplicity of homeostatic mechanisms that protect the medulla. For instance, rats can be salt depleted then given a non-steroidal anti-inflammatory drug and radiocontrast. The combination produces acute tubular necrosis, whereas two of the three does not [18].

Can acute tubular necrosis be prevented? Volume expansion and salt loading, which reduce the work of urine concentration and stimulate medullary vaso-dilatation, are vital in preventing critical medullary ischaemia. Synergy between hypovolaemia and toxic insults (e.g. gentamicin) results from the increased renal concentration of toxins in medullary tubules at a time when tubular reabsorption is increased and oxygen supply is reduced [1]. Establishing a diuresis, and thus reducing the tubular concentration of toxins, will protect against the onset of acute tubular necrosis. Although experimental work provides a rationale for the clinical use of frusemide, recent data suggest that it confers no benefit over saline infused alone. Similarly, mannitol may prevent cell swelling, promote urine flow, release vasodilatory mediators and even act as an antioxidant, but clinical studies have not shown any reproducible benefit, either for it or for dopamine, in the prevention or amelioration of acute tubular necrosis [13].

Nevertheless, there are encouraging developments that focus on repair and regeneration. The work cited on the role of ICAM-1 inhibition is very exciting, and studies on tubular cell recovery and regeneration are promising. A number of growth factors (epidermal growth factor, hepatocyte growth factor, insulin-like growth factor-1), when given to animals with renal ischaemia, reduce the extent of injury and accelerate recovery [19]. Clinical trials of insulin-like growth factor-1 are in progress.

References

1. Brezis M, Rosen S. Hypoxia of the renal medulla – its implications for disease. N Engl J Med 1995; 332: 647–55

2. Neild GH. Endothelial and mesangial cell dysfunction in acute renal failure. In: Bihari D, Neild GH (eds) Acute renal failure in the intensive therapy unit. London: Springer-Verlag, 1990: 77–89

3. Dinour D, Agmon Y, Brezis M. Adenosine: an emerging role in the control of renal medullary oxygenation? Exp Nephrol 1993; 1: 152–7

4. Thurau K, Boylan JW. Acute renal success. The unexpected logic of oliguria in acute renal failure. Am J Med 1976; 61: 308–15

5. Woolfson RG, Millar CGM, Neild GH. Ischaemia and reperfusion injury in the kidney: current status and future direction. Nephrol Dial Transplant 1994; 9: 1529–33.

6. Zager RA. Sepsis-associated acute renal failure: some potential pathogenetic and therapeutic insights. Nephrol Dial Transplant 1994: 9 Suppl. 4: 164–7

7. Kashgarian M, Siegel NJ, Ries AL, DiMeola HJ, Hayslett JP. Hemodynamic aspects in development and recovery phases of experimental postischemic acute renal failure. Kidney Int 1976; 10: S160–8

8. Mason J, Welsch J, Torhorst J. The contribution of vascular obstruction to the functional defect that follows renal ischaemia. Kidney Int 1987; 31: 65–71

9. Better OS, Stein JH. Early management of shock and prophylaxis of acute renal failure in traumatic rhabdomyolysis. New Engl J Med 1990; 322: 825–9

10. Kelly KJ, Williams WW, Colvin RB, et al. Intercellular adhesion molecule-1 deficient mice are protected against ischaemic renal injury. J Clin Invest 1996; 97: 1056–63

11. Granger DN, Korthuis RJ. Physiologic mechanisms of postischaemic tissue injury. Ann Rev Physiol 1995; 57: 311–32.

12. Kelly KJ, Williams WW, Colvin RB, Bonventre JV. Antibody to intercellular adhesion molecule 1 protects the kidney against ischemic injury. Proc Natl Acad Sci USA 1994; 91: 812–16

13. Thadhani R, Pascual M, Bonventre JV. Acute renal failure. New Engl J Med 1996; 334: 1148–60

14. Ratcliffe PJ, Moonen CTW, Holloway PAH, Ledingham JGG, Radda GK. Acute renal failure in hemorrhagic hypotension: cellular energetics and renal function. Kidney Int 1986; 30: 355–60

15. Weinberg, JM, Buchanan DN, Davis JA, Abarzua M. Metabolic aspects of protection by glycine against hypoxic injury to isolated proximal tubules. J Am Soc Nephrol 1991; 1: 949–58

16. Weinberg JM, Davis JA, Roeser NF, Venkatachalam, MA. Role of increased cytosolic free calcium in the

pathogenesis of rabbit proximal tubule cell injury and protection by glycine or acidosis. J Clin Invest 1991; 87: 581–90

17. Schrier RW, Arnold PE, van Putten VJ, Burke TJ. Cellular calcium in ischaemic acute renal failure: role of calcium entry blockers. Kidney Int 1987; 32: 313–21

18. Heyman SN, Brezis M, Reubinoff CA, et al. Acute renal failure with selective medullary injury in the rat. J Clin Invest 1988; 82: 401–12

19. Hammerman MR, Miller SB. Therapeutic use of growth factors in renal failure. J Am Soc Nephrol 1994; 5: 1–11

Chronic renal failure

10

G. H. Neild

Introduction

Definition

Severe renal failure is recognised by consistently high plasma urea and creatinine concentrations. The degree of renal failure can be arbitrarily divided into mild, moderate or severe, based on the plasma creatinine (Table 10.1). It is convenient (and accurate) to consider the value of glomerular filtration rate or creatinine clearance as a percentage of normal (i.e. 20 ml/min is equivalent to 20% of normal).

Aetiology

There are many causes of renal failure. The cause will vary depending on age and to some extent on ethnic origin and geographical location. For instance, a paediatric population waiting for a renal transplant will be dominated by those with nephro-urological malformations. An elderly population will be dominated by renovascular disease and diabetes. In third world countries, glomerulonephritis remains a major cause of renal failure.

Table 10.2 shows a typical range of the diseases causing renal failure in an adult population in the UK. As an increasingly elderly population is accepted for dialysis, the percentages change and hypertension and diabetes become more prevalent. In the USA, these two diagnoses alone account for more than 50% of all new dialysis patients [1].

Incidence and epidemiology

In the UK, around 80 per 1 million population are accepted on to dialysis programmes each year. This is

Table 10.1 Degrees of renal failure

Renal failure	Glomerular filtration rate (ml/min)	Creatinine ($\mu mol/l$)
Mild	20–50	150–300
Moderate	10–20	300–700
Severe	<10	>700

Table 10.2 Aetiology of chronic renal failure

	Percentage
Glomerulonephritis	28
Scarred kidneys (reflux nephropathy) and malformations of the urinary tract	17
Diabetes mellitus	16
Uncertain	13
Polycystic kidney disease	10
Hypertension and renovascular disease	8
Hereditary nephritis	1
Others	7

an increase from the recommended target of 60 per million in 1991. The target was increased after an audit in five different parts of the UK showed that many patients were not being considered for dialysis, and that 80 per million was a consistent figure in all parts of the UK for those generally considered as suitable for dialysis [2]. This figure underestimates the need in inner cities where there are large ethnic populations. For reasons that are still not clear, renal failure is four to six times more common in Asians and Afro-Caribbeans, compared with the white (Caucasian) population. This increased disease burden is true for hypertension, diabetes and non-diabetic forms of chronic renal failure [3].

In the USA, the figure is more than 100 new patients per 1 million population each year and reflects the larger percentage of the non-white population. In all countries, the incidence rises exponentially with age, and by 80 years of age, end-stage renal failure will occur in approximately 800 per million population [1].

Presentation/symptoms

Progressive renal failure due to disease of the kidney is often insidious and asymptomatic. Symptoms attributable to the kidney failure per se are not specific (Table 10.3) and do not usually occur until 80–90% of kidney function is lost.

The predominant early symptoms of uraemia, such as fatigue, lethargy and tiredness, are attributable to the anaemia of renal failure and improve when the anaemia is corrected by blood transfusion or the recombinant hormone erythropoietin.

Table 10.3 Uraemic symptoms

Early (due to anaemia)
  Malaise, lethargy, tiredness
  Shortness of breath on exertion

Late (due to uraemic toxins)
  Itching (pruritis)
  Loss of appetite (anorexia)
  Nausea and vomiting

Variable (related to abnormal calcium, phosphate)
  Muscle weakness
  Bone and joint pain

Severe (after dialysis should have been started)
  Pericarditis
  Impaired mental performance, drowsiness, stupor, coma
  Rapid respiration (tachypnoea) due to acidosis

Intrinsic kidney disease is most commonly due to progressive glomerular disease, which is invariably associated with proteinuria, and usually some haematuria, hypertension and a tendency to retain salt and water. In contrast, some progressive disease is predominantly due to tubulo-interstitial disease and this is typically seen when there is a primary urological disease or dysplasia. Tubular disease is characterised by minimal proteinuria, early loss of renal concentrating ability, a tendency to salt wasting (therefore no peripheral oedema), early onset of acidosis and normal blood pressure.

Signs

There are few specific signs of uraemia:

1. Patients may be pale because of anaemia and, if both anaemia and renal failure are severe, often have a yellow tinge to their skin.
2. Patients tan easily in the sun and the pigmentation fades more slowly than normal.
3. If the renal failure is long standing since childhood, the patient may be of small stature (in relation to other family members).
4. There may be excoriation of the skin from scratching.

Pathophysiology

This section first discusses the universal mechanisms that lead to progressive, inexorable renal failure. Secondly, the consequences of loss of kidney tissue are reviewed.

Mechanisms of progressive renal failure

Not all kidney disease is progressive, but once the kidney is sufficiently damaged, for any reason, then progressive loss of the remaining nephrons is almost inevitable and is associated with a progressive glomerulosclerosis [4].

Different diseases progress at different rates. The prognostic factors are predominantly:

1. hypertension,
2. magnitude of proteinuria.

The most important development in the past decade is the recognition that careful control of blood pressure slows the rate of loss of renal function [5, 6].

Moderately severe renal failure that progresses inexorably is due to progressive glomerular disease. This is invariably associated with proteinuria and hypertension. Thus, there is a final common pathway even when, for example, the original cause of scarred kidneys was urological.

Glomerular capillary hypertension and glomerular hyperfiltration injury

Our understanding of these important mechanisms is based almost exclusively on a reproducible experimental model in which rats have five-sixths or more of their renal mass ablated. Following nephrectomy, the 'remnant kidney' initially hypertrophies and hyperfiltrates in an attempt to improve the glomerular filtration rate. Subsequently, over a number of months, the animals develop increasing proteinuria, hypertension and progressive renal failure with a glomerular lesion that is characterised histologically by focal and segmental glomerulosclerosis [7].

Following the initial nephrectomy, a predictable sequence of glomerular haemodynamic events occurs. Renal blood flow per glomerulus increases, and the glomerular capillary hydrostatic pressure increases, leading to a great increase in single nephron glomerular filtration rate or 'hyperfiltration'. This glomerular capillary hypertension appears to be the central event in the mechanism of progressive glomerular injury. The mechanism by which this capillary hypertension causes injury and focal and segmental glomerulosclerosis is less certain. Nevertheless, there is good evidence that the hypertension leads to endothelial damage, which in turn causes platelet adhesion, fibrin formation and subsequent sclerosis. In favour of this mechanism is the ability of various anticoagulant and antiplatelet regimens to reduce the injury and protect the kidney. Secondly, there is increasing evidence that glomerular epithelial cell injury occurs and contributes to the sclerosis [7].

In these animals, a low-protein diet is effective at reducing this injury and is associated with a fall in single nephron glomerular filtration rate, capillary flow and pressure [4]. It has also been shown that treatment of this model with an angiotensin-converting enzyme inhibitor is able to prevent the development of the proteinuria, focal and segmental glomerulosclerosis and renal failure, whereas conventional hypotensive drugs, which are equally effective at reducing systemic blood pressure, have no beneficial effect on the disease process [8, 9]. The explanation for this is that while all hypotensive agents will tend to lower glomerular capillary pressure through a reduction in afferent arterial pressure, only angiotensin-converting enzyme inhibitors are able to lower the glomerular pressure independently of systemic pressure by their ability to reduce efferent arteriolar tone.

There is now conclusive evidence in progressive renal disease that reducing systemic blood pressure slows the rate of loss of glomerular filtration rate [5]. Moreover, angiotensin-converting enzyme inhibitors are more effective than other hypotensive agents at reducing the loss of glomerular filtration rate and reducing proteinuria [10–12].

Consequences of progressive renal failure

The kidney not only excretes toxins and regulates salt and water balance (Table 10.4), but is an important source of hormones and enzymes that regulate:

1. the normal production of red cells by the bone marrow (erythropoiesis);
2. calcium and phosphate homeostasis and normal bone mineralisation;
3. blood pressure.

Failure of these systems leads to the endocrine problems associated with renal failure (Table 10.5).

Table 10.4 Roles of the kidney

Excretion of toxic metabolites
Regulation of salt and water balance
Regulation of acid–base balance

Hormonal role promoting:
   erythropoietin – which stimulates red cell production
   renin – which regulates blood pressure
   enzymes to activate vitamin D
   uncharacterised factor – which lowers blood pressure

Table 10.5 Complications of uraemia

Endocrine
   Hypertension
   Accelerated atherosclerosis
   Anaemia
   Renal bone disease (osteodystrophy)
   Acidosis

Toxic
   Skin: pruritis
   Gastrointestinal system: anorexia, nausea, vomiting
   Cardiovascular system: pericarditis
   Peripheral nervous system: neuropathy
   Central nervous system: convulsions, coma

Uraemic toxins

The principal role of the kidney is to excrete the metabolic products of nitrogen catabolism. The two conventional markers that are routinely measured as indices of renal function are urea and creatinine.

Urea

The plasma urea is more prone to daily variation, particularly in hospital. It depends on the amount of protein catabolism by a healthy liver. Higher values will occur with high protein intake, or in sick people when there is a greatly increased catabolism of body protein. Lower values will occur with low protein intake or with liver disease.

Creatinine

The advantage of creatinine as a measure of renal function is that the amount produced (from muscle) is very constant. However, the amount produced depends on the patient's muscle mass. Thus, children and small, elderly people will have low values. Normal ranges for children vary with age; for 10-year-olds, values are 40–75 µmol/l. Only the meatiest of men will have values at the so-called upper limit of normal (i.e. about 120 µmol/l). Thus, a 60-kg lady of 60 years with a creatinine of 125 µmol/l has an estimated clearance of 47 ml/min (Figure 10.1), while a 30-year-old male of 80 kg with a creatinine of 125 µmol/l has an estimated clearance of 86 ml/min.

In reality, laboratories quote a wide range for all comers (50–125 µmol/l), which causes great confusion to doctors if they are not aware of the implications.

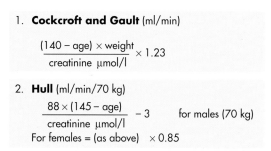

1. **Cockcroft and Gault** (ml/min)

$$\frac{(140 - age) \times weight}{creatinine\ \mu mol/l} \times 1.23$$

2. **Hull** (ml/min/70 kg)

$$\frac{88 \times (145 - age)}{creatinine\ \mu mol/l} - 3 \quad \text{for males (70 kg)}$$

For females = (as above) × 0.85

Figure 10.1 *Formulae for estimating creatinine clearance.*

Thus, the urea and creatinine are both pointers to renal insufficiency, but the creatinine is used on a day-to-day basis to *follow* renal function.

Please note that when either the urea or creatinine is above normal, the glomerular filtration rate is already reduced by 50%.

The nature of toxins

Urea and creatinine are not themselves toxic. The toxins that give rise to the symptoms and complications of chronic renal failure are poorly characterised and there are very many of them. They are clearly related to protein catabolism as symptoms will improve on a low-protein diet and are made worse by a high-protein diet. The majority of toxins are filtered by the glomerulus and are therefore removed by dialysis, but some are protein bound, depend normally for excretion on tubular secretion, and are therefore not readily removed by dialysis.

Compounds increased in uraemia include guanidines (methylguanidine, guanidinosuccinic acid), products of nucleic acid catabolism, amines from gut bacteria, phenoles, carbohydrate derivatives (myoinositol, mannitol, sorbitol) and large numbers of unknown molecules of sizes 500 to 5000 Da known as 'middle molecules' [13].

The regulation of salt and water balance

The kidney's principal role is to filter the plasma. In a healthy young adult kidney, approximately 120 ml of this plasma is filtered per minute, i.e. 120 ml of ultrafiltrate is produced per minute. This means that in one hour 7200 ml (120 × 60) of ultrafiltrate are produced; in 24 hours, 173 litres (7.2 × 24) are produced. Because we only produce 1–2 litres of urine a day, there is obviously a very efficient system of recovery, or tubular fluid reabsorption.

A normal daily urine volume of, say, 1.7 litres would mean that only 1% of the ultrafiltrate was excreted, while 99% was reabsorbed. The 99% is all the 'good things' that need to be recovered, i.e. water, salts, sugar, amino acids. The toxic metabolites remain in the tubules and are excreted in the urine.

Water

The medullary component of the tubules is responsible for the ability to concentrate the urine by reabsorbing water, as well as diluting the urine in response to a water load. Both these abilities are progressively lost until urine of a fixed concentration is produced in end-stage renal failure.

The ability to concentrate urine requires several mechanisms to be intact including:

1. the countercurrent system normally generates a very high interstitial osmolality in the medulla;
2. the descending tubule and collecting ducts are impermeable to water in the presence of vasopressin.

In chronic renal failure, several factors disrupt these mechanisms. Damage to the medulla causes a progressive loss of the hypertonic interstitium, damage to tubules causes resistance to antidiuretic hormone ('nephrogenic diabetic insipidus'), and an increasing solute load per remaining nephron causes an obligatory solute diuresis.

The inability to concentrate urine in the presence of dehydration is one of the earliest symptoms in tubular disease and leads to symptoms of nocturia and polyuria.

Sodium

As renal function decreases, hormonal mechanisms increase the fraction of filtered sodium excreted from less than 1% in normals up to 30% in end-stage renal failure. Thus sodium balance and extracellular fluid volume are maintained until the glomerular filtration rate is <10 ml/min [14, 15]. Eventually, the kidney cannot maintain the homeostasis and the extracellular fluid increases, leading to hypertension and dependent oedema, or in severe cases pulmonary oedema. When discussing extracellular fluid homeostasis, sodium is a

shorthand for sodium *and* chloride. It is the retention of chloride anions that leads to volume overload and hypertension.

In renal (tubulo-interstitial) disease in which medullary damage predominates, there can be an inability to conserve sodium chloride. Such patients are usually normotensive, do not develop oedema and may require salt supplementation.

Potassium

Potassium is excreted into the urine by tubular secretion. This occurs principally in the distal tubule, where sodium exchanges for potassium in the presence of aldosterone. Most patients can maintain potassium homeostasis down to a glomerular filtration rate of 5 ml/min, but capacity to increase excretion is limited and severe hyperkalaemia can occur with a sudden reduction of glomerular filtration rate [15, 16].

Acidosis raises plasma potassium by potassium ion transfer out of cells (in exchange for hydrogen ions), and prevents tubular secretion of potassium (as hydrogen will be exchanged preferentially for sodium in the distal tubule). Conversely, correction of acidosis can lead to a rapid fall in plasma potassium.

In some forms of renal disease (particularly diabetes and amyloid), there may be inappropriately raised potassium for the degree of renal impairment. This is usually due to relative deficiency of aldosterone ('hyporeninaemic hypoaldosteronism') and responds to supplementation with fludrocortisone.

The regulation of acid–base balance

The kidney is responsible for acid–base homeostasis, a key role of which is the excretion of non-volatile

Table 10.6 Uraemic acidosis I

Failure to excrete non-volatile acids
Failure of bicarbonate ion reabsorption (proximal renal tubular acidosis)
Failure of hydrogen ion secretion (distal renal tubular acidosis)
Failure of ammonia synthesis (distal renal tubular acidosis)

acids [15, 17] (Table 10.6). Non-volatile acids are principally derived from the metabolism of sulphur-containing amino acids (methionine and cystine).

The kidney maintains acid–base balance by:

1. the reabsorption of filtered bicarbonate;
2. hydrogen ion excretion and acidification of urinary buffers (mainly filtered monobasic phosphate salts, HPO_4^{2-});
3. the generation and secretion of ammonia from the proximal tubule (which traps urinary H^+ as NH_4^+).

In this way, homeostasis is generally maintained down to glomerular filtration rates of 20 ml/min. When renal disease is principally due to tubular damage, acidosis can occur early in renal insufficiency.

Although it has been recognised for many years that chronic acidosis may cause osteomalacia and particularly rickets in children, a number of other sequelae are now recognised (Table 10.7).

Anaemia

One of the earliest features of chronic renal failure is anaemia [18], which is multifactorial but predominantly due to a failure of renal erythropoietin synthesis. The renal cells responsible for erythropoietin synthesis have been identified as interstitial cells present in the renal cortex.

Anaemia in severe chronic renal failure is also due to reduced red cell survival, increased blood loss from the gastrointestinal tract associated with an increased bleeding tendency, and uraemic suppression of erythropoiesis. Typically, there is a normochromic normocytic anaemia.

Table 10.7 Uraemic acidosis II

Reduced cardiac output
Increased muscle catabolism
Reduced bone mineralisation and growth
Osteomalacia
Increased urinary and faecal calcium ion excretion
Inhibition of 1-α-hydroxylase

The effects of the anaemia are partly compensated for by a shift in the oxygen-dissociation curve to the right due to increased concentration of 2,3-diphosphoglycerate and phosphates in red cells.

Hypertension

There are two principal mechanisms that lead to hypertension in renal disease:

1. salt and water retention leading to an expansion of extracellular fluid;
2. renal damage leading to activation of the renin–angiotensin system.

In addition, there is evidence that the kidney produces a lipid mediator that lowers blood pressure. It is certainly remarkable the way in which hypertension can regress following a successful renal transplant. There is also increasing interest in the role of endothelium-derived vasorelaxant factors that counteract the resting sympathetic tone of blood vessels. The most potent and significant of these is nitric oxide and there is evidence that in uraemia this ability of the normal vessel to produce nitric oxide is reduced or the action of nitric oxide is antagonised, which leads to an increase in resting tone and hypertension.

Renal bone disease

Renal bone disease is a mixture of hyperparathyroidism, osteomalacia and osteoporosis. Typically, hyperparathyroidism predominates. A fourth but rare component is the radiological appearance of osteosclerosis. In dialysis patients, or patients who have received aluminium hydroxide as phosphate binders, aluminium toxicity can play a role [19].

Hyperparathyroidism

Three separate forces activate the parathyroid glands to cause secondary hyperparathyroidism.

1. The earliest metabolic derangement in chronic renal failure is phosphate retention due to a reduction in glomerular filtration of PO_4^{2-}. The rise in plasma PO_4^{2-} causes a reciprocal fall in plasma calcium, and directly activates the parathyroids to release more hormone (parathyroid hormone). The increase in parathyroid hormone acts on the

tubules to increase urinary phosphate excretion and correct the rise in plasma phosphate.

2. As the kidney fails, there is simultaneous loss of the renal tubular enzyme 1-α-hydroxylase and thus falling plasma levels of 1,25-dihydroxycholecalciferol (calcitriol), and therefore plasma calcium. If untreated, this leads to the state of 'vitamin D-resistant rickets' (osteomalacia). Reduction in 1,25-dihydroxycholecalciferol is a powerful stimulus to parathyroid hormone release, which in turn activates the failing enzyme.

3. Hypocalcaemia directly activates the parathyroids to produce more parathyroid hormone. Parathyroid hormone also has a direct effect on the enzyme 1-α-hydroxylase, which is responsible for the final activation of vitamin D to calcitriol. This activation will act to correct the hypocalcaemia.

Thus, there is a complex interplay of kidney, parathyroid gland and gut attempting to maintain calcium homeostasis. The parathyroid glands have vitamin D receptors to which calcitriol binds and the latter is a potent inhibitor of parathyroid hormone synthesis. The glands also have calcium-sensing receptors and calcium inhibits parathyroid hormone synthesis. In contrast, phosphate activates parathyroid hormone synthesis. The situation becomes more complex in renal failure as the sensitivity and density of these parathyroid receptors change in response to the prevailing milieu.

The management of secondary hyperparathyroidism has been made much easier by the availability of sensitive and specific assays for the intact hormone (as opposed to previous assays for metabolites, which are retained in chronic renal failure). A rise in parathyroid hormone is the earliest detectable metabolic derangement in chronic renal failure and starts to occur even with glomerular filtration rates of 50–60 ml/min.

Osteomalacia

The natural history of progressive renal failure is of progressive vitamin D resistance (see above). Restriction of dietary calcium, or a diet or lifestyle that promotes vitamin D deficiency, will exacerbate the problem, thus in Asian patients osteomalacia may be the predominant form of renal bone disease. Osteomalacia is also caused by chronic metabolic acidosis, when the bones take on a major role as a buffer for the acid.

Osteoporosis

Osteoporosis is a natural part of the ageing process, but may be exacerbated in renal patients by premature ovarian failure, long-term use of glucocorticosteroids, chronic ill-health associated with immobility, hypercatabolism, or injudicious protein/calcium dietary restriction.

Today, based on our understanding of all these processes, we have very effective treatment to prevent bone disease:

(a) early restriction of dietary phosphate;

(b) the use of phosphate binders (calcium carbonate, aluminium hydroxide) to reduce the gut adsorption of phosphate;

(c) the use of analogues of calcitriol that will increase plasma calcium and inhibit parathyroid hormone secretion;

(d) when appropriate, the correction of acidosis with oral sodium bicarbonate.

Hyperlipidaemia

The uraemic state itself causes hypertriglyceridaemia and hypercholesterolaemia. Moreover, many patients have other risk factors for hyperlipidaemia, including hypertension and hyperinsulinaemia (particularly common in non-white ethnic groups), diabetes, drugs used to treat hypertension (diuretics), other drugs (steroids), and unfitness.

Bleeding tendency

In severe uraemia, there is an increased bleeding tendency, although this is not apparent until the creatinine is usually in excess of 600 μmol/l. The defect is due to the impairment of normal platelet adhesion to damaged endothelium. In addition, platelet function is abnormal and, ex vivo, platelets are hyperaggregable in response to aggregating agents.

In uraemia, it is becoming increasingly acknowledged that there is a generalised defect in normal endothelial function, with evidence of impaired activity of endothelium-derived nitric oxide.

Atherosclerosis

The commonest cause of death in dialysis and transplant patients is cardiovascular disease as a consequence of premature and accelerated atherosclerosis. There are many factors, some well defined, others less clear. They can be divided into two groups (Table 10.8).

On the one hand, there are the usual factors, which are overrepresented in renal failure patients and are very similar to those associated with hyperlipidaemia and hypertension. On the other hand, there are factors that are uniquely uraemic and ill-defined. It is still not clear whether haemodialysis or continuous ambulatory peritoneal dialysis imposes a greater burden and risk of atheroma. The uraemic factors probably relate to the abnormal endothelial function that is present plus the increased oxidative stress that occurs. The latter will cause, in particular, an increase in oxidatively modified low-density lipoproteins.

Clinical practice

Estimating kidney function

Glomerular filtration rate

The gold standard for the accurate measurement of kidney function is the glomerular filtration rate. In clinical practice, at specialist centres, this is measured by giving a single intravenous injection of a small inert molecule that is freely filtered by the glomerulus and not reabsorbed (or secreted) by the tubules. EDTA is usually used – linked to a radio-isotope ([51]chromium). Blood is taken from the other arm, after three and four hours, and the glomerular filtration rate can be calculated from the rate of loss of EDTA from the circulation.

Creatinine clearance

Accurate measurement of the glomerular filtration rate is not possible for most centres, and instead the creatinine clearance is measured. If done carefully on one or two occasions, an accurate answer will be obtained, but the method is prone to error.

Patients are asked to collect all the urine they pass in a 24-hour period. The timing is important as it is part of the equation to calculate the answer. The collection could last for 18 or 36 hours as long as that time is noted – invariably, however, the figure 24 hours is used in the calculation. The answer is usually expressed as ml/min. Creatinine clearance declines slowly with age. Normal values for young people are 100–130 ml/min; for the elderly they are 70–90 ml/min. It is convenient (and accurate) to translate directly the creatinine clearance (or glomerular filtration rate) as a percentage of normal function, i.e. 70 ml/min is best thought of as kidney function of 70% of normal.

Clues that the collection is shorter than 24 hours, or incomplete, are that the total volume is obviously low (normal 1–2 litres), or that the 24-hour excretion of creatinine is low (normal 7–18 mmol/24 h). Because of these errors and the obvious disadvantage of collecting large volumes of urine, several formulae have been developed that can estimate the creatinine clearance [20, 21]. These all use the reciprocal creatinine (1/creatinine), the patient's age, sex and weight (see Figure 10.1).

Investigations for chronic renal failure

Blood biochemistry

By definition, the urea and creatinine are raised. One expects plasma potassium, phosphate to be high and bicarbonate and calcium to be low.

With long-standing untreated renal failure, there is often bone disease due to overactivity of the parathyroid gland (hyperparathyroidism) and the serum parathyroid hormone is invariably raised, and the alkaline phosphatase, an enzyme derived from bone, is

Table 10.8 Uraemia and atherosclerosis

Burden of risk factors
Hypertension
Hyperlipidaemia
Unfit
Therapy (including steroids)
Uraemic factors
Endothelial injury
Increased oxidative stress
Platelet dysfunction

generally raised (depending on the severity of bone disease).

Haematology

Apart from a normochromic normocytic anaemia, there are no specific features. Patients with severe renal failure have an increased tendency to bleed – even though their blood clots normally and their platelet count is normal.

Radiology

Chest X-ray is required as a baseline to assess the lungs and the size of the heart and to exclude pericardial effusion around the heart. With intrinsic renal disease, ultrasound will show two small kidneys with greatly increased 'echogenicity' due to the amount of fibrosis inside the kidney. X-rays (usually just of the hand) will show the changes of hyperparathryoidism if they are present.

Progression of renal failure

Almost all kidney diseases progress with time, although different diseases progress at different rates. Generally, the rapidity of progress is faster if blood pressure is high or the amount of protein excreted in the urine is high.

Serial measurement of plasma creatinine is the most useful way in which progression of kidney disease can be monitored. Plasma creatinine rises exponentially with deteriorating renal function (i.e. with time). However, if the creatinine is plotted as a reciprocal against time or as the $\log_{10}$, then the change in creatinine becomes linear and most patients follow a predictable course according to their reciprocal creatinine (although some patients' rate of progress fits a log plot better). This means that reasonably accurate predictions of when end-stage renal failure is likely to occur can be made from extrapolating these slopes.

All efforts should be made to treat the underlying disease, but assuming that nothing more can be done to this effect, then reducing the blood pressure to normal or low normal values has been shown to slow the rate of progression of kidney disease, in some cases dramatically.

Patients should be monitored regularly and it has been observed that this alone slows the rate of progression of renal failure. Patients with mild chronic renal failure should be seen at least every six months; patients with moderate renal failure every two to four months; and patients approaching dialysis may need to be seen every three to four weeks.

At clinic attendances:

1. the weight should be measured (for assessment of nutrition and fluid status);
2. the blood pressure should be measured lying and standing;
3. blood tests should include urea, creatinine, bicarbonate, calcium, phosphate and alkaline phosphatase as well as haemoglobin.

Treatment and diet

Diet

Protein intake

There is evidence that a very low-protein diet may slow the rate of progression. Unfortunately, the degree of protein restriction (0.6 g of protein per kg body weight per day) is difficult or impossible for most patients to adhere to and there is a danger of malnutrition in overzealous patients. Conversely, a high-protein diet may accelerate the rate of progression. It is therefore sensible to advise moderation in protein intake, usually of around 1 g of protein per kg body weight per day.

Symptoms of severe renal failure attributable to uraemic toxins will often improve when the protein intake is reduced.

Potassium

Potassium in the diet may be a problem as it can cause hyperkalaemia. Patients should be advised about which foods are rich in potassium and should avoid an excess of them.

Salt

Many patients will have problems excreting salt from their diet and are advised to take a low-salt intake. This will also reduce the risk or severity of hypertension. With predominantly tubular disease, patients can exhibit signs of chronic hypovolaemia and feel much better when they are encouraged to increase their salt intake – even if this unmasks hypertension that subsequently requires treatment.

Phosphate

To minimise bone disease, the level of phosphate in the blood should be controlled and kept in the middle of the normal range. Dietary phosphate restriction is difficult to achieve and absorption of phosphate is reduced by giving 'phosphate binders'. These are compounds such as calcium carbonate or aluminium hydroxide that are taken with the food and form an insoluble phosphate salt, which should not be absorbed [22].

Treatment

Blood pressure

It is imperative that the blood pressure is kept normal or low-normal. There are increasing data to suggest that angiotensin-converting enzyme inhibitors are most effective not only at controlling the blood pressure but at slowing the rate of progression and reducing the proteinuria. However, great care must be taken in starting these drugs in patients with renal failure. It is likely that these drugs will reduce the kidney function by 10–15% and there is usually little to be gained by starting them once the creatinine is above 400 µmol/l. At this level there is a danger that the drugs will simply precipitate uraemic symptoms.

Acidosis

With severe renal failure, it is inevitable that the plasma bicarbonate is at or below the lower level of normal. When severe, or occurring with less severe degrees of renal insufficiency (such as with urological patients), it should be corrected by giving oral sodium bicarbonate until the plasma level is back in the normal range.

Bone disease

It is always better to treat renal bone disease sooner rather than later. Nowadays, the serum parathyroid hormone level can be easily measured, and supplementation with analogues of active vitamin D (such as 1-alpha calcidol) should be given once the parathyroid hormone starts to rise.

Treating the underlying disease

The underlying kidney disease should always be treated when possible, and care taken that extra problems such as bladder outflow obstruction have not occurred.

Nephrotoxic drugs

Nephrotoxic drugs and non-steroidal anti-inflammatory drugs should be avoided.

References

1. USRDS 1994 Annual Data Report. IV. Incidence and causes of treatment ESRD. Am J Kidney Dis 1994; 4(Suppl.2): S48–56
2. Roderick PJ, Ferris G, Feest TG. The provision of renal replacement therapy in England 1993–5 and Wales 1995. Part I. Report to the Renal Assoc Executive, 1997, 1–13
3. Roderick PJ, Raleigh VS, Hallam L, Mallick NP. The need and demand for renal replacement therapy in ethnic minorities in England. J Epidemiol Community Health 1996; 50: 334–9
4. Brenner BM, Meyer TW, Hostetter TH. Dietary protein intake and the progressive nature of kidney disease: the role of hemodynamically mediated glomerular injury in the pathogenesis of progressive glomerular sclerosis in aging, renal ablation, and intrinsic renal disease. N Engl J Med 1982; 307: 652–9
5. Klahr S, Levey AS, Beck GJ, et al. The effects of dietary protein restriction and blood-pressure control on the progression of chronic renal disease. New Engl J Med 1994; 330: 877–84
6. Lazarus JM, Bourgoignie JJ, Buckalew VM, et al. Achievement and safety of a low blood pressure goal in chronic renal disease. The Modification of Diet in Renal Disease Study Group. Hypertension 1997; 29: 641–50
7. El Nahas AM. Mechanisms of experimental and clinical renal scarring. In: Davison AM, Cameron JS, Grunfeld J-P, Kerr DN, Ritz E, Winearls CG, eds. Oxford Textbook of Clinical Nephrology. 2nd ed. Oxford: Oxford University Press, 1998: 1749–88
8. Zatz R, Dunn BR, Meyer TW, Anderson S, Rennke HG, Brenner BM. Prevention of diabetic glomerulopathy by pharmacological amelioration of glomerular capillary hypertension. J Clin Invest 1986; 77: 1925–30

9. Anderson S, Rennke HG, Brenner BM. Therapeutic advantage of converting enzyme inhibitors in arresting progressive renal disease associated with systemic hypertension in the rat. J Clin Invest 1986; 77: 1993–2000

10. Bjorck S, Mulec H, Johnsen SA, Norden G, Aurell M. Renal protective effect of enalapril in diabetic nephropathy. Br Med J 1992; 304: 339–43

11. Lewis EJ, Hunsicker LG, Bain RP, Rohde RD. The effect of angiotensin-converting-enzyme inhibition on diabetic nephropathy. The Collaborative Study Group. N Engl J Med 1993; 329: 1456–62

12. The GISEN Group (Gruppo Italiano di Studi Epidemiologici in Nefrologia). Randomised placebo-controlled trial of effect of ramipril on decline in glomerular filtration rate and risk of terminal renal failure in proteinuric, non-diabetic nephropathy. Lancet 1997; 349: 1857–63

13. Hoerl WH. Genesis of the uraemic syndrome. In: Davison AM, Cameron JS, Grunfeld J-P, et al eds. Oxford Textbook of Clinical Nephrology. 2nd ed. Oxford: Oxford University Press, 1998: 1821–36

14. Kumar S, Berl T. Sodium. Lancet 1998; 352: 220–8

15. Rose BD, Rennke HG. Renal pathophysiology – the essentials. Baltimore: Williams and Wilkins, 1994

16. Halperin ML, Kamel KS. Potassium. Lancet 1998; 352: 135–40

17. Gluck SL. Acid-base. Lancet 1998; 352: 474–9

18. Macdougall IC, Eckardt K-U. Haematological disorders. In: Davison AM, Cameron JS, Grunfeld J-P, et al eds. Oxford Textbook of Clinical Nephrology. 2nd ed. Oxford: Oxford University Press, 1998: 1935–54

19. Reichel H, Druecke TB, Ritz E. Skeletal disorders. In: Davison AM, Cameron JS, Grunfeld J-P, et al eds. Oxford Textbook of Clinical Nephrology. 2nd ed. Oxford: Oxford University Press, 1998: 1954–1981

20. Cockcroft DW, Gault MH. Prediction of creatinine clearance from serum creatinine. Nephron 1976; 16: 31–41

21. Hull JH, Hak LJ, Koch GG, et al. Influence of range of renal function and liver disease on predictability of creatinine clearance. Clin Pharmacol Ther 1981; 29: 516–21

22. Weisinger JR, Bellorin-Font E. Magnesium and phosphorus. Lancet 1998; 352: 391–6

Structure and function of the lower urinary tract

11

A. R. Mundy

Introduction

Before starting, the reader should be aware of certain problems in discussing the subject.

First of all, a great deal is known (relatively speaking) about the microscopic structure of the bladder, urethra and pelvic floor, but as one works back proximally through the innervation of the lower urinary tract to the spinal cord and up to the brain, and as one turns more from structure to function, so knowledge of the subject becomes exponentially less.

Secondly, much of the published research on the lower urinary tract has been done on animals other than humans and there are considerable species differences that make interpretation of such work very difficult.

Thirdly, in the same vein, many of the experimental studies have been done after neuronal ablation or otherwise in circumstances that are very far from physiological. Extrapolation from ablative pathophysiology in experimental animals to normal physiology in humans is also problematic.

Fourthly, many experimental studies have been based on the identification of receptors for neurotransmitters, or on the demonstration by radioimmunoassay of the presence of neurotransmitters themselves or have attempted to infer the presence of a physiologically significant mechanism from the presence of one component of a presumed 'reflex arc'. One or two examples will show the fallacy of such an extrapolation. Firstly, one of the most significant medical advances in recent years has been in the development of beta adrenergic receptor-active drugs for the treatment of bronchospasm, but there is no significant beta sympathetic innervation to the human lung. Receptors are present that may be therapeutically manipulated, but they have no apparent physiological significance. Secondly, and more obviously, 'receptors' can be identified in human platelets but no-one imagines that platelets have an innervation.

Finally, it should be appreciated that just because a reflex mechanism exists does not mean that that mechanism is active, let alone important in normal circumstances. Thus, a reflex may be present or elicitable or evident in disease, but it does not necessarily mean that it is active or important in health.

These various points should be borne in mind when reading about studies of the structure and function of the lower urinary tract. Equally, it is hoped that the reader will forgive the author for the speculation that will creep in to provide a reasonably smooth narrative when substance is lacking.

The discussion begins distally in the bladder and urethra and then moves proximally, considering structure first and function second but integrating both as far as possible.

The structure of the bladder and urethra

The bladder consists of three layers: an epithelial layer, a muscular layer and an adventitial layer, which on its posterior aspect is covered with peritoneum. The adventitial layer is circumscribed by two fascial layers – the first on the anterior and lateral aspect of the bladder and the second on the dome and posterior aspect of the bladder – the two fusing together anteriorly and laterally to form what Uhlenhuth [1] described as the superior hypogastric wing (Figure 11.1), which runs laterally to the external iliac vessels and anteriorly on to the anterior abdominal wall, ensheathing the medial umbilical ligaments and the urachus. The same two layers form the anterior layer of the sheath around the ureters and the superior and inferior vesical vessels posterolaterally in what Uhlenhuth described as the inferior hypogastric wing (Figure 11.2). Posteriorly, the sheet of fascia that covers the dome and posterolateral aspect of the bladder sweeps back onto the posterolateral pelvic side wall

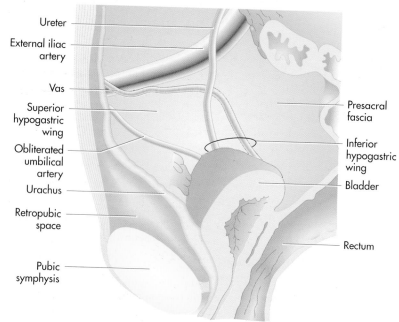

Figure 11.1 *Diagram of the distribution of pelvic fascia to show the superior hypogastric wing. (Modified from Mundy AR. Urodynamic and reconstructive surgery of the lower urinary tract. Edinburgh: Churchill Livingstone, 1993.)*

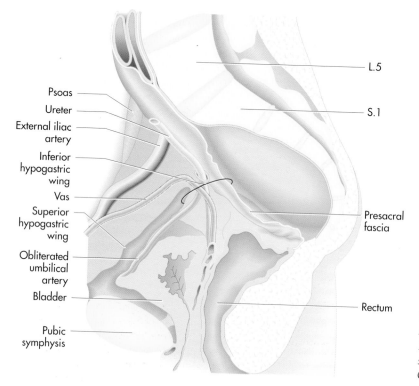

Figure 11.2a *Diagram of the pelvic fascia to show the inferior hypogastric wing. (Modified from Mundy AR. Urodynamic and reconstructive surgery of the lower urinary tract. Edinburgh: Churchill Livingstone, 1993.)*

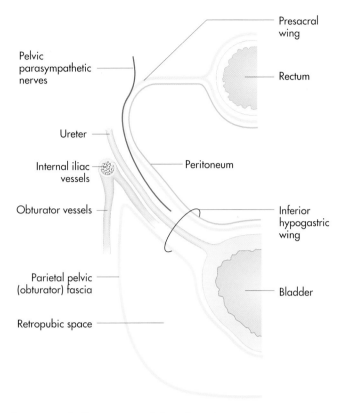

Pelvic parasympathetic nerves

Presacral wing

Rectum

Ureter

Internal iliac vessels

Peritoneum

Obturator vessels

Inferior hypogastric wing

Parietal pelvic (obturator) fascia

Bladder

Retropubic space

Figure 11.2b *Cross-section of the inferior hypogastric wing to show its structure, origin, disposition and contents. (Modified from Webster G, Kirby R, Chilton CP, King L, Goldwasser B (eds) Reconstructive Urology. Cambridge, MA: Blackwell Scientific Publications, 1993.)*

and to ensheath the rectum as Uhlenhuth's presacral fascia (Figure 11.3). These fascial layers and the neurovascular structures that they ensheath hold the bladder in place, as does the urethra, and the prostate in males, with which the bladder is continuous. The urethra and prostate have their attachments too, notably the endopelvic fascia, which tethers them to the pelvic side wall and the periurethral component of the levator ani muscle in males (it is vestigial in females) and the posterior vaginal wall in females, to which the female urethra is intimately related (Figure 11.4).

There are other supporting structures that are thought to be important in lower urinary tract function, particularly in the female.

First and foremost, in the female, are the pubourethral ligaments, which sling the full length of the urethra but particularly the proximal urethra from the inferior pubic area (Figure 11.5). These have been particularly studied by Zacharin [2] and his findings have since been confirmed by others, and all of these authors have sought somehow to link a deficiency in these ligaments to the genesis of stress incontinence.

The homologous structures in the male are the puboprostatic ligaments, which have become of particular interest since the development by Walsh [3]

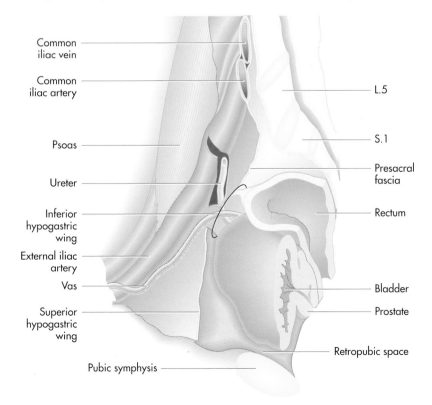

Common iliac vein

Common iliac artery

L.5

S.1

Psoas

Presacral fascia

Ureter

Inferior hypogastric wing

Rectum

External iliac artery

Vas

Bladder

Superior hypogastric wing

Prostate

Retropubic space

Pubic symphysis

Figure 11.3 *Diagram of the pelvic fascia to show the distribution of the presacral fascia. (Modified from Mundy AR. Urodynamic and reconstructive surgery of the lower urinary tract. Edinburgh: Churchill Livingstone, 1993.)*

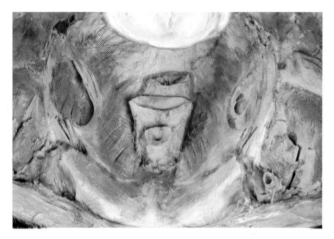

Figure 11.4a *The relationship of the urethra to the anterior vaginal wall. (Taken from Gosling JA, Dixon JS, Humpherson JR. The functional anatomy of the urinary tract. Edinburgh: Churchill Livingstone, 1983.)*

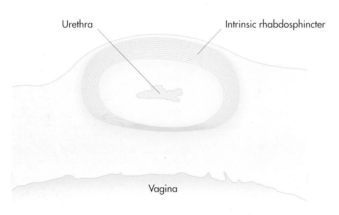

Figure 11.4b *Cross-section to show the integration of the urethra, below the bladder neck within the anterior vaginal wall. (Modified from Mundy AR. Urodynamic and reconstructive surgery of the lower urinary tract. Edinburgh: Churchill Livingstone, 1993.)*

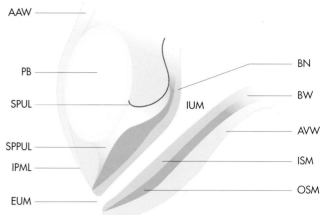

Figure 11.5 *The orientation of the pubourethral ligaments. AAW = anterior abdominal wall; PB = pubic bone; BN = bladder neck; BW = bladder wall; AVW = anterior vaginal wall; ISM = inner smooth muscle; OSM = outer striated muscle; IUM = internal urinary meatus; EUM = external urinary meatus; SPUL = superior pubourethral ligament; SPPUL = subpubic pubourethral ligament; IPML = inferior pubomeatal ligament. (Modified from Chilton CP. The urethra. In: Webster G, Kirby R, Goldwasser B, King L, (eds) Reconstructive Urology. Cambridge, MA: Blackwell Scientific Publications, 1993.)*

of his technique of radical retropubic prostatectomy.

One supporting structure identified in the anatomical and more traditional urological literature, the existence of which is now disputed, is the so-called urogenital diaphragm. Described as the layer upon which the prostate sits [4], it has proved elusive to others [5] and probably does not exist as a separate entity.

The urothelial layer is a multilayered transitional epithelium that is continuous with the ureters above and the prostatic urethra below. Under the light microscope, the urothelium is similar in the bladder and the prostatic urethra, but there are differences on scanning electron microscopy that become more marked the further one proceeds down the urethra

towards the bulbar segment where it changes to a columnar epithelium. The urothelium has numerous so-called tight junctions (see Chapter 1), which make it impermeable to fluids and solutes.

The smooth muscle of the bladder, which accounts for most of the thickness of the bladder wall, is called the detrusor layer. There have been various attempts to identify specific bundles of muscle within the bladder wall [6], largely in order to substantiate a hypothetical mechanism to account for the opening of the bladder neck at the initiation of voiding, but there is no good evidence that such layering exists [7]. The bladder should be considered as a single homogenous layer of relatively large muscle bundles in a relatively small amount of connective tissue. These muscle bundles have no particular orientation (Figure 11.6). As one approaches the bladder base from above down, there is the triangular region of the trigone between the two ureters and the internal urinary meatus, where there is a flimsy additional superficial layer of smooth muscle quite separate from the underlying smooth muscle, which is typical detrusor. This additional trigonal layer is derived from the ureters and shows several distinct characteristics. The muscle fibres form bundles that

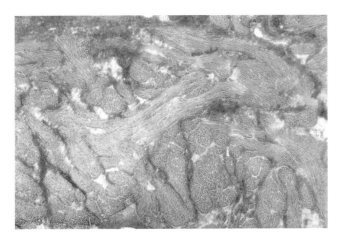

Figure 11.6 *Low-power microscopy of the detrusor stained with Masson's trichrome to show the orientation of the smooth muscle bundles. (Taken from Gosling JA, Dixon JS, Humpherson JR. The functional anatomy of the urinary tract. Edinburgh: Churchill Livingstone, 1983.)*

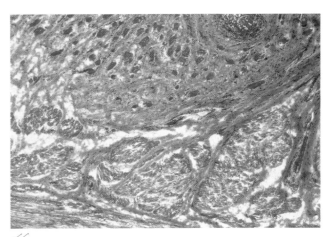

Figure 11.7a *Low-power microscopy of the detrusor stained with Masson's trichrome to show the distribution of the smooth muscle bundles in relation to the trigone superficially, compared with the detrusor proper, more deeply. (Taken from Gosling JA, Dixon JS, Humpherson JR. The functional anatomy of the urinary tract. Edinburgh: Churchill Livingstone, 1983.)*

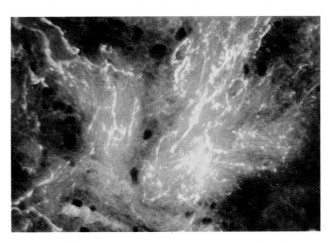

Figure 11.7b *Immunofluorescent microscopy study to show the presence of adrenergic nerves in the trigone. (Taken from Gosling JA, Dixon JS, Humpherson JR. The functional anatomy of the urinary tract. Edinburgh: Churchill Livingstone, 1983.)*

are much smaller with a higher connective tissue component and a fairly dense adrenergic innervation [8] (Figure 11.7). The trigonal muscle was once thought also to have a role in opening the bladder neck, but this too has not been substantiated. As one approaches closer to the bladder neck, the disposition and orientation of the detrusor change uniformly around it. The muscle bundles get smaller, there is a relatively greater amount of connective tissue, and the orientation of the muscle bundles becomes more uniform, to loop obliquely around the bladder neck (Figure 11.8).

Below the bladder neck in both sexes, the muscle bundles continue to be relatively small in size and interspersed with a relatively larger connective tissue component and they continue to show an oblique looping arrangement around the urethra. The vascular component of the wall increases by comparison with the bladder, particularly in females [9]. In the male, the prostate forms an additional component at this level, and at the upper part, where the prostate and the bladder neck merge, there is the pre-prostatic sphincter in which adrenergically innervated smooth muscle bundles form a distinct sphincter around the urethra to prevent retrograde ejaculation [8] (Figure 11.9). It should be emphasised that this adrenergically innervated smooth muscle component – the pre-prostatic sphincter – which is present in males but not in females, is a genital sphincter and not the bladder neck urinary sphincter mechanism in the strict sense, which is presumably the same in both sexes.

The pre-prostatic sphincter and the trigone are the only areas to show a distinct adrenergic innervation, otherwise the only adrenergic neurons in the bladder are those that supply the blood vessels [8]. This is not to say that there are not adrenergic receptors present; indeed, there are alpha receptors in the bladder base and beta receptors elsewhere in the bladder dome [10], but there is no evidence that there is a functionally important innervation to these receptors in the normal individual. Further down the urethra at the apex of the prostate in males and in the mid-urethra in females, there is the urethral sphincter mechanism,

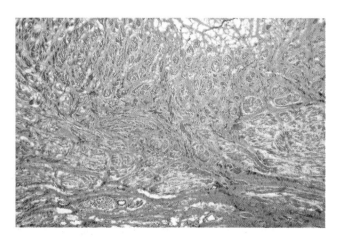

Figure 11.8a *Low-power microscopy of the detrusor stained with Masson's trichrome to show the distribution of the smooth muscle bundles at the bladder neck. (Taken from Gosling JA, Dixon JS, Humpherson JR. The functional anatomy of the urinary tract. Edinburgh: Churchill Livingstone, 1983.)*

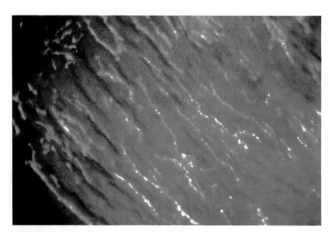

Figure 11.8b *Immunofluorescent microscopy to show the presence of adrenergic nerve fibres in the bladder neck. (Taken from Gosling JA, Dixon JS, Humpherson JR. The functional anatomy of the urinary tract. Edinburgh: Churchill Livingstone, 1983.)*

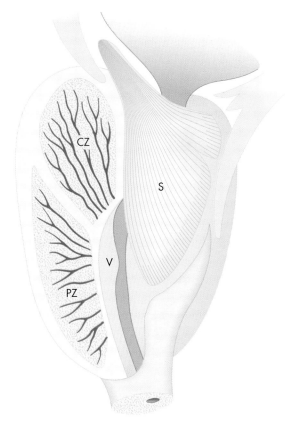

Figure 11.9 *A diagram to show the pre-prostatic sphincter. CZ = central zone; PZ = peripheral zone; S = pre-prostatic sphincter; V = verumontanum.*

sometimes called the 'distal sphincter mechanism' to distinguish it from the proximal sphincter mechanism, which is the other name for the bladder neck. Whereas there is a readily identifiable sphincter mechanism in the 'sphincter active' area of the urethra in both sexes, there is no anatomically identifiable sphincter mechanism at the bladder neck in either sex (using the term bladder neck in its strictest sense – as distinct from the pre-prostatic sphincter). The urethral sphincter mechanism has three components (Figure 11.10). The innermost is the urethral smooth muscle and the middle layer is the striated muscle

component within the urethral wall. These two components within the urethral wall itself are separated from the third component, which is the periurethral component of the levator ani, or pubouretheral sling, which is slung around the urethra in much the same way as the puborectal sling is disposed round the rectum [11]. These two sling components, the pubourethral and the puborectal slings, are distinct from and below the diaphragmatic layer of the levator ani [12] (Figure 11.11). They both form substantial components of their respective sphincter mechanisms and they share several common features.

The urethral sphincter mechanism

Of the three layers of the urethral sphincter mechanism, two are relatively quickly dealt with. The outermost layer – the pubourethral sling – is the levator ani

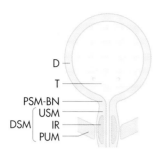

Figure 11.10 *Diagrammatic representation of the components of the urethral sphincter mechanism. D = detrusor; T = trigone; PSM-BN = proximal sphincter mechanism-bladder neck; DSM = distal sphincter mechanism; USM = urethral smooth muscle; IR = intrinsic rhabdosphincter; PUM = peri-urethral musculature.*

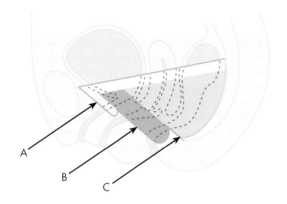

Figure 11.11 *Illustration of the various components of levator ani showing separate sling and diaphragmatic components. A = pubo-urethral sling; B = pubo-rectal sling; C = levator diaphragm.*

component most closely related to the urethra [11]; it is typical striated muscle; it has typical striated muscle innervation; it is relatively insignificant in the female compared to the male because of the presence of the vagina; and it is activated along with the rest of the levator ani under 'stress conditions', acting specifically on the urethra at such times to augment urethral occlusion pressure.

The urethral smooth muscle is dealt with relatively quickly for an entirely different reason: we know very little about its function. It appears to have a predominantly cholinergic innervation but less dense than in the bladder [8]. When the striated muscle of the urethral sphincter mechanism is paralysed, the urethral smooth muscle continues to produce a high-pressure zone, which suggests that it is tonically active [12] – whereas the bladder smooth muscle is phasically active – and recent experimental studies suggest that

this tonic smooth muscle contraction may be relaxed by nitric oxide [13, 14]. Current opinion is that this nitric oxide-related relaxant mechanism in this area of the urethra, is at least partly responsible for the urethral relaxation that occurs when the bladder contracts at the onset of voiding.

It appears that it is the striated muscle component within the urethral wall that is the most important component for continence. It is sometimes called the intrinsic rhabdosphincter [8]. This striated muscle is unusual in a number of ways [8]. It is orientated predominantly anteriorly in both the vertical and horizontal planes and is relatively deficient posteriorly, giving it, overall, a signet ring distribution (Figure 11.12). This is clearly seen microscopically in both sexes (Figure 11.13). The reason for this is not clear, but it is common experience that the easiest way of stopping water flowing through a hosepipe is to kink it rather than to squeeze it circumferentially. It may be that the distribution of the fibres of the intrinsic striated muscle of the urethra produces a kinking rather than a circumferential compression when it contracts, for this sort of reason, but this is entirely conjectural. This intrinsic striated muscle sphincter is composed of relatively very small muscle fibres when compared with typical striated muscle; the fibres themselves are disposed in small muscle bundles within a very much greater connective tissue component than is seen in typical striated muscle (Figure 11.14); the muscle fibres themselves are stuffed with mitochondria; there are no muscle spindles; and there are several distinct histochemical staining characteristics of these muscle fibres, most notably a uniform staining with acid-stable myosin adenosine triphosphatase (ATPase) [15] (Figure 11.15). By contrast, the typical striated muscle of the pubourethral sling that is immediately adjacent to the intrinsic rhabdosphincter shows larger muscle fibres in larger muscle bundles, with little connective tissue, fewer mitochondria, muscle spindles present and a mixed pattern of staining for acid-stable myosin ATPase (Figure 11.16). Furthermore, whereas the nerve supply to the levator ani originates in typical cell bodies in the motor cell nuclei of the anterior horn of the sacral spinal cord, the cell bodies of the fibres that innervate the intrinsic rhabdosphincter appear to arise in a nucleus more medially situated in the sacral anterior horn, as do the fibres innervating the anal sphincter mechanism, and this spinal cord nucleus is known as spinal nucleus X, sometimes called Onuf's nucleus [16] (Figure 11.17). The fibres from Onuf's nucleus to the intrinsic rhabdosphincter run out of the anterior primary rami and the nerve fibres run initially with the nervi erigentes, which are the preganglionic parasympathetic neurons. They run with these fibres through the pelvic plexuses and down with the postganglionic parasympathetic neurons into the urethra [8].

Whether this is the sole innervation of the intrinsic rhabdosphincter or whether there is a separate component arising from the pudendal nerve is not clear [17], but after pudendal neurectomy or pudendal nerve blockade, the urethral sphincter mechanism is intact so there is clearly a source other than the pudendal nerve.

These characteristics of the intrinsic rhabdosphincter are very unusual but not unique; the intrinsic laryngeal muscles are very similar in structure and in the nature of their innervation.

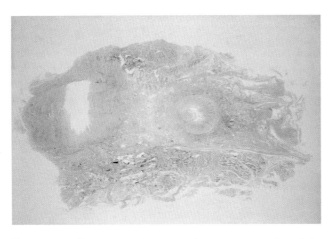

Figure 11.12 Low-power microscopy of a transverse section of the male sphincter-active urethra to show the 'signet ring' distribution of the intrinsic rhabdosphincter. (Anterior to the right of the figure.)

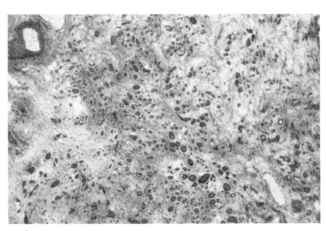

Figure 11.14 Low-power microscopy of the intrinsic rhabdosphincter to show the relative distribution of muscle bundles and connective tissue. (Taken from Gosling JA, Dixon JS, Humpherson JR. The functional anatomy of the urinary tract. Edinburgh: Churchill Livingstone, 1983.)

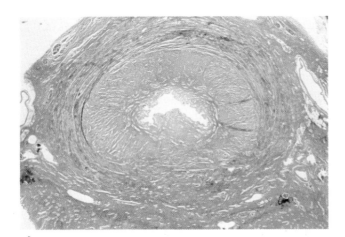

Figure 11.13 Low-power microscopy of a transverse section of the female sphincter-active urethra to show the 'signet ring' distribution of the intrinsic rhabdosphincter. (Anterior to the top of the figure.)

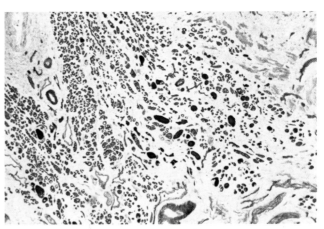

Figure 11.15 Low-power histochemistry of the intrinsic rhabdosphincter to show the distribution of acid-stable myosin ATPase. (Taken from Gosling JA, Dixon JS, Humpherson JR. The functional anatomy of the urinary tract. Edinburgh: Churchill Livingstone, 1983.)

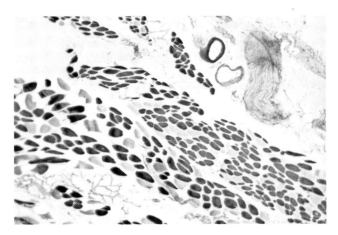

Figure 11.16 *Low-power histochemistry of the typical striated muscle, in this case the pubourethral sling, to show the distribution of acid-stable myosin ATPase. (Taken from Gosling JA, Dixon JS, Humpherson JR. The functional anatomy of the urinary tract. Edinburgh: Churchill Livingstone, 1983.)*

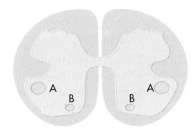

Figure 11.17 *Diagram to show the separate origin of the innervation of the intrinsic rhabdosphincter from Onuf's nucleus as distinct from the site of origin of typical striated msucle from anterior horn cells. A = α motorneuron group; B = Onuf's nucleus.*

The innervation of the bladder and urethra

Four separate neuronal pathways to the lower urinary tract have been alluded to (Figure 11.18). The principal one is derived from cell bodies in the intermediolateral column of the second, third and fourth sacral segments of the spinal cord. These are preganglionic parasympathetic fibres that run out of the anterior primary rami of S2, S3 and S4 and then separate out from the somatic component which runs to the sacral plexus, to run as the nervi erigentes to the pelvic plexuses. These preganglionic parasympathetic neurons end by synapsing in ganglia on the cell bodies of the postganglionic parasympathetic nerves, which then run to the bladder and to the urethra (and more

proximally to the rectum and the genital structures). In humans, 50% of the ganglia of the pelvic plexus are in the adventitial tissue around the base and posterolateral aspects of the bladder and 50% are within the bladder wall itself [8]. For this reason it is, strictly speaking, technically impossible to denervate the bladder because the 50% within the bladder wall itself will still remain and there will therefore still be reflex activity, even if this is not physiologically significant. A more semantically correct term would therefore be decentralisation rather than denervation when discussing the stripping of the nerves from around the outside of the bladder.

The somatic nerve fibres that arise from Onuf's nucleus and that travel with the otherwise autonomic parasympathetic nerve fibres of the nervi erigentes and pass ultimately to the intrinsic rhabdosphincter have already been mentioned.

The third component is the sympathetic nerve component that arises from the intermediatolateral column of the 10th, 11th and 12th thoracic and the 1st and 2nd lumbar segments of the spinal cord.

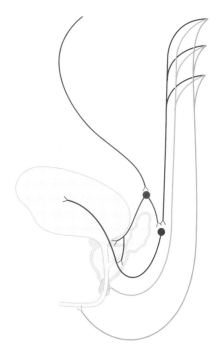

Figure 11.18 *Diagram to show the four components of innervation of the lower urinary tract. (—) Sympathetic; (—) parasympathetic; (—) somatic innervation of intrinsic rhabdosphincter; (—) pudendal nerve. (Taken from Gosling JA, Dixon JS, Humpherson JR. The functional anatomy of the urinary tract. Edinburgh: Churchill Livingstone, 1983.)*

These preganglionic sympathetic fibres and their postganglionic sympathetic derivatives travel as the hypogastric nerves, which innervate the trigone, the blood vessels of the bladder and the smooth muscle of the prostate in males, including the pre-prostatic sphincter. They also have postganglionic branches that end in the parasympathetic ganglia [8], where they exert an inhibitory effect that is described in detail below.

Finally, there is the pudendal nerve component, also arising from S2, S3 and S4, in this instance from typical anterior horn motor neuron cell bodies, which innervates the urethra and the pelvic floor musculature and provides afferent innervation to the urethra.

By comparison with typical anatomical 'nerves' such as the obturator nerve, the femoral nerve and even the sciatic nerve, the total mass of the autonomic nerves in the pelvis is large. The autonomic nerves are not as discrete and easily identifiable as the somatic nerves referred to, disposed as they are as a sheet within the fascial layers that invest the rectum, the genital structures and the lower urinary tract, but if the nerve fibres are dissected out and considered as a whole, their volume is considerable. It is this sheer mass that protects pelvic autonomic function from extensive damage during pelvic surgery such as hysterectomy or rectal resection, but they are nonetheless vulnerable to traction injuries during such procedures [18], as of course they are in females during childbirth.

Functional aspects of the innervation of the bladder and urethra

Cholinergic nerves cannot be stained directly for microscopical study – only indirectly by staining for acetylcholinesterase, the enzyme that breaks down acetylcholine at the neuromuscular junction. Staining for acetylcholinesterase shows a dense 'presumptive-cholinergic' innervation of the detrusor smooth muscle (Figure 11.19) with a nerve to muscle cell ratio of about 1:1, and a less dense cholinergic innervation of the urethral smooth muscle [8]. Under the electron microscope, the terminal branches of the parasympathetic neurons within the bladder wall are seen to contain varicosities (Figure 11.20). These varicosities are there because of the presence of numerous vesicles within the terminal neuron at that point and these

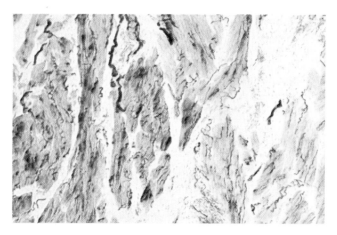

Figure 11.19 Low-power microscopy of the muscle wall after staining with acetylcholinesterase to show the distribution of presumptive cholinergic nerves in the bladder wall. (Taken from Gosling JA, Dixon JS, Humpherson JR. The functional anatomy of the urinary tract. Edinburgh: Churchill Livingstone, 1983.)

vesicles contain neurotransmitter substances. Alongside the varicosity is the specialised area of the smooth muscle that constitutes the receptor site, although this is not very specialised by comparison with the receptor site – the neuromuscular junction – in striated muscle. Adjacent smooth muscle cells are connected by so-called 'regions of close approach', like gap junctions in effect, which could, at least theoretically, allow electrotonic spread of activity from one smooth muscle cell to the next and which thereby confer so-called 'cable properties' on the smooth muscle fibres. This would supplement the spreading neuronal stimulus as a sort of 'parallel pathway', and help to ensure a uniform simultaneous contraction of all the bladder smooth muscle cells at the time of voiding.

Vesicles are of two main types [19]: small clear vesicles and larger vesicles with a dense core. The small clear vesicles are thought to contain so-called 'fast' neurotransmitter substances, which are released directly into the area between the neuron and the adjacent neuron across a synapse, or the adjacent smooth muscle cell across a neuromuscular junction (Figure 11.21) to open ligand-gated ion channels on the receptor site that will initiate an action potential. Outside the central nervous system, the commonest neurotransmitter to be found in these small clear vesicles is acetylcholine and the commonest receptor is the nicotinic acetylcholine receptor, although acetylcholine does not exclusively act as a fast neurotransmitter to open ligand-gated ion channels in this way. In the central nervous system, gamma-aminobutyric acid (GABA) is also found in small clear vesicles [20].

Large, dense-cored vesicles contain so-called 'slow' neurotransmitters [20], which are called 'slow' because they are released non-specifically from around the area of the varicosity (Figure 11.22) rather than specifically into the receptor site; and because they generally act by binding to G-protein-linked receptors (see Chapter 1) and initiating smooth muscle contraction through second messengers systems. This is so-called 'pharmacomechanical' coupling of the neuronal stimulus to smooth muscle contraction, as distinct from the 'electromechanical' coupling initiated by the binding of ligand-gated ion channels by fast neurotransmitters.

A single nerve impulse will empty about half the vesicles in a varicosity, each of which will release about 5000 molecules of acetylcholine as a quantum. These vesicles empty their contents in response to a rise in cytosolic calcium within the varicosity as a result of the opening of membrane calcium channels induced by the neuronal electrical impulse (voltage-gated calcium channels), causing an influx of extracellular calcium [21].

There are other ways of demonstrating the primacy of parasympathetic cholinergic activity in the excitatory innervation of the bladder other than by showing its density on light microscopy and electron microscopy. The most convincing way is by the physiological study of strips of detrusor smooth muscle in an organ bath (Figure 11.23). The organ bath keeps the muscle strip at the right temperature, sufficiently oxygenated and in the right fluid medium to keep it viable sufficiently long for adequate study. The excitatory nerve supply to the muscle fibres within the muscle strip is stimulated by using an electrical impulse. If the strength and amplitude are optimised and the frequency of the electrical stimulus is then varied, a frequency-response curve is produced between about 0.5 Hz and 20 Hz, above which the response rate plateaus until the electrical impulse is of sufficiently high frequency to cause damage (Figure 11.24). This response can be abolished by the application of tetrodotoxin, which is a sodium channel blocker which therefore blocks nerve conduction [21]. (Tetrodotoxin is

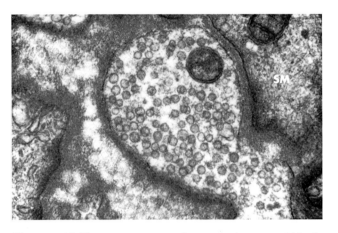

Figure 11.20 Electron microscopy of a terminal neuron within the detrusor smooth muscle layer to show a varicosity containing small clear vesicles containing acetylcholine. (Taken from Gosling JA, Dixon JS. Anatomy of the bladder, urethra and pelvic floor. In: Mundy AR, Stephenson TP, Wein AJ (eds) Urodynamics – principles, practice and application. Edinburgh: Churchill Livingstone, 1984.)

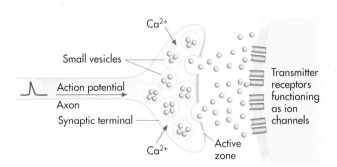

Figure 11.21 Diagram of a nerve ending and neuromuscular junction to show the release of so-called 'fast' neurotransmitters into the neuromuscular junction. (Modified from Goodman SR. Medical cell biology. Philadelphia: JB Lippincott, 1994.)

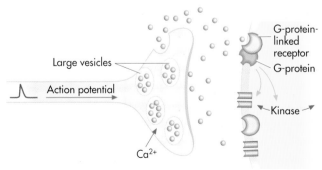

Figure 11.22 Diagram of a nerve ending and neuromuscular junction to show the release of so-called 'slow' neurotransmitters from around the neuromuscular junction. (Modified from Goodman SR. Medical cell biology. Philadelphia: JB Lippincott, 1994.)

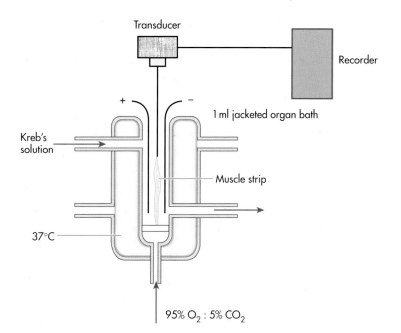

Figure 11.23 *Diagrammatic representation of an organ bath experiment. (Modified from Mundy AR, Thomas PJ. Clinical physiology of the bladder, urethra and pelvic floor. In: Mundy AR, Stephenson TP, Wein AJ (eds) Urodynamics – principles, practice and application. 2nd edition. Edinburgh: Churchill Livingstone, 1994.)*

extracted from the liver of the puffer fish – called fugu in Japan – and will be known as such to James Bond afficionados.) If a frequency-response curve is plotted after the application of tetrodotoxin, there will be a very small response at higher frequencies that is not nerve mediated but due to direct stimulation of the smooth muscle cell membrane itself. If the frequency-response curve is performed after the application of atropine at a sufficient dose to give complete cholinergic blockade, then the only response left will be the same as that after tetrodotoxin (Figure 11.25). In other words, in the normal human specimen (stressing both adjectives), there is no excitatory component left after atropine blockade and there is no 'atropine-resistant' component to excitatory neurotransmission. Normal excitatory neurotransmission in the human bladder is exclusively muscarinic cholinergic [22–24]. In other mammals, it is a completely different story. In some small mammals, there may be as much as 30% of the frequency-response curve that is atropine resistant. This is thought to be due to the presence of an alternative excitatory neurotransmitter that, in most animal species showing this type of excitatory neurotransmission, is thought to be adenosine triphosphate (ATP) [20]. This is thought to give rise to the type of bladder contraction responsible for the excretion of a small amount of urine for the purposes of territorial marking. In those animals that exhibit territorial

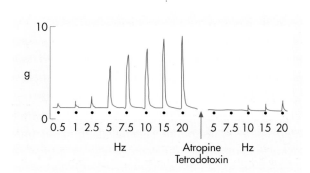

Figure 11.24 *A frequency-response curve before and after tetrodotoxin showing a very small residual contraction that is not nerve mediated and due to direct smooth muscle stimulation. (Modified from Mundy AR, Thomas PJ. Clinical physiology of the bladder, urethra and pelvic floor. In: Mundy AR, Stephenson TP, Wein AJ, (eds) Urodynamics – principles, practice and application. 2nd edition. Edinburgh: Churchill Livingstone, 1994.)*

marking, it seems likely that a normal voiding detrusor contraction is cholinergic in origin, whereas the small-volume 'squirt' of urine excreted for territorial marking is under so-called purinergic (ATP-mediated) innervation.

This is not to say that ATP cannot be made to cause contraction of human detrusor smooth muscle. It has indeed been shown to do so [21], but it does not appear to be a component of normal human voiding. It may, however, be a cause of abnormal detrusor function in detrusor instability and hyperreflexia.

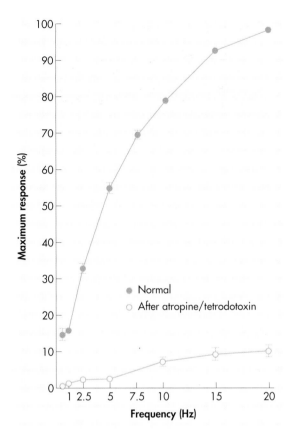

Figure 11.25 *A frequency-response curve before and after atropine in a human showing a very small residual response. In this case it is a graphical representation of the percentage response. (Modified from Mundy AR, Thomas PJ. Clinical physiology of the bladder, urethra and pelvic floor. In: Mundy AR, Stephenson TP, Wein AJ (eds). Urodynamics – principles, practice and application. 2nd edition. Edinburgh: Churchill Livingstone, 1994.)*

Excitation–contraction coupling

Reference has already been made to the two types of excitation–contraction coupling: electromechanical coupling, in which an electrical impulse causes the release of a neurotransmitter that binds to a ligand-gated ion channel, which causes membrane depolarisation and contraction and onward spread of the impulse by the generation of an action potential; and pharmacomechanical coupling, in which a G-protein-linked receptor is bound and there is release of a second messenger – inositol triphosphate (IP_3) – which causes the release of intracellular calcium from calcium stores [25], mainly in the endoplasmic reticulum, which in turn causes contraction and also opening of ligand-gated ion channels in the cell membrane

and generation of an action potential. In either case, intracellular calcium rises and is bound by calmodulin, a ubiquitous intracellular calcium-binding protein, which is thereby activated. This in turn activates myosin light chain kinase, which activates myosin, causing it to bind to actin, and this produces the so-called 'power stroke' in which the actin and myosin filaments shorten, leading to contraction [26] (Figure 11.26).

The relative importance of electromechanical coupling and pharmacomechanical coupling in the human bladder is not clear, but it is thought that they are probably equally important. Either way, the most important factor is the occurrence of a rise of cytosolic calcium levels. In electromechanical coupling, the calcium comes initially from outside the cell, firstly in response to membrane depolarisation, which opens voltage-sensitive calcium channels, and secondly in response to the calcium binding of calcium-gated calcium channels. In pharmacomechanical coupling, the calcium initially comes from intracellular calcium stores via a G-protein-linked receptor and a second messenger system using IP_3 as the second messenger. Both of these processes are described in detail and illustrated in Chapter 1.

The G-protein-linked receptor that is activated by cholinergic neurons in pharmacomechanical coupling is the muscarinic acetylcholine receptor. The muscarinic receptor is a typical seven-span transmembrane receptor in which the extracellular receptor domain confers specificity and the intracellular domain between the fifth and sixth transmembrane domains contains the binding site for the particular G-protein activated by ligand binding (Figure 11.27).

There are three types of muscarinic receptors: M1, M2 and M3. The highest percentage of receptors in the bladder are of the M2 type, accounting for more than 80% [27], but physiologically these are the least important and it is the M3 muscarinic receptor that is most important for bladder physiology [28] (Figure 11.28).

The final pathway of excitatory neurotransmission in the lower urinary tract is therefore as follows. Preganglionic parasympathetic nerve activity causes the release of acetylcholine in the parasympathetic ganglia. Acetylcholine activates the nicotinic receptors of

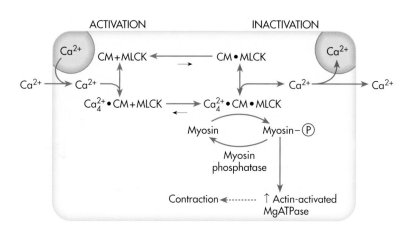

Figure 11.26 *Diagram of the biochemical basis of smooth muscle contraction. MLCK = myosin light-chain kinase; CM = calmodulin.*

the postganglionic neurons, which are ligand-gated ion channels (for which the ligand is acetylcholine). The postganglionic neurons also release acetylcholine at their terminals, which in their case are neuromuscular junctions within the detrusor. On the smooth muscle cell membranes, the acetylcholine receptors are muscarinic receptors, of which the most important are M3 receptors, which are G-protein-linked receptors. These cause the generation of inositol triphosphate from membrane phospholipids, which in turn causes the release of calcium from intracellular calcium stores. This has two principal effects: firstly, bound to calmodulin, it causes smooth muscle contraction by pharmacomechanical coupling and, secondly, it opens calcium-gated calcium channels in the plasma membrane. This causes an influx of extracellular calcium to perpetuate the contraction and to replenish intracellular calcium stores.

Mention has been made of the presence of other types of receptors such as ATP (purinergic) receptors in the bladder as a whole and adrenergic receptors, which are more specifically localised – beta receptors in the dome and alpha receptors in the base and in the urethra. It has been argued, however, that although receptors are present, there is no significant innervation except to the blood vessels, the trigone and, in males, the preprostatic sphincter in healthy humans, although there may be in disease or in other animals.

Adrenergic receptors are also G-protein-linked receptors, but here the effector protein is the enzyme adenylate cyclase, which is switched on by the alpha receptor G-protein and switched off by the beta receptor. Adenylate cyclase generates cyclic adenosine monophosphate (cAMP), which is a second messen-

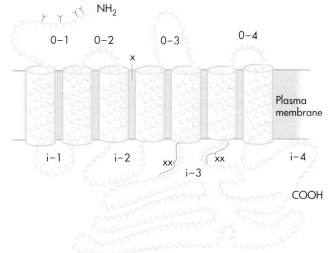

Figure 11.27 *Diagrammatic representation of a muscarinic receptor.*

ger which, in general, has the opposite effect of the calcium–calmodulin complex. Cyclic AMP tends to inhibit smooth muscle contraction and reduce intracellular calcium.

The contractile apparatus

The contractile apparatus of striated muscle is clearly defined by the striations visible under the light microscope that have been shown to be interlinking fibres of actin and myosin. Smooth muscle also contracts because of the relationship between actin and myosin, but the disposition of these fibres is not as clearly defined as in striated muscle and is not visible by light microscopy.

Under the electron microscope, 'dense bodies' are visible that are the closest smooth muscle gets to revealing its contractile apparatus (Figure 11.29). How-

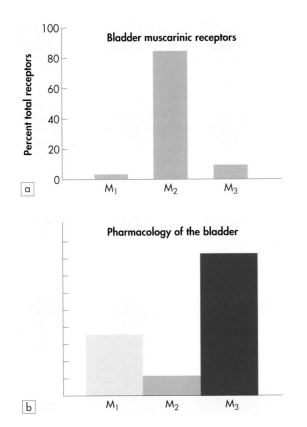

Figure 11.28 *The relative distribution of M1, M2 and M3 receptors: (a) by number, (b) by pharmacological importance.*

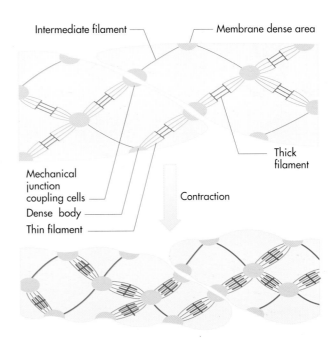

Figure 11.29 *Diagram to show dense bodies in smooth muscle on electron microscopy. (Modified from Goodman SR. Medical cell biology. Philadelphia: JB Lippincott, 1994.)*

ever, the principle of action is the same as in striated muscle except less well organised and less efficient. The calcium–calmodulin complex in smooth muscle activates the enzyme myosin light chain kinase, which causes the myosin fibres to straighten out and align themselves with actin fibres and form cross-linkages through the myosin heads.

Phosphorylation causes the myosin heads to flex in relation to their tails and this causes the myosin fibres to move over the actin fibres (or vice versa). The effect of this is for the contractile apparatus to shorten, thereby generating contractility (Figure 11.30). The flexion of the myosin head is known as the 'power stroke'.

Dephosphorylation switches off this process and relaxation occurs passively as a result.

Relaxant mechanisms

Until recently, most of the relaxant mechanisms in the bladder were thought to be quite simply related to

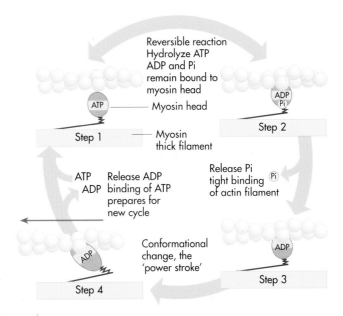

Figure 11.30 *The process of smooth muscle contraction. Step 1: the binding of ATP to myosin disrupts the binding of actin to myosin. Step 2: the hydrolysis of ATP to ADP allows actin to make contact with myosin. Step 3: the release of phosphate associated with the hydrolysis of ATP to ADP causes the actin to bind tightly to myosin. Step 4: tight binding of actin to myosin causes a conformational change (flexion) of the myosin head known as the 'power stroke'. (Modified from Goodman SR. Medical cell biology. Philadelphia: JB Lippincott, 1994.)*

reversing the contractile mechanisms. They were also, therefore, calcium related, in this instance by inhibitions of calcium influx, extrusion of intracellular calcium or facilitation of intracellular sequestration of calcium. All of the stimulatory effects of IP$_3$ and calcium tend to be reversed by cAMP and so anything that increased intracellular cAMP would cause relaxation.

In the last few years, however, a new relaxant mechanism has been identified that is thought to be much more important, particularly in the bladder neck and urethra. This is nitric oxide [13, 14] – an unlikely neurotransmitter as it is a gas. Nitric oxide is synthesised from L-arginine under the influence of nitric oxide synthase. It acts through cyclic guanosine monophosphate-dependent phosphorylation – dephosphorylation of myosin light chains. It has been shown to induce relaxation of muscle strips from the bladder neck and urethra on electrical stimulation and it is in these areas that nitric oxide synthase is principally concentrated. This electrically induced relaxation is dependent on extracellular calcium influx through voltage-gated calcium channels. This seems a little strange at first sight – that both contraction in response to muscarinic receptor activation and relaxation, through the action of nitric oxide, are mediated by a rise in intracellular calcium. It suggests that normally there is a balance between calcium-induced contraction and calcium-induced relaxation and it may be that the balance is tipped either way in relation to the exact site of intracellular calcium availability [13], although the details are not yet clear.

Other neurotransmitters

To classify as a neurotransmitter, a potential candidate must satisfy certain stringent criteria. In the last 15 years or so, numerous compounds have been identified as potential neurotransmitters, many of which fail to satisfy these criteria but nonetheless appear to be involved in the process of neurotransmission, either as neurotransmitters or as neuromodulators [20].

A further observation is that many of these compounds seem to be related to nerves that show the characteristics of cholinergic or adrenergic neurons. In other words, the putative neurotransmitter or neuromodulator appears to be 'co-localised' with a known 'classical' transmitter or with another putative neurotransmitter [20].

Several of these putative neurotransmitters are peptides, which have been grouped together as neuropeptides. This group includes substance P [29, 30], vasoactive intestinal polypeptide [31, 32] and neuropeptide Y, to name but a few. Substance P is thought to be involved in afferent neurotransmission [30]. Vasoactive intestinal polypeptide relaxes detrusor smooth muscle [31] and has been shown in some studies to be co-released with acetylcholine. Similarly, neuropeptide Y has been co-localised in adrenergic neurons. This concept of co-localisation, co-release and co-transmission is interesting as it provides a means of modifying the effects of neural activity either temporally or spatially. Thus, the same nerves could produce two transmitters with different effects, both being simultaneously released but with one predominating in one area and the other in the other area. For example, an excitatory and an inhibitory transmitter, if co-released, might cause bladder contraction if the former predominated in the bladder and relaxation of the bladder neck if the latter predominated at that site. This neuromodulatory activity could have other effects which would less dramatically act to 'fine tune' the actions of the lower urinary tract.

The afferent innervation of the bladder

This chapter has so far concentrated almost exclusively on the efferent innervation of the bladder, contractile and relaxant. The afferent innervation is obviously equally important, but is less well understood. Afferent impulses arise from the nerve plexus in the lamina propria underneath the urothelium and from within the muscle layer itself and presumably also from the adventitia. Afferent nerve endings have been identified but their nature is poorly understood. Substance P is thought to be a sensory neurotransmitter and there is some evidence to support this view, but again the mechanism is not well understood. What is clear, from the work of Nathan [33], is that there are three types of sensation arising from the bladder (Figure 11.31). The first and most general sensation of bladder filling arises from receptors throughout the bladder. The afferent fibres run with the parasympathetic nerves back to the sacral cord, where there is some local synapsing on preganglionic parasympathetic cell bodies in the intermediolateral column of the sacral cord, but the majority of afferent neurons run in the ascending tracts of the spinal cord and up to the pons, where they synapse with preganglionic neurons in the nucleus locus coeruleus in the rostral pons. Other fibres pass up to the cerebral cortex to give rise to sensory awareness. This type of afferent stimulus gives rise to a volume-related awareness of bladder filling that is easily suppressed.

Less easily suppressed is the next type of bladder sensation, which is stimulated by definite fullness of the bladder. This is a stimulus that arises in the trigonal area and the afferent impulses are transmitted in neurons that run with the sympathetic nerves up to the thoracolumbar cord. Once again, there are local relays in the cord, but most fibres run up in the ascending tracts to the pons and to the cerebral cortex to give awareness.

Finally, there is the feeling of severe urgency and the sense that voiding is imminent. This sensation cannot be overlooked. It arises in the urethra and the afferent fibres run with the pudendal nerve, again giving rise to local relays in the sacral cord, but with most fibres running in the ascending tracts to the pons and to the cerebral cortex.

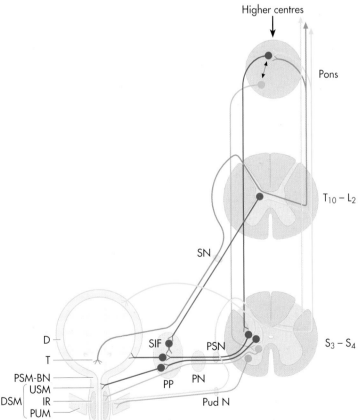

SN   = sympathetic nerves
PSN = parasympathetic nerves
O   = Onuf's nucleus
PN   = pelvic nerves
Pud N = pudendal nerve
PP   = pelvic plexus
SIF = small intensely fluorescent cells

Figure 11.31 *The nervous pathways concerned with the three different types of sensation from the lower urinary tract; (—) from the bladder, (—) from the trigone, (—) from the urethra and pelvic floor. (Modified from Mundy AR, Thomas PJ. Clinical physiology of the bladder, urethra and pelvic floor. In: Mundy AR, Stephenson TP, Wein AJ (eds). Urodynamics – principles, practice and application. 2nd edition. Edinburgh: Churchill Livingstone, 1994.)*

Within the spinal cord, the ascending and descending fibres all run in an equatorial plane through the spinal canal, as also shown by Nathan [34] (Figure 11.32). The medial tracts are visceral efferent, the intermediate tracts are somatic efferent to the intrinsic rhabdosphincter and the pelvic floor, and the most lateral fibres lying at the periphery of the cord between the corticospinal and the spinothalamic tracts are visceral afferent. The location of these tracts in relation to the urinary tract was found by postmortem studies of patients who had undergone the neurosurgical procedure of percutaneous cordotomy during life for relief for severe visceral pain, usually malignant in origin.

The nature of the neurotransmitters in both the afferent and efferent pathways of the spinal cord [35] is largely unknown [36]. Excitatory dopaminergic and muscarinic pathways and inhibitory GABA-ergic, glycinergic and encephalinergic pathways have been identified in experimental animals.

Cerebral control of voiding

Within the brain, there are five areas that are concerned with continence and voiding (Figure 11.33).

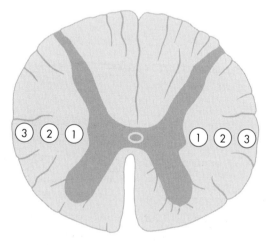

Figure 11.32 *The orientation within the spinal cord of the pathways related to lower urinary tract function. 1 = autonomic efferent; 2 = somatic efferent; 3 = afferent. (Modified from Mundy AR, Thomas PJ. Clinical physiology of the bladder, urethra and pelvic floor. In: Mundy AR, Stephenson TP, Wein AJ (eds). Urodynamics – principles, practice and application. 2nd edition. Edinburgh: Churchill Livingstone, 1994.)*

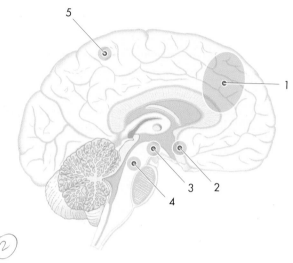

Figure 11.33 *Five areas of the brain concerned with lower urinary tract function. 1 = medial aspect of frontal lobe; 2 = septal and pre-optic nuclei; 3 = hypothalamus; 4 = nucleus locus coeruleus (Barrington's Pontine Micturition Centre); 5 = para-central lobule. (Modified from Mundy AR, Thomas PJ. Clinical physiology of the bladder, urethra and pelvic floor. In: Mundy AR, Stephenson TP, Wein AJ (eds). Urodynamics – principles, practice and application. 2nd edition. Edinburgh: Churchill Livingstone, 1994.)*

The first has already been alluded to – the nucleus locus coeruleus in the rostral pons where afferent nerves synapse on the cell bodies of efferent nerve fibres. There are two connections of importance at this site. The first is the synapse by which means an adequate afferent impulse gives rise to an efferent impulse that will generate a detrusor contraction that is sufficient in amplitude and duration to cause complete bladder emptying. The second connection that occurs at this site co-ordinates this contraction with relaxation of the bladder outflow in order to given unobstructed voiding. The details of these two mechanisms and their co-ordination are unclear; it is, however, quite clear that this is the site where both these actions – generation of a normal voiding contraction and reciprocal relaxation of the sphincter mechanism – occur and are co-ordinated. If there is such a thing as a 'micturition centre', then this is it [37].

Clearly, as this is largely an autonomic event, parasympathetically mediated, the hypothalamus is important, and this is the second of the five centres. The third is the paracentral lobule of the cerebral cortex, which is responsible for the control of the pelvic floor musculature. The importance of this centre becomes manifest in spastic conditions such as congenital cerebral palsy, in which failure of relaxation can cause quite severe voiding difficulties. The normal physiological role of other related areas of the brain, such as the basal ganglia, is not clear although diseases that affect these areas such as Parkinson's disease and multiple system atrophy have obvious adverse effects.

At the junction of the diencephalon and telencephalon are the septal and pre-optic nuclei where the 'associated acts' of both micturition and defecation (and, for that matter, coition) are co-ordinated [38]. In some animals, such as the cat, these associated acts of voiding are quite elaborate, but in the human being they are restricted to fixation of the diaphragm and anterior abdominal wall musculature.

Finally, there is the area in the medial aspect of the frontal lobe that, although described initially as an inhibitory area [39], seems to facilitate or inhibit voiding according to circumstances. Thus, it would appear, this area of the frontal lobe can facilitate the nucleus locus coeruleus to cause voiding when the bladder is only partially full and afferent activity is therefore subthreshold. This is the way in which the bladder can be emptied before going to bed or before undertaking a long journey to avoid, perhaps, the need to void during the night or the journey. Equally, if afferent activity has reached a threshold level but there is a good programme on the television, then this area of the frontal lobe can suppress the need to void until a more appropriate time.

The details of our understanding of the spinal cord mechanisms involved in voiding are sparse – in the brain, our knowledge of the mechanisms involved in continence and voiding is scant indeed.

The normal bladder filling–voiding cycle

So far, a summary has been given of our anatomical and physiological knowledge peripherally in the bladder and urethra themselves and then centrally within the nervous system. It has been seen that the most important 'reflex arcs' are mediated through the nucleus locus coeruleus in the rostral pons; that excitatory neurotransmission in the human is exclusively cholinergic, and specifically muscarinic in origin; that relaxation of the bladder neck and urethral smooth muscle is probably mediated through the action of nitric oxide; and that the intrinsic rhabdosphincter is the most important component of the sphincter mechanism for continence and must be reciprocally relaxed through a co-ordinating mechanism in the rostral pons for normal voiding to occur. However, these issues and the other matters discussed to not explain all that we need to know about normal continence and voiding.

It is apparent during a normal filling and voiding cycle of a cystometrogram, with synchronous measurement of pressure within the sphincter-active urethra (Figure 11.34), that bladder pressure stays almost completely unchanged throughout filling to a normal capacity despite an increasing afferent stimulus. There is, however, a small but definite rise in intraurethral pressure that is volume related. Then, just before or synchronous with the onset of voiding, there is a drop in intraurethral pressure, matched by a cessation of the electromyographic activity of the intrinsic rhabdosphincter, after which or synchronous with which detrusor pressure starts to rise [12]. This rise in pressure is then sustained until the bladder is empty, by which time detrusor pressure has returned to normal and urethral resistance has risen back to normal. The cycle then starts over again.

What keeps the bladder pressure low during filling?

This ability of the bladder to keep its pressure almost unchanging irrespective of bladder volume and afferent stimulation is known as compliance. The bladder is highly compliant: it shows very little change in pressure for a substantial change in volume. A steady rise in pressure during filling, which is sometimes seen when the bladder wall is 'stiff' due to disease, is known as low compliance or poor compliance.

The exact nature of normal bladder compliance is not clear but it can be observed to be present in the bladder postmortem, at least up to a certain filling volume [40]. This has been explained on the basis of the physical characteristics of the protein fibres that

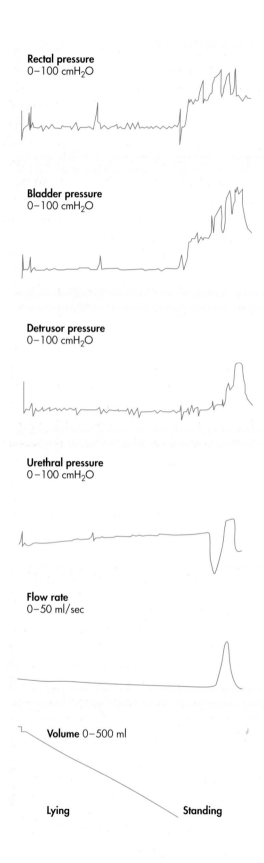

Rectal pressure
0–100 cmH$_2$O

Bladder pressure
0–100 cmH$_2$O

Detrusor pressure
0–100 cmH$_2$O

Urethral pressure
0–100 cmH$_2$O

Flow rate
0–50 ml/sec

Volume 0–500 ml

Lying   Standing

Figure 11.34 *Synchronous urethral and bladder pressure studies to show the urethra pressurised during bladder filling and pressure fall before the onset of detrusor contraction. (Modified from Mundy AR, Thomas PJ. Clinical physiology of the bladder, urethra and pelvic floor. In: Mundy AR, Stephenson TP, Wein AJ (eds). Urodynamics – principles, practice and application. 2nd edition. Edinburgh: Churchill Livingstone, 1994.)*

constitute the cellular and connective tissue structures of the bladder wall. They can be imagined as being coiled in the collapsed bladder and filling simply uncoils them, at least until 100–200 ml of filling has occurred (Figure 11.35). Detrusor smooth muscle cells have a striking ability to change their length without any change in tension. They may lengthen as much as fourfold during bladder filling, in a linear relationship with increasing bladder radius.

Our understanding of what happens over and beyond this elastic component and a certain 'visco-elastic' property of the bladder is due to the work of de Groat and his co-workers, who have studied this mechanism in great detail in the cat [41]. In a series of elegant experiments, de Groat has shown that there is

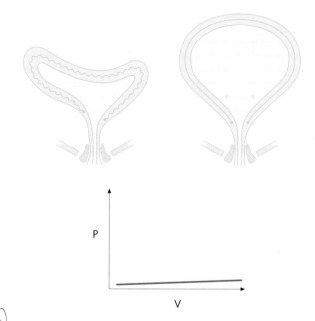

Figure 11.35 *The contribution of passive properties of the bladder wall to normal bladder compliance. (Modified from Mundy AR, Thomas PJ. Clinical physiology of the bladder, urethra and pelvic floor. In: Mundy AR, Stephenson TP, Wein AJ (eds). Urodynamics – principles, practice and application. 2nd edition. Edinburgh: Churchill Livingstone, 1994.)*

a 'gating' mechanism in the parasympathetic ganglia of the pelvic plexuses, which means that subthreshold activity in the preganglionic neurons is not transmitted to postganglionic efferent neurons (Figure 11.36). There is also an inhibitory interneuron mechanism within the spinal cord that helps to keep afferent impulses from being transmitted onwards until they reach a critical level. At low levels of afferent activity, the inhibitory interneurons prevent the transmission of impulses from the afferent nerves to the preganglionic efferent nerves. As afferent activity builds up, the inhibitory interneurons are progressively inhibited and impulses start to appear in the preganglionic efferent neurons, but the gating mechanism prevents these from being transmitted to the postganglionic efferent neurons until preganglionic efferent activity has reached a critical 'threshold' level. When this level is reached, a barrage of impulses is then transmitted down the postganglionic efferent neuron to the bladder, which therefore contracts (Figure 11.37).

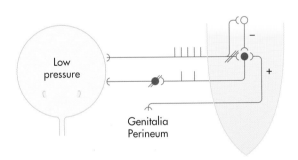

Figure 11.36 *The 'gating' mechanism by which, with minor degrees of activity in the afferent and preganglionic efferent nerves, there is no transmission to postganglionic efferent nerves.*

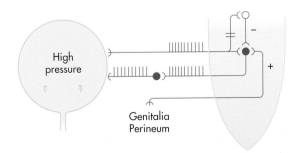

Figure 11.37 *The 'gating' mechanism showing that, with threshold afferent and preganglionic efferent activity, efferent activity is transmitted to postganglionic neurons.*

In addition, there are the inhibitory effects of the sympathetic neurons that have postganglionic branches ending on parasympathetic ganglion cells, as mentioned earlier in the chapter. The afferent fibres are presumably those that arise in the trigone, conveying fullness of the bladder and running up to the thoracolumbar cord, where the local relay gives rise to efferent sympathetic activity that tends to inhibit neurotransmission across the parasympathetic ganglia of the pelvic plexuses, thereby enhancing de Groat's gating mechanism (Figure 11.38).

What causes the rise in urethral pressure during bladder filling?

This appears to be due to local reflex activity within the sacral cord by which afferent impulses from the bladder cause a local reflex rise in efferent activity to the urethral smooth muscle. It is thought to be spinal because it persists after complete spinal cord transection above the level of the sacral segments. Other than that, the mechanism is unclear.

What causes the fall in urethral pressure at the onset of voiding?

The mechanism of this is not clear either, but it has regularly been observed that intraurethral pressure drops to a degree that indicates that both the smooth and the striated components of the urethral sphincter mechanism are relaxed [12]. Cessation of rhabdosphincter electromyogram activity synchronous with the fall in urethral pressure has also been observed to support this conclusion. This possibly explains why the most urgent sense of a very full bladder is more a urethral than a bladder sensation, transmitted through the pudendal nerve. It seems, in fact, that the urethral sphincter mechanism is reflexly opening and only voluntary contraction of the pelvic floor and suppression of the micturition reflex can stop it occurring. It seems, therefore, that at this point there has been threshold activation of the efferent cell bodies in the nucleus locus coeruleus and only positive intervention by higher centres to suppress the

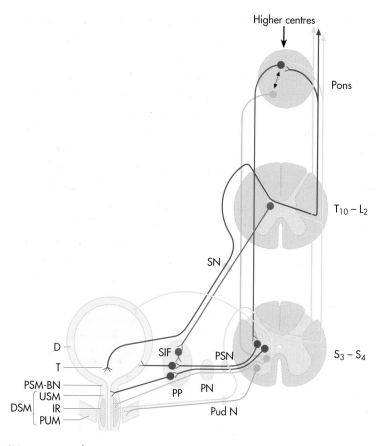

Higher centres

Pons

$T_{10} - L_2$

SN

$S_3 - S_4$

D

SIF

PSN

T

PSM-BN

USM

DSM   IR

PUM

PP   PN

Pud N

SN   = sympathetic nerves
PSN   = parasympathetic nerves
PN   = pelvic nerves
Pud N = pudendal nerve
PP   = pelvic plexus
SIF   = small intensely fluorescent cells

Figure 11.38 The action of sympathetic fibres (—) on parasympathetic ganglia. (Modified from Mundy AR, Thomas PJ. Clinical physiology of the bladder, urethra and pelvic floor. In: Mundy AR, Stephenson TP, Wein AJ (eds). Urodynamics – principles, practice and application. 2nd edition. Edinburgh: Churchill Livingstone, 1994.)

process can prevent the urethra relaxing and stop reflex detrusor contraction from following.

How does the bladder neck open?

There have been several theories to account for this. It used to be thought that there was a reciprocal innervation of the bladder by the parasympathetic system and of the bladder neck by the sympathetic system and that when the one caused contraction the other caused relaxation [42] (Figure 11.39), but that was discounted when the role of the sympathetic system in the lower urinary tract was effectively ruled out, as discussed above. With the recent discovery of the role of nitric oxide, however, this reciprocal innervation theory might well be resuscitated. Nitric oxide may be

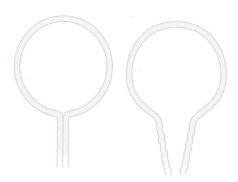

Figure 11.39 Diagrammatic representation of the theory of 'reciprocal innervation'.

co-transmitted with acetylcholine and it may be that the acetylcholine component causes contraction of the detrusor smooth muscle, whereas at the bladder neck and in the urethra there is a more dominant nitric oxide effect released from the same type of neurons, which causes bladder neck and urethral relaxation. This does not explain the relaxation of the intrinsic rhabdosphincter, but if one presupposes that relaxation of the rhabdosphincter is a necessary precondition for detrusor contraction to occur, then bladder neck and urethral smooth muscle relaxation at the onset of detrusor contraction is all that is left to explain.

Another explanation popularised by Lapides [43] (Figure 11.40) was that the bladder neck and the urethral musculature were continuous and fixed like a system of guy ropes at the urogenital diaphragm. Contraction therefore caused shortening, which therefore caused opening of the bladder neck. This theory was never widely held and was eventually discounted by the demonstration that the urogenital diaphragm did not exist.

The next theory to explain bladder neck opening was Hutch's 'base plate' theory [44] (Figure 11.41). This was based on the importance of the trigonal musculature and of certain bands of detrusor smooth muscle that acted to trip open the base plate of the bladder neck, but the presence of such layers and bands has never been demonstrated convincingly by anybody else and so this theory, too, has been discounted.

There is the simple hydrokinetic observation that there is only actually one way out of the bladder and that is through the bladder neck, so that when the detrusor contracts the force is likely to be transmitted in that direction (Figure 11.42). It may well be that this simplistic point of view is at least in part correct, perhaps in conjunction with the reciprocal relaxation theory modified to incorporate the action of nitric oxide rather than the sympathetic nervous system. In addition, it should be noted that it has been observed in spinal cord-injured patients fitted with a sacral anterior root stimulator that the bladder neck can be made to open and close separately from events in the main body of the detrusor, indicating that there may be a separate innervation to the bladder neck (Giles Brindley, personal communication). Clearly, as it can only be demonstrated in this way and then only under certain circumstances and in some patients, this innervation cannot readily be dissected out from innervation of the bladder as a whole, but again it would tend to support the reciprocal innervation theory, with the co-release of nitric oxide in the sphincter-active area to

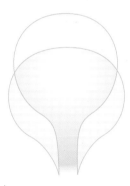

Figure 11.40 *Diagrammatic representation of Lapides' theory of bladder neck opening.*

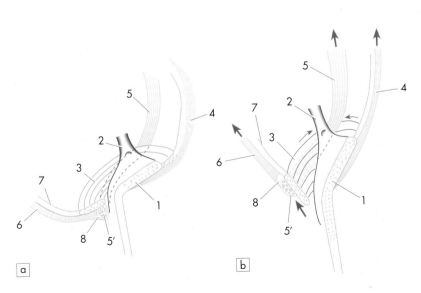

a

b

Figure 11.41(a, b) *Diagrammatic representation of Hutch's theory of bladder neck opening. Figures refer to hypothetical muscle bundles identified by Hutch. (Modified from Hutch JA. Anatomy and physiology of the bladder, trigone and urethra. London: Butterworths, 1972.)*

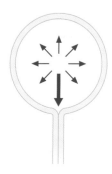

Figure 11.42 *A simple hydrokinetic explanation of bladder neck opening.*

explain opening coincident with cholinergic-mediated detrusor contraction.

Vesico-urethral reflexes

As many as 12 so-called 'micturition reflexes' have been described, largely following the descriptions by Barrington earlier this century [37] and by Kuru more recently [45]. Some of these are only active in experimental animals subject to various neural ablation procedures and at least one of them is the genital reflex of closing off the bladder neck to ensure antegrade ejaculation. Some have been observed in animals but not in humans. So far in this chapter, reference has been made to four reflexes (Figure 11.43). The first is the afferent impulse routed up to the pons to cause the parasympathetic efferent contraction of the bladder of sufficient amplitude and duration to give complete bladder emptying; and the second is that which causes reciprocal relaxation of the intrinsic rhabdosphincter to allow unobstructed voiding. The third is the local spinal reflex increase in urethral pressure during bladder filling. The fourth reflex is the one that causes sympathetic inhibition of parasympathetic ganglionic transmission in the pelvic plexuses with more advanced degrees of bladder filling.

There is, therefore, one local sacral reflex causing a rise in urethral pressure during filling, and one thoracolumbar reflex causing sympathetic inhibition of ganglionic transmission in the parasympathetic innervation to the bladder, thereby supporting de Groat's gating mechanism that keeps the bladder quiescent during filling. Then, there are the two pontine reflexes,

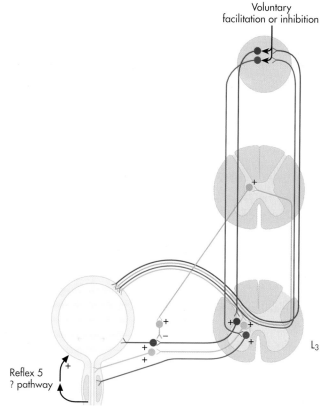

Figure 11.43 *Diagram to show the bladder reflexes described in this chapter. Reflex 1 (—); Reflex 2 (—); Reflex 3 (—); Reflex 4 (—). (Modified from Mundy AR, Thomas PJ. Clinical physiology of the bladder, urethra and pelvic floor. In: Mundy AR, Stephenson TP, Wein AJ (eds). Urodynamics, principles, practice and application. 2nd edition. Edinburgh: Churchill Livingstone, 1994.)*

the one to cause a bladder contraction of adequate amplitude and duration and the second to co-ordinate this with reciprocal relaxation of the intrinsic rhabdosphincter.

In addition, there is a reflex facilitation that occurs during a detrusor contraction that is mediated by afference in the pudendal nerve. The mechanism for this is unclear, but Brindley has noted that after pudendal blockade, the force of detrusor contraction is considerably reduced [46], hence the afferent pathway can be identified as pudendal but the rest of the reflex is unclear.

This is not to say that other reflexes do not exist and particularly that other reflexes do not exist in disease, but these are the only ones that can be positively identified as being important in health.

Summary

It will be apparent to the reader that there is a great deal to be learnt about the structure and even more about the function of the lower urinary tract, particularly about the spinal and supraspinal mechanisms that control it.

The fundamental features are that during bladder filling, intravesical pressure changes very little despite the bladder filling by 400 ml or more, and this 'compliance' is achieved by a 'gating' mechanism that prevents afferent neuronal activity being transmitted to postganglionic efferent activity until that afferent activity reaches a critical level. Critical afferent activity is transmitted by ascending spinal pathways that synapse on cell bodies in the nucleus locus coeruleus in the rostral pons in addition to providing conscious awareness of bladder filling. When afferent activity to the nucleus locus coeruleus, subject to suprapontine facilitation or inhibition, reaches a threshold level, efferent activity is initiated, mediated through the pelvic parasympathetic nerves and muscarinic receptors. This causes a detrusor contraction of sufficient amplitude and duration to give complete bladder emptying and a synchronous co-ordinated reciprocal relaxation of the urethral sphincter mechanism to allow unobstructed voiding until the bladder is empty. It seems clear that excitatory neurotransmission in the normal human detrusor is exclusively cholinergic, and it is becoming increasingly clear that reciprocal relaxation of the urethral sphincter is a prerequisite for detrusor contraction, and that the synchronous relaxation of the bladder neck and urethral smooth muscle is probably mediated by nitric oxide, which is co-transmitted with acetylcholine from postganglionic parasympathetic neurons. Unfortunately, although this fundamental mechanism appears reasonably clear, a lot of the details are lacking at present.

References

1. Uhlenhuth E, Hunter DT, Loechel WE. Problems in the anatomy of the pelvis. Philadelphia: Lippincott, 1953
2. Zacharin RF. The anatomical supports of the female urethra. Obstet Gynaecol 1968; 32: 754–9
3. Walsh PC. Radical retropubic prostatectomy. In: Walsh PC, Gittes RF, Perlmutter AD, Stamey TA (eds) Campbell's urology. 5th ed. Philadelphia: WB Saunders, 1986: 2769–71
4. Redman JF. Anatomy of the genitourinary system. In: Gillenwater JR, Grayhack JT, Howards SS, Duckett JN (eds) Adult and pediatric urology. 3rd ed. Philadelphia: Mosby, 1996, pp. 3–61
5. Kaye KW, Milne N, Creed K, Van-der-Werf B. The urogenital diaphragm external urethral sphincter and radical prostatectomy. Austr NZ J Surg 1997; 67: 40–4
6. Hutch JA. Anatomy and physiology of the bladder, trigone and urethra. London: Butterworths, 1972
7. Gosling J. The structure of the bladder and urethra in relation to function. Urol Clin N Am 1979; 6: 31–8
8. Dixon J, Gosling J. Structure and innervation in the human. In: Torrens M, Morrison FB (eds) The physiology of the lower urinary tract. London: Springer Verlag, 1987. pp. 3–22
9. Raz S, Caine M, Zeigler M. The vascular component in the production of intraurethral pressure. J Urol 1972; 108: 93–6
10. Sundin T, Dahlstrom A, Norlen L, Svedmyr N. The sympathetic innervation and adrenoreceptor function of the human lower urinary tract in the normal state and after parasympathetic denervation. Invest Urol 1977; 14: 322–8
11. Chilton CP. The urethra. In: Webster G, Kirby R, King L, Goldwasser B (eds) Reconstructive urology. Cambridge, MA: Blackwell Scientific Publications, 1993: 59–73
12. Tanagho EA. The anatomy and physiology of micturition. Clin Obstet Gynaecol 1978; 5: 3–26
13. James MJ. Relaxation of the human detrusor. University of Nottingham, MD Thesis, 1993
14. Bridgewater M, MacNeil HF, Brading AF. Regulation of tone in pig urethral smooth muscle. J Urol 1993; 150: 223–8
15. Gosling JA, Dixon JS, Critchely HOD, Thompson SA. A comparative study of the human external sphincter and periurethral levator ani muscles. Br J Urol 1981; 53: 35–41
16. Schroder HD. Onuf's nucleus X: a morphological study of a human spinal nucleus. Anat Embryol 1981; 162: 443–53
17. Zrara P, Carrier S, Kour NW, Tanagho EA. The detailed neuroanatomy of the human striated urethral sphincter. Br J Urol 1994; 74: 182–7

18. Mundy AR. An anatomical explanation for bladder dysfunction following rectal and uterine surgery. Br J Urol 1982; 54: 501–4

19. Burnstock G. Autonomic innervation and transmission. Br Med Bull 1979; 35: 255–62

20. Burnstock G. The changing face of autonomic transmission. Acta Phsysiol Scand 1986; 126: 67–91

21. Brading AF. Physiology of the urinary tract smooth muscle. In: Webster G, Kirby R, King L, Goldwasser B, (eds) Reconstructive urology. Cambridge, MA: Blackwell Scientific Publications, 1993: 15–26

22. Brindley GS, Craggs MD. The effect of atropine in the urinary bladder of the baboon and of man. J Physiol 1975; 255: 55P

23. Kinder RB, Mundy AR. Atropine blockade of nerve-mediated stimulation of the human detrusor. Br J Urol 1985; 57: 418–21

24. Sibley GA. An experimental model of detrusor instability in the obstructed pig. Br J Urol 1985; 57: 292–8

25. Iacovou JW, Hill SJ, Birmingham TA. Agonist-induced contraction and accumulation of inositol phosphates in the guinea pig detrusor: evidence that the muscarinic and purinergic receptors raise intracellular calcium by different mechanisms. J Urol 1990; 144: 775–9

26. McConnell JD. Activation of smooth muscle contractile elements. Neurourol Urodyn 1990; 9: 303–6

27. Wall SJ, Vasuda RP, Li M, Wolfe BB. Development of an antiserum agonist in 3 muscarinic receptors: distribution of M3 receptors in rat tissues and clonal cell lines. Mol Pharmacol 1991; 40: 783–9

28. Egen RM, Whiting RL. Muscarinic receptor subtypes: a critique of the current classification and a proposal for a working nomenclature. J Autonom Pharmacol 1986; 6: 323–44

29. Alm P, Alumets J, Brodin E, et al. Peptidergic (substance P) nerves in the genito-urinary tract. Neurosci 1978; 3: 419–25

30. Maggi C, Barbanti G, Santicoli P, et al. Cystometric evidence that Capsaicin-sensitive nerves modulate the afferent branch of the micturition reflex in humans. J Urol 1989; 142: 150–4

31. Gu J, Restorick J, Blank M, et al. Vasoactive intestinal polypeptide in the normal and unstable bladder. B J Urol 1983; 55: 645–7

32. Alm P, Alumets J, Hakenson R, Sundler F. Peptidergic (vasoactive intestinal peptide) nerves in the genito-urinary tract. Neurosci 1977; 2: 751–4

33. Nathan PW. Sensations associated with micturition. Br J Urol 1956; 28: 126–31

34. Nathan PW. The central nervous connections of bladder. In: Chisholm GD, Williams DI (eds) Scientific foundation of urology. London: Heinemann, 1976

35. MacMahon SB, Morrison JFB. Spinal neurones with long projections activated from the abdominal viscera of the cat. J Physiol 1982; 332: 1–20

36. Sillen U. Central neurotransmitter mechanisms involved in the control of urinary bladder function. Scand J Urol Nephrol 1980; Supplement 58.

37. Barrington FJF. The effect of lesions on the hind and midbrain on micturition in the cat. Q J Exp Physiol 1915; 15: 181–202

38. Hess WR. The functional organisation of the diencephalon. London: Grune & Stratton, 1957

39. Andrew J, Nathan PW. Lesions of the anterior frontal lobes and disturbances of micturition and defecation. Brain 1964; 87: 233–61

40. Tang PC, Ruch TC. Non-neurogenic basis of bladder tonus. Am J Physiol 1955; 181: 249–57

41. De Groat WC. Physiology of the urinary bladder and urethra. Ann Int Med 1980; 92: 312–15

42. Denny-Brown D, Robertson EG. On the physiology of micturition. J Physiol 1933; 56: 149–90

43. Lapides J. Structure and function of the internal vesical sphincter. J Urol 1958; 80: 341–53

44. Hutch J. A new theory of the anatomy of the internal urinary sphincter and the physiology of micturition. Invest Urol 1965; 3: 36–58

45. Kuru M. Nervous control of micturition. Physiol Rev 1965; 45: 425–94

46. Brindley GS, Craggs MD. The pressure exerted by the external sphincter of the urethra when its motor nerve fibres are stimulated electrically. Br J Urol 1974; 46: 453–62

J. P. Pryor

Normal male sexual function is considered to be essential for good health and it is important to remember that psychological factors impinge upon all elements of it. This chapter concentrates on erectile function and fertility but commences with discussion of the hormone testosterone, which is of paramount importance with regard to male sexual function.

Testosterone metabolism

The Y chromosome (Figure 12.1) determines that an embryo will develop into a male and is essential for normal sexual function. It contains fewer genes than other chromosomes but it is important for male sexual function as it has the sex (or testis) determining gene (SRY) [1] which controls gender by triggering the formation of a testis in the male embryo, and the azoospermic factor (AZF) group of genes [2], which are associated with spermatogenesis.

The cells in the primitive genital ridge differentiate in the presence of the SRY gene during the seventh week of fetal life into Leydig and Sertoli cells (Figure 12.2). The Leydig cells produce testosterone, initially under the influence of maternal chorionic gonadotrophin and then pituitary gonadotrophins. This causes mesonephric (Wolffian) duct differentiation to become the seminal vesicles, vasa deferentia and the body and tail of the epididymes. Testosterone, in the presence of intracellular 5α-reductase, is converted into dihydrotestosterone in the genital sinus and accounts for external virilisation of the penis and scrotum. The Sertoli cells produce a glycoprotein, Müllerian inhibiting factor, which causes regression of the paramesonephric (Müllerian) ducts and also stimulates the first phase of testicular descent. Müllerian inhibiting factor may now be measured and has clinical implications [3]. The second stage is androgen dependent and additional roles are played by the genitofemoral nerve and calcitonin-related peptide. An

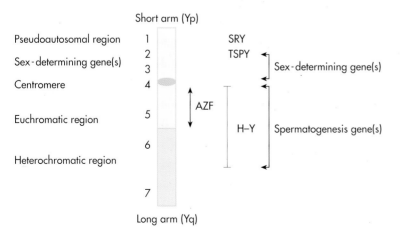

Figure 12.1 *The Y chromosome is critical for the normal male sexual determination.*

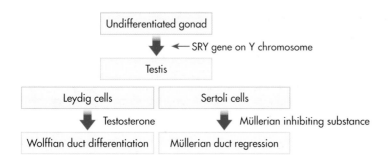

Figure 12.2 Male genital development in the fetus.

understanding of these factors helps to explain abnormalities of gender and testicular maldescent [4].

Testosterone is the most important circulating androgen in men and is bound to sex hormone-binding globulin and albumin. The latter binds to all steroids with low affinity, whereas the former is a glycoprotein, synthesised in the liver, and with a high affinity but low capacity for testosterone. In men, 60% of the circulating testosterone is bound to sex hormone-binding globulin, 38% to albumin and the remaining 2% is free. Free and albumin-bound testosterone constitute the bioavailable functions of circulating testosterone, but some sex hormone-binding globulin-bound testosterone may be found in the prostate and testes.

The biosynthesis of testosterone (Figure 12.3) takes place in the Leydig cells. Steroidogenesis is stimulated through a cyclic adenosine monophosphate (cAMP)/ protein kinase C mechanism, which mobilises cholesterol substrate and promotes the conversion of cholesterol through pregnanilone, dihydroepiandrosterone, androstenedione to testosterone. Testosterone is converted to dihydrotestosterone by 5α-reductase within the target organ.

Hypothalamic–pituitary–testicular axis

Anterior pituitary gonadotrophin secretion is controlled by hypothalamic gonadotrophin-releasing hormone released into the pituitary portal circulation by axon terminals in the median eminence of the hypothalamus. These neurosecretory neurons are responsive to a wide variety of sensory inputs as well as to gonadal negative feedback. Gonadotrophin-releasing hormone stimulates both luteinising hormone and follicle-stimulating hormone secretion from the anterior pituitary gland. These hormones consist of about 115 amino acids, have a molecular weight of

about 30 000 Da and are produced by the gonadotrophic cells of the adenohypophysis. There is still some debate as to whether there are one or two releasing hormones for follicle-stimulating hormone and luteinising hormone. The gonadotrophin-releasing hormone precursor gene has been identified and mapped to the chromosome 8p [5]. In the adult male, this hormone is released episodically into the pituitary portal circulation at a frequency of about every 140 minutes; each volley of gonadotrophin-releasing hormone elicits an immediate release of luteinising hormone, producing the typical pulsatile pattern of luteinising hormone in the systemic circulation [6]. Though also secreted episodically, follicle-stimulating hormone and testosterone pulses are not apparent in normal men because of the slower secretion of newly synthesised rather than stored hormone, and the longer circulating half-lives. The intermittent mode of gonadotrophin-releasing hormone stimulation within a narrow physiological range of frequency is obliga-

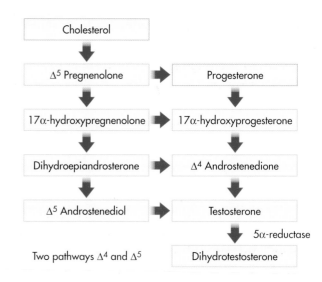

Figure 12.3 The metabolic pathway for androgen production.

tory for sustaining the normal pattern of gonado-trophin secretion. Continuous or high-frequency gonadotrophin-releasing hormone stimulation para-doxically desensitises the pituitary gonadotro-phin response because of depletion of receptors and refractoriness of postreceptor response mechanisms.

Testosterone exerts the major negative feedback action on gonadotrophin secretion. Its effect is predominantly to restrict the frequency of gonado-trophin-releasing hormone pulses from the hypothal-amus to within the physiological range. Testosterone also acts on the pituitary to reduce the amplitude of luteinising hormone response to gonadotrophin-releasing hormone; this may require the local conver-sion of testosterone to oestradiol in the pituitary. These inhibitory actions are best seen in agonadal or castrated males in whom high-frequency and high-amplitude luteinising hormone pulsatile secretion prevails. Feedback inhibition of pituitary follicle-stimulating hormone synthesis is also affected by testosterone, particularly at high concentrations, as well as the recently purified glycoprotein Sertoli cell product, inhibin [7]. It is believed that tubular damage associated with Sertoli cell dysfunction and a conse-quently reduced capacity for inhibin secretion is the cause for the follicle-stimulating hormone rise, with normal luteinising hormone, commonly found in infertile men.

Testosterone levels vary throughout life. There is a relatively high level in late fetal life, which falls to a very low level throughout childhood. Puberty is asso-ciated with a surge in testosterone production that remains high until late adult life. The fall in testos-terone levels after the age of 55 is not sudden but the mean plasma testosterone level in healthy men falls by about 0.17 nmol/annum [8]. The fall may be more in men with intercurrent disease or adverse social circumstances.

The action of androgens

Androgens are essential for normal male sexual differ-entiation and function, and a deficiency results in a failure of sexual development (see Chapter 23), delayed or absent puberty, and other clinical syndromes (Table 12.1). In men, there is no sudden fall in androgen secretion to cause a male menopause. The decline in

Table 12.1 Testosterone deficiency

Primary (hypergonadotrophic hypogonadism)

Congenital testicular agenesis
   Klinefelter's syndrome
   Sterogenic enzyme defects
   Testicular maldescent
Acquired
   Bilateral orchidectomy
   Bilateral torsion testis
   Bilateral orchitis
   Radiotherapy/chemotherapy

Secondary (hypogonadotrophic hypogonadism)

Congenital
   Idiopathic (e.g. Kallmann's syndrome)
   Fertile eunuch
Acquired
   Pituitary lesions:
      trauma
      surgery
      tumour (N.B.: hyperprolactinaemia)
      haemochromatosis

testosterone levels may be associated with partial androgen deficiency in the ageing male, but the mental changes occurring in the mid-fifties are likely to be the result of social stresses rather than of hormonal deficiency [8]. Androgen replacement may be with testosterone patches applied to the skin daily, or oral medication, a two-weekly to three-weekly injection of testosterone esters (Sustenon) or the implantation of a testosterone pellet (six monthly).

Erection

The key to understanding erection and erectile dys-function is to realise that they are dependent upon the relaxation of cavernous smooth muscle. Cyclic guanosine monophosphate (cGMP) and cAMP are the second messengers for the development of cavernous smooth muscle relaxation and they are both inacti-vated by phosphodiesterases. Inhibition of the phosphodiesterase would therefore enhance the action of cAMP and cGMP. During relaxation of the smooth muscle cell, there is a net loss of calcium ions.

Nitric oxide is the key substance causing smooth muscle relaxation [9, 10]. It is synthesised from L-arginine and oxygen in a reaction under the control of nitric oxide synthase. It stimulates activity of the enzyme guanylate cyclase to increase the conversion of guanosine triphosphate (GTP) to cGMP, which in turn causes the relaxation of the smooth muscle. The release of nitric oxide has been shown to follow nerve stimulation to cause the relaxation of smooth muscle, and the relaxation of smooth muscle can be blocked by substances binding nitric oxide or blocking guanylate cyclase activity. Nitric oxide is also released from the endothelium lining the trabecular smooth muscle spaces. The stimulation for this might be the increase in blood flow at the start of erection and the sheer forces resulting from this.

In erectile dysfunction, there is evidence to suggest that both neuronal release of nitric oxide and the smooth muscle responsiveness to nitric oxide may be impaired. The ability of smooth muscle to relax is also impaired in hyperprolactinaemia and androgen deficiency. The latter may account for the decline in rigidity and increased incidence of erectile dysfunction associated with ageing.

It is the action of drugs on the cavernous smooth muscle (Figure 12.4) that has led to our understanding of the physiology of erection. Papaverine acts by inhibiting the action of phosphodiesterases and this prolongs the effectiveness of cAMP and cGMP. A similar mode of action occurs with sildenafil [11, 12], but this drug has the advantage of being active when taken orally. Alprostadil (synthetic prostaglandin E1) acts by stimulating the production of adenylate cyclase, which causes increased conversion of adenosine triphosphate (ATP) to cAMP [13, 14]. A fuller review of the pharmacology of smooth muscle may be found elsewhere [15] and a classification of therapeutic options is given in Table 12.2 [16].

Table 12.2 Classification of treatments for erectile dysfunction[1]

Central initiator	Apomorphine
Peripheral initiator	Papaverine Prostaglandin E1
Central conditioner	Trazadone Testosterone Yohimbine?
Peripheral conditioner	Testosterone Sildenafil
Miscellaneous	Vacuum devices Penile revascularisation Veno-occlusive dysfunction Penile prosthesis

[1] See Heaton et al. [16]

Neurological control of erection

In 1863, Eckhard demonstrated in the dog that stimulation of the parasympathetic nervi erigentes would induce a penile erection, but it was another 75 years before it was shown that stimulation of the sympathetic nerves causes shrinkage of the penis. Erection and flaccidity are under the control of the autonomic nervous system and this includes the non-adrenergic non-cholinergic neural mechanisms.

Afferent impulses from the genitalia via the dorsal penile nerves pass through the pudendal nerves to the dorsal roots of S2, S3 and S4 of the spinal cord. Information is transmitted upwards through the spinal thalamic tracts to the thalamus and sensory cortex. Other afferent impulses (visual, auditory, olfactory and tactile) may also serve to initiate erectile activity.

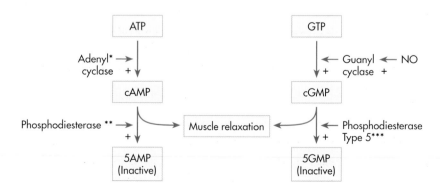

Figure 12.4 *The action of drugs to cause relaxation of penile smooth muscle in penile erection. * PGE1 and vaso-active intestinal polypeptide (VIP) stimulate; ** papaverine inhibits; *** sildenafil inhibits.*

It has been customary to differentiate between reflexogenic erections (arising from genital sensation) and psychogenic erections but such a division serves little purpose. It does, however, serve to emphasise that following spinal cord injuries higher than T9, erections are the result of a local reflex arc, and that with lower lesions, erections may occur as a result of efferent impulses through the thoracic sympathetic outflows. There is some evidence to suggest that sympathetic stimulation that is normally considered to cause smooth muscle contraction and flaccidity may in some circumstances be associated with erectile activity [17].

The central co-ordinating centre for erectile activity is considered to be the medial pre-optic area, which is contiguous with the hypothalamus. Efferent impulses pass via the medial forebrain bundle to the spinal cord, with sympathetic outflow through segments T11 to L4. These fibres constitute the pre-aortic plexus, which passes via the superior and inferior hypogastric plexuses to the pelvic plexus and thence to the genital organs. The parasympathetic fibres pass in the intermediate lateral bundle and outflow through sacral segments 2, 3 and 4 in preganglionic pelvic nerves (nervi eregentes) to the pelvic plexus and thence to the erectile tissue through the cavernous nerves.

The importance of oxytocin neurons in the hypothalamus remains uncertain, but stimulation of these neurons may provoke erections. The initial experiments with apomorphine – a dopamine agonist – found it to be erectogenic, and further research has found means of avoiding the side-effects of yawning and vomiting from the drug [18].

Peripheral nerve mechanisms and neurotransmitters

The autonomic nervous system consists of cholinergic (parasympathetic) and adrenergic (sympathetic) nervous systems. Recently, the presence of non-adrenergic non-cholinergic fibres has been identified with numerous other neuropeptide transmitters. Vasoactive intestinal polypeptide is the most important of these and it is co-localised with neuronal nitric oxide synthase in cavernosal nerves and pelvic ganglia. The precise role of vasoactive intestinal polypeptide and other peptides such as neuropeptide Y and calcitonin

gene-related peptide remains unclear, but they may serve to modulate erection and flaccidity [10]. The control of cavernous smooth muscle demands the integration of external nerve impulses with an internal signalling mechanism between muscle cells [19].

It has also been suggested that variations in oxygen tension in the corpus cavernosus play an active role in regulating penile erection through the release of nitric oxide. The oxygen tension in the cavernous tissue is low during penile flaccidity and nitric oxide synthesis is inhibited. The oxygen tension rises during erection with the inflow of blood, and nitric oxide synthesis is stimulated and muscle relaxation is facilitated [20].

Haemodynamics of erection

During erection, the penis enlarges and becomes hard. The vascular changes may be divided into different phases, five of which were described by Lue [21].

Latent phase

The start of an erection is preceded by relaxation of arterial and cavernous smooth muscle. This leads to a fall in vascular resistance, with a resulting rapid inflow of blood into the cavernous spaces. For a short period there is no increase, or even a slight fall, in the intracorporeal pressure. This period of isometric filling of the sinusoidal spaces is associated with the highest flow rate of the whole erectile process and may be more than double the resting value. During this phase there is only slight elongation and fullness of the penis.

Tumescence phase

As the inflow of blood continues, it becomes associated with increasing cavernous pressure. When the intracavernous pressure rises above diastolic pressure, flow occurs only during systole. This phase is characterised by rapid expansion and elongation of the penis to its full size. The duration of this phase is age dependent and is influenced by the strength of stimulation.

Full erection phase

The continued inflow of blood, and distension of the sinusoidal spaces, compresses the subtunical plexus against the non-compliant tunica albuginea. This impedes the outflow of blood through the emissary veins [22], and the intracavernous pressure rises further. A stage of full erection is reached when the intracorporeal pressure equals mean systolic pressure. The pressure remains steady during this phase, indicating that the rate of arterial inflow is lower than during the tumescence phase and equals the venous outflow.

Rigid erection phase

Penile rigidity is achieved by contraction of the ischiocavernosus smooth muscles and this raises the intracavernous pressure to well above systolic blood pressure [23]. There is no flow in the cavernosus artery at this stage and, at the same time, there is further obstruction of the venous channels and flow in them also approaches zero. Consequently, for a short period of a few minutes, the corpora cavernosa become functionally dead spaces with hardly any inflow or outflow. This phase occurs naturally during sexual intercourse or masturbation and its duration is limited by muscle fatigue, which obviates the risk of tissue ischaemia.

Detumescence phase

This commences with the relaxation of the ischiocavernosus muscles, but detumescence is also an active process due to the contraction of the cavernosal smooth muscle under sympathetic nervous stimulation. This contraction expels blood from the sinusoidal spaces and it is accompanied by arterial vasoconstriction to reduce the inflow to the resting level. The penis becomes smaller and shorter and eventually flaccid.

The changes described above all take place in the corpora cavernosa, but similar changes take place in the corpus spongiosus, including the glans penis. However, the pressure rise is not so great as there is no limiting investing layer of tunica albuginea. Furthermore, the venous outflow into the deep dorsal vein is unimpeded. There is a valvular mechanism in these veins [24, 25] and it may be that these are regulated by non-adrenergic mechanisms – possibly neuropeptide Y [26]. There is some compression of the deep dorsal vein between the overlying stretched skin and the expanded corpora during full erection. This raises pressure in the glans and increases its engorgement and fullness. There is a further increase in venous resistance with contraction of the ischiocavernosus and bulbocavernosus muscles during the rigid phase of erection.

Physiological changes in erection associated with ageing

Specific age-related changes are difficult to quantify as any changes may be the result of intercurrent pathology. It would seem that older men find it more difficult to initiate and sustain an erection. Physical stimulation may be required and any distraction may lead to a loss of erection. The erection is less rigid and, following ejaculation, there is a longer period before it is possible to obtain another erection.

Fertility

Male fertility depends upon the satisfactory integration of a series of physiological events starting with sperm production and ending with fertilisation of the oocytes (Table 12.3) This process may be interrupted voluntarily, by pathological changes, or by adverse factors in the female partner. The essence of fertility management is to establish a prognosis, or the chance of the partner conceiving in a given period of time, and in order to make such a prognosis it is necessary to have a sound understanding of the pathophysiology of infertility.

During childhood, the testes are small and the seminiferous tubules are solid, cord-like structures containing primitive spermatocytes and Sertoli cells. The seminiferous tubules gradually acquire a lumen as the spermatocytes differentiate after the age of six years. Testicular and penile sizes increase greatly at puberty, driven by hormonal changes, with an increase in plasma levels of both luteinising hormone and follicle-stimulating hormone. The hormonal control of the testes has already been mentioned in the control of testosterone secretion. Testosterone is essential for spermatogenesis but the control of spermatogenesis is by follicle-stimulating hormone, which acts through the Sertoli cells to stimulate the germ cells to manufacture sperm. Inhibin is a protein, not a steroid, produced by the Sertoli cells once spermatogenesis

Table 12.3 Sequence of events leading to fertilisation

Event	Test (assay)	
Spermatogenesis	Testis biopsy	Semen analysis
Acquisition of motility	Semen analysis	CASA
Migration through female tract	Penetration tests	
Capacitation		
Hyperactive motility	CASA	HOPT
Membrane integrity	HSA	
Zona pellucida binding	HZA	
Acrosome reaction	HZA	HOPT
Zona pellucida penetration	HZA	HOPT
Sperm head decondensation		HOPT
Fusion with oocyte DNA		

CASA, computer analysis of sperm number and quality test; HOPT, heterologous oocyte penetration test; HSA, hypo-osmotic swelling assay; HZA, hemizoma assay.

proceeds to the spermatocyte stage and is the feedback mechanism to regulate follicle-stimulating hormone production.

Spermatogenesis is a complex process of cellular changes that are divided into three groups. The spermatogenic cycle in the testis is about 16 days in duration, but the total time from the commencement of spermatogenesis to the expulsion of spermatozoa in the semen is approximately 72 days. In the first phase of spermatogenesis, the spermatogonia undergo cell division to produce type-A spermatogonia, which in turn produce intermediate and then type-B spermatogonia. Recognition of these spermatogonia is difficult with ordinary light microscopy. In the second phase of spermatogenesis, the spermatogonia divide to produce spermatocytes, which undergo division with halving of the number of chromosomes. The secondary spermatocytes divide in the final stage of spermatogenesis to produce spermatids and then spermatozoa. During spermiogenesis (the third stage), the rounded spermatocytes become elongated and recognisable as sperm, with an acrosomal cap, a midpiece and a tail. The Sertoli, or supporting, cells serve to capture hormones that nourish the germ cells. Sertoli cells rest on the basement membrane of the seminiferous tubules and have multiple cytoplasmic extensions into the lumen of the tubules between the germinal cells. The contents of the seminiferous tubules are outside the body and special tight cell junctions exist adjacent to the Sertoli cells. These junctions allow passage of fluid into the seminiferous tubules. The Sertoli cell is thought to contribute to the blood–testis barrier.

Spermatogenesis is usually assessed by histological examination of a small portion of the testis using a fixative that does not cause shrinkage of the seminiferous tubules. Bouin's solution is favoured in many centres, and the tissues are sliced and stained according to preference. The histological findings should be described and there is some merit in using a semiquantitative technique such as that described by Johnsen [27].

Hormonal control of spermatogenesis

The hormonal control of spermatogenesis requires the actions of pituitary gonadotrophins luteinising hormone and follicle-stimulating hormone (Figure 12.5). There is general agreement that both these hormones are needed for the initiation of spermatogenesis during puberty. However, the specific role and relative contribution of the two gonadotrophins in maintaining spermatogenesis are unclear [28]. Luteinising hormone stimulates Leydig cell steroidogenesis, resulting in increased production of testosterone. Normal spermatogenesis is absolutely dependent on testosterone but its mode of action and the amount required remain uncertain. Specific androgen receptors have not been demonstrated in germs cells but are present in Sertoli and peritubular cells. This implies that the actions of androgens on spermatogenesis

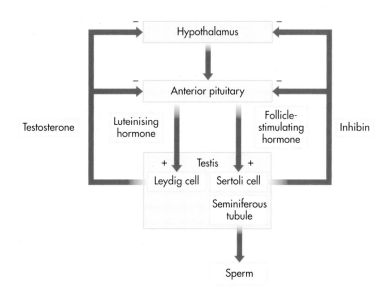

Figure 12.5 *Hormonal regulation of testicular function.*

must be mediated by somatic cells in the seminiferous tubules. The concentration of testosterone in the testis is 50 times higher than that in the peripheral circulation. There is thus a gross over-abundance of testosterone within the normal adult testis and any T-related abnormalities must be due to defects in steroid utilisation rather than supply. Follicle-stimulating hormone initiates function in immature Sertoli cells prior to the onset of spermatogenesis by stimulating the formation of the blood–testis barrier, secretion of tubular fluid and other specific secretory products via follicle-stimulating hormone receptors that activate intracellular cAMP. Once spermatogenesis is established in the adult testis, Sertoli cells become less responsive to follicle-stimulating hormone. It is uncertain whether follicle-stimulating hormone maintains spermatogenesis by increasing spermatogonial mitosis or by decreasing the number of cells that degenerate at each cell division. Testosterone is essential for the subsequent stages from meiosis to spermiogenesis.

Spermatozoa

Spermatozoa have a dense oval head with an acrosomal cap, a midpiece and a tail. These highly specialised structural features reflect the unique functional activities of the spermatozoon. The acrosome contains enzymes essential for fertilisation, the tail contains the mechanism for motility, and these combine to deliver the paternal contribution of genetic information in the nucleus to the egg to initiate the development of a new individual. The head is made up largely of highly condensed nuclear chromatin, constituting the haploid chromosome complement, and it is covered on its anterior half by a membrane-enclosed sac of enzymes, the acrosome. The area of the sperm head immediately behind the acrosome is important as it is this part that attaches and fuses with the egg. The motor apparatus of the tail is the axoneme, which consists of a central pair (doublets) of microtubules of non-contractile tubulin protein enclosed in a sheath linked radially to nine outer pairs of microtubules. Each doublet is also joined by nexin bridges to its neighbour via two ATPase-rich dynein protein arms. Lack of these dynein arms is associated with Kartagener's syndrome of bronchiectasis, sinusitis and situs inversus. Energy for sperm motility is provided by the sheath of mitochondria in the midpiece of the tail through a second messenger system involving the calcium-mediated calmodulin-dependent conversion of ATP to cAMP and interaction with the ATPase of the dynein.

Disorders of spermatogenesis

Impaired spermatogenesis may occur for a variety of reasons. Patients with primary testicular failure usually have elevated levels of plasma follicle-stimulating hormone and small testes. Secondary testicular failure is usually characterised by low or sometimes normal levels of follicle-stimulating hormone due to hormonal abnormalities.

Primary testicular failure (hypergonadotrophic hypogonadism)

This condition is characterised by small testes, impaired spermatogenesis and elevated levels of follicle-stimulating hormone which may or may not be accompanied by androgen deficiency [29].

Genetic abnormalities

Chandley [30] found the overall incidence of chromosome abnormalities to be 2.2% in 2372 men attending an infertility clinic, but it rose to 15.4% of those men with azoospermia. The most common abnormality was Klinefelter's syndrome (XXY), which accounted for nearly half of the abnormalities. More recent studies have related defective spermatogenesis with abnormalities of the gene in the Y chromosome (see Figure 12.1) but some spermatogenesis may still occur even in the absence of the *AZF* gene [31, 32].

Testicular maldescent

Argument persists as to whether the failure of testicular descent is due to an intrinsic defect in the testis or to multiple external factors. There is no good evidence that an intra-abdominal testis will make sperm, and the occurrence of spermatogenesis following bilateral orchidopexy for a truly undescended testis is uncertain. Such testes usually have normal numbers of Leydig cells but atrophy and/or fibrosis of the germinal epithelium. The incidence of carcinoma of the testis is increased in adults with undescended testes [33]. Carcinoma was found in 25% of abdominal testes compared to only 0.5–1% in men having a testicular biopsy as part of their evaluation for subfertility/infertility [34].

Bilateral Sertoli cell-only syndrome

In this condition, seminiferous tubules are lined by Sertoli cells with a complete absence of any spermatogenic epithelium. With the advent of intracytoplasmic sperm injection, it is now realised that even when testicular biopsies show bilateral Sertoli cell only, the patient may have foci of spermatogenesis and even have sperm in the ejaculate [35].

Acquired testicular failure

Anoxia, due to testicular torsion or acute epididymo-orchitis, mumps orchitis, radiotherapy or chemother-apy, may damage the testis to a varying extent. The histological appearances vary from focal loss of spermatogenesis, a variable amount of fibrosis or even the appearances of Sertoli cell-only syndrome.

Secondary testicular failure (hypogonadotrophic hypogonadism)

In this condition, the defect is due to a deficiency of hypothalamic-releasing or pituitary hormones. The latter may be part of an overall pituitary deficiency, a loss of both gonadotrophic hormones, a loss of luteinising hormone (fertile eunuch syndrome), an isolated deficiency of follicle-stimulating hormone or due to excessive production of prolactin.

Recognition of hypogonadotrophic hypogonadism is important as it is the sole cause of azoospermia that is amenable to hormonal treatment.

Sperm maturation

Spermatozoa are functionally immature and immotile when they pass from the testis into the caput epididymis and the maturation process continues as they pass through the epididymis. The epididymis [36] is under adrenergic and androgen control and the epithelium actively reabsorbs testicular fluid and also secretes a hyperosmolar fluid rich in glycerophosphorylocholine, inositol and carnitine. The specific transport of these compounds across the epithelium creates a favourable fluid environment whereby progressive motility and fertilising capacity of the spermatozoa are normally acquired. Thus, the cytoplasmic droplets decrease in size and move distally along the midpiece, the acrosome membrane swells, the epididymal glycoproteins are incorporated into the plasma membrane, S–S bonds are formed in the sperm tail cytoskeleton, and cAMP content increases. The normal site of sperm storage is in the cauda epididymis, and spermatozoa are only found in the seminal vesicles in ejaculatory duct obstruction [37].

Ejaculation

The processes of orgasm and ejaculation are closely associated and usually occur synchronously when sexual activity is associated with a sufficient degree of stimulation. Orgasm is dependent on intact pudendal nerves through which the pelvic floor ischiocavernosus and bulbocavernosus muscles are stimulated to contract rhythmically. This is associated with emotional changes and with the emission of semen into the prostatic urethra, closure of the bladder neck and propulsion of the semen out of the urethra. The bulk of the ejaculate consists of secretions of the seminal vesicles (65%) and prostate (30%). The seminal vesicle secretions are rich in fructose, prostaglandins and coagulates, whereas the prostatic fluid contains protolytic enzymes that liquefy the coagulated proteins of the ejaculated semen and are rich in citric acid, acid phosphatase and zinc. Men with ejaculatory duct obstruction have a characteristically low-volume (0.3–1.0 ml), acid (pH 6.5) semen with an absence of fructose and spermatozoa. Similar semen abnormalities are also found in men with congenital bilateral vasal aplasia – a condition often found in cystic fibrosis [38].

It is usual to divide ejaculation into three phases. The first phase consists of the emission of seminal fluid into the urethra. This is under sympathetic control and is associated with contraction of the epididymes and vasa and is followed by contraction of the seminal vesicles and subsequently the prostate. The order of ejaculation may be studied using the split ejaculate technique, by cinephotography, or video. In the second phase of ejaculation, the bladder neck is closed to resist retrograde flow into the bladder and there is contraction of the posterior urethra. In the third phase, the external sphincter closes and there is rhythmic contraction of the bulbospongiosus along the urethra. The precise level for the centre controlling ejaculation is uncertain, but it is probably in the hypothalamus. Ejaculation is triggered when the sensory stimuli reach sufficient intensity. The effector mechanism is through the thoracic sympathetic outlets and the sympathetic chains. The preganglionic fibres for the genital system exit via the bifurcation of the aorta to synapses at short adrenergic fibres that terminate in alpha receptors within the smooth muscle cells of the epididymes, vasa and seminal vesicles.

Disorders of ejaculation are discussed elsewhere [39].

Seminal analysis

Seminal analysis is an important element of fertility assessment. Routine seminal analysis should be standardised and performed as recommended by the World Health Organisation [40]. Unfortunately, there is no agreement as to the criteria for normal fertility and a man with 5 million sperm of good progression in an ejaculate is probably fertile. It is important to consider all aspects of the semen test whilst assessing fertility.

Computer analysis of sperm number and quality and other special tests of sperm function (see Table 12.3) are valuable research tools but have no place in routine fertility management. The outcome of in-vitro fertilisation is the best functional assessment of spermatozoa that is currently available.

Fertilisation

At the site of fertilisation, capacitated sperm with intact acrosomes penetrate the cumulus to reach the outer zona. Mechanical shearing forces generated by the characteristic flagellar movements of the capacitated sperm are probably the main mechanism responsible for cumulus penetration. Surface hyaluronidase (possibly escaping from the acrosomal membrane) may facilitate cumulus penetration but is not essential.

Binding of sperm to zona triggers the acrosome reaction, which is an essential step in the fertilisation process because only acrosome-reacted sperm can penetrate the zona pellucida and fuse with the oolemma. During the acrosome reaction, the outer acrosome membrane fuses progressively with the inner plasma membrane at a number of sites and vesiculates, forming exit pores (fenestrations) through which the acrosome enzyme matrix is released.

The proteins contained in semen serve to buffer the acidity of the vaginal secretions. Few, perhaps 200, of the many millions of ejaculated sperm are functionally competent and capable of fertilising oocytes. Only those sperm with good progressive motility are capable of transversing the cervical canal and entering the uterine cavity to reach the middle third of the fallopian tube where fertilisation usually occurs. In the female genital tract, spermatozoa undergo the process of capacitation whereby the protective coating of proteins on the sperm head, which was acquired during passage through the epididymis, is lost. The plasma membrane of the sperm head is destabilised and the sperm movement changes, with vigorous beating of the sperm tail with poor progression and marked undulation of the sperm head. This facilitates the penetration of the cumulus of the egg, which is further aided by surface hyaluronidase of the sperm. Binding of the sperm to the egg triggers the acrosome reaction, which is an essential step in the fertilisation process since only acrosome-reacted sperm can penetrate the zona pellucida and fuse with the oolemma. Defects in the sperm quality and/or fertilising capacity may be overcome by the direct microinjection of a single sperm into each egg. This technique of intracytoplasmic sperm injection has revolutionised infertility management [41].

Infertility

Infertility occurs when a woman fails to conceive after 12 months of unprotected coitus, and the essence of management is to assess and improve the prognosis (the percentage chance of conception within the next 12 months). The age of the woman and the duration of infertility (Table 12.4) are of as much importance in establishing the prognosis as the diagnosis of specific defects in the female and male partners [42]. Some of the male factors have already been discussed, but others are summarised in Table 12.5 [43, 44].

Table 12.4 Percentage chance of spontaneous conception during the subsequent 12 months of couples attending an infertility clinic[1]

Motile sperm concentration (million/ml)	Duration of infertility (years)			
	1	2	4	8
0	0	0	0	0
0.5	16	12	9	6
1	25	19	14	9
2	34	26	19	13
5	36	28	21	14
>10	37	28	21	14

[1] See Hargreave and Elton [42].

Table 12.5 Aetiologies of male infertility

Diagnosis	WHO[1] 1979–1982 (%)	Melbourne[2] 1979–1980 (%)
Unrecognised	48.3	47.9
Idiopathic azoo/oligozoospermia	16.1	
Idiopathic astheno-teratozoospermia	16.8	7.3
Varicocoele	17.2	25
Genital tract infection	4.0	
Sperm autoimmunity	1.6	5
Congenital (crypto-orchidism) chromosomal disorders	2.1	1.9
Genital tract obstruction	1.8	10.8
Systemic/iatrogenic	1.3	1.0
Coital disorders	1.0	0.5
Gonadotrophin deficiency	0.6	0.6

[1] See reference 43.
[2] See reference 44.

References

1. Editorial. The secret of sex? Lancet 1990; 2: 348–9
2. De Kretsner DM, Burger HG. The Y chromosome and spermatogenesis. N Engl J Med 1997; 336: 576–8
3. Forest MG. Serum Müllerian inhibiting substance assay – a new diagnostic test for disorders of gonadal development. N Engl J Med 1997; 336: 1519–21
4. Charnette TD, Sugita Y, Hutson JM. Genital abnormalities in human and animal models reveal the mechanisms and hormones governing testicular descent. Br J Urol 1997; 79: 99–112
5. Hayflick JS, Adelman JP, Seeberg PH. The complete sequence of human gonadotrophin releasing hormone gene. Nucl Acid Res 1989; 17: 6403–4
6. Wu FCW, Taylor PL, Sellar RE. Luteinising hormone releasing hormone pulse frequency in normal and infertile men. J Endocrinol 1989; 123: 149–58
7. McLachlan RI, Robertson DM, de Kretser DM, Burger HG. Inhibin – a non-steroidal regulator of pituitary follicle stimulating hormone. Baillières Clin Endocrinol Metab 1987; 1: 89–112
8. Gooren LJG. The age-related decline of androgen levels in men: clinically significant. Br J Urol 1997; 18: 763–8
9. Andersson K-E, Wagner G. Physiology of penile erections. Physiol Rev 1995; 75: 191–236
10. Pickard R. The role of nitric oxide and other neurotransmitters in erectile function. Curr Opin Urol 1996; 6: 347–51

11. Boolell M, Allen MJ, Ballard DA, *et al.* Sildenafil: an orally active type 5 cyclic GMP-specific phosphodiestene inhibitor for the treatment of penile erectile dysfunction. Int J Impot Res 1996; 8: 47–52

12. Boolell M, Gepi Attee S, Gingell JC, Allen MJ. Sildenafil, a novel effective oral therapy for male erectile dysfunction. Br J Urol 1996; 78: 257–61

13. Lea AP, Bryson HM, Balfour JA. Intracavernous Alprostadil: a review of its pharmacodynamic and phamacokinetic properties and therapeutic potential in erectile dysfunction. Drugs Aging 1996; 8: 56–74

14. Porst H. The rationale for prostaglandin E₁ in erectile failure: a survey of world wide experience. J Urol 1996; 155: 802–15

15. Saenz de Tejada I, Moncada I. Pharmacology of penile smooth muscle. In: Porst H (ed) Penile disorders. Berlin: Springer-Verlag, 1997: 125–43

16. Heaton JPW, Adams MS, Morales A. A therapeutic taxonomy of treatments for erectile dysfunction: an evolutionary imperative. Int J Impot Res 1997; 9: 115–21

17. Brindley GS, Sauerwein D, Hendry WH. Hypogastric stimulation for obtaining semen from paraplegic men. Br J Urol 1989; 64: 72–7

18. Heaton JPW, Morales A, Adams MA, Johnston B. Resolution of erectile failure after oral treatment with apomorphine. Urology 1995; 45: 200–3

19. Christ GJ, Richards S, Winkler A. Integrative erectile biology: the role of signal transduction and cell-to-cell communication in coordinating corporal smooth muscle tone and penile erection. Int J Impot Res 1997; 9: 69–84

20. Kim N, Vardi Y, Padma-Nathan H, Daley J, Goldstein I, Saenz de Tejada I. Oxygen tension regulates the nitric oxide pathway. Physiological role in penile erection. J Clin Invest 1993; 91: 3006–12

21. Lue TF. Mechanism of penile erection in the monkey. Semin Urol 1986; 4: 217–24

22. Wespes E, Schulman CC. Study of human penile venous system and hypothesis on its behaviour during erection. Urology 1990; 36: 68–72

23. Lavoisier P, Courtois F, Barres D. Correlation between intracavernous pressure and ischiocavernosus muscle in man. J Urol 1986; 136: 936–9

24. Fitzpatrick TJ, Cooper JF. A cavernosogram study on the valvular competence of the human deep dorsal vein. J Urol 1975; 113: 497–9

25. Fitzpatrick TJ. The penile intercommunicating venous valvular system. J Urol 1982; 127: 1099–100

26. Crowe R, Burnstock G, Dickinson IK, Pryor JP. The human penis: an unusual penetration of NPY-immunoreactive nerves within the medial muscle coat of the deep dorsal vein. J Urol 1991; 145: 1292–6

27. Johnsen SG. Testicular biopsy score count – a method for registration of spermatogenesis in human testis. Normal values and results in 335 hypogonadal males. Hormones 1970; 1: 2–25

28. Sharpe RM. Testosterone and spermatogenesis. J Endocrinol 1987; 113: 1–2

29. Pryor JP, Cameron KM, Collins WP, Hirsh AV, Mahony JDH, Pugh RCB. Indications for testicular biopsy or exploration in azoospermia. Br J Urol 1978; 50: 591–4

30. Chandley AC. Chromosomes. In: Hargreave TB (ed) Male infertility. 2nd edition. Berlin: Springer-Verlag, 1994: 149–64

31. Reijo R, Alagappan RK, Patrizio P, Page DC. Severe oligozoospermia resulting from deletions of azoospermia factor gene on Y chromosome. Lancet 1996; 347: 1290–3

32. Pryor JL, Kent-First M, Muallem A, *et al.* Microdeletions in the Y chromosome of infertile men. N Engl J Med 1997; 336: 534–9

33. Ford TF, Parkinson MC, Pryor JP. The undescended testis in adult life. Br J Urol 1985; 57: 181–4

34. Pryor JP, Cameron KM, Chilton CP, *et al.* Carcinoma in situ in testicular biopsies from men presenting with infertility. Br J Urol 1983; 55: 780–4

35. Silber SJ, Van Stirtegheim AC, Devroey P. Sertoli cell only revisited. Hum Reprod 1995; 10: 1031–52

36. Cooper TG. The epididymal influence on sperm maturation. Reprod Med Rev 1995; 4: 141–61

37. Jarrow JP. Seminal vesicle aspiration in the management of patients with ejaculatory duct obstruction. J Urol 1994; 152: 899–901

38. Oates RD, Amos JA. The genetic basis of congenital bilateral absence of the vas deferens and cystic fibrosis. J Androl 1994; 15: 1–8

39. Pryor JP. Ejaculatory disorders. In: Whitfield H, Hendry WF, Kirby R, Duchett J (eds) Textbook of genitourinary surgery. 2nd edition. Oxford: Blackwell, 1998: 1503–9

40. World Health Organisation. WHO laboratory manual for the examination of human semen and sperm mucous interaction. 3rd edition. Cambridge: Cambridge University Press, 1992

41. Palermo G, Joris H, Devroey P, Steirtegheim AC. Pregnancies after intracytoplasmic injection of single spermatozoon into an oocyte. Lancet 1992; 340: 17–18

42. Hargreave TB, Elton RA. Is conventional semen analysis of any use? Br J Urol 1983; 55: 780–4

43. Cates W, Farley TMM, Rowe PJ. Worldwide patterns of infertility: is Africa different? Lancet 1985; ii: 596–8

44. Baker HWG. Clinical evaluation and management of testicular disorders in the adult. In: Burger H, de Kretser DM (eds) The testis. 2nd edition. New York: Raven Press, 1989: 419–40

The prostate and benign prostatic hyperplasia

13

M. Emberton and A. R. Mundy

The prostate

The average urologist spends about 30% of his or her time dealing with problems related to the prostate. Surprisingly, for a structure that attracts so much of our attention, we know very little about why the prostate is there and what it does. It is one of four accessory sex glands or pairs of glands; the other three are the seminal vesicles, Cowper's glands and the glands of Littre. If we know little about the prostate, we know even less about the others. The seminal vesicles, which are secretory glands and not storage organs for semen as their name implies, contribute substantially to the volume of seminal fluid and produce one or two substances that we know about, notably fructose and glyceryl phosphocholine. However, the other two structures are something of a mystery.

We do know that the prostate is intimately related anatomically to the bladder neck and plays an integral part in ensuring antegrade ejaculation. We know it contains a substantial amount of smooth muscle as well as glandular tissue and that this smooth muscle is under alpha-adrenergic control and is thought somehow to be involved in the process of seminal emission prior to ejaculation. We know that the prostate contributes various substances to the ejaculate, some of which are present in unusually high concentrations, notably zinc, citrate and polyamines. We know that its development and function are under hormonal control; in other words, it is a secondary sex organ.

We do not know, however, what part if any the prostate plays in continence in normal individuals; the mechanism of emission and ejaculation is uncertain (in humans); and we do not know why the prostatic secretion contains so much zinc, citrate and polyamines, nor what the roles are of these and the various other substances that the prostate secretes.

The structure of the prostate

The prostate has been described as having a lobar structure, firstly, because of the endoscopic appearance of 'lobes' in patients with benign prostatic hyperplasia and in the pathological specimen after retropubic prostatectomy, and secondly, on embryological grounds in which the prostate is seen to develop from five distinct ductal systems [1]. More recently, the morphology of the prostate has been described on the basis of the predisposition of parts of its structure to various pathological processes, and to McNeal we owe our current understanding of the structure of the prostate (Figure 13.1) [2–5].

McNeal noted that the nodules of benign prostatic hyperplasia began in the periurethral glandular area within the collar of the preprostatic sphincter in the supramontanal part of the prostate. Subsequently, he noted that these microscopic nodules were principally concentrated just below the distal margin of the preprostatic sphincter, and he named that area the transitional zone. The transitional zone only accounted for about 2% of the glandular tissue of the normal prostate but accounted for much more as the hyperplastic nodules coalesced, became macroscopic and tended to displace the normal prostate away from the urethra.

McNeal noted that about 25% of prostatic cancer originated within the transitional zone, whereas 75%

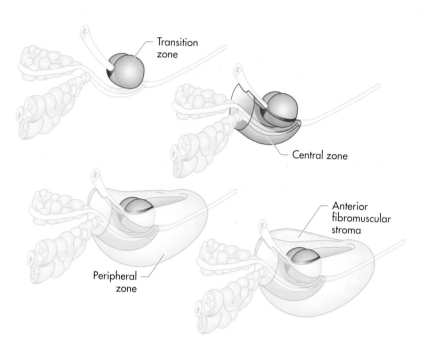

Figure 13.1 Zones of the prostate.

of cancers and almost all instances of prostatitis arose in the so-called peripheral zone. The peripheral zone forms a posteriorly and inferiorly orientated cup that encloses the central zone, through the centre of which are transmitted the ejaculatory ducts. McNeal noted the comparative absence of disease in the central zone by comparison with the other glandular areas of the prostate and likened it to the seminal vesicles, which are also comparatively free of disease. He speculated further that both these structures might arise embryologically from the Wolffian ducts and he noted some histological similarities between the central zone and the seminal vesicles to support this contention [5].

Completing the anterior aspect of the substance of the prostate where the peripheral zone peters out on either side is the anterior fibromuscular stroma of the prostate. Most of the glandular tissue of the prostate is in the peripheral zone, which accounts for 65% of the total, the remaining 25% of the glandular tissue of the prostate being in the central zone. It is not known whether the three zones of glandular tissue – transitional, central and peripheral – have different secretory functions.

Embryological development of the prostate

As mentioned above, the seminal vesicles (and possibly the central zone of the prostate) arise from the Wolffian ducts along with the vasa and their ampullae

and the epididymes. Their development is under the control of testosterone. However, the prostate develops from urogenital sinus mesenchyme and its development is under the control of dihydrotestosterone. This difference of embryological origin and hormonal control may account for the observation that, whereas the prostate is commonly involved in disease, the structures of Wolffian duct origin rarely are.

Endocrinology of the prostate

The prostate develops and functions in response to dihydrotestosterone, which is produced within the prostate cells themselves from circulating testosterone (Figure 13.2). The circulating testosterone is derived from testicular secretion; the testis produces 6–7 mg a day under the influence of luteinising hormone, which in turn is produced by the pituitary in response to the pulsatile release of luteinising hormone-releasing hormone from the hypothalamus. Testosterone is insoluble in water and is carried in the circulation bound principally to sex hormone-binding globulin, with only a tiny free fraction. However tiny it is, the free testosterone is the important component, and because it is a small, lipid-soluble molecule, it transfers across the lipid cell membrane with ease to be converted by 5-alpha reductase into the active component dihydrotestosterone.

The adrenal produces androgens that can be con-

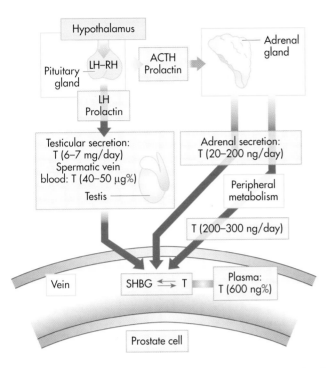

Figure 13.2 *Endocrinological influences on the prostate. Pulsatile release of luteinising hormone-releasing hormone (LH-RH) from the hypothalamus causes the release of luteinising hormone (LH) from the anterior pituitary, which circulates to the Leydig cells of the testis, which produce testosterone (T). Testosterone circulates from the testis bound to sex hormone-binding globulin (SHBG) and is available to the prostate. Circulating testosterone has a negative-feedback inhibition of the hypothalamic release of luteinising hormone-releasing hormone. Adrenal secretion and peripheral aromatisation are other sources of circulating androgens.*

verted to testosterone, and there is a mechanism for the peripheral conversion of various substrates into testosterone, but the vast majority of testosterone is derived from testicular secretion and without testicular testosterone the prostate undergoes involution.

The enzyme 5-alpha reductase within the prostatic cell is crucial in producing the active androgen, dihydrotestosterone. There are two types of 5-alpha reductase, of which type 2 is the more important, and it is blocked by the 5-alpha reductase inhibitor finasteride, which has recently been introduced therapeutically for the treatment of benign prostatic hyperplasia [6]. It is a deficiency of this enzyme also that is responsible for the intersex state first noted by Imperato-McInley in the Dominican Republic in which apparently normal girls change to boys at puberty [7].

Dihydrotestosterone exerts its effect by binding to the androgen receptor and then translocating to the

nucleus to bind with DNA and initiate transcription. Binding of dihydrotestosterone to the androgen receptor causes a confirmational change of the androgen receptor, thereby exposing its hormone-responsive element, which binds to its target DNA to initiate transcription (Figure 13.3).

Both the epithelial cells and the stromal cells are capable of producing dihydrotestosterone as both contain the 5-alpha reductase enzyme [8]. Similarly, both epithelial and stromal cells contain androgen receptors. However, it appears that dihydrotestosterone is principally formed in epithelial cells and although some of this acts within the epithelial cell nuclei to initiate the transcription of DNA that is responsible for the secretory activity in the prostate, most of the dihydrotestosterone formed in epithelial cells diffuses to the stromal cells where most of the androgen receptors are found. In stromal cells, the binding of dihydrotestosterone to the androgen receptor principally stimulates the stromal nuclei to produce growth factors and these growth factors drive both the epithelial cells and the stromal cells themselves to grow and develop [9, 10].

It is this interaction between the stroma and the epithelium that is thought to account not only for

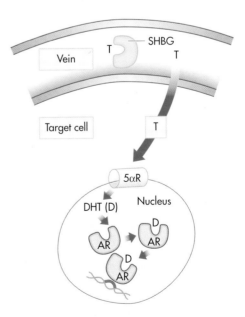

Figure 13.3 *Testosterone (T) dissociates from its protein binding and translocates across the cell membrane. Intracellularly, it is converted to dihydrotestosterone (DHT) and binds to the androgen receptor (AR), from where it translocates to the nucleus.*

development and for normal function but also, when the interaction is deranged, for the process leading to benign prostatic hyperplasia.

Thus, several processes are active within the prostate. The endocrine effect of testosterone leads to the intracrine effect of dihydrotestosterone, which generates the autocrine and paracrine effects of growth factors on both the stroma and the epithelium of the prostate (Figure 13.4). These growth factors, responsible for the autocrine and paracrine effects, act principally during the G1 phase of the cell cycle and have various effects, mainly stimulatory but in some instances inhibitory, leading generally to the entry of the cell into the S phase and ultimately then to mitosis.

The normal adult prostate should not be thought of as being an entirely static structure. There is a turnover of cells throughout life and this turnover is heterogenous [11]. Those glandular cells further out in the periphery of the gland away from the urethra show little in the way of secretion and most in the way of mitotic activity within the prostate, resembling basal or stem cells. At an intermediate level along the prostatic duct, the epithelial cells show less mitosis

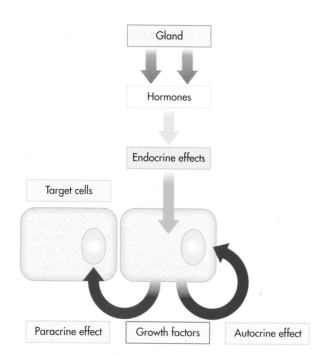

Figure 13.4 *The effect of androgens in the stroma is to cause the release of growth factors that have an autocrine effect on themselves and a paracrine effect on epithelial cells.*

but almost all of the secretory activity of the prostate. These two types of acinar cells are tall and columnar and show no evidence of cell death. More centrally, close to the urethra, the epithelial cells are lower, flatter and without any secretory activity, and programmed cell death (apoptosis) is readily visible. In relation to these different epithelial cell types there are differences in the underlying extracellular matrix that probably reflect the driving force for epithelial differentiation [12]. In addition, there are the neuroendocrine cells described below.

Growth factors in the prostate

It has been known for many years that prostatic cells could only proliferate in vitro in the presence of serum. The factors that were present in serum were not present in plasma and so it seemed that whatever was necessary to stimulate cell growth in vitro was derived from the process of blood coagulation and most probably liberated from platelets. Thus, one of the first 'growth factors' to be identified was called platelet-derived growth factor. Various other factors were subsequently identified as being 'growth factors' for various different cell types in vitro and have derived their names from the circumstances under which they were isolated. These substances may have effects other than being 'growth factors' and most have many different roles in stimulating cellular growth both in vitro and in vivo (see Chapter 1).

Other factors that are known to be important in the normal growth and development in the prostate have been: (a) derived from the mouse submaxillary gland (epidermal growth factor); (b) shown to have a very characteristic and strong tendency to bind to heparin (fibroblast growth factor, one of the so-called heparin-binding growth factors); or (c) biochemically related to pro-insulin (insulin-like growth factor). Hence the origin of names that are somewhat confusing to the uninitiated.

Typically, growth factors are grouped into families of factors having similar effects and there is an epidermal growth factor family, a fibroblast growth factor family, a transforming growth factor-β family (transforming growth factor-α – somewhat confusingly – is a member of the epidermal growth factor family), and the insulin-like growth factor family. There are other growth factor families as well, but these are the ones that are thought to be important in the normal prostate.

Of these various growth factors, the most important stimulatory ones are epidermal growth factor and transforming growth factor-α, both of which are derived from the epidermal growth factor family, and basic fibroblast growth factor of the fibroblast growth factor family. Of these, basic fibroblast growth factor and epidermal growth factor are thought to account for 80% and transforming growth factor-α for 20% of the stimulatory growth factor effect in health [13]. The other important growth factor is transforming growth factor-β, whose effects are complex but generally inhibitory [14].

Other growth factors such as insulin-like growth factor are thought to be principally 'permissive' in the same sense that androgens are permissive. Insulin-like growth factor and testosterone have to be present in vivo and in vitro but adding more and more of either does not produce a corresponding parallel proliferation of the prostate in vitro, whereas adding epidermal growth factor, transforming growth factor or basic fibroblast growth factor does. The effects of some of these factors are only or principally apparent at different stages of development. Epidermal growth factor and basic fibroblast growth factor are predominant in the adult (developed) prostate. On the other hand, transforming growth factor and another member of the fibroblast growth factor family, acidic fibroblast growth factor, are principally evident in fetal life [15].

The role of the prostate in continence

One could be forgiven for thinking that the prostate has a major role in continence by virtue of its situation around the bladder neck, but of course the female of the species manages perfectly well without it.

In individuals of either sex there is a change in the orientation of the smooth muscle bundles of the detrusor as they approach the region of the bladder neck, with a tendency to become more oblique in disposition, smaller and more finely interspersed in a more dense connective tissue framework (Figure 13.5) [16]. In males, but not in females, there is a quite definitely circular/oblique orientation of smooth muscle

bundles around the area just below the bladder neck and within the substance of the prostate, with a dense adrenergic innervation that can be demonstrated by immunofluorescence (Figure 13.6) [17]. Elsewhere in the bladder in both sexes and in the female urethra, alpha-adrenergic innervation is only seen in relation to blood vessels, although alpha-adrenergic receptors may be more widely distributed. This ring of smooth muscle around the supramontanal prostatic urethra, between the bladder neck and the site of drainage of the prostatic ducts and ejaculatory ducts into the urethra, is called the preprostatic sphincter. It is present to ensure antegrade ejaculation (see below).

Elsewhere within the prostate, particularly within the prostatic capsule but distributed throughout the

Figure 13.5 *The orientation of smooth muscle bundles at the bladder neck to form the preprostatic sphincter.*

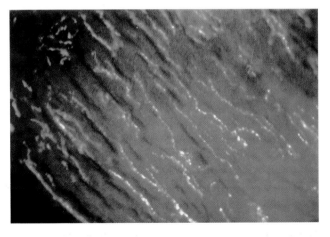

Figure 13.6 *Immunofluorescence photomicrograph to show the presence of noradrenergic nerves interspersed between the smooth muscle bundles at the bladder neck.*

stroma, there are smooth muscle cells that amount to about 50% of the total mass of the stroma of the prostate [18]. These cells also have (mainly) an alpha-adrenergic innervation [19].

Classical pharmacological studies were able to distinguish between alpha- and beta-adrenergic activities and, more recently, between alpha-1 receptors (postjunctional alpha adrenoceptors that mediate the effector response) and alpha-2 receptors (prejunctional alpha adrenoceptors that regulate neurotransmitter release). Further, pharmacological alpha-1 subtypes are now distinguished by the selective antagonistic effects of certain blockers. Recently, the International Union of Pharmacology published a new classification of alpha receptors. This was needed to clarify the confusing nomenclature that was being used to describe native as distinct from cloned receptors [20]. Suffice it to say that all three alpha-1 receptor subtypes have been identified in human prostatic stroma but the predominant one is the alpha-1A subtype. Unfortunately, none of the alpha blockers in use today has much selectivity for the alpha-1A subtype. The most selective at present seems to be indoramin [21], but its other pharmacological effects (antihistaminic, local anaesthetic and cardiodepressant) limit its potential clinical usefulness.

This adrenergic innervation is not the only form of innervation to the prostate however; it is not even the only innervation of prostatic smooth muscle cells. There is a cholinergic innervation and there are a number of different non-adrenergic non-cholinergic nerve or receptor types as well. The latter include serotonin (5-hydroxytryptamine), dopamine beta hydroxylase, vasoactive intestinal polypeptide, neuropeptide Y, leu-encephalin, met-encephalin, calcitonin gene-related peptide and substance P [22]. What these are all doing is by no means clear.

The majority of the adrenergic receptors are of the alpha adrenergic type, 98% of which are located within the stroma, of which 90% are of the alpha-1 subtype. Only 10% of alpha receptors and neurons are of the alpha-2 subtype. Of the alpha-1, the alpha-1A type accounts for 60% and it is these that are the cells that have been targeted pharmacologically by drugs such as indoramin, terazosin and doxazosin in an attempt to reverse some of the features of bladder outflow obstruction due to benign prostatic hyperplasia [21]. The cholinergic innervation is thought to control epithelial secretion [23].

Some of the non-adrenergic non-cholinergic substances listed above are present in so-called 'neuroendocrine cells' [24]. The principle neuroendocrine cell types are cells that secrete serotonin and thyroid-stimulating hormone. Other cells contain calcitonin or the calcitonin gene-related peptide and somatostatin. It is not clear what these do, but they are thought to be involved in the regulation of secretion or cell growth. The function of the other neurons or receptors is completely unknown; they may not actually have any function. As has been pointed out elsewhere in this volume, the presence of neurons does not necessarily imply the presence of receptors for those neurons and vice versa, and even if both are present, that does not necessarily mean that there is a neural pathway, and if there is, it does not necessarily follow that that pathway has a physiological significance even if it has a pathological significance.

Thus, there is no evidence that the prostate plays any active role in continence, although in disease it may interfere with normal continence. There is no evidence that the male bladder neck in the strict sense is any different from the female bladder neck except that it simply has a preprostatic sphincter superimposed on the common bladder neck pattern. All the evidence is that the prostatic smooth muscle and its innervation and the other nerve supply to the prostate are involved in glandular secretion and the process of emission.

Emission and ejaculation

Ejaculation in human beings remains a mystery, in part as it is so difficult to study because of the problems of sexual sensibilities. In animals this is less of a problem; indeed, because of the financial implications of breeding in animal husbandry, ejaculation in some species has been studied in considerable detail.

We have known for some time from so-called 'split ejaculate' studies in humans that spermatozoa and prostatic fluid are ejaculated first, followed by seminal vesicle fluid later [25]. We also know that ejaculation is antegrade in the presence of a competent bladder neck despite the competence of the urethral sphincter mechanism, which therefore must be overcome actively or reflexly to enable ejaculation to occur. It is also common male experience that voiding is difficult with an erection and for a while after ejaculation.

The latter has been shown to be due to tightening of the 'bladder neck' – more accurately, of the pre-prostatic sphincter – on erection, which becomes more marked in the period leading up to ejaculation. This has been shown both on urethral pressure profile studies, which show enhancement of the pressure zone produced by the bladder neck (Figure 13.7), and on transrectal ultrasound studies, which demonstrate the preprostatic sphincter quite clearly and which show it to become more marked in the pre-ejaculatory period [26].

The next step, also shown on transrectal ultra-sound [26] (and radiographically in some animal species), is the transportation of spermatozoa from the ampullae of the vasa into the prostatic urethra. This process of filling of the inframontanal prostatic urethra, below the occluding preprostatic sphincter, is known as emission, as distinct from the process by which the seminal fluid is transported to the outside world, which is ejaculation. The mechanism for this is not clear. Once it occurs, ejaculation is imminent.

Next is a contraction of the prostatic smooth muscle including the preprostatic sphincter, which is presumably under alpha-1A adrenergic control.

Synchronously but not in any co-ordinated fashion, there is a sequence of five or six contractions of the bulbo-spongiosius muscle. The first generally occurs before any of the seminal fluid has entered the bulbar urethra, and the last occurs after pulsatile ejaculation ceases. The mechanism for this is not clear either, nor is the means by which the urethral sphincter mechanism is overcome. It used to be thought that it was overcome passively by the sheer pressure that prostatic emission generates. But the recent transrectal ultrasound studies referred to above suggest that this is probably not the case. Urethral sphincter studies to look for a relaxation mechanism have not been useful

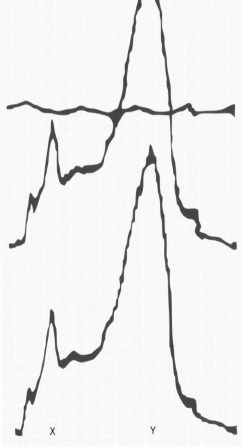

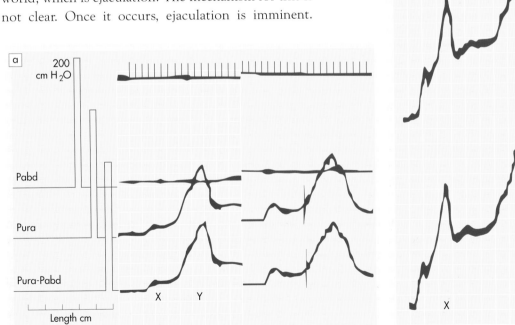

Figure 13.7 (a) A urethral pressure profile of the bladder neck (where x is the site of the bladder neck and y is the site of the urethral sphincter mechanism). (b) A urethral pressure profile during erection to show the enhanced pressure zone at the bladder neck.

in providing an alternative explanation. In any case, a postulated urethral sphincter relaxation mechanism would tend to flounder on the observation that after transurethral resection, men are not incontinent during sexual activity when the bladder neck mechanism has been ablated.

Once emission and ejaculation have begun, there is further contraction of the prostate and of the seminal vesicles until the process is complete.

There is therefore an important role for the prostate in the process of emission leading to ejaculation, irrespective of the content of prostatic secretion added.

The physiological function of prostatic secretion

In an average ejaculate, 2 ml are contributed by the secretion of the seminal vesicles, 0.5 ml is contributed by the secretion of the prostate, and Cowper's glands and the glands of Littre contribute 0.1 ml [27]. The contribution of the sperm cells themselves is insignificant. Although the function of these various secretions is not clear, epididymal sperm can fertilise an ovum but not as well as ejaculated sperm, so presumably their function is to maximise the potential for fertilisation. This may be by having a protective effect during the onward journey of the sperm until its contact with the ovum, or an effect to enhance motility and sperm survival more directly, or a role to increase the fertilising effect of the sperm when it reaches the ovum. There are various pieces of evidence to support a role in each of these three areas, but details are distinctly lacking.

These various secretions also have a protective role in the lower urinary tract itself. The sheer presence of the fluid provides lubrication both of the urethra itself and, through the pre-ejaculatory fluid, for penetration, although penetration has often occurred long before most human males produce pre-ejaculatory fluid. Nonetheless, this may at least be the role of the glands of Littre. It would be nice to think they were there for some purpose!

A protective effect on the lower urinary tract by the biological effects of some of the components of seminal fluid may be more important, indeed much more important than just the mechanical washing of the urethra. In fact, it has been argued that the principle function of the prostate and the other sexual secondary sex organs is to protect the integrity of the spermatozoa. Zinc has a strong antimicrobial action, spermine less so. Immunoglobulins of various types could have a similar biological role. All this is, however, unproven.

One substance known to enhance the fertilising capacity of ejaculated sperm cells after ejaculation is fertilisation-promoting peptide, which is structurally similar to thyrotrophin-releasing hormone [28]. Its mode of action is unknown, nor is it known whether there are other compounds with a similar action. Epidermal growth factor has a high concentration in seminal fluid, second only to colostrum in fact, and it may be that this reflects a role in fertilisation.

Numerous compounds are produced by the prostate, most of which have no obvious function. Acid phosphatase splits glycerylphosphocholine produced by the seminal vesicles to produce glycerylphosphate ultimately and it may be that glycerylphosphate is important in sperm protection. It may be more than just coincidental that in a laboratory setting glycerine is used for this sort of purpose. Polyamines are the strongest known cationic substances in nature and they may have an important role in transcription and translation [29]. Alternatively, these two observations may be no more than just coincidence. Prostate specific antigen is a serine protease that has a role in sperm liquefaction [30]. Sperm coagulation and liquefaction have an important role in small mammals such as rats and mice but their role in humans is unclear.

More interesting perhaps, because of their high concentration within the prostate, are zinc and citrate. Citrate is present in 240–1300 times the concentration found elsewhere [31], and zinc is present in about 30 times the concentration elsewhere [32]; it seems likely that there is a reason for this and for the uniquely high concentrations of polyamines. There appears to be a close correlation between all three, and it has long been suspected that citrate is there as a ligand for zinc [33]. It is thought that the zinc is there to help maintain the quaternary structure of sperm chromatin [34] in addition to the biological protective effect mentioned above. It now seems likely that the complex of zinc and citrate and polyamines forms a structure that has electrochemical neutrality and therefore buffers the citrate [35], although this does seem an extremely energy-inefficient way of achieving this effect. An alternative, or additional, explanation is that the complex is there not just to protect the zinc (so to speak) but to hold the citrate there [36]. The optimum pH for the activity of acid phosphatase is much lower than the natural pH of seminal fluid and if acid phosphatase does indeed have an important biological role, this may be facilitated by the availability of large amounts of citrate. This, however, is pure speculation at present.

One of the problems is that most of these substances have only been investigated from the point of view of their concentrations in disease to serve as a marker for a disease state rather than to investigate their physiological role. Until the thrust of research is redirected, the function of these various components of prostatic and seminal vesicular secretion will continue to remain obscure.

Benign prostatic hyperplasia

Having discussed some of the aspects of our current understanding of the prostate in health, we now turn to a consideration of the disorders of the prostate seen in benign prostatic hyperplasia.

The general impression generated in many reviews is that benign prostatic hyperplasia is a generalised and diffuse disease of the prostate that occurs as a result of some sort of hormonal derangement that leads to hyperplasia of the prostate producing enlargement of the gland as a whole, which in turn leads to compression of the prostatic urethra and a progressive occlusion of the bladder outflow and the clinical syndrome of 'prostatism'. None of this is true.

Benign prostatic hyperplasia is very unusual in that it only occurs in human beings and dogs. The same is true of carcinoma of the prostate. Despite this and the fact that both diseases are common, most authorities suggest that there is no direct link between the two diseases [37]. Recently, however, there has been a suggestion that the two are related: that a series of

genetic 'hits' gives rise to benign prostatic hyperplasia, and further 'hits' to prostate cancer [38]. Benign prostatic hyperplasia is therefore an early stage in the development of prostate cancer in this hypothesis.

Benign prostatic hyperplasia seems to be a disease (also like carcinoma of the prostate) that any human male can expect to get if he lives long enough with functioning testes and assuming his prostate was normal to start off with. It is clearly important, therefore, to distinguish between the clinical condition associated with the histological disease of benign prostatic hyperplasia and other clinical conditions affecting the lower urinary tract in ageing males.

The recent interest in symptom scores and in the effects of ageing on the bladder in individuals of either sex seems to make it clear that there are symptoms arising from the lower urinary tract, and particularly from the bladder, that are related to ageing that need to be distinguished from those symptoms related to histological benign prostatic hyperplasia in males. Furthermore, many of the features of the benign prostatic hyperplasia clinical symptom complex are difficult to explain in relation to histological benign prostatic hyperplasia alone. Acute retention can be explained when it is secondary to urinary tract infection, severe constipation or sympathetic stimulation in hypothermia and psychological stress, but otherwise its nature is somewhat elusive, although it may be due to prostatic infarction or some other prostatic 'vascular accident' [39]. The 'urge' symptom complex related to secondary detrusor instability is more easy to explain [40], but bladder decompensation is more difficult given our present knowledge of clinical benign prostatic hyperplasia and the experimental effects of obstruction on bladder function [41], unless this is related more to the coincidentally ageing bladder than to benign prostatic hyperplasia per se. It is, in fact, difficult to explain how benign prostatic hyperplasia causes obstruction at all. Squeezing on a hose pipe is a very inefficient way of stopping the water emerging from the end, and a very marked restriction of the calibre of the hose pipe has to be produced before there is any overt change in flow. Obstruction by urethral constriction is easily understood in relation to urethral stricture disease but it is much more difficult to argue for a similar effect in the prostatic urethra in benign prostatic hyperplasia when a large resectoscope can be passed through and into the bladder with ease. It may therefore be that it is distortion of the prostatic urethra that is more important in producing outflow obstruction than compression or constriction, as it is distortion of a hose pipe by kinking that is more likely to stop flow.

Aetiology

It has already been mentioned that the only proven risk factors for developing benign prostatic hyperplasia are ageing and the presence of functioning testes [42], assuming that the prostate was normal to start off with – in other words, if 5-alpha reductase was present to convert testosterone to dihydrotestosterone and there were functioning androgen receptors for the dihydrotestosterone to bind to.

Various factors have been investigated such as dietary factors, alcohol and cirrhosis of the liver [43], all of which may affect androgen–oestrogen balance, but there is no substantial evidence to support any of these contentions. The only evidence for any other factor is for an inherited predisposition to develop the disease at a younger than usual age, which runs in families [44].

Pathogenesis

It has also been pointed out that androgens (in other words, functioning testes) were permissive for prostatic growth and development in health, and the same is true for the prostate in vitro. Androgens (and insulin-like growth factor and other 'factors') have to be present for the prostate to grow, but once the critical 'permissive' concentration has been reached, there is no extra growth produced by adding more.

Also discussed above was the concept of a stromal–epithelial interaction in which testosterone production by the epithelial cells leads to the elaboration of growth factors by the stromal cell that act in both an autocrine and paracrine fashion to produce further growth and differentiation in both the stroma and the epithelium. This stromal–epithelial interaction was most clearly demonstrated by Cunha (Figure 13.8), who implanted embryonic urogenital sinus mesenchyme and adult bladder epithelial cells from a normal mouse under the renal capsule of a nude mouse and showed that the urogenital sinus mesenchyme induced prostatic epithelial differentiation of the bladder epithelium [45]. Cunha also showed that normal prostatic differentiation could be induced from the bladder epithelium taken from a mouse with

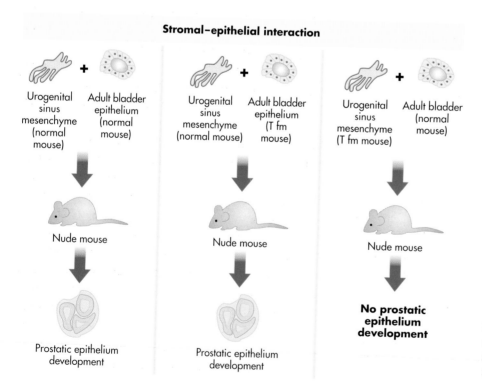

Figure 13.8 Cunha's experiments showing the importance of stroma (in this case urogenital sinus mesenchyme) in epithelial differentiation.

androgen receptor deficiency as long as the urogenital sinus mesenchyme was taken from a normal mouse. Prostatic epithelial differentiation did not occur when the urogenital sinus mesenchyme was taken from a mouse with androgen receptor deficiency whatever the androgen receptor status of the bladder epithelium. In this way, Cunha demonstrated the importance of the androgen receptor in the prostatic stroma (derived from urogenital sinus mesenchyme) as well as the importance of the stromal–epithelial interaction in producing epithelial and glandular development.

In benign prostatic hyperplasia, the stromal: epithelial ratio increases [18]. Normally, it is something in the region of 2:1, but in benign prostatic hyperplasia it increases to 3 or 4:1. As mentioned above, there is a substantial smooth muscle component to the stroma in health and in benign prostatic hyperplasia, but the majority of the stroma is made up of connective tissue such that about 50% of benign prostatic hyperplasia is connective tissue, 25% is smooth muscle and 25% is epithelium [19].

The first discernible sign of benign prostatic hyperplasia is the presence of microscopic nodules of fibromuscular hyperplasia with a variable epithelial cell component. These nodules are found initially in the transition zone just below the smooth muscle collar of the preprostatic sphincter (Figure 13.9) [46]. The transition zone is found on either side of the urethra and nodules in this area are a mixture of glandular and epithelial hyperplasia. The nodules of benign prostatic hyperplasia also form, with lesser frequency, in the periurethral glandular tissue within the smooth muscle collar of the preprostatic sphincter. Here, they form principally posteriorly and have no epithelial or

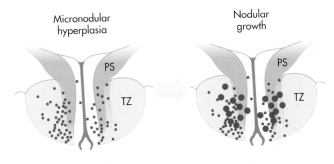

Figure 13.9 *The siting of early nodules in benign prostatic hyperplasia: just below and within the collar of the preprostatic sphincter (PS) in the general area of the transitional zone (TZ).*

glandular component [47, 48]; they are pure connective tissue nodules. In these nodules, there are changes visible that are most unusual, notably fibroblasts transforming themselves into smooth muscle cells. It was this observation that led McNeal to suggest that the nodules of benign prostatic hyperplasia, wherever they occurred, were the result of an 'embryonic re-awakening' as a consequence of localised changes in the normal stromal–epithelial interaction [46, 49].

The so-called lateral lobes of benign prostatic hyperplasia are derived from micronodule formation and coalescence and further growth within the transition zone, whereas the so-called middle lobe is derived from nodule formation and development within the periurethral glandular sleeve posteriorly. The remainder of the prostate – as has been well recognised for many years – is compressed outwards to form a false capsule posteriorly [50].

In other words, benign prostatic hyperplasia is not a diffuse and generalised disease of the prostate but is a highly localised disease of the smallest area of the prostate (the transition zone and the periurethral gland area). There is no evidence that it is related either directly to a derangement of androgen metabolism or to an androgen–oestrogen imbalance, given that it occurs at a time when serum androgen levels are steadily decreasing and oestrogen levels are steadily increasing, and that only a small proportion of the prostate as a whole is affected [51].

Whereas the description 'embryonic re-awakening' may not be entirely accurate, the disease does seem to be related to an abnormal stromal–epithelial interaction confined to this small area of the prostate, in which both increased cell growth and reduced cell death – that is to say, programmed cell death (apoptosis) – are equally important components [52]. It was mentioned above that along the prostatic duct, from the urethra out to the periphery, the most distal glands were dividing whilst the most proximal ones (nearest the urethra) were undergoing apoptosis. The epithelial cells of the more distal or peripheral glands, which have been noted to be more mitotically active, seem to be related to underlying smooth muscle cells that are vimentin positive, whereas those that are proximal or central, which tend to show apoptosis, are related to smooth muscles that are actin positive [12, 53].

Perhaps vimentin-positive smooth muscle cells tend to be more stimulatory, whereas those that are actin positive produce inhibitory growth factors or growth factors that tend to promote apoptosis. Alterations in growth factor expression have, indeed, been identified in benign prostatic hyperplasia, although it is not yet possible to say with confidence that these growth factors are the cause of this histological condition, that they are confined to the transition zone and are not found elsewhere within the prostate, and that they alone are responsible for the changes seen in benign prostatic hyperplasia.

Most of the work on growth factors in the prostate has been very recent; new work is being published all the time, and the picture is far from clear and changing. Nonetheless, what follows is a summary of what currently appears to be true at the time of writing [54].

Most of the growth factors alluded to above act to increase gene expression, although the transforming growth factor beta family is notable for generally producing inhibition. Most growth factors act through single-pass transmembrane receptors with tyrosine kinase activity that, through a transduction pathway, induce mitogent-activated protein kinases, which produce the increase in gene expression.

In the normal prostate, the main stimulatory growth factors are epidermal growth factor and transforming growth factor alpha, the former being principally active in adults and the latter in growth and differentiation of the prostate. Neither of these appears to play any part in benign prostatic hyperplasia, although the epidermal growth factor expression appears to be reduced [55]. Another growth factor family with an important role in the normal prostate is the fibroblast growth factor family. Like transforming growth factor alpha, acidic fibroblast growth factor is predominantly active in growth and differentiation [15]. It is basic fibroblast growth factor that is the main stimulatory growth factor of this group in adults. All members of the fibroblast growth factor family have a variety of actions on a variety of different cell types, including producing angiogenesis and remodelling the extracellular matrix by producing modulating proteases and inducing the synthesis of fibronectin [14, 56]. Members of the fibroblast growth factor family are abundant in the extracellular matrix, where they bind heparin avidly. Basic fibroblast growth factor is interesting because it is not secreted; it is only released from cells by injury or cell death, although it may, of course, have intracrine activity [57]. However, there is another member of this family, called keratinocyte growth factor [58]. This is a truly paracrine substance that is secreted only by stromal cells but for which there are only receptors on epithelial cells. It may be that some of the simulatory activity previously ascribed to basic fibroblast growth factor is, in fact, more related to keratinocyte growth factor. Both basic fibroblast growth factor and keratinocyte growth factor appear to have a role in benign prostatic hyperplasia as both show increased expression [59].

The transforming growth factor-β family is the family of growth factors that are generally inhibitory for epithelial cells. It is more true to say that they may be inhibitory or stimulatory depending on the cell type, the state of differentiation and the circumstances [14, 60], but in general they are inhibitory for epithelial cells and stimulatory for stromal cells. They also increase angiogenesis and extracellular matrix formation [61, 62]. This family is interesting, firstly because these growth factors have receptors that are serine/threonine kinases rather than tyrosine kinases, which are usual with growth factor receptors [62], and secondly, because they can inhibit the transition from the G1 phase to the S phase of the cell cycle and thereby override the action of mitogens, including the growth factors alluded to above [14, 63].

There are five isoforms of transforming growth factor alpha, but only three have been found in mammals (1–3) and only alpha-1 and alpha-2 have been investigated in benign prostatic hyperplasia. Transforming growth factor alpha-1 is negatively regulated by androgen: a fall in androgen leads to increased expression of the growth factor, and vice versa [62]. It also seems that basic fibroblast growth factor and keratinocyte growth factor expression is regulated by transforming growth factor β [14]. As a result, fibroblast growth factor expression is regulated by androgen indirectly by the androgen effect on transforming growth factor alpha expression.

The fibroblast growth factors – basic fibroblast growth factor and keratinocyte growth factor – are stimulatory growth factors and transforming growth factors alpha-1 and alpha-2 are inhibitory. Stromal cells produce both fibroblast growth factors and transforming growth factor alpha-1 [14, 58]. Epithelial cells produce transforming growth factor alpha-2 [64]. Basic fibroblast growth factor acts on both epithelial cells and stromal cells but principally on stromal cells because that is where it is released. Keratinocyte growth factor, on the other hand, can only act on epithelial cells because only epithelial cells have receptors for it. The transforming growth factors alpha-1 and alpha-2 act on both epithelial and stromal cells (Figure 13.10).

Thus, keratinocyte growth factor stimulates and transforming growth factor beta inhibits epithelial cells, and basic fibroblast growth factor stimulates and transforming growth factor beta inhibits stromal cells and, in the normal prostate, a steady state exists in which each pair is in balance. It is believed [65] that in benign prostatic hyperplasia, the fibroblast growth factors tend to override the transforming growth factor alphas and there is therefore a proliferation of epithelial and stromal cells and, in addition, because of the effect on extracellular matrix components, an increased activity there as well.

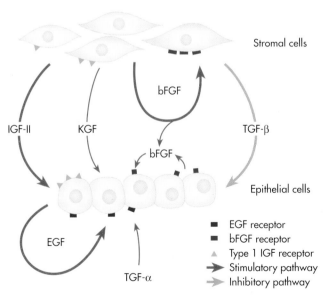

Figure 13.10 *The interaction of growth factors in benign prostatic hyperplasia. bFGF, basic fibroblast growth factor; IGF-II, insulin-like growth factor II; KGF, keratinocyte growth factor; TGF-β, transforming growth factor beta; TGF-α, transforming growth factor alpha; EGF, epidermal growth factor.*

If one assumes that this hypothesis is true, there is still a need to identify the cause of the changes outlined above. It has been suggested that declining androgen levels could account for the increasing expression of transforming growth factor alpha [66], but that would not explain the localised nature of the disease process. An alternative explanation is that repeated microtrauma or inflammation produced by repeated (lifelong) voiding and ejaculation, acting, as they do, on the point of angulation of the prostatic urethra, which is where the transition zone is situated, lead to cell damage at that site, which in turn leads to the release of basic fibroblast growth factor, which starts the whole process off.

Whether or not the details given above and the hypothesis outlined in the last few paragraphs prove ultimately to be true, it is quite clear that benign prostatic hyperplasia is not a diffuse generalised disease of glandular epithelium due to androgen imbalance within the glandular epithelium or due to an altered androgen:oestrogen ratio. It is a focal, stromal-induced disease affecting the transition and peri-urethral zones, producing micronodule formation by a stromal–epithelial interaction that appears to be mediated by growth factors. Androgen appears to act through transforming growth factor alpha expression to regulate the expression of other growth factors. The micronodules enlarge and coalesce, perhaps with an altered balance between cell growth and programmed cell death, which is also mediated by growth factor activity. This, in turn, produces an effect on the prostatic urethra, possibly by distortion, to produce bladder outflow obstruction. This, however, is only one of the symptom complexes found in ageing patients who have histological benign prostatic hyperplasia, and in some, non-obstructive benign prostatic hyperplasia may well produce symptoms by means that are not entirely clear. Others, possibly as a result of a 'vascular accident' within the prostate, or otherwise due to sympathetic stimulation or superadded obstruction by external compression in constipation, or by epithelial oedema in urinary infection, develop acute retention. Others develop detrusor instability as a consequence of the secondary changes induced by obstruction in the detrusor cells, although many patients with benign prostatic hyperplasia will have detrusor instability coincidentally as a result of this. Still others, possibly as a result of the coincidence of benign prostatic hyperplasia in conjunction with the impaired detrusor contractility that is commonly seen with the ageing bladder, develop detrusor decompensation and the symptom complex that leads ultimately to chronic retention and overflow incontinence. In some of these patients, the obstructive element causes high intravesical pressures, leading to structural and functional abnormalities of the upper urinary tract and thus to renal impairment and renal failure.

It should again be stated that some of the changes outlined in the last paragraph are hypothetical and unproven, but are nonetheless more likely to be accurate than the rather simplistic ideas hitherto promulgated on the basis of 'prostatic enlargement', 'urethral compression' and 'obstruction' leading to 'prostatism'.

Urodynamic aspects

It has already been suggested that benign prostatic hyperplasia may be asymptomatic or symptomatic, and that symptoms may arise purely and simply from the condition itself by virtue of its effects on the prostate alone or from its secondary obstructive effect on the prostatic urethra. Mention has been made of the secondary effects that obstruction can have on the previously normal bladder, leading to detrusor instability, and on the ageing bladder, hastening the process begun by ageing and leading through progressive degrees of detrusor decompensation to chronic retention with overflow; and that in the latter category high intravesical pressures can lead to obstructive changes in the upper tracts leading ultimately to renal failure. Also mentioned have been those factors that can act in benign prostatic hyperplasia to cause acute retention.

Symptom severity, which is increasingly being defined by symptom scores [67–69], can be used as selection criteria for surgery. When symptom scores are high, 90% of men will experience substantial improvement in symptoms after surgery, even in the absence of proven urodynamic obstruction [70, 71]. In addition, the symptoms of benign prostatic hyperplasia in obstructed patients seem to be relieved by thermotherapy and other recent 'alternative treat-

ments' for this condition without any effect on flow [72].

Urinary symptoms may equally be the result of detrusor instability that has developed as a consequence of obstruction, in which case the patient may have both obstructive and irritative symptoms, and they might equally be relieved by transurethral resection of the prostate if relief of the obstruction causes the detrusor to return to normal function.

Unfortunately, those same urinary symptoms may occur as a result of 'idiopathic' detrusor instability that the patient has developed for some entirely different reason, and the fact that he might coincidentally have histological benign prostatic hyperplasia is irrelevant. Such a patient will not benefit from transurethral resection of the prostate because the instability will persist.

Similarly, a patient with a poorly contractile bladder may have it in association with, or even, perhaps, as a consequence of, outflow obstruction due to benign prostatic hyperplasia and might therefore benefit from transurethral resection of the prostate. But, equally, the poorly contractile bladder may be an age-related phenomenon and coincidental benign prostatic hyperplasia may not be causing any symptoms, in which case transurethral resection of the prostate would not be helpful [73, 74].

Clearly, therefore, benign prostatic hyperplasia is not always obstructive but may nonetheless cause symptoms, generally of an irritative nature, and, equally, those symptoms may occur for other reasons than benign prostatic hyperplasia, generally arising in the bladder smooth muscle as an age-related or other phenomenon causing detrusor instability or impaired detrusor contractility or a combination of the two.

Somehow, these different phenomena have to be dissected out to determine the cause of a patient's symptoms and to decide how best to treat him; and urodynamic studies of various different types are the means by which this is done in clinical practice.

Historically, only bladder outflow obstruction was considered of any significance. Indeed, 50 years ago, treatment was only considered in the presence of urinary retention or when there was evidence of impaired function of the upper urinary tract and kidneys. More recently, detrusor instability has been recognised as an entity, but even so, detrusor instability and bladder decompensation leading to chronic retention and overflow incontinence were both thought of only as consequences of obstruction rather than conditions that might arise per se. Irritative symptoms in the absence of obstructive instability were largely ignored. It is only the recent interest in symptom scores, in alternative treatments for benign prostatic hyperplasia that reduce symptoms without any effect on urodynamic variables, and in the effect of ageing on the bladder that has led to a reconsideration of this historical attitude. Nonetheless, the attitude that only obstruction mattered has established the primacy of the pressure–flow relationship in the objective assessment of benign prostatic hyperplasia in clinical practice.

Urinary obstruction can be regarded as being present when intravesical pressure has to be raised in order to maintain the urinary flow rate. When an elevated intravesical pressure can no longer maintain the urinary flow rate, the flow rate begins to decline. Thus, in the first stage of obstruction, voiding detrusor pressure is raised above the upper limit of normal (which is about 50 cmH$_2$O) but the peak urinary flow rate is still greater than 15 ml/s, which is the lower limit of normal. In the second stage of obstruction, the peak urinary flow rate drops below 15 ml/s.

This relationship between pressure and flow was likened by Griffiths [75] to the Hill equation, which was a well-established and widely accepted means of describing the relationship between the force of contraction and the speed of shortening of skeletal muscle. Griffiths, by relating detrusor pressure to flow rate in what he called the 'bladder output relation', showed that the two relationships were very similar. He also introduced the concept of the 'urethral resistance relationship' by relating flow rate to detrusor pressure throughout the period of a voiding detrusor contraction [76]. In this way, he was able to distinguish graphically (Figure 13.11) between an obstructed system, in which pressure was high and flow was low, and an unobstructed system, in which pressure was low and flow was high. In practice, rather than plot the continuous relationship graphically, Abrams and Griffiths [77] devised a nomogram on which could be plotted the single point of detrusor pressure at maxi-

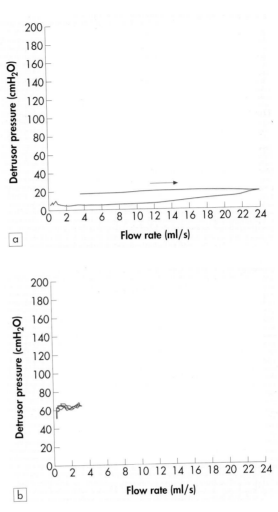

Figure 13.11 *(a) A dynamic pressure–flow plot during voiding to illustrate normal emptying with low pressure and high flow. (b) A dynamic pressure–flow plot of so-called compressive bladder outflow obstruction due to benign prostatic hyperplasia – with high pressure and low flow.*

mum urinary flow rate (Figure 13.12). Several other physicists, notably Schafer, have devised more sophisticated techniques for the analysis of pressure–flow data, but they are all based on the same principles [78, 79].

The two main reasons why physicists are continuing to analyse this pressure–flow relationship are, firstly, to be able to express it in a single term rather than as a relationship between two variables, particularly if this could be determined non-invasively, and, secondly, to minimise the equivocal zone.

The desire to find a non-invasive way of extrapolating the pressure–flow relationship is obviously commendable but has so far been unsuccessful.

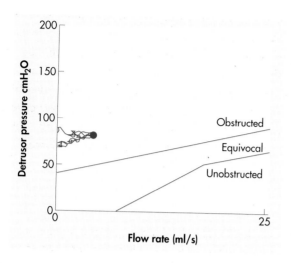

Figure 13.12 *An obstructive pressure–flow plot, similar to Figure 13.11b, superimposed on the Abrams–Griffiths nomogram. Normally, only the detrusor pressure at maximum flow (the dot) would be marked on the plot – this figure illustrates the principle.*

Nonetheless, in the interests of patient comfort and as it is a quick, simple, cheap and easy test to use, the problem has been circumvented in routine clinical practice by measuring flow rate alone and by inferring the pressure–flow relationship from this measurement [77]. In this way, most unobstructed patients with normal flow rates can be saved from ineffective and inappropriate obstruction-relieving surgery. Unfortunately, a low flow rate is not exclusively due to high pressure–low flow outflow obstruction; a low flow rate may also be due to a poorly contracting detrusor.

Poor detrusor contractility also accounts for most of the equivocal results on pressure–flow analysis. Poor detrusor contractility characteristically shows normal or low detrusor pressure and low flow, and this is very common, with an incidence that increases with age. Indeed, as a general rule, all men over the age of 80 have a maximum flow rate of less than 10 ml/s [80].

Thus, we appear to have three independent variables determining the clinical picture – symptoms, benign prostatic hyperplasia and bladder outflow obstruction – each of which, as has been said, may be confounded by two age-related abnormalities of detrusor contractility – impaired detrusor contractility and detrusor instability. Irritative symptoms in men with or without benign prostatic hyperplasia

correlate strongly with the presence of detrusor instability on urodynamic evaluation [81], and this presumably accounts, at least in part, for the observation that symptom scores are the same in an unselected population of elderly women (in whom detrusor instability is equally common) as they are in an unselected population of elderly men [82]. By contrast, objectively demonstrable obstruction correlates poorly with symptoms [83], presumably because obstructive symptoms are less 'bothersome', although those with bothersome obstructive symptoms who have objectively demonstrable obstruction, rather than low pressure–low flow bladders due to impaired detrusor contractility, do best after transurethral resection of the prostate [84].

Detrusor instability is clearly an important factor in the patient with benign prostatic hyperplasia, whether it is a secondary consequence of obstruction or coincidental. Nocturia and daytime urgency and frequency are the commonest reasons why elderly men seek medical attention [85], and although there are other causes of these symptoms, detrusor instability is the commonest reason for all these symptoms being present together.

It is generally thought that most instances of detrusor instability in patients with benign prostatic hyperplasia are secondary to obstruction, and that 70% or so will improve symptomatically after transurethral resection of the prostate because the obstruction has been relieved, allowing the detrusor to recover and the pathophysiological changes to reverse. Various experimental studies support this view [86], although they have failed to show complete recovery after relief of obstruction, only a tendency to improve. The alternative view is that detrusor instability in these patients is an entirely age-related phenomenon in both sexes that coincidentally develops at the same time as benign prostatic hyperplasia in men, and that the reason why so many men improve after transurethral resection of the prostate is related to denervation (or de-afferentation, to be more accurate) produced by this surgical procedure [87, 88].

Impaired detrusor contractility is more problematic. Like detrusor instability, this is common in the elderly of both sexes and is a regular cause of dissatisfaction in male patients who have undergone transurethral resection of the prostate because they were thought to be obstructed [89]. Unlike detrusor instability, which regularly seems to resolve after this operation, impaired detrusor contractility rarely, if ever, improves. This is the first reason for suggesting that impaired detrusor contractility is an independent age-related condition rather than secondary to obstruction, as has always been assumed. The second reason is that experimental models of obstruction cause a thick-walled, trabeculated, high-pressure, unstable bladder and not chronic retention [90]. Thus, the view that impaired contractility – causing residual urine initially, progressing eventually to chronic retention with overflow incontinence – arises as a result of decompensation of the detrusor in the face of continuing obstruction after an initial phase of compensation seems flawed. It may be that if obstruction is superimposed on impaired detrusor contractility, the consequences are correspondingly more severe, and it may be that these patients are prone to high-pressure retention and renal impairment as a result. Either way, impaired detrusor contractility is common in elderly men and women, and may be complicated by superadded detrusor instability in some [91], suggesting that in many, if not all, males with benign prostatic hyperplasia, impaired contractility is an independent variable unrelated to obstruction in its cause.

And so the diagnostic quandary persists. Obstruction is still the only problem that can reliably and predictably be treated, and urodynamic studies that measure both detrusor pressure and urinary flow during voiding are still the only way to diagnose obstruction reliably. With a clinical problem that is so common, this poses logistic problems and, as obstruction is only one part of the picture, the problems are compounded. Nonetheless, a normal flow rate will virtually exclude obstruction and such patients might be treated by any of the various non-surgical treatments currently available and discussed in detail elsewhere. Otherwise, these patients might benefit from simple reassurance and discussion. Those with a reduced flow rate and a little or no residual urine can confidently be diagnosed as obstructed and treated accordingly. Those with a substantial residual urine volume (250 ml or more on repeated assessment) may have an obstructive component to their symptoms but are more likely to have impaired detrusor contractility, and the likelihood of this increases as the residual urine volume and the patient's age increase, and the likelihood that transurethral resection of the prostate will help these patients symptomatically or objectively decreases accordingly. There are various caveats to these generalisations, but at least they form a basis for considering the problems in clinical practice.

References

1. Lowsley O. The development of the human prostate gland with reference to the development of other structures at the neck of the urinary bladder. Am J Anat 1912; 13: 299–346

2. McNeal JE. The zonal anatomy of the prostate. Prostate 1981; 2(1): 35–49

3. McNeal JE. The prostate gland: morphology and pathology. Monogr Urol 1983; 4: 3–6

4. McNeal JE. The prostate gland: morphology and pathobiology. Monogr Urol 1988; 9: 3–4

5. McNeal JE. Normal histology of the prostate. Am J Surg Pathol 1988; 12: 619–33

6. Gormley G, Stoner E, Bruskewitz R, et al. The effect of finasteride in men with benign prostatic hyperplasia. N Engl J Med 1992; 327: 1185–91

7. Wilson J, Griffin J, Russell D. Steroid five alpha reductase (II) deficiency. Endocr Rev 1993; 14: 577–93

8. Schweikert H, Totzauer P, Rohr H, Bartschi G. Correlated biochemical and stereological studies on testosterone metabolism in the stromal and epithelial compartment of human benign prostatic hyperplasia. J Urol 1985; 134: 403–7

9. Camps J, Chang S, Hsu T, et al. Fibroblast-mediated acceleration of human epithelial tumour growth in vivo. Proc Natl Acad Sci USA 1990; 87: 75–9

10. Cunha G, Battle E, Young P, et al. Role of epithelial–mesenchymal interactions in the differentiation and spacial organisation of visceral smooth muscle. Epith Cell Biol 1992; 1: 76–83

11. Bruchovski N, Lesser B, Van Doorn E, Craven S. Hormonal effects of cell proliferation in rat prostate. Vitamin Horm 1975; 33: 61–102

12. Lee C, Sensibar J, Dudek S, et al. Prostatic ductal system in rats: regional variation in morphological and functional activities. Biol Reprod 1990; 43: 1079–86

13. Begun F, Story MT, Hopp K, et al. Regional concentration of basic fibroblast growth factor in normal and

benign hyperplastic human prostates. J Urol 1995; 153: 839–43

14. Story MT, Hopp KA, Meier DA, *et al.* Influence of transforming growth factor beta 1 and other growth factors on basic fibroblast growth factor level and proliferation of cultured human prostate-derived fibroblasts. Prostate 1993; 22: 183–97

15. Taylor TB, Ramsdell JS. Transforming growth factor alpha and its receptor are expressed on the epithelium of the rat prostate gland. Endocrinology 1993; 113: 1306–8

16. Gosling JA, Dixon DS. The structure and innervation of smooth muscle in the wall of the bladder neck and proximal urethra. Br J Urol 1975; 47: 549–52

17. Hedlund H, Anderson K, Larsson B. Alpha adrenoceptors and muscarinic receptors in the isolated human prostate. J Urol 1985; 134: 1291–3

18. Bartsch G, Muller H, Oberholzer M, Rohr H. Light microscopic and stereological analysis of the normal human prostate and of benign prostatic hyperplasia. J Urol 1979; 122: 487–91

19. Shapiro E, Hartanto V, Lepor H. The response to alpha blockade in benign prostatic hyperplasia is related to the percent area density of prostate smooth muscle. Prostate 1992; 21: 297–307

20. Bylund D, Eikenberg D, Hieble J, *et al.* International Union of Phamacology nomenclature of adrenoceptors. Pharmacol Rev 1994; 45: 703–9

21. Forray C, Bard J, Wetzel J, *et al.* The alpha-1 adrenergic receptor that mediates smooth muscle contraction in the human prostate has the pharmacological properties of the cloned human alpha-1c subtype. Mol Pharmacol 1994; 45: 703–9

22. Gu J, Polak J, Probert L, *et al.* Peptidergic innervation of the human male genital tract. J Urol 1983; 130: 386–91

23. Lieberman C, Nogimori T, Wu CF *et al.* Acta Endocrinol (Copenh) 1989; 120: 134–42

24. Crowe, R, Chapple C, Burnstock G. The human prostate gland: a histochemical and immunohistochemical study of neuropeptides, serotonin, dopamine beta hydroxylase and acetylcholinesterase in autonomic nerves and ganglia. Br J Urol 1991; 68: 53–61

25. Brindley, G. Pathophysiology of erection and ejaculation. In: Hendry W, Whitfield H (eds). A textbook of genitourinary surgery. London: Churchill Livingstone, 1988: 1083–94

26. Gil-Vernet J, Alvarez-Vijande R, Gil-Vernet J Jr. Ejaculation in men: a dynamic endorectal ultrasonographical study. Br J Urol 1994; 73; 442–8

27. Tauber PF, Zaneveld LJD, Propping D, Schumacher GF. Components of human split ejaculate. J Reprod Fertil 1975; 43: 249–67

28. Kennedy AM, Morrell JM, Siviter RJ, Cockle SM. Fertilisation promoting peptide in reproductive tissues and semen of the male marmoset. Mol Reprod Dev 1997; 47(1): 113–19

29. Williams-Ashman HG, Cannellakis ZN. Polyamines in mammalian biology and medicine. Perspect Biol Med 1979; 22: 421–53

30. Lilja H. Structure and function of prostatic and seminal vesicle-secreted proteins involved in the gelatin and liquefaction of human semen. Scand J Lab Invest 1988; 48(Suppl): 13–17

31. Coffey DS. Physiology of male reproduction: the biochemical and physiology of the prostate and seminal vesicles. In: Harrison JH, Gittes RF, Perlmutter AD *et al.* (eds) Cambell's urology, Vol. 1, 4th edition. Philadelphia: WB Saunders, 1978: 61–94

32. Fair WR, Wehner N. The prostatic antibacterial factor: identity and significance. In: Marberger H (ed) Prostatic disease, Vol. 6. New York: Alan R Liss, 1976: 383

33. Grayhack JT, Kropp KA. Changes with aging in prostatic fluid: citric acid and phosphatase and lactic dehydrogenase concentration in man. J Urol 1965; 56: 6–11

34. Kvist U. Reversible inhibition of nuclear chromatin decondensation (NCD) ability of human spermatozoa induced by prostatic fluid. Acta Physiol Scand 1980; 109: 73–8

35. Kvist U. Importance of spermatozoal zinc as temporary inhibitor of sperm nuclear chromatin decondensation ability in man. Acta Physiol Scand 1980; 109: 79–84

36. Kvist U, Kjellberg J, Bjorndahl L, Santir JC, Arver S. Seminal fluid from men with agenesis of the Wolffian ducts: zinc binding properties and effects on sperm chromatin stability. Int J Androl 1990; 13: 245–52

37. Greenwald P, Kirmes V, Polan A, Dick V. Cancer of the prostate among men with BPH. J Natl Cancer Inst 1974; 355: 53–6

38. Carter H, Plantadosi S, Isaacs J. Clinical evidence for and implications of the multistep development of prostate cancer. J Urol 1990; 143: 742–6

39. Spiro L, Labay G, Orkin L. Prostatic infarction: role in acute urinary retention. Urology 1974; 3: 345–7

40. Cuchi A. The development of detrusor instability in prostatic obstruction in relation to sequential changes in voiding dynamics. J Urol 1994; 51: 1342–4

41. Levin R, Longhurst P, Monson F, *et al.* Effect of bladder

outlet obstruction on the morphology, physiology and pharmacology of the bladder. Prostate 1990; 3 (Suppl.): 9–26

42. Glynn R, Campion E, Bouchard G, Silbert J. The development of benign prostatic hyperplasia among volunteers in the normative aging study. Am J Epidemiol l985; 121(1): 78–90

43. Adlercreutz H. Western diet and Western diseases: some hormonal and biochemical mechanisms and associations. Scan J Clin Invest 1990; 50 (Suppl.): 3–23

44. Sanda M, Beatty T, Stautzman R. Genetic susceptibility of benign prostatic hyperplasia. J Urol 1994; 151: 115–19

45. Cunha G, Battle E, Young P, et al. Role of epithelial–mesenchymal interactions in the differentiation and spatial organisation of visceral smooth muscle. Epith Cell Biol 1992; 1: 76–83

46. McNeal JE. Origin and evolution of benign prostatic enlargement. Invest Urol 1978; 15: 340–5

47. Eble JN, Tejada E. Prostatic stromal hyperplasia with bizarre nuclei. Arch Pathol Lab Med 1991; 115: 87–9

48. Leong SS, Vogt PF, Yu GM. Atypical stroma with muscle hyperplasia of the prostate. Urology 1988; 31: 163–7

49. McNeal JE. The pathobiology of nodular hyperplasia. In: Bostwick DG (ed) Pathology of the prostate. New York: Churchill Livingstone, 1990: 31–6

50. Franks LM. Benign nodular hyperplasia of the prostate: a review. Ann R Coll Surg Engl 1954; 14: 92–106

51. Partin AW, Oesterling JE, Epstein JI, et al. Influence of age and endocrine factors on the volume of benign prostatic hyperplasia. J Urol 1991; 145: 405–9

52. Isaacs JT. Antagonistic effect of androgen on prostatic cell death. Prostate 1984; 5: 545–7

53. Sensibar JA, Griswold MD, Sylvester SR, et al. Prostatic ductal system in rats: regional variation in localisation of an androgen-repressed gene product, sulphated glycoprotein-2. Endocrinology 1991; 128: 2091–102

54. Steiner MS. Review of peptide growth factors in benign prostatic hyperplasia and urological malignancy. J Urol 1995; 153; 1085–96

55. Gregory H, Willshire IR, Kavanagh JP, et al. Urogastrone-epidermal growth factor concentrations in prostatic fluid of normal individuals and patients with benign prostatic hypertrophy. Clin Sci 1986; 70: 359–63

56. Folkman J, Klagsbrun M, Sane J, et al. Heparin-binding angiogenic protein – basic fibroblast growth factor – is stored within the basement membrane. Am J Pathol 1988; 130: 393–400

57. Ku PT, D'amore P. Regulation of fibroblast growth factor (bFGF) gene and protein expression following its release from sublethally injured endothelial cells. J Cell Biochem 1995; 58: 328–43

58. Yan G, Fukabovi Y, Nikolaropoulos S. Heparin-binding keratinocyte growth factor is a candidate for stromal to epithelial andromedin. Mol Endocrinol 1992; 6: 2123–8

59. Yan G, Fukabovi Y, McBride G, et al. Exon switching and activation of stromal and embryonic fibroblast growth factor (FGF)–FGF-receptor genes in prostate epithelial cells accompany stromal independence and malignancy. Mol Cell Biol 1993; 13: 4513–22

60. Sporn MB, Roberts AB. TFT-beta: problems and prospects. Cell Regul 1990; 1: 875–82

61. Brogli E, Wu T, Namiki A, Isner JM. Indirect angiogenic cytokines upregulate VEGF and bFGF gene expression in vascular smooth muscle cells, whereas hypoxia upregulates VEGF expression only. Circulation 1994; 90: 649–52

62. Roberts AB, Sporn MB. Physiological actions and clinical applications of transforming growth factor-beta (TGF-β). Growth Factors 1993; 8: 1–9

63. Timme TL, Truong LD, Merz VL, et al. Mesenchymal epithelial interactions and transforming growth factor beta expression during mouse prostate morphogenesis. Endocrinology 1994; 134: 1039–45

64. Millan FA, Denhez F, Kondaiah P, Akhurst RJ. Embryonic gene expression patterns of TGF beta-1, beta-2 and beta-3 suggest different development functions in vivo. Development 1991; 111: 131–43

65. Sporn MB, Roberts AB. Interactions of retinoids and transforming growth factor beta in regulation of cell differentiation and proliferation. Mol Endocrinol 1991; 5: 3–7

66. Katz AE, Benson MC, Wise GL, et al. Gene activity during the early phase of androgen-stimulated rat prostatic regrowth. Cancer Res 1989; 49; 5889–94

67. Boyarski S, Jones G, Paulson DF, et al. A new look at bladder neck obstruction by the Food and Drug Administration regulators: guidelines for the investigation of benign prostatic hypertrophy. Trans Am Assoc Genitourin Surg 1977; 68: 29–32

68. Madsen PO, Iversen P. A point system for selecting operative candidates. In: Hinman F Jr (ed) Benign prostatic hypertrophy. New York: Springer-Verlag, 1983: 763–5

69. Barry MJ, Fowler FJ, O'Leary MP, *et al*. The American Urological Association symptom index for benign prostatic hyperplasia. J Urol 1992; 148: 1549–57

70. McConnell JD, Barry MJ, Bruskewitz RC *et al*. Benign prostatic hyperplasia: diagnosis and treatment. In: Clinical practice guidelines, No. 8. Rockville, MD: US Department of Health and Human Services, 1994: 99–103

71. Emberton M, Neal DE, Black N, *et al*. The effect of prostatectomy on symptom severity and quality of life. Br J Urol 1996; 77: 233–47

72. Tubaro A, Ogden C, de la Rosette J, *et al*. The prediction of clinical outcome from thermotherapy by pressure flow study. Results of a European multicentre study. World J Urol 1994; 12: 352–6

73. Neal DE, Styles RA, Powell PH, Ramsden PD. Relationships between detrusor function and residual urine in men undergoing prostatectomy. Br J Urol 1987; 60: 560–6

74. George NJR, Feneley RCL, Roberts JBM. Identification of the poor risk patient with prostatism and detrusor failure. Br J Urol 1986; 58: 290–5

75. Griffiths DJ. Urodynamics: the mechanics and hydrodynamics of the lower urinary tract. Medical physics handbook 4. Bristol: Adam Hilger, 1980

76. Griffiths DJ. Urethral resistance to flow: the urethral resistance relation. Urol Int 1975; 30: 28

77. Abrams PH, Griffiths DJ. The assessment of prostatic obstruction from urodynamic measurements and from residual urine. Br J Urol 1979; 51: 129–34

78. Van Mastrigt R, Rollema HJ. Urethral resistance and urinary bladder contractility before and after transurethral resection as determined by the computer program CLIM. Neurol Urodyn 1988; 7: 226–30

79. Schafer W. Principles and clinical application of advanced urodynamic analysis of voiding function. Urol Clin North Am 1990; 17: 553–66

80. Jorgensen JB, Jensen KME, Morgensen P. Age-related variation in urinary flow variables and flow cure patterns in elderly males. Br J Urol 1992; 69: 265–71

81. Olssen CA, Goluboft ET, Chang DT, Kaplan SA. Urodynamics and the etiology of post-prostatectomy incontinence. J Urol 1994; 151: 2063–5

82. Lepor H, Machi G. Comparison of AUA symptom index in unselected males and females between fifty-five and seventy-nine years of age. Urology 1993; 42: 36–40

83. Barry MJ, Cockett ATK, Holtgrewe HL, *et al*. Relationship of symptoms of prostatism to commonly used physiological and anatomical measures of the severity of benign prostatic hyperplasia. J Urol 1993; 150: 351–6

84. Abrams P. In support of pressure flow studies for evaluating men with lower urinary tract symptoms. Urology 1994; 44: 153–5

85. Roberts RO, Rhodes T, Panser LA. Natural history of prostatism: worry and embarrassment of firm urinary symptoms and health care-seeking behaviour. Urology 1994; 43: 621–8

86. Malkowiez SB, Sein AJ, Elbadawi A, *et al*. Acute biochemical and functional alterations in the partially obstructed rabbit urinary bladder. J Urol 1986; 136: 1324–9

87. Susset JG. The effect of aging and prostatic obstruction on detrusor morphology and function. In: Hinman C (ed) Benign prostatic hypertrophy. New York: Springer Verlag, 1985: 653–65

88. Luutzeyer W, Hannapel J, Schafer W. Sequential events in prostatic obstruction. In: Hinman C (ed) Benign prostatic hypertrophy. New York: Springer Verlag, 1985: 693–700

89. Schafer W, Rubben H, Noppeney R, Deutz FJ. Obstructed and unobstructed prostatic obstruction. A plea for urodynamic objectivation of bladder outflow obstruction in benign prostatic hyperplasia. World J Urol 1989; 6: 198–203

90. Dixon J, Gilpin C, Gilpin S, *et al*. Sequential morphologic changes in the pig detrusor in response to chronic partial urethral obstruction. Br J Urol 1989; 64: 385–90

91. Coolsaet BRLA, Blok C. Detrusor properties related to prostatism. Neurourol Urodyn 1986; 5: 435–41

Energy sources in urology

14

T. H. Lynch and J. M. Fitzpatrick

Surgical diathermy

History

In 1890, the Italian surgeon Bottini presented the first recorded results of the transurethral use of cautery on the neck of the bladder and prostate. D'Arsonoval recognised the effects of muscle contractions with low frequency and then the development of heat in the tissues with higher frequencies. In 1911, in the USA, Clark developed a spark-gap generator, and in the 1920s, WT Bovie (a physicist) and Harvey Cushing (a neurosurgeon) designed the first surgical diathermy machine having the capability of both cutting and haemostasis.

Although the word diathermy – a Greek derivative meaning 'through heat' – has become a household word, it is a misnomer because heating is only at the points of application as the alternating current passes through the tissues.

Diathermy machines work in the range of radio frequencies used by radio stations. It was for this reason that their use was withdrawn during the Second World War except in properly screened operating theatres, and these machines were also used effectively to interfere with the German frequency generators used to direct night-time bombing raids.

Basic principles

Diathermy machines convert ordinary 240-volt alternating current into high-frequency current, which is conducted through the body. The operating frequency varies from 300 to 3000 kHz. This high frequency produces sufficient heating for cutting or diathermy without causing muscle contractions. Spark-gap gener-

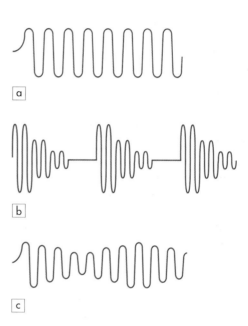

Figure 14.1 *(a) Pure sine wave alternating current: cutting current with minimal tissue damage and no haemostatis. (b) Undamaged interrupted current coagulation. (c) Blended current: cuts with coagulation; mild haemostatis.*

ators were in common usage in the past, whereas transistorised generators are more the norm today.

It is the interruption of the sine wave that is responsible for coagulation and, if the interval between shorter bursts is increased, then more effective coagulation is achieved (Figure 14.1). If the bursts are increased in length with a consequent decrease in the interval, the current will be more cutting until a pure sine wave is achieved, giving the purest cutting. By altering this wave form, any combination of coagulation and cutting can be achieved, thus giving a blend. Increased amplitude of current is required to make up for periods of inactivity during the gap.

The blended current is used when surrounding tissue destruction is required such as with resection of bladder tumours. The benefits here are twofold: deeper destruction of tumour and greater coagulation of deeper blood vessels. This can also be helpful for transurethral resection of the prostate for carcinoma of the prostate to destroy deeper malignant tissue.

Isolated output systems are in common usage today. These machines allow little or no current to flow to earth and provide a high degree of safety if there is a fault in the circuit. Even with these isolated systems, diathermy current can pass to earth if the plate is left accidentally on the diathermy machine or left in contact with the table.

With the earthed system, the current can pass through an alternative route back to the unit, such as through electrocardiogram leads or patient contact with the table, leading to severe burns.

Active electrode and patient plate
There are different types for different requirements. The basic idea is that the active electrode is made small enough to concentrate the heat at a point where it is needed and the passive electrode large enough to dissipate the heat produced (a minimum conduction area of $70 \, \text{cm}^2$ ($10 \, \text{inches}^2$) is recommended).

If both the active electrode and the patient plate were of the same size, then a heating effect of equal intensity would be produced. If both electrodes are small, then a burn will be produced at both electrodes. The most serviceable plate in use is the aluminium foil plate, which requires no cream. For transurethral surgery, it can be placed under the buttocks or on the thigh.

This active electrode may be activated by foot or by hand.

Clinical application

When a short-wave current passes through living tissue and back to the generator via the indifferent electrode, one of three specific functions is produced: coagulation, fulguration or cutting (Figure 14.2).

Coagulation
If the intensity and/or time of application is increased, a point is reached at which coagulation is achieved due

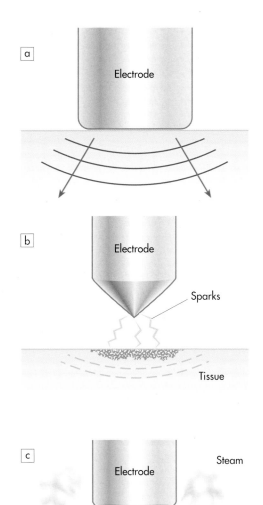

Figure 14.2 (a) Coagulation: the electrode is in contact with the tissue, and coagulation spreads radially. (b) Fulguration: there is a gap between the electrode and tissue, and coagulation is followed by fulguration. (c) Cutting: a thin layer of steam produced by the current separates the electrode from the tissue: haemostatis is minimal.

to direct heating of the tissues. This causes spasm of the muscular vessel wall, explaining why diathermy is more effective on arteries than on veins. The current also changes the polarity of the plasma, leading to thrombus formation, and causes the drying out of cells. Electrodes should be placed directly on the vessel in order to minimise surrounding dead tissue, which would give a greater risk of infection and secondary haemorrhage when the slough separates. The practice of passing the diathermy roller over the bed of the prostate should be discouraged for this same reason.

Fulguration

As the intensity or the time is increased, extensive charring of the tissues is seen. Although used by some surgeons to achieve quicker haemostasis, it should be avoided as fulgurating diathermy results in much deeper tissue destruction, which delays healing. Fulguration is of use, however, for the destruction of tumours in the bladder and rectum.

Cutting

At maximum power, a further stage is reached whereby a continuous arc passes from the electrode to the tissues, producing a high quality of heat per second that vaporises the body cells, with consequent cutting.

Underwater cutting can only be achieved with a pure sine wave, as previously discussed, and greater energy output is required than in open surgery. Diathermy requirements are between 125 and 250 W for normal cutting and 40 and 75 W for coagulation.

Machines are generally standarised to a maximum of 400 W output power. Output power remains the same for any given patient but may vary between patients, depending on differing impedance between the fat and the thin. Fat has a high resistance to current.

With certain generators, the arc will not develop if the loop is in contact with the tissues.

The object should be to obtain a good, clean cut with minimal local tissue damage causing adherence of tissue debris, thus the current should be little more than the minimum required.

A small amount of diathermy also takes place, producing less bleeding and tissue trauma than when a scalpel is used.

Dangers and precautions

The aim of diathermy safety should be to prevent mains voltage from entering the patient circuit. For this current to be lethal, it must find a path to earth through the patient; thus, all equipment should be earth free. The following are useful points.

1. Diathermy should be used with care on pedunculated structures such as the penis or a testis removed from the scrotum. The vessel could coagulate at the narrowest part of the pedunculated structure: the so-called channelling effect.

2. Flammable anaesthetic gases (ether and cyclopropane) are no longer a real problem as they are rarely used. Nonetheless, sparks are prohibited within 25 cm of the anaesthetic gases, as directed by the Department of Health.

3. Electrocution is rare with regularly serviced machines.

4. It is possible for surgical diathermy to ignite alcohol given off by skin preparation that may pool in areas such as the umbilicus or the vagina. For this reason, care should be taken to dry the skin following cleansing. A mixture of gases including oxygen may accumulate in the bladder at the time of resection, particularly of bladder tumours. If these gases are allowed to accumulate, a small explosion may occur, which has been known to rupture the bladder. With continuous irrigation systems, the bladder should be 'vented' from time to time during a long resection.

5. The greatest hazard is the thermoelectrical burn. The cause of such burns is nearly always poor plate-to-patient contact, inadvertent activation of the foot switch, or a break in the cable. If the plate becomes marginally dislodged during a procedure and the surgeon has to turn up the power to get the same effect, the patient may get a nasty burn at the site of the plate.

In general, the isolated diathermy unit offers a certain degree of safety over the earthed system. With the former, the current is greatly reduced or cut off completely, alerting the theatre staff to check the connections. With an earthed system, the current will find an alternative route back to the unit, such as through the stirrups or arm rest, and a burn will occur at this site.

6. When the effectiveness of a diathermy machine is not optimal, the temptation is to turn up the power. However, this should not be done until possible faults have been checked:
   (a) a faulty foot switch connection,
   (b) a faulty active electrode,
   (c) poor patient/plate contact,

(d) a cable problem,

(e) internal failure of the diathermy machine.

7. Diathermy burns with earthed machines may occur at the site of electrocardiogram leads if the current should pass out through these leads. This is usually prevented from happening by:

   (a) not placing electrocardiogram leads between the operative site and the patient plate;

   (b) ensuring that the electrocardiogram machine has a radiofrequency filter fitted to the monitor, preventing the passage of current through it;

   (c) incorporating a 10 000-ohm resistor in the extremity of each lead, which can prevent burns if the indifferent electrode is broken.

8. A noise of activation is incorporated into all diathermy machines to overcome the risk of inadvertent activation and consequential burning of a patient. In general, there is a different noise for different applications.

9. The cable from the patient plate generally has two cores. This cable carries a small circulating current in addition to the main current and if there is any loss of continuity, an alarm will sound and the current is automatically cut off.

10. The diathermy plate should be big enough, as previously discussed, and not folded for any reason. Shave the underlying hair to allow for good contact and make sure the area is dry before and during use. Place the plate as close to the operative site as possible.

11. Ensure that all metallic parts of cables are earth free and insulated.

12. Saline should not be used for transurethral resection as it conducts current and no local cutting or diathermy effect will be seen. If saline is used inadvertently and the surgeon turns the diathermy machine up to get the desired cutting effect, the machine may be irreparably damaged; 1.5% glycine is probably the safest and simplest solution to use.

Surgical diathermy and other theatre equipment

Much of the other equipment used in theatre is earthed and may therefore be hazardous unless specifically protected. Metallic parts of light cables and video cameras that attach to endoscopes are earth free, making them safe for use.

Pacemakers

Modern pacemakers show little or no response to diathermy machines and transurethral resection can generally be performed without harm to most patients if the electrodes are placed at a distance from the pacemaker. There are, however, two types of pacemaker that can give rise to problems:

1. the demand pacemaker, which takes over only if the ventricular rate falls below a certain predetermined level;

2. the synchryonous P wave pacemaker for heart block, which picks up the P wave and provides a stimulus to the ventricles after an appropriate P–R interval.

Problems peculiar to transurethral resection

Although surgical diathermy is used extensively in surgical practice today, there is no area in which it is used more than in transurethral surgery. The finer the electrode used, the cleaner and more effective the cut. However, these fine electrodes can bend very easily. If the loop is too thick, if clean, brisk sweeps are not taken through the tissues, or if the power is too low, then tissue will stick to the electrode. Although resectoscope sheaths or their tips are generally made from insulating material, this is not an absolute requirement because the surface area of a 24 Ch sheath is approximately 35 cm^2 and this is perfectly adequate to disperse the current without causing any damage to the urethra or surrounding structures.

The advantages of the all-metal sheath are:

1. a smaller circumference is required for the same luminal size as the thickness of the metal is smaller;

2. it gives a cleaner cut at the end of resection as the arc is in direct contact with the sheath.

Bipolar diathermy

Both the active and the return electrodes (patient plate) are combined within one electrode. A patient plate is not required as no current passes through the patient. A disadvantage is that cutting is virtually impossible.

Lasers

Laser stands for the light amplification by stimulated emission of radiation. Normal atoms exist with their electrons in a low-energy configuration. If external energy is applied, these atoms can be forced into a higher energy level (Figure 14.3). This higher energy level is unstable and these atoms quickly revert to a lower energy configuration and in so doing emit energy in the form of photons of light. The non-parallel light is dissipated, whereas the parallel light is reflected back and forth by mirrors within the laser cavity (Figure 14.4). These photons of light may cause further atoms to rise to a higher energy level, releasing further photons. This process causes the light to become amplified.

Thus, a laser generates a parallel, monochromatic beam of light. Lasers differ primarily in the wavelength of the light emitted by the active medium. Laser wavelengths cover the entire visible portion of the electromagnetic spectrum as well as wavelengths in the ultraviolet and infrared portions. With certain wavelengths, the beam can be propagated along a flexible fibre with little energy loss. The light may be delivered in the form of a continuous wave (more common in urology) or in the form of multiple pulses known as pulsed lasers.

The absorption of tissues varies according to the wavelength. Regardless of the method of delivery, the tissue effects may be characterised as thermal, mechanical or photochemical. The more common lasers in use in urology are the carbon dioxide laser, the argon laser and the neodymium-yttrium aluminium-garnet laser (Nd:YAG). High-power lasers such as holmium:YAG and KTP:YAG are now commercially available. The pulsed-dye laser usually refers to a laser lithotriptor and is discussed in the section on stones (Chapter 8).

Effects of laser

Thermal effect
If normal body temperature is increased from 37°C to 60°C, no change in tissue structure is discernible. However, above 60°C, tissue coagulation begins. This results in cell death with no loss in the integrity of the tissue. Above 100°C, carbonisation and vaporisation occur.

Mechanical effect
A low-energy laser with a short pulsed duration can produce mechanical fragmentation of a stone, which is discussed later in this chapter.

Photochemical effect
Low-power laser energy light can activate photochemically a drug such as haematoporphyrin derivative, which then becomes cytotoxic and causes cell death. After systemic administration of the drug, it is retained by malignant cells rather than normal tissue. The exact method of cellular death is uncertain.

Types of laser
The name of each laser type refers to the medium used.

Carbon dioxide laser
Carbon dioxide molecules are the active medium and emit light with a wavelength of 10 600 nm in the infrared portion of the spectrum. The energy is

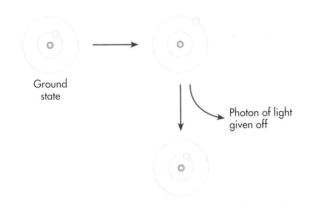

Figure 14.3 *Atoms are forced into a higher energy level, which is unstable. These atoms quickly revert to a lower energy level and emit photons of light.*

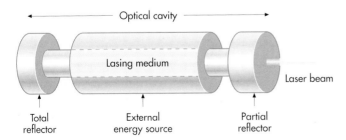

Figure 14.4 *Diagrammatic representation of a laser.*

absorbed almost entirely by water, thus its effects do not penetrate deeply and it produces intense heat and vaporisation at the point of impact. This surface heating allows it to be used as a type of surgical scalpel and it is particularily useful for various lesions of the external genitalia.

Argon laser

Transmission has a blue-colour emission between 488 and 514 nm. It is poorly absorbed by water and selectively absorbed by melanin and haemoglobin, and is therefore useful for pigmented lesions and those with a high blood perfusion. Its tissue penetration is about 1.0 nm and it can be readily transmitted down a flexible scope, making it useful for superficial bladder tumours. Because the argon laser will pass through clear peritoneal tissues, it is an excellent laser to vaporise endometriotic lesions.

Neodymium-Yttrium Aluminium-Garnet (Nd:YAG) laser

The Nd:YAG laser is the most versatile and widely used laser in urology. The medium is a solid crystal of yttrium aluminium garnet containing neodymium, which emits a wavelength of 1060 nm in the infrared region. As the beam is invisible, its point of impact is defined by a low-power helium neon laser. It is poorly absorbed by water and body pigments and thus penetrates up to a depth of 5 mm, with a large area around the point of contact becoming heated. This makes it useful for the treatment of bladder tumours.

The Potassium-Titanyl Phosphate (KTP) crystal laser

The KTP crystal laser is generated by passing an Nd:YAG beam through a crystal, which doubles the frequency and halves the wavelength to 532 nm. Unlike the Nd:YAG, this laser has a clearly visible green beam but, like the argon laser, has a shallow depth of penetration (0.3–1 mm) compared to the Nd:YAG laser. Like the argon and the Nd:YAG lasers, it can be passed down the laparoscope.

Holmium Yttrium Aluminium Garnet (Ho:YAG) laser

Holmium is a rare-earth element, which, when doped in YAG, can emit laser radiation at a wavelength of 2.1 μm, with normal pulse duration of 250 ms. Thermal tissue damage is moderate, with good haemostasis, when used in the pulse mode at low pulse repetition rates.

Dye lasers

Early in laser technology, the search was on to find a device that could be tuned over a broad range of wavelengths. The dye laser was the solution to this problem, producing wavelengths in the visible part of the spectrum. These lasers are tunable. The 'dye' used is an organic dye such as is used to colour fabrics, food or other material. This dye has to be excited by another light source (another laser or flash lamp). If used in the pulsed mode, this laser can be used for stone fragmentation. The dye in these lasers must be changed at regular intervals, making them somewhat difficult and expensive to maintain.

Clinical applications

In surgery, there are only a few circumstances in which the laser can perform any surgical procedure more effectively than diathermy. Lasers have been used in almost all areas of urology, with varying degrees of success.

Although the first three types of laser have been reported to be of use for lesions of the external genitalia, the Nd:YAG seems to be superior. The largest experience appears to be with condylomata of the external genitalia and penile carcinoma.

As the carbon dioxide laser lacks a suitable delivery system and is absorbed by water, it is not suitable for endoscopic use except for meatal condylomata. The Nd:YAG is more suitable for endoscopic use such as for urethral strictures and superficial bladder tumours. It can be used with the flexible cystoscope and does not require a general anaesthetic. In theory, invasive tumours could also be treated successfully as laser irradiation leaves the bladder wall intact, thus allowing full-thickness treatment. The Nd:YAG laser can also be used for treating upper tract lesions.

The most common use of laser in urology has been for the treatment of benign prostatic hyperplasia, as discussed in Chapter 13.

Photodynamic therapy

A photosensitising agent is administered intravenously and is taken up by malignant tissues and cleared from most other tissues. Between 48 and 72 hours later, light is used to excite the photosensitiser in the presence of oxygen. A short-lived, unstable, excited state is produced, which causes cell injury and ultimately death. Although laser is a convenient mode of delivery of light, it is not a prerequisite for photodynamic therapy.

Safety with surgical lasers

All lasers used in a hospital should be the responsibility of one individual. As hazard analysis is an evolving process, it is important to understand and interpret the significance of changes relating to exposure limits that should not be exceeded.

The area where the laser is being used should be clearly marked with laser warning notices and the theatre doors should be locked when the laser is in use. The area must also be completely obscured by black curtaining to a point above eye level. Any possible surface that may reflect the laser light must be covered.

The retina is the most vulnerable to laser irradiation from 400 to 1400 nm, which spans both the visible and the near infrared spectrum. Momentary exposure will cause thermal lesions. A burn into the periphery of the retina may cause a small scotoma (blind spot), which may not be detected. If the individual is looking directly at the laser beam, a foveal burn may be sustained, destroying the centre of vision. A burn to the optic nerve can render that eye blind. In addition to these field defects, haemorrhage and debris in the vitreous can permanently impair vision. Beyond wavelengths of 1400 nm, a corneal burn may be sustained, causing permanent scarring. If the burn is minor, it will disappear within two days, which is the turnover time for corneal epithelium.

Protective eye wear should be worn and checked regularly for scratches. It is important to check that the eye wear is the correct type to protect against laser output. The eye wear should also fit well around the eyes, leaving no room for gaps through which a stray beam could reach the eye.

Staff should also be instructed not to look directly at the laser beam.

There is a greater chance of an accidental burn to the skin than to the eye. For visible and infrared radiation, the damage mechanism in skin is thermal, whereas for ultraviolet wavelengths the erythematous reaction is photochemical in nature.

Therapeutic applications of ultrasound in urology

Generation of ultrasound

Ultrasound waves are generated by electrically inducing a deformation in a solid, the particles of which are made to oscillate within the frequency of the applied ultrasonic energy – the piezoelectric effect. These vibrations produce the mechanical sound waves, which are sinusoidal in shape with alternating positive and negative deflections.

The wavelength used in clinical practice is sufficiently short to enable it to be brought to a tight focus within the body. With low output power, good resolution can be obtained for diagnostic purposes, whereas higher energy ultrasound can produce heating and cavitation.

Ultrasound waves cannot travel through a vacuum and because they lie above the frequency audible to the human ear (20 kHz), they cannot be heard. Being mechanical in nature, ultrasound waves do not ionise the medium as X-rays and gamma rays do.

The effects of ultrasound are either mechanical or thermal, and the underlying principle of diagnostic ultrasound is that short bursts of ultrasound are passed into the patient, and differing acoustic impedances give off different echoes, which are translated into images.

Thermal effects of ultrasound

In diagnostic ultrasound systems, the amount of heat dissipated has been shown to be very small. However, with the use of high intensities, significant temperature elevations can be achieved for therapeutic purposes.

A beam of high-intensity ultrasound can be brought to a focus at a selected depth within the body. This focused beam can be used to damage tissues. (For further discussion, see the section on energy sources on the prostate in Chapter 13.)

Mechanical effects of ultrasound

The mechanical effects of ultrasound are employed in contact lithotripsy, ultrasound tissue dissection and extracorporeal shock wave lithotripsy. Pyrotherapy is the therapeutic effect of extracorporeal ultrasound on tissue. (The use of ultrasound for the fragmentation of stones is discussed further in the section on stones, Chapter 8).

Ultrasound dissection

If the vibration of ultrasound probes exceeds 50 μm, the soft tissues can be disintegrated upon contact. The benefit of this is that there is minimal damage to the surrounding structures. This technology has been used in ophthalmology to assist with cataract extraction with minimal damage to the sclera. Its use in urology is limited, but has been reported in nephron-sparing surgery and it has been tested experimentally for bladder tumours and benign prostatic hyperplasia.

Ultrasonic tissue tripsy (pyrotherapy)

A combination of the negative pressure of a shock and increasing frequency of the shock can cause considerable cavitation (mechanical effect) with the focal zone of an ultrasound wave. Bubbles form within the focal zone, which eventually collapse, causing a significant increase in local temperature (thermal effect). The energy source is an adaptation of a lithotripter and early animal and human studies have been undertaken to ablate prostatic and renal tissue.

Energy sources used on the prostate

Newer treatment options for benign prostatic hyperplasia are constantly being evaluated and most newer methods rely on some form of heat damage to the prostate using different delivery systems to ablate prostatic tissue. These heat therapies have taken the form of transrectal and transurethral hyperthermia (42 °C to 45 °C), transurethral thermotherapy (>45 °C), thermoablation (>70 °C) and transurethral vaporisation.

The devices used can generate very high temperatures using lasers, high-intensity focused ultrasound waves, electrocauterisation and radio frequency (Table 14.1).

Table 14.1 Changes that living tissue undergoes depending on temperature

Temperature (°C)	Tissue changes
43–45	Tissue retracts
>50	Reduced enzymatic activity
50–60	Protein coagulates
90–100	Tissue dessication
>100	Water in tissue boils and evaporates
>150	Tissue carbonises
>300	Tissue vaporises

Electrodiathermy

Electrocautery is the most common energy source used on the prostate and is employed for the gold standard transurethral resection of the prostate. The basics of electrocautery are discussed in the first section of this chapter.

Electrovaporisation

Electrovaporisation uses a high current density to destroy tissue and has been used for several years by gynaecologists to treat endometriosis. It uses the existing electrosurgical equipment and requires no additional technical skills to be acquired by the urologist.

Several different shapes of electrodes from a variety of manufacturers are available but all have the same basic principle: they all have either ridges or spikes projected above the surface of a roller ball (Figure 14.5) that serve as points of high-power density. Vaporisation occurs when these projections come into contact with the tissues. The large area of the grooved construction causes coagulation. Vaporisation is caused by sparking from the ridges, where high current accumulates because of the small surface area. In addition, steam is trapped between the grooves, enhancing the depth of both vaporisation and coagulation.

The power settings must be increased by 25–75% over standard settings for transurethral resection, with

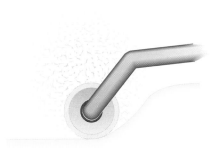

Figure 14.5 *A roller ball with ridges or spikes for electrovaporisation.*

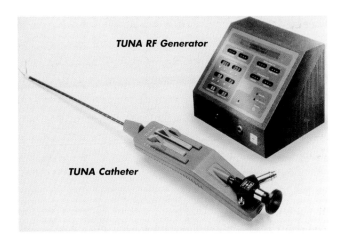

Figure 14.6 *A radiofrequency generator and transurethral needle ablation catheter.*

settings of about 230–250 W for pure cut and 60–80 W for coagulation.

Dessication, coagulation, steaming and vaporisation are all important for electrovaporisation. The initial dessication results in cellular dehydration. Coagulation causes protein bonds to form, creating a gelatinous structure. Blood vessels and lymphatics are thrombosed. Dessicated and coagulated tissues result in the accumulation of heat, leading to charring and carbonisation. During vaporisation, water changes to steam, increasing the temperature from 37 °C to 100 °C.

If low power is used initially, the increased charring and carbonisation (rather than vaporisation) will cause less vaporisation of subsequent passes of the electrode due to increased tissue impedance. It is preferable to use a higher voltage initially and, once fibres of the capsule have been identified, the power can be turned down to increase coagulation and promote haemostasis.

Transurethral needle ablation

One of the latest technologies in thermoablation is transurethral needle ablation, which uses low-level radiofrequency energy to ablate tissue. The tissues heat up as they resist the flow of a radiofrequency current. The radiofrequency energy is delivered through a specially designed catheter device, allowing selective placement of needle antennae to ablate the prostate.

Equipment

The TUNA system consists of a powered radiofrequency generator and a transurethral needle abla-

tion catheter (Figure 14.6). The generator delivers low-power (15 ± 3 W) radiofrequency energy at 482 ± 1 kHz.

The transurethral needle ablation catheter is 24 cm long and 22 Fr. in diameter. A direct viewing fibre-optic unit is introduced through its centre and it is advanced into the prostatic urethra under direct fibre-optic vision.

The catheter tip contains two needles that are deployed at an acute angle to each other and at 90° to the catheter tip (Figure 14.7). Each needle has a retractable shield to protect the urethral wall and control lesion geometry. The needles and the shields are advanced and retracted by controls on the catheter handle and can be rotated to either lateral lobe of the prostate.

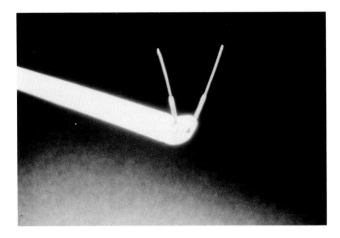

Figure 14.7 *The catheter tip contains two needles that are deployed at an acute angle to each other and at 90° to the catheter tip.*

Needle deployment is determined by taking the transverse measurement of each lateral lobe of the prostate as assessed by transrectal ultrasound. The needles should be kept at a minimum of 6 mm from the prostatic capsule.

Temperature

Temperature distribution is determined by the radius of the electrode and by the increase in temperature next to the electrode surface. The electrode's tip length determines the length of the lesion. Other parameters such as lesion current, power, voltage and build-up time also influence lesion size. The radiofrequency current and power required to achieve a given temperature may vary, depending on tissue impedance, vascularity and thermal conductivity.

A thermosensor is located at the end of both shields to monitor prostate temperature near the lesion. Another thermocouple is located on the tip of the catheter to monitor urethral temperature.

A constant and steady rise in temperature over a 5-minute treatment is expected and the temperatures often reach 500 °C or greater at the proximal edge of the lesion (shield temperature). Power output is monitored every 30 seconds and increased by 1 W if the temperature on either shield increases by less than 3 °C. Power is increased to a maximum of 11 W.

Tissue impedance is also recorded at 30-second intervals during power application. If the impedance increases during treatment, the power is decreased until it stabilises. This ensures that tissue is not charred, and a larger necrotic lesion is not produced.

Method of action

Although the mechanism of action of transurethral needle ablation is not clearly understood, earlier feasibility studies demonstrate that this treatment creates well-defined necrotic lesions within the prostate (Figure 14.8), while sparing the urethra and adjacent organs such as the rectum and bladder. Pathological studies have shown that necrotic lesions are produced and that this coagulative necrosis subsequently changes to a retractile fibrous scar. This process could result in a decrease in the volume of the treated area, although the

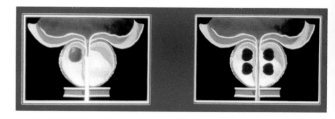

Figure 14.8 *Transurethral needle ablation treatment creates well-defined necrotic lesions within the prostate.*

entire prostatic volume is minimally changed, or a decrease in the tonus of the periurethral tissues through destruction of adrenoceptors, with effects on both dynamic and static components of obstruction, or some other mechanism within the prostatic urethra.

Lasers

Currently, there are several lasers and laser-delivery systems available. These include the initial side-firing fibres that were available to treat benign prostatic hyperplasia: the transurethral ultrasound-guided laser-induced prostatectomy (TULIP), the BARD urolase, and the contact tip laser.

The TULIP device consists of a right-angle fibre with a dilating balloon. It is guided to the prostate per urethra by ultrasound, and the balloon compresses the prostate to allow for greater penetration of the tissue. The balloon material is transparent to Nd:YAG light. The device is then pulled out at 1 mm/s, with several passes being made after rotation.

The urolase is a bare fibre passed under cystoscopic control and is thus often called visual laser-assisted prostatectomy (VLAP).

Although various protocols are available, the procedure is generally performed using 40–60 W of power from a Nd:YAG laser.

Direct contact fibres using a diode laser can also be passed under cystoscopic control, as can interstitial fibres.

The use of the Nd:YAG laser to photocoagulate the capsule of a malignant prostate after transurethral resection has also been reported. Lasers can also be used for the endoscopic destruction of ureteric calculi.

Hyperthermia and thermotherapy

Several devices have been introduced to heat the prostate either transrectally or transurethrally. They were first used in patients with prostate cancer but are now employed for patients with benign prostatic hyperplasia. The International Consensus Conference organised by the World Health Organisation on benign prostatic hyperplasia held in 1991 defined thermotherapy as being intraprostatic temperatures above 45 °C and hyperthermia as being below 45 °C. Because of the poor symptomatic relief, the Second International Consultation on benign prostatic hyperplasia recommended that hyperthermia should be abandoned.

The apparatus consists of a (915 MHz, 1296 MHz) microwave generator with a microwave radiometer for temperature measurement. For urethral application, an antenna is introduced with a Foley-type catheter, which is maintained at a constant temperature by flowing water. The Foley balloon is used to ensure accurate placement during treatment and a computer is required to regulate the treatment.

The problem of measuring heat emitted has been overcome by microwave radiometry, enabling total temperature control of the tissue being treated. The physical basis of this is that the heat emits spontaneous electromagnetic radiation – the so-called thermal noise power – which is directly related to the body temperature. This noise power gives information corresponding to the average temperature of the entire volume of prostate being heated.

Rectal versus transrectal route

Using standard equipment, the maximum penetration of the microwave is less than 2 cm, which causes maximum deposition to the peripheral zone when delivered rectally and not to the transition zone, which is the area of benign enlargement. Thus, although microwave thermotherapy can be delivered by the urethral or endorectal route, the former is preferred simply because of its proximity to the transitional zone.

Lesions induced

The transmission of microwaves or radiofrequency waves appears to be the most effective way to produce local heat damage. The penetration of the electromagnetic waves produced depends on their frequency, the duration of treatment and the vascularity of the tissue being treated. Low-frequency waves give a deeper and more uniform penetration.

The variation in temperatures recorded in different prostates is presumably due to tissue composition and vascularisation. In general, heat damage to malignant prostates is greater than to benign glands and this can partly be explained by the vascularity of the gland. Malignant glands are less vascular, thus the heat cannot be dissipated as quickly and a local destructive effect is maintained for longer.

The microwave antenna produces an electromagnetic field that causes oscillation of ions in the tissue or a change in the magnetic orientation of the molecules, which is converted to heat.

The lesions induced vary with the temperature delivered to the prostate. At temperatures below 40 °C, no appreciable effect is noted on either benign or malignant prostates. In a series of patients whose prostates were removed after thermotherapy treatment, histological examination revealed necrotic lesions at temperature levels of 47 °C (corresponding to an intraprostatic temperature of 55–60 °C). In those patients in whom the prostate was not removed, there was endoscopic evidence six weeks later of necrosis and cavitation.

Peak rectal and urethral temperatures are measured throughout the thermotherapy procedure. Coagulative necrosis is achieved by thermotherapy at 915 or 1296 MHz at temperatures above 45 °C.

It is still not clear how exactly thermotherapy affects the symptoms of patients with benign prostatic hyperplasia. A potential effect is the shrinkage of tissue, thus decreasing outflow resistance. Patients' irritative symptoms may be improved by its effect on the autonomic nervous system. Another theory is that repeated heating causes an alteration in the compliance of the prostate and bladder neck.

High-intensity focused ultrasound

In diagnostic ultrasound systems, the amount of heat dissipated has been shown to be very small. However, with the use of high intensities, significant temperature elevations can be achieved for therapeutic purposes.

A beam of high-intensity ultrasound can be brought to a focus at a selected depth within the body. Maximum damage is achieved to all cellular elements within this focused beam and thermal damage to the intervening tissues is spared. This form of energy is known as high-intensity focused ultrasound.

In the early 1950s, high-intensity focused ultrasound was used to destroy small volumes of brain tissue and later work demonstrated its benefits in treating liver tumours in experimental animals. Animal studies in which it was applied transrectally to the prostates of dogs demonstrated the formation of prostatic cavities between two hours to three months after treatment. More recently, ultrasound probes have been designed for transrectal use in humans.

New rectal probes have been designed to deliver high-intensity focused ultrasound to the prostates of men with benign prostatic hyperplasia with the aim of causing coagulative necrosis and in the hope of lessening bladder outflow obstruction. These probes may also incorporate a small ultrasound imaging probe (Figure 14.9). The source of energy is a piezoceramic transducer. The rectal probes used are 13.13 cm in length and 2.95 cm in diameter. The transducer is oval shaped (22 cm × 30 cm), with a curved surface without acoustic lens. The specific focal lengths are 3, 3.5 and 4 cm and the specific one used is determined by the size of the gland, as assessed by transurethral ultrasonography, with larger glands requiring larger focal lengths. For air-free contact of the high-intensity focused ultrasound beam to the rectal wall, a condom is placed over the probe and degassed water is used to inflate it.

Mechanism of action
High-intensity focused ultrasound produces its effects in two ways. Firstly, the ultrasound wave is focused at a particular point, the energy being converted into heat energy with temperatures in the region of 80–1000 °C. These temperatures can be attained in less than 4 seconds and dissipate quickly and, as a consequence, no diffusion of heat into the surrounding tissues is detectable. Secondly, as a result of intracellular water being forced into the gaseous phase by the ultrasound waveforms, bubbles are formed within the tissue, causing coagulative necrosis and hence

cavitation. The term 'cavitation' is applied to the histological changes, which also include collagen denaturation and various enzymatic changes.

The lesion affected by one cycle measures 2 × 2 × 10 mm and the computer adjusts the area of treatment with each cycle to include each area in the predefined treatment zone. Each cycle consists of 16 seconds comprising 4 seconds of therapy and 12 seconds to allow for combined cooling, transducer movement and image update. The length of treatment varies with the size of the gland, larger glands taking longer to treat.

Clinical application
High-intensity focused ultrasound has been used for the treatment of benign prostatic hyperplasia and has resulted in small improvements in flow and symptom score. Using the technique of transrectal delivery of energy as opposed to a transabdominal approach allows for greater accuracy of in-depth thermoablation. Also, it has the advantage that treatment is contact free, allowing tissue to be coagulated without urethral or intraprostatic manipulation.

High-intensity focused ultrasound may have a role to play in destroying localised prostate cancer. Currently, its wider clinical application is limited by its relatively short focal length, which prevents its use for deeper structures. It is expected that future developments with the equipment may broaden its clinical application.

Cryotherapy
Cryotherapy was abandoned over 20 years ago for the treatment of benign prostatic hyperplasia due to the significant morbidity associated with it. The introduction of ultrasound imaging for the accurate placement of multiple probes within the prostate and monitoring of the ice ball has decreased the incidence of complications, including rectal fistulae, incontinence and impotence. Interest in this technology has thus been rekindled and its potential use in the treatment of localised prostate cancer is currently undergoing investigation.

A minimum of five prostatic probes are placed perineally so as to encircle the urethra and preserve the rectum. If there is tumour extending laterally,

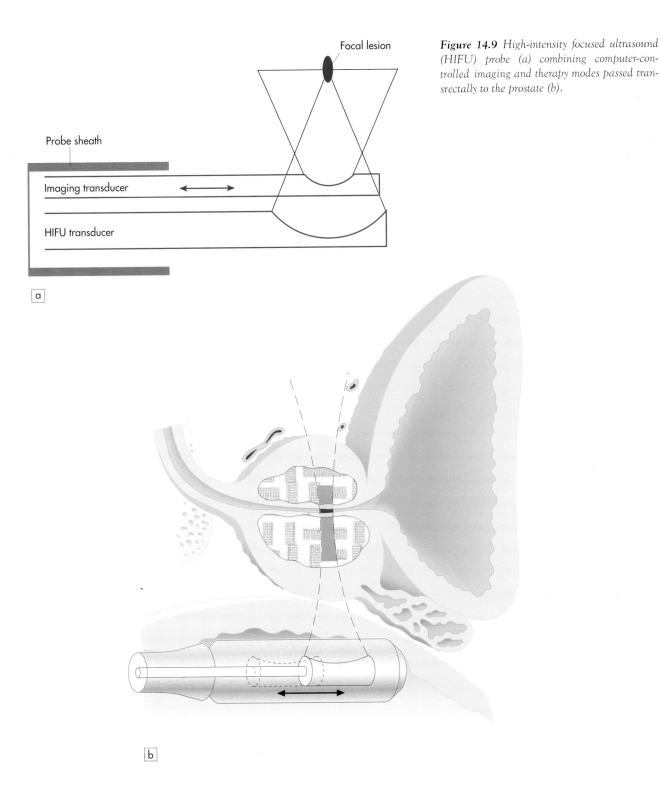

Figure 14.9 *High-intensity focused ultrasound (HIFU) probe (a) combining computer-controlled imaging and therapy modes passed transrectally to the prostate (b).*

extra probes can be placed to deal with this. A urethral warming device is placed across the prostatic urethra to protect it. The prostate is frozen to approximately −10 °C for 10 to 20 minutes and then allowed to thaw, at which time its echogenicity on transrectal ultrasound returns to normal.

At present, the poor results obtained do not warrant the addition of cryotherapy to the armamentarium of the urologist in the fight against localised prostate cancer. The use of percutaneous cryoprobes has also been described for hepatic and renal tumours.

Energy sources used to fragment stones

The treatment of renal tract stones has been revolutionised by the advent of multiple minimally invasive technologies.

Extracorporeal shock wave lithotriptors

Full credit for the development of extracorporeal shock wave lithotriptors must go to the Dornier Company and the University of Munich, whose collaboration between 1974 and 1980 culminated in the first lithotripter for clinical use, the HM-1 (Human Model No. 1). The first patient was treated in February 1980 and by 1984 the HM-3 became commercially available after 1000 patients had been treated. Shock waves are generated outside the body and are brought to a focus within the body.

Types of shock wave generators
The main commercially available types of shock wave generators are spark gap, piezoelectric and electromagnetic (Table 14.2).

Spark gap
The spark gap generator is a spark gap formed by two electrodes that sits in a liquid medium and is powered by a high-kilovoltage generator. The temperature of the water rises rapidly to very high temperatures and a compressive pressure pulse results from the expansion of the heated gases. This is followed some time later by a negative pressure pulse as the gas bubble contracts. The shock waves generated must be coordinated with the electrocardiogram to prevent arrhythmias.

Piezo-electric
A high-frequency, high-voltage pulse excites a piezo-electric substance, which changes its shape and size. This movement of the ceramic crystal produces a pressure wave. The number of crystals used in the lithotripter generator depends on the manufacturer (Wolf, approximately 3000; EDAP, approximately 300); the crystals are placed in a concave reflector to focus the shock wave on the stone. The pressure wave leaving the disc is large, allowing a wide entry zone on the skin, thus minimising the discomfort experienced. The short focal length allows the wave to be focused on a kidney stone. No cardiac arrhythmias are produced by this technology. The ceramic crystals have a limited life span due to mechanical damage. They are also used for diagnostic ultrasound.

Table 14.2 Types of commercially available shock wave generators

Manufacturer	Machine	Shock wave generation	Patient coupling	Localisation	Portable
Siemens Medical Systems	Lithostar	Electromagnetic	Water membrane	X-ray	No
EDAP	LT-01	Piezo-electric	Water membrane	Ultrasound	No
Wolf	Piezolith 2300	Piezo-electric	Water/direct contact	Ultrasound	Yes
Dornier	Various	Underwater electrode	Water bath/ cushion	X-ray (ultrasound for newer machines)	No
Technomed	Sonolith 3000	Underwater electrode	Partial water bath	Ultrasound	Yes

Electromagnetic

An electric current travelling through a wire generates an electric field. With an electromagnetic lithotriptor, a flexible membrane is repelled to create a pressure wave. The shock wave thus generated is brought to a focus by an acoustic lens. A water cushion is coupled to the skin to transmit the shock wave into the body. The Siemens Lithostar was the first electromagnetic generator to use this technology.

Stone localisation

The stone may be localised by ultrasound or fluoroscopy or a combination of both.

The advantages of ultrasound localisation are that radiolucent calculi and those too small to visualise fluoroscopically are often detected. It also allows for real-time monitoring of stone fragmentation. The initial costs and maintenance charges are usually lower than for fluoroscopy, with less radiation exposure.

However, ultrasound is not useful for the localisation of ureteric calculi unless a lower ureteric stone can be seen through a full bladder. It is thus not ideal for in-situ fragmentation. It is also a more difficult skill to attain.

With X-ray imaging, two fluoroscopes are mounted in the long axis of the patient at a 45° angle to the patient and at a 90° angle to each other. Some machines use a C arm for stone localisation.

The placement of stents or nephrostomy drains often helps in the localisation of the stone.

Fragmentation

When a shock wave strikes a stone, the pressure front is split and a series of pressure waves moves off into the substance of the stone. A reflected component moves back towards the shock wave source, causing a high-pressure gradient, which causes the outer surface of the stone to disintegrate. The wave that travels through the stone is reflected at the distant surface and again meets 'itself' head on, creating another pressure gradient with further disintegration of the stone (Figure 14.10).

Clinical factors

The requirement for anaesthesia is due more to the way that the wave is focused than to the energy source.

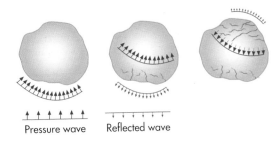

Figure 14.10 *Stone fragmentation.*

A small final focus with a large area at skin entry so as to disperse the energy is the optimal situation.

It is not really known how many shock waves the kidney can tolerate. Haematuria is almost universal and is probably due to parenchymal injury rather than to a stone fragment traumatising the urothelium. Such bleeding is generally short lived and resolves spontaneously. Imaging studies have demonstrated some transient swelling of the kidneys immediately after treatment due to subcapsular and perinephric fluid collections.

Contact lithotripsy

This method of endoscopic stone fragmentation differs from electrohydraulic lithotripsy and laser lithotripsy in that contact is required and stone fragmentation takes place by drilling.

Mechanism

The basic principle is the piezoelectric excitation of crystals in the transducer tip making it expand and contract. This ultrasound energy propels a steel probe, which acts like a jackhammer. This causes vibration of the tip, with a longitudinal amplitude in the range of $20\,\mu m$ in addition to some lateral vibration. Increasing the frequency causes the tip to vibrate at higher speeds. The instrument consists of a transducer with an external generator. Probes are made in various sizes for endoscopic use.

Better contact between probe and stone leads to greater efficiency and worn probes should be discarded. As probes heat up very quickly, they are generally cooled with continuous irrigation. The probe is thus hollow to allow for suction of the fluid, which has the advantage that small particles are also sucked away.

Hard stones may be difficult to break and a combination of ultrasound lithotripsy and electrohydraulic lithotripsy may be helpful, with the former making a small hole in the stone initially and then the latter fragmenting it. There are minimal effects on the surrounding tissue due to the short amplitude of the probe (20 μm).

Laser fragmentation of calculi

The laser has been used to fragment stones since 1968, but the earlier machines could not be used clinically due to the local tissue heat generated during stone fragmentation and the fact that fibre-optic scopes were also damaged.

The pulsed dye laser, which emits a green light of wavelength 504 nm, was found to be effective at fragmentation and could be used through miniaturised instruments. The optimum pulse duration is 1 ms, with five to ten pulses per second (5–10 Hz).

The tip is placed in contact with the stone, which absorbs the energy and forms a plasma that rapidly expands. This creates a shock wave, which breaks the stone as the compression and tension forces pass through it with minimal thermal effect. For maximal effect, the probe has to be placed directly on the stone. Q-switched Nd:YAG lasers can produce stone disruption by inducing a breakdown in the fluid surrounding a stone.

The safety of the pulsed dye laser (504 nm) has to do with the short pulse duration. At 1 ms, this is minimal for a small amount of haemoglobin to absorb the light. In the presence of blood, the amount of light absorbed can be significant and can cause damage to the ureteral wall. Safety is also due to the fact that the probe is placed directly on the stone, away from the ureter and under direct vision. Tissue heating does not appear to be a problem with the pulsed dye laser. The average number of pulses is approximately 500 and even if all the energy was absorbed, this would only heat 1 ml of water by 6.25 °C. This heat can be removed easily by continuous irrigation.

Electrohydraulic lithotripsy

Electrohydraulic lithotripsy and laser lithotripsy are two methods of shock generation that share the same principles of stone fragmentation with electro-magnetic shock wave lithotripsy (ESWL). Shock waves can be generated close to (intracorporeal) or distant from (extracorporeal) a stone. A localised shock wave on or very close to a stone is created and is used endoscopically, either via a nephroscope for the kidney or the bladder or via a ureteroscope for the ureter. A high voltage is discharged between two underwater electrodes, causing an 'explosion'.

The fluid medium is thus vaporised, creating a bubble that spreads out at the speed of sound, resulting in a shock wave. A stone is broken up in the same fashion as described with ESWL. Normal saline is the best medium for electrohydraulic lithotripsy.

Electrohydraulic lithotripsy differs from ultrasonic lithotripsy in that any proximity to the urothelium can cause damage, thus good visualisation must be obtainable at all times.

Radiation biology

Historical basis of radiation

Radiation has been present through the evolution of life, but the extent to which we are subjected to extra radiation, largely for medical purposes, has changed dramatically.

X-rays were first discovered in 1895 by the German physicist Wilhelm Conrad Roentgen, who made the first radiograph of the hand of his colleague Herr Kolliger.

Controversy exists as to who was first to use X-rays therapeutically. In 1887, Professor Freund demonstrated before the Vienna Medical School the disappearance of a hairy mole by the use of X-rays.

In the wake of the Second World War and the use of atomic weapons on Hiroshima and Nagasaki, research into radiobiology developed rapidly. A most significant milestone was the development of the first mammalian cell survival curve in 1956.

Physical and biological basis of radiation

Excitation is defined as the raising of the energy of an electron in an atom or molecule to a higher energy level. When this extra energy increase is sufficient to eject an electron from the atom or molecule, the process can be referred to as an ionising event. An important characteristic of this ionising event is the localised release of large amounts of energy (radiation).

Gamma rays and X-rays are both types of electromagnetic radiation that differ only in the way in which they are produced. They are both indirectly ionising, which means that they do not produce damage directly. When they are absorbed in the medium through which they pass, they give up their energy to produce fast-moving electrons, thereby causing chemical and biological damage. Gamma rays are emitted by radioactive isotopes; they represent the excess energy that is given off as the unstable nucleus breaks up and decays in its efforts to reach a stable form. X-rays are generated in an electrical device that accelerates electrons to high energy and then stops them abruptly on a target, which is usually made of tungsten or gold. Part of the kinetic energy of these electrons is converted into photons of X-rays.

The unit of dose in current use is the gray (Gy) which is defined to be an energy absorption of 1 joule per kilogram.

It is generally accepted that the most important attacking species responsible for molecular disruption in irradiated biological material is the hydroxy radical, which attacks at specific vital sites of the cell.

Many forms of cellular damage are induced by radiation. These include reproductive death, interphase death, division delay, chromosome aberrations, mutation and transformation. Radiation is potentially toxic to all mammalian cells. Ionising radiation can damage every molecule in a cell, but DNA is by far the most sensitive target molecule.

After irradiation, cell death is not detectable until the cells attempt to divide. If the initial dose has been low, the cells may divide several times before coming to a halt, whereas with higher doses death occurs after the first division.

J. P. Blandy

History

Endoscopic surgery began with attempts to shine light into the bladder using the light of an oil lamp and a head mirror, rather like that used by old-fashioned laryngologists. For a brief period this was succeeded by the invention of the cystoscope by Nitze [1], a Viennese instrument maker, who used a heated platinum loop as its light source, with all the dangers of burning the bladder despite his water-cooling system. Finally, Edison's invention of the incandescent electric lamp in 1879 was to change things. The lamp was soon miniaturised and adapted by Nitze and Leiter to the cystoscope in 1886. Electric light cystoscopy had begun.

In the UK, it was Hurry Fenwick who took the trouble to visit Nitz and Leiter, learned how to use the new instrument, wrote books about it, and introduced many adaptations including ureteric catheters, biopsy forceps, and a device for coagulating the prostate [2]. Thanks to Fenwick, endoscopy became a key part of urology, and thanks to the cystoscope, urology became a specialty of its own, though it was not fully separated from general surgery for another century.

The design of the cystoscope changed very little between 1886 and 1951. The author's generation of urologists was brought up to use an instrument that Nitze would have recognised. It consisted of a thin tube containing a series of glass lenses, separated by a second set of annular spacers holding them apart at measured distances. It was difficult to grind the tiny lenses with precision, and stray images occurred from their surface, with the result that there was often degradation of the peripheral image and poor contrast (Figure 15.1).

The light was provided by a tiny 'bijou' lamp, which had the irritating property of burning out just when it was most necessary to have a good view, or whenever there was a surge in the electric current. Changing the little lamp required removal and reinsertion of the instrument, and from time to time it was common for the patient to receive a mild electric shock when the current was turned on. Cystoscopy was generally performed under local urethral anaesthetic and took skill and confidence on the part of the surgeon, and fortitude on the part of the patient.

Harold Hopkins

In 1950 everything changed, thanks to the genius of one man, the late Professor Harold Hopkins, whose invention of the zoom lens might well be regarded as

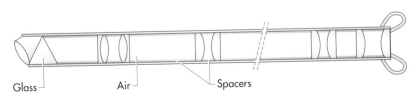

Figure 15.1 *Section of a classical Nitze cystoscope. The glass lenses are separated by spacers.*

achievement enough for one lifetime (Figure 15.2). The story is an unusual one, and is worth telling again [3, 4]. It began with a chance encounter at a dinner party between Harold Hopkins and Dr Hugh Gainsborough, a gastroenterologist at St George's Hospital, London. In those days, the gastroscope consisted of a brass tube about a yard in length with a slightly flexible end. Passing the instrument down the oesophagus into the stomach was rather like swallowing a sword: it took great skill and carried considerable risks of injury to the teeth and oesophagus. The view was very limited, and there was the same tiresome problem of failure of the lamp that bedevilled cystoscopy. Gainsborough discussed his difficulties with Hopkins and Hopkins went away to think about the problem.

It was three years later that two letters appeared in the New Year's edition of *Nature* in 1954 from Van Heal of Delft, and from Hopkins and his research student, Kapani at Imperial College, in London [5]. Both groups had succeeded in transmitting images down a bundle of transparent fibres coated with a layer with a different refractive index. This was not an entirely new idea: John Logie Baird, the inventor of television, had experimented with the system some 20 years before [6], but the difficulty had always been to ensure that the fibres were aligned exactly. Hopkins solved this problem by winding the glass fibres on a wheel, gluing them together at one point, and cutting them there.

The letter from Hopkins and Kapani was noticed

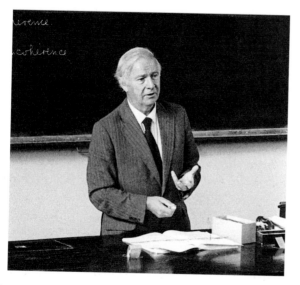

Figure 15.2 *Professor Harold H. Hopkins* FRS.

by Basil Hirschowitz, a South African gastroenterologist then working in London with Sir Francis Avery Jones [3]. Hirschowitz visited Hopkins, and made attempts to construct a gastroscope using ordinary glass fibres, but found that the image was too green. Later, he teamed up with Dr William Peters, the Professor of Physics at Ann Arbor, Michigan, and one of his research students, Lawrence Curtis. Finally, he developed a clinically useful flexible gastroscope using glass fibres of optical quality developed by Dow Corning. The instrument was commercially available by 1960. Curiously, flexible endoscopy was not applied to urology for a considerable time, and the reason for this is that Hopkins had turned his attention to the rigid cystoscope for an entirely different purpose.

Mr JG Gow, a urologist of Liverpool, and a keen amateur photographer, was concerned at the increasing number of carcinomas of the bladder referred to him, and was anxious to document them by colour photography. Gow sought the help of his local university department of physics, and was put in touch with Hopkins [3, 4]. Gow obtained a grant from the Medical Research Council, and Hopkins took on a research student to look into the matter. Hopkins calculated that in order to get a colour photograph of the inside of the bladder it would be necessary to increase the light transmission of the conventional cystoscope by a factor of 50. However much he tampered with the existing telescope design, he did not think he could do better than double the light transmission; a radical new idea was needed. It was only after another two years that he came up with the idea of the rod-lens telescope.

Using air spaces as the lenses, there was no need to take up any room inside the cystoscope for the spacers. The rods could be ground and aligned with greater precision. At once, the light transmission was increased more than twofold. A further and greater increase was obtained by two layers of antireflective coating at each end of the rod, which increased the light transmission 80 times (Figure 15.3).

But the illumination was still obtained by means of a filament lamp at the end of the cystoscope. Hopkins experimented with a number of alternative methods of illuminating the cystoscope, including one device that made use of an arc lamp and a solid quartz rod

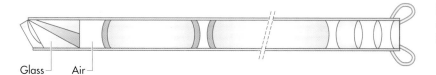

Glass — Air —

Figure 15.3 Section through a Hopkins rod-lens cystoscope. (From a drawing made by Professor Hopkins for the author.)

attached to the cystoscope, which the author remembers well when he brought it to be tried out at St Paul's Hospital, London, in 1963, where unfortunately nobody took it seriously: it was certainly very hot and noisy. Despite these difficulties, Gow was able to obtain a number of excellent photographs of the interior of the bladder, and some of these were demonstrated by Hopkins at a conference on medical photography in Dusseldorf in 1963 [4].

By chance, Karl Storz, who ran an instrument company in Tuttlingen in South Germany, got to hear about these photographs, and telephoned Professor Hopkins, who answered him in perfect German. Storz was already using a system of transmitting light by glass fibres in a range of retractors and other instruments, which he called the cold light. Unlike the English instrument makers, Storz was willing to back his judgement and invest a large sum of money in the development of a series of endoscopes under Hopkins' supervision. Hopkins brought to the task a number of new theoretical techniques of optical design and electronic computers. At last the genius of Hopkins and the imagination of Storz were combined in an instrument containing the Hopkins optical system and the Storz cold light. By 1967, the first Storz–Hopkins instrument was demonstrated to the world of urology at the International Society of Urology in Munich in 1967.

It is hard for young urologists today to understand just what a revolution this was; and it is even harder for older urologists to understand why the Storz–Hopkins system took so long to be introduced into our hospitals. Whatever the reason, urologists were now provided with a cystoscope for which the only limit to the amount of light that could be shone into the bladder was the brightness of the external source, while the precision of the lenses gave the image the quality of a first-rate microscope.

Until then, transurethral resection was performed with conventional telescopes illuminated by a bijou lamp that was even smaller than that in use in the ordinary cystoscope. The view was poor, and made much poorer when there was any bleeding, so that the operator inevitably called for the battery to be turned up, with the result that the lamp would blow. By the time the lamp had been changed, the bladder might be full of clot. Teaching transurethral resection was slow and difficult [7].

Teaching attachments

Again, Hopkins applied his intellect to the problem. The most obvious teaching attachment was a simplified version of his flexible gastroscope attached to the end of the cystoscope, but the image was always rather speckled, as if seen through ground glass. He then developed a more sophisticated system using swivelling prisms with either three or five arms, which not only allowed the pupil to see clearly every step of the operation, but could be attached to a television camera and, for the first time, enabled a large audience to watch. Teaching courses based on this new endoscopic television system were set up in Munich, London and Copenhagen. Within a few years, transurethral resection of the prostate and of tumours of the bladder had almost completely displaced open surgery. The generation that had struggled so hard to make transurethral resection accepted and indeed respectable is apt to smile wryly when it hears it referred to as the gold standard.

Today, there is a very wide range of endoscopes all based on the Storz–Hopkins principles and, thanks to them, it has been possible to develop a whole new field of minimally invasive surgery that was inconceivable without them. In urology, different procedures call for different angles of view, and in transurethral resection a rather curious vestige has persisted from the old filament-lit endoscopes. Because the lamp had to be placed at the tip of the

resectoscope, the lens was angled at 30° and the generation of surgeons who learned transurethral resection
with this device insisted on having their Storz–Hopkins
telescopes with a similar angle. Those who begin to
learn the operation today often find it easier to keep
their sense of orientation if they use a telescope
that looks straight ahead – the so-called 0° telescope
(Figure 15.4).

Which telescope to resect with – 0° or 30°

There was another curious anomaly that resulted
from the design of the conventional cystoscope. In
general, it was provided with a right-angled lens at the
end, and was introduced into the bladder blindly. A
generation of urologists was brought up never to look
at the urethra. It was only when Storz–Hopkins 0°

telescopes became available that it became customary
to pass the cystoscope under direct vision but, within
a few more years, diagnostic cystoscopy had been
taken over by the flexible cystoscope.

The flexible cystoscope

Some attempts had been made to use the small-calibre
flexible endoscope, designed for examining the common bile duct, in urology [8]. The rather dim ground-
glass image was so much inferior to the brilliance of
the Storz–Hopkins telescope that it was very slow to
be adopted, especially when one could buy five
Hopkins telescopes for the price of a single flexible
endoscope. It was, however, economics that forced the
London Hospital team into taking it seriously.
Around 1980, like other busy urological departments, this team was faced with a log-jam of patients

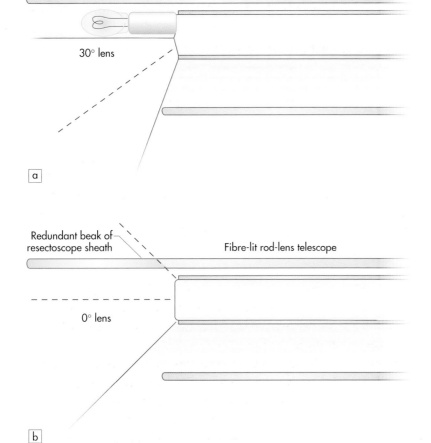

Conventional lamp-lit telescope

30° lens

a

Redundant beak of
resectoscope sheath

Fibre-lit rod-lens telescope

0° lens

b

Figure 15.4 *The vestigial 30° telescope had its
origin in the need to avoid the bijou lamp (a).
Beginners find it easier to keep their orientation if
they use a 0° or direct-viewing telescope (b), but
this needs a sheath without a long beak.*

requiring check cystoscopy for bladder cancer. The number was growing exponentially, thanks in part to an increase in the number of these cases, and in part to their improved survival. Chris Fowler, who had come to the department from a background in gastroenterology and had considerable experience with gastroscopy, was convinced that the flexible endoscope could solve this log-jam. He conducted a pilot study to demonstrate that recurrences would not be missed by the flexible cystoscope and, having convinced the author, set about teaching the team how to use the instrument. Within a few months, the technique was adopted as the routine method in the clinic, to the delight of the patients and with enormous savings [9].

For cystoscopy, the small-calibre flexible choledochoscope was not ideal, and Fowler set about making a series of modifications to its design, in collaboration with the Japanese instrument maker Olympus. A longer and more rigid insertion tube was designed to make it easier to pass the instrument, and the radius of the bending portion was increased to allow the observer to curve the cystoscope on itself and examine the bladder neck from the inside. Fowler insisted on making the instrument watertight so that it could be sterilised by immersion in antiseptic. An irrigation channel and a working channel were adapted to fill the bladder, pass a ureteric catheter or a double-J stent, obtain a biopsy, and coagulate tumours with the neodymium YAG laser [10].

Sterilisation

There remain certain unsolved problems. Probably the most important of these concerns the sterilisation of endoscopic equipment. Heat is still the only thoroughly effective means of sterilisation, but few modern rod-lens telescopes can be repeatedly autoclaved without sustaining damage, and the leisurely cycle of the conventional steam autoclave calls for the duplication of much expensive equipment if more than one case is to be dealt with on an operating list. 'Pasteurisation' by means of a water-bath heated to 70°C is known to kill off all vegetative forms of pathogenic bacteria, and spore-bearing micro-organisms are almost irrelevant in urology. But even the lesser heat

of the pasteurising bath is apt to damage some rod-lens telescopes and all flexible instruments. As a result, urologists have returned to the use of antiseptic solutions for routine disinfection of endoscopes. Here, the problems have always been (a) how to be sure that the fluid has reached the hidden crevices in taps and hinges, and (b) to find an effective antiseptic fluid. Today, 2% activated glutaraldehyde is most commonly used [11], but requires special precautions if ancillary staff are not to suffer serious respiratory allergic effects, and it must be thoroughly washed off the instrument if it is not to cause chemical irritation to the patient's urethra or the surgeon's eye. Because of this somewhat unsatifactory state of affairs, the quest for better methods of sterilisation continues.

Gas sterilisation using ethylene oxide or formaldehyde is very effective against all forms of bacteria, and can reach hidden crevices in instruments. Unfortunately, the mixture of ethylene oxide and air is explosive and calls for elaborate precautions and, because the gas dissolves in plastic equipment, it must 'air' for 24 hours, so delaying the turn around of instruments. Moreover, both ethylene oxide and formaldehyde must be used at the temperature of 80°C to be effective, a temperature that may damage delicate equipment.

Closed circuit television

Although television was developed for teaching endoscopic surgery, it has so many advantages in transurethral resection that many urologists now prefer to operate 'off the screen' rather than looking down the eyepiece of the telescope. Among the many advantages two stand out: first, it avoids the awkward craning of the neck that has caused cervical spondylosis in so many urologists [12] and, secondly, it avoids at least some of the splashes of blood that get into the face, eyes or mouth on some 70% of occasions [13]. For teaching young surgeons, endoscopic television is, in the author's opinion, essential.

Today, chip cameras are so sensitive and their colour rendering so good that there is no point in investing in a three-tube camera, with the necessity of using a jointed Hopkins teaching arm.

Nor is it absolutely necessary to purchase a

specially bright light source but, if one can afford a dedicated light source that is electronically linked with the camera, the image on the screen will be of uniform brightness rather than showing occasional very bright flashes interspersed with deep gloom, which can be so tiresome to the observer, especially during the resection of a bladder cancer. The junction between camera and telescope must allow the camera to stay in one position while the telescope rotates, otherwise the image will rotate in an infuriating way, making it very difficult to keep correct orientation, and for this reason a beam-splitter is preferable to a chip camera attached rigidly to the eyepiece. When teaching, it is a great advantage to use a continuous flow resectoscope, adjusted so that a constant volume of irrigant remains inside the bladder. This avoids frequent interruption of the operation to evacuate the bladder.

The monitor used by the surgeon need not be large, and it should be placed at a convenient height above the table during the operation. A second larger monitor placed elsewhere in the operating theatre allows pupils and nursing staff to see what is going on. Before buying anything, insist on a demonstration in your own operating theatre, using your own diathermy equipment, otherwise you may find the image ruined by interference, to avoid which can take hours of expensive expert's time.

A video-recording system is an optional extra that everyone buys and uses for the first few enchanted months. After that it is seldom used. When demonstrating a technique, an audience learns far more by watching the operation 'live' rather than on an edited tape. If you insist on recording your operation on tape, then make sure you have added a colour bar for the whole length of the tape: without this, subsequent editing becomes almost impossible to do neatly. An unedited tape is seldom possible to watch without extreme boredom, and to edit videotape well needs a considerable investment both in time and in equip-

ment. For most surgeons, it will be wiser to hire the use of an editing suite as and when it is needed.

Finally, take trouble to look after the equipment. This means a safe place where it can be locked away when not in use, but, even more important, it means fitting locks or notices that will discourage knob-twiddling. It is amazing how much expensive damage can be done by the passing amateur who cannot resist adjusting the set for you.

References

1. Nitze M. Eine neue Beobachtungs – und Untersuchungsmethode für Harnröhre, Harnblase und Rectum. Wien Med Wochenschr 1897; 29: 649–52
2. Burckhardt E. Atlas of electric cystoscopy. Edited and translated by EH Fenwick. London: Churchill, 1893
3. Smith JC. Tribute to Harold Hopkins and his contribution to medicine. 1995
4. Hopkins HH. Personal communication. 1986
5. Hopkins HH, Kapani NS. A flexible fibrescope using static scanning. Nature 1954; 173: 39–41
6. Baird JL. British Patent Specification No 20 969/27. London: HM Patent Office, 1927
7. Blandy, JP. Transurethral resection. London: Pitman, 1971: 15–16
8. Blandy JP, Fowler CG. Lower tract endoscopy. Br Med Bull 1986; 42: 280–3
9. Fowler CG, Badenoch DF, Takar DR. Practical experience with flexible fibrescope cystoscopy in outpatients. Br J Urol 1984; 56: 618–21
10. Fowler CG, Boorman LS. Outpatient treatment of superficial bladder cancer. Lancet 1986; 1: 38
11. Babb HR, Bradley CR, Deverill CEA, Ayliffe GAJ, Melikian V. Recent advances in the cleaning and disinfection of endoscopes. J Hosp Infect 1981; 2: 329–40
12. Whitaker RH, Green NA, Notley RG. Is cervical spondylosis an occupational hazard for urologists? Br J Urol 1983; 55: 585–7
13. McNicholas TA, Jones DJ, Sibley GN. AIDS: the contamination risk in urological surgery. Br J Urol 1989; 63: 565–8

Cancer, tumour suppressor genes and oncogenes

16

D. E. Neal

Cancer

An understanding of cancer is important to the urologist, not only because it is common, but also because its study provides insight into normal and abnormal cellular function. One in five adults die of cancer (Table 16.1) and about 30–50% of common solid epithelial tumours are advanced and incurable when first detected clinically. So far as urological tumours are concerned, prostate, bladder and kidney cancers are common, and although testis cancer is rare, it is important because even when advanced it is frequently curable and because it occurs in young men with an otherwise full life expectancy.

It is thought that every individual cancer arises from a single cell following a set of genetically determined events. The evidence for this monoclonal origin lies in findings, firstly, that all cells in a tumour often contain specific point mutations in genes that would be unlikely to arise by chance in several cells, and secondly, that in women, in whom one X chromosome is inactivated in a mosaic and apparently random fashion throughout the body, one particular X chromosome is inactivated throughout the tumour.

Chemical carcinogenesis

Many different chemicals have been shown to be carcinogenic (Table 16.2). The best-known historical example is that of scrotal cancer: Percival Pott demonstrated through epidemiological observations that boys who had been employed as chimney sweeps were likely to develop this disease as adults. He hypothesised that chemicals in soot caused the problem.

Tobacco use (mainly cigarette smoking) was later shown to be clearly associated with cancers of the mouth, larynx, trachea, lung, kidney and bladder.

Further evidence of a chemical cause for bladder cancer was found by Rehn in 1894 when he recorded a series of tumours occurring in workers in aniline dye factories. Hueper was subsequently able to show that 2-naphthylamine was carcinogenic in dogs, and further investigation has demonstrated that the compounds listed in Table 16.3 may also be carcinogenic. Occupations that have been reported to have a significantly high risk of bladder cancer are shown in Table 16.4.

Historically, chemicals were classified into those that produced mutations in DNA on first application (initiators) but which of themselves were usually insufficient to cause cancer unless there was further exposure to the initiator or unless initiator application was followed by a promoter. Promoters are compounds that do not cause cancer, however often they are applied, but that will cause the development of a cancer when there have been previous applications of an initiator. Promoters include chemicals such as phorbol esters, which stimulate protein kinase C. Protein kinase C phosphorylates several proteins on serine and threonine residues and activates mitogen-activated protein kinase – which is also activated by the ras pathway (see below).

Most carcinogens are genotoxic and cause damage to DNA. It is thought that there is also a class of non-genotoxic carcinogens that, in mice, cause peroxisome proliferation and that may activate agents which interfere with the cell cycle or apoptosis. It is uncertain whether this mechanism is active in humans.

Table 16.1 Cancer incidence and death in the USA and England and Wales

Type of cancer	New cases per year	Percentage	Deaths per year	Percentage
Total	1 170 000	100	528 300	100
Mouth and pharynx	29 800	3	7 700	1
Colon and rectum	152 000	13	57 000	11
Stomach	24 000	2	13 600	3
Pancreas	27 700	2	25 000	5
Lung	170 000	15	149 000	28
Breast	183 000	16	46 300	9
Malignant melanoma	32 000	3	6 800	1
Prostate	165 000	14	35 000	7
Ovary	22 000	2	13 300	3
Cervix	13 500	1	4 400	1
Uterus	31 000	3	5 700	1
Bladder	52 300	4	9 900	2
Kidney				
Haematopoietic	93 000	8	50 000	9
Central nervous system	18 250	2	12 350	2
Testis				
Sarcomas	8 000	1	4 150	1

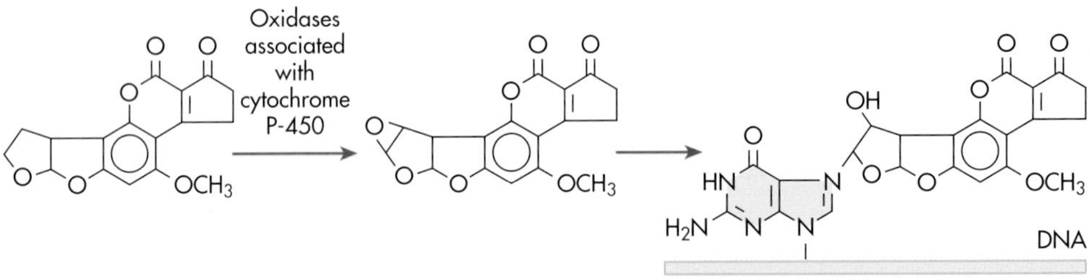

Figure 16.1 *Metabolic activation of a carcinogen. Many chemical carcinogens have to be activated by a metabolic transformation before they will cause mutations by reacting with DNA. The compound illustrated here is aflatoxin B1, a toxin made from a mould (Aspergillus flavus oryzae) that grows on grain and peanuts when they are stored under humid tropical conditions. It is thought to be a contributory cause of liver cancer in the tropics and is associated with specific mutations of the p53 gene.*

Table 16.2 Common causes of human cancer

Ionising radiation (haematopoietic cells, bone)
Sunlight (malignant melanoma, squamous cell carcinoma of the skin
Familial genetic causes (certain types of breast, colon, kidney and prostate cancer)
Familial cancer predispositions due to altered activity in detoxyfying or activating enzymes such as N-acetyl transferase 2 and glutathione transferase M (bladder, lung and colon cancer)
Chemicals from occupation and smoking (bladder, larynx and lung cancer)
Chronic inflammation (squamous cell carcinoma arising in a chronic ulcer, schistosomal bladder cancer, tumours in ulcerative colitis and adenocarcinoma arising in a Barrett's oesophagus)
Viral infection DNA viruses: penile and cervical cancer (papovavirus), liver cancer (Hep B and C), Epstein–Barr (Burkitt's lymphoma, nasopharyngeal cancer); RNA viruses: human T cell leukaemia (HTLV-1), Kaposi's sarcoma (HIV-1)
Common factors to most human cancers include damage to several genes (rather than one) resulting from mutations. insertions or deletions in certain genes known as oncogenes or tumour suppressor genes

Table 16.3 Compounds associated with bladder cancer

2-Naphthylamine
4-Aminobiphenyl
Benzidine
Chlornaphazine
4-Chloro-o-toluidine
o-toluidine
4,4'-Methylene bis (2-chloraniline)
Methylene dianiline
Benzidine-derived azo dyes

Genetic polymorphisms

Many genotoxic carcinogens are inactive and require to be converted into active agents by acetylation or hydroxylation (Figure 16.1). Mammalian cells have developed a complex system for detoxifying external biologically active chemicals known as xenobiotics. These enzymes also detoxify drugs and carcinogens and include:

enzymes of the cytochrome P450 system (Cyp), which are found on the microsomal fraction of cells (mainly in the liver);
glutathione transferases, which couple glutathione to water-insoluble chemicals and which are classified into families (α, β, μ, π);
N-acetyl transferase type 1 and 2 (NAT1 and NAT2).

Some individuals are more at risk than others following exposure to a carcinogen because of genetic polymorphisms. This arises because each individual carries two alleles for each gene, but within a population there may be many alleles. Some combinations will lead to an individual having enzymes that may be

Table 16.4 Occupations associated with bladder cancer

Textile workers
Dye workers
Tyre rubber and cable workers
Petrol workers
Leather workers
Shoe manufacturers and cleaners
Painters
Hairdressers
Lorry drivers
Drill press operators
Chemical workers
Rodent exterminators and sewage workers

more or less active than those found in other individuals. Polymorphic genes of interest in bladder cancer include *NAT1*, *NAT2*, glutathione transferase M1 and π (*GSTM1* and *GSTπ*) and several cytochrome P450s, including *CYP2D6* (debrisoquine hydroxylase) and *CYP1A1*. Individuals who have high levels of *NAT2* or *GSTM1* may be less likely to develop cancer following exposure to smoking because they can detoxify the mutagen, whereas those with high levels of *CYP2D6* may be more likely to develop cancer because they convert inactive to active forms of the mutagen. Similarly, some individuals may be generally resistant to carcinoma formation because they have polymorphisms that produce protective compounds. It should be noted that some enzymes will have a dual effect; for instance, *NAT2* in the liver will detoxify some carcinogens but may activate others, explaining the paradoxical observation that fast acetylators are less likely to develop bladder cancer but may be more likely to develop colon cancer. *NAT1* is found in high levels in the bladder urothelium, and non-toxic metabolites produced by *NAT2* in the liver and excreted in the urine can be taken into the urothelial cell and converted by *NAT1* into active carcinogens, which produce genotoxic damage in the bladder cell.

Cancer is a multistep process

Human cancer requires several mutations to occur before a tumour develops clinically. One factor supporting this view is that cancer incidence increases markedly with age, which would be unlikely to be the case if tumours simply arose following a single gene mutation, which would be more likely to occur randomly throughout life. Recent molecular biological studies have supported the view that cancer only arises when there has been an accumulation of several genetic events.

Cancer genes

Several tumours have a strong genetic component including: retinoblastoma (*Rb* gene), Wilms' tumour (*WT* gene), familial forms of prostate cancer (unknown gene, maybe on chromosome 1), breast cancer (*BRCA1* and *BRCA2* genes and mutations in *p53*

in Li-Fraumeni families), familial adenomatosis polyposis (*APC* gene), hereditary non-polyposis colon cancer (*MSH1* gene) and von Hippel–Lindau disease (*VHL* gene). These tumours have proven to be instructive because in most cases they appear to be inherited clinically in a dominant fashion. Nevertheless, biochemically, these genes act in a recessive fashion because, although the disease is caused by an inherited mutation in one allele of a tumour suppressor gene, cancer only develops when the other normal allele becomes deleted or mutated by chance (Figure 16.2). Why tumours in such patients appear only in certain tissues remains uncertain when tumour suppressor genes are inactivated in most cells.

Other tumours can arise in patients whose DNA repair machinery is deficient (xeroderma pigmentosa, ataxia telangiectasia and hereditary non-polyposis colon cancer).

DNA repair genes

Mismatch repair

Patients with hereditary non-polyposis colon cancer have tumours in the genome of which there is a large number of microsatellites. Microsatellites are short (two to four nucleotides: e.g. CACA on one strand and GTGT on the other), non-coding, tandem repeats of DNA that are found throughout the genome and that show pronounced polymorphism. Abnormalities in microsatellites have been found in Huntingdon's chorea, the fragile X syndrome and in spinobulbar atrophy in which, over several generations, there is a progressive expansion of the nucleotide repeats in the genes of interest. This leads to disease, but it is found that, with each succeeding generation, there is an increased severity of the disease because the microsatellites become longer. This phenomenon is called genetic anticipation. In hereditary non-polyposis colon cancer, microsatellite instability is thought to be the result of failure of correction of replication errors that arise during cell division. This is caused by hereditary defects in enzymes that are responsible for the repair of these replication mismatch errors. These enzymes include MSH2, MLH1, GTBP, PMS1 and PMS2.

Nucleotide excision repair

Abnormal nucleotide insertions can occur during DNA replication and are excised by mechanisms that are deficient in xeroderma pigmentosa.

Cellular characteristics of cancer

Not all features of cancer cells are caused directly by abnormal genes; some abnormalities are due to the failure of regulation of genetically normal genes. These epigenetic events include: up-regulation of enzymes that can dissolve the basement membrane (e.g. cathepsins and plasminogen activators) and may predispose the cell to metastasise; changes in expression of cell surface molecules (e.g. HLA antigens) that may allow the cancer cell to escape detection by the body's immunosurveillance mechanism; molecules responsible for intercellular adherence may be lost, leading the cell to be more likely to metastasise (e.g. E-cadherin); up-regulation of growth factors or their receptors allowing the cell to become self-reliant, e.g. epidermal growth factor (EGF) and its receptor (EGFr); and up-regulation of molecules that detoxify anticancer drugs (e.g. the multitumour suppressor gene *MDR1*).

Oncogenes

What have sometimes been referred to as 'recessive oncogenes' are now more commonly called tumour suppressor genes. Many DNA viruses produce proteins that directly perturb the function of tumour suppressor genes (e.g. large T antigen of SV40, which binds p53 and Rb; E6 and E7 of the papilloma virus, which bind p53 and Rb; the E1A protein of adenovirus, which binds Rb).

The term oncogene was originally used to describe those genes carried by viruses (most of them being retroviruses) that were found to be the cause of transmissible forms of cancer in animals. These retroviral oncogenes (*v-oncs*) were closely related to normal host cellular genes called proto-oncogenes. Cellular oncogenes found in cancer (*c-oncs*) were shown to be normal proto-oncogenes that had become 'activated' by a variety of mechanisms, including point mutations, deletion, insertional mutagenesis, translocation and over-expression – often associated with gene amplification. The initial techniques involved in identifying these genes (transfection of tumour DNA and NIH

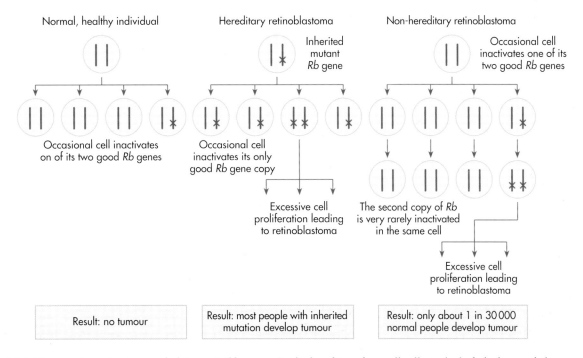

Figure 16.2 *The genetic mechanisms underlying retinoblastoma. In the hereditary form, all cells in the body lack one of the normal two functional copies of a tumour suppressor gene, and tumours occur where the remaining copy is lost or inactivated by a somatic mutation. In the non-hereditary form, all cells initially contain two functional copies of the gene, and the tumour arises because both copies are lost or inactivated through the coincidence of two somatic mutations in one cell.*

Table 16.5 Some oncogenes

Oncogene	Proto-oncogene	Scource of virus	Virus-induced tumour
abl	Tyrosine kinase	Mouse	Leukaemia
erbB	Tyrosine kinase (EGFr, c-erbB2 etc.)	Chicken	Erythroleukaemia
fes	Tyrosine kinase	Cat	Sarcoma
fms	Tyrosine kinase (M-CSM factor)	Cat	Sarcoma
fos	AP-1 protein	Mouse	Osteosarcoma
jun	AP-1 protein	Chicken	Fibrosarcoma
raf (MAP-kinase, kinase, kinase)	Serine kinase activated by ras	Chicken	Sarcoma
myc	Transcription factor	Chicken	Sarcoma
H-ras	GTP (G)-binding protein	Rat	Sarcoma
K-ras	G-protein	Rat	Sarcoma
rel	NFκB transcription factor	Turkey	Reticuloendotheliosis
sis	Platelet-derived growth factor	Monkey	Sarcoma
src	Tyrosine kinase	Chicken	Sarcoma

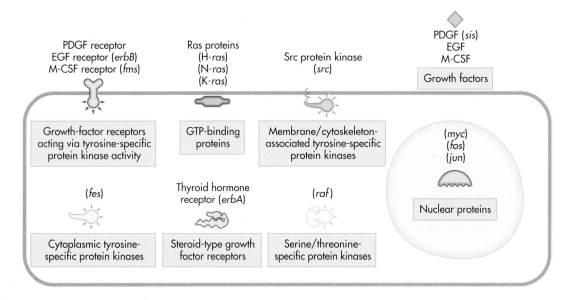

Figure 16.3 The activities and cellular locations of the products of the main classes of known proto-oncogenes. Some representative proto-oncogenes in each class are indicated in brackets.

3T3 fibroblasts) tended to select dominantly acting transforming genes, which are now generally known as 'oncogenes'.

As the number of known oncogenes increased and their functions became known, they were classified into families, defined by their normal cellular counterparts. They include growth factors and their receptors, nuclear regulators of gene transcription and DNA replication, and signal transduction proteins that couple cell surface receptors and the nucleus. More than 60 oncogenes have now been identified (Table 16.5). The types of oncogenes and some of their functions are shown in Figure 16.3. Their transfection into cells causes transformation (Table 16.6).

A cellular proto-oncogene can be converted to an oncogene in a variety of ways:

insertion of a section of DNA into the promoter of the gene (insertional mutagenesis, e.g. Wnt-1);
deletion (conversion of EGFr to v-erbB-2);
translocation or chromosomal re-arrangement (Philadelphia chromosome: Figure 16.4);
point mutation (H-ras);
gene amplification (EGFr in brain tumours).

G-proteins and ras

Proteins that bind and hydrolyse guanosine trisphosphate (GTP) are found commonly in the cell and play a crucial role in cell signalling. When GTP (which is found in large excess in the cell compared with guanosine diphosphate [GDP]) is bound to such G-proteins, the protein becomes activated and initiates a cascade

Table 16.6 Characteristics of the transformed cell

Plasma membrane abnormalities
Increased transmembrane transport (e.g. glucose and calcium)
Excessive endocytosis and blebbing
Increased mobility

Adhesion molecules
Decreased adhesion
Failure of organisation of actin into stress fibres
Reduced fibronectin expression
Increased expression of enzymes such as cathepsin and plasminogen activators

Growth
Grows to high density (lack of density-dependent inhibition)
Decreased requirement for added growth factors
Anchorage-independent growth
Immortal
Can cause animal tumours

of events. However, GTP-binding proteins also rapidly hydrolyse GTP to GDP, thereby rendering themselves inactive. Other proteins can control the activity of GTP binding to such proteins, including one called GTPase activating protein (GAP), which binds to G-proteins inducing them to convert GTP to GDP and become inactive. Another protein, called guanine nucleotide releasing protein (GNRP), binds to G-proteins inducing them to release GDP and bind GTP (which is present in large amounts in the normal cell), converting it into an active form. G-proteins are classified into:

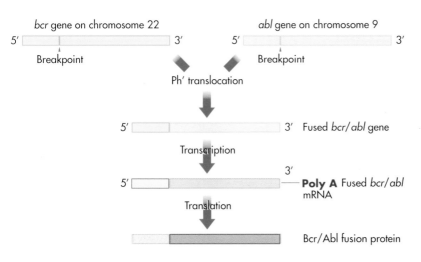

Figure 16.4 *The translocation between chromosomes 9 and 22 responsible for chronic myelogenous leukaemia. The smaller of the two resulting abnormal chromosomes is called the Philadelphia chromosome, after the city in which the abnormality was first recorded.*

monomeric G-proteins (e.g. ras, rac and rho)

hetero-trimeric G-proteins (often directly coupling cell surface receptors to intracellular receptors, e.g. adrenoceptors or muscarinic acetylcholine receptors to adenyl cyclase and phospholipase C respectively).

The ras family

The human *ras* gene family consists of three closely related genes – H-*ras*, K-*ras* and N-*ras* – which encode 21-kDa signal transduction G-proteins involved in the transmission of signals from cell surface receptors. Ras proteins belong to the monomeric family of G-proteins, as distinct from the trimeric family that couples cell surface receptors (e.g. adrenergic receptors) to intracellular events. Other monomeric G-proteins include the rho and rac families, which, like ras proteins, are involved in the relay of signals from the cell membrane. Activation of *ras* by mutation occurs as a result of a single amino acid change as a consequence of single nucleotide mutations. Activated H-*ras* has been found in bladder carcinomas, Ki-*ras* in lung and colon carcinomas, and N-*ras* in haematological malignancies. H-*ras* is a monomeric G-protein. In its mutated (H-*ras*) form, it contains a single point muta-

tion leading to the conversion of a glycine to a valine residue at codon 12. Mutated H-*ras* is constitutively active whether GTP is bound or not.

Ras helps to link activated tyrosine kinase receptors to downstream events by acting as a molecular switch. It is in the 'off' position when bound to GDP and in the 'on' position when bound to GTP. Some tyrosine kinase receptors phosphorylate themselves on tyrosine residues, which then bind to other proteins that have SH2 domains that dock to phosphorylated tyrosine residues. These proteins with SH2 domains then link to other proteins (e.g. Sos) that activate *ras*. Activated *ras* initiates a serine/threonine phosphorylation cascade that eventually activates a kinase called mitogen-activated protein kinase. Eventually, such activation stimulates the action of a number of transcription factors, including jun and elk-1 (Figure 16.5). Figure 16.5 also shows another important point: namely, that protein kinase C can also activate mitogen-activated protein kinase.

Hetero-trimeric G-proteins

A large number of membrane-bound receptors function by activating downstream trimeric G-proteins, which initiate a phosphorylation cascade stimulating certain enzymes. The trimeric G-proteins consist of

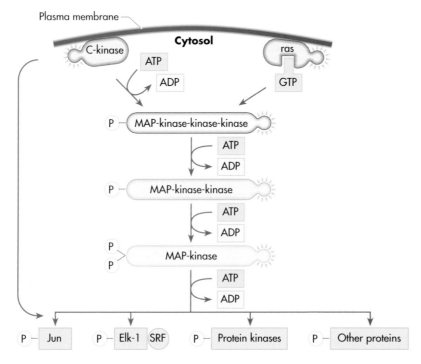

Figure 16.5 *The serine/threonine phosphorylation cascade activated by ras and C-kinase. In the pathway activated by receptor tyrosine kinases via ras, the MAP-kinase-kinase-kinase is often a serine/threonine kinase called raf, which is thought to be activated by the binding of activated ras. In the pathway activated by G-protein-linked receptors via C kinase, the MAP-kinase-kinase-kinase can either be raf or a different serine/threonine kinase. A similar serine/threonine phosphorylation cascade involving structurally and functionally related proteins operates in yeasts and in all animals that have been studied, where it integrates and amplifies signals from different extracellular stimuli. Receptor tyrosine kinases may also activate a more direct signalling pathway to the nucleus by directly phosphorylating, and thereby activating, gene regulatory proteins that contain SH2 domains.*

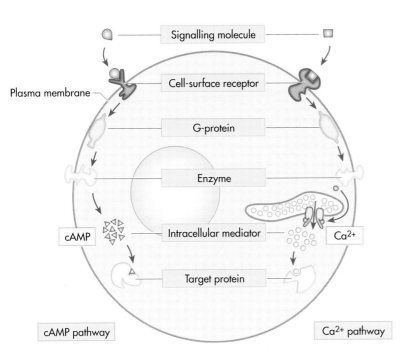

Figure 16.6 *Two major pathways by which G-protein-linked cell-surface receptors generate small intracellular mediators. In both cases, the binding of an extracellular ligand alters the conformation of the cytoplasmic domain of the receptor, causing it to bind to a G-protein that activates (or inactivates) a plasma membrane enzyme. In the cyclic AMP (cAMP) pathway, the enzyme directly produces cyclic AMP. In the Ca²⁺ pathway, the enzyme produces a soluble mediator (inositol trisphosphate) that releases Ca²⁺ from the endoplasmic reticulum. Like other small intracellular mediators, both cyclic AMP and Ca²⁺ relay the signal by acting as allosteric effectors: they bind to specific proteins in the cell, altering their conformation and thereby their activity.*

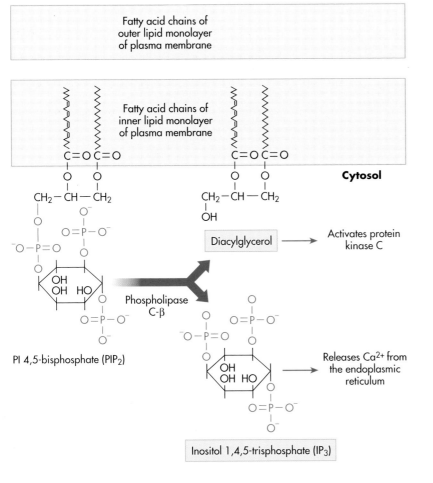

Figure 16.7 *The hydrolysis of PIP₂. Two intracellular mediators are produced when PIP₂ is hydrolysed: inositol trisphosphate (IP₃), which diffuses through the cytosol and releases Ca²⁺ from the endoplasmic reticulum, and diacylglycerol, which remains in the membrane and helps activate the enzyme protein kinase C. There are at least three classes of phospholipase C – β, γ, and δ – and it is the β class that is activated by G-protein-linked receptors. It will be seen later that the γ class is activated by a second class of receptors, called receptor tyrosine kinases, that activate the inositol phospholipid signalling pathway without an intermediary G-protein.*

three parts (α, β and γ) that disassemble when activated; the α subunit bound to GTP activates nearby enzymes such as adenyl cyclase, which synthesises cyclic adenosine monophosphate (cAMP) (Figure 16.6), or phospholipase C, which forms inositol trisphosphate and diacylglycerol from inositol bisphosphate found in the cell membrane (Figure 16.7). Inositol trisphosphate causes calcium release from various intracellular stores, and diacylglycerol activates protein kinase C, which is a serine/threonine kinase (Figure 16.8) that, as pointed out above, can also stimulate mitogen-activated protein kinase.

Examples of receptors linked via G-proteins to phospholipase C include the muscarinic receptor. Activation of the muscarinic receptor causes an increase in transmembrane calcium flux and also a release of inositol trisphosphate, which further releases calcium from the endoplasmic reticulum. Receptors linked via G-proteins to adenyl cyclase include the β adrenergic receptor (stimulation of cAMP) and the α2 receptor (inhibition of cAMP). The α1 receptor stimulates phospholipase C as well as inhibiting adenyl cyclase. Thus, although a wide variety of receptors is coupled to different G-proteins, the exact consequences of receptor activation depend on the specific G-protein that couples the receptor to downstream intracellular signalling mechanisms (Figure 16.9).

Tyrosine kinase growth factor receptors

Many cell surface receptors for growth factors contain a tyrosine kinase domain as part of the protein, which is similar to the *src* family of oncogene tyrosine kinase (including Src, Yes, Fgr, Lck, Lyn, Hck and Blk) and which contains SH2 domains facing the internal portion of the cell. Other growth factor receptors are closely associated with separate tyrosine kinase proteins that are not an intrinsic part of the receptor protein itself. Most of the transforming growth factor receptors (EGFr; IGF-Ir; NGFr; PDGFr, FGFr and VEGFr) contain an intrinsic tyrosine kinase domain, with the exception of that for transforming growth factor beta which contains a serine/threonine kinase. When activated by ligand binding, tyrosine kinase receptors autophosphorylate at several phosphorylation sites and can then act as docking sites for a small set of intracellular proteins that recognise tyrosine-associated phosphate sites via their SH2 domains (e.g. Sos and GRB2). Activation of the EGFr produces dimerisation of the receptor, autophosphorylation of tyrosine residues and phosphorylation of target proteins. EGFr activation is linked to the *ras* signal transduction pathway via two proteins (Sos and GRB2) which, when EGFr is activated, link via raf (mitogen-activated protein kinase-kinase-kinase) to the downstream signals of the *ras* pathway such as mitogen-activated protein kinase.

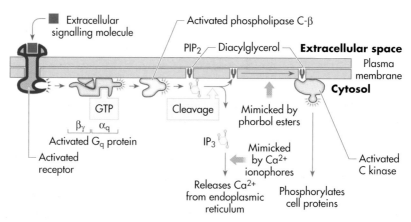

Figure 16.8 *The two branches of the inositol phospholipid pathway. The activated receptor binds to a specific trimeric G-protein (G_q), causing the α subunit to dissociate and activate phospholipase C-β, which cleaves PIP_2 to generate IP_3 and diacylglycerol. The diacylglycerol (together with bound Ca^{2+} and phosphatidylserine – not shown) activates C kinase. Both phospholipase C-β and C kinase are water-soluble enzymes that translocate from the cytosol to the inner face of the plasma membrane in the process of being activated. The effects of IP_3 can be mimicked experimentally in intact cells by treatment with Ca^{2+} ionophores, while the effects of diacylglycerol can be mimicked by treatment with phorbol esters, which bind to C kinase and activate it.*

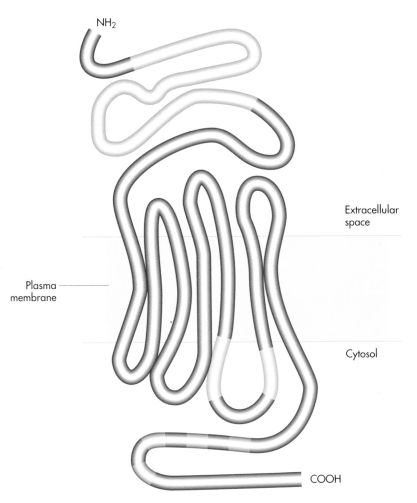

NH₂

Extracellular space

Plasma membrane

Cytosol

COOH

Figure 16.9 *A schematic drawing of a G-protein-linked receptor. Receptors that bind protein ligands have a large extracellular ligand-binding domain formed by the part of the polypeptide chain shown in grey. Receptors for small ligands such as adrenaline have small extracellular domains, and the ligand-binding site is usually deep within the plane of the membrane, formed by amino acids from several of the transmembrane segments. The parts of the intracellular domains that are mainly responsible for binding to trimeric G-proteins are shown in orange, while those that become phosphorylated during receptor desensitisation (discussed later) are shown in red.*

In many growth factor receptors, ligand binding induces dimerisation, a conformational change takes place, and the tyrosine kinase domain is activated. Some mutated growth factor receptors are constitutively active, whereas other receptors can become activated in the absence of ligand if the receptor protein is found at very high levels. Such receptors can also form hetero-dimers (e.g. c-erbB2 with c-erbB3 or with c-erbB1 [EGFr]).

Epidermal growth factor and epidermal growth factor receptor

Epidermal growth factor is a 53-amino acid peptide with mitogenic activity whose action is mediated by binding to a membrane-bound receptor. It was originally isolated from murine submaxillary gland extracts and its distribution is widespread, with high levels in milk, prostatic fluid and urine. The detection of high levels in urine prompted studies of EGFr levels in bladder cancer.

The EGFr is a 175-kDa transmembrane protein with an extracellular epidermal growth factor-binding domain, a small hydrophobic region that spans the plasma membrane, and an intracellular domain that has tyrosine kinase activity as well as target tyrosine residues for autophosphorylation. The EGFr (c-erbB1 gene) has considerable sequence homology with the gp65^{erbB} protein from the avian erythroblastosis virus. The EGFr is also the target for the peptide growth factor transforming growth factor alpha (TGF-α), which is synthesised by a wide range of common epithelial tumours including transitional cell carcinomas of the urinary bladder, renal and prostate cancer.

EGFr are distributed throughout the body and are present on normal fibroblasts, corneal cells, kidney cells, basal prostate epithelium and basal urothelium.

Increased expression of EGFr protein is transforming in some cell lines, and some human solid tumours, including transitional cell carcinomas, have increased levels of EGFr protein. This appears to be achieved by a variety of mechanisms, including gene amplification, up-regulation of mRNA, increased translation or post-translational modification of the protein.

c-erbB2

The proto-oncogene c-erbB2 (also known as *neu* or HER2) encodes a transmembrane glycoprotein that is related to the EGFr. Several groups have reported a candidate ligand for the c-erbB2 receptor, and elucidation of its structure – neu differentiation factor (NDF) or Heregulin-α (HRG-α) – reveals it to be an additional member of the EGF family. Two further members of the erb-B receptor family are HER3/p160^{erbB3} and HER4/p180^{erbB4}. Recent evidence suggests, however, that Heregulin is the physiological ligand for c-erbB3, and that for c-erbB2 is as yet unidentified.

Fibroblast growth factor

The fibroblast growth factors (FGFs) are a family of peptides related by sequence similarity that have been implicated in the regulation of cell proliferation, angiogenesis, embryonal development, differentiation and motility. The family includes acidic fibroblast growth factor (aFGF; FGF1), basic fibroblast growth factor (bFGF; FGF2), *int2* (FGF3), *hst* (FGF4), FGF5, *hst2* (FGF6), keratinocyte growth factor (KGF; FGF7), androgen-inducible growth factor (AIGF; FGF8) and FGF9. These factors bind with varying degrees of specificity to a family of tyrosine kinase receptors. bFGF has been shown to transform mouse fibroblasts in vitro, and *int2* (FGF3) is the human homologue to one of the common integration sites of mouse mammary tumour virus (MMTV), and *hst* (FGF4) is the most frequently detected human transforming gene after *ras* in the NIH 3T3 assay. These two genes were reported to be amplified in 3/43 (7%) of bladder tumours and 41/238 (17%) of breast carcinomas.

Basic FGF has been identified in both benign and malignant human prostate. Immunohistochemistry has identified FGF-2 predominantly in prostatic stroma but also in epithelial cells. FGF-1 is also pre-

sent in the prostate but at a lower level than FGF-2. In addition, using a prostate stromal cell culture model, there is evidence for the interaction of FGF-2 and TGF-β₁, resulting in positive and negative proliferative effects respectively. Besides potential autocrine loop activation, FGFs may also contribute to the pathophysiology of the prostate via paracrine activity. FGF-7, or KGF, is synthesised and secreted by stromal cells, being thought to act on FGF-receptor-bearing epithelial cells, resulting in cellular proliferation. It is also interesting to note that, in a transgenic mouse system, over-expression of FGF-3 (*int*-2) changes in the prostate of the male progeny were dramatic and involved only hyperplasia, without evidence of malignant transformation.

The fibroblast growth factor receptors (FGFrs) share structural similarities in both the extracellular domains tht bind FGFs and the intracellular domains that activate the signal transduction pathway. The four FGFrs, FGF-1 to FGF-4, display different binding affinities for the different FGFs. FGF-1 binds to all four receptors while FGF-2 is more restricted and only binds to the first three FGFrs. Receptor/receptor interactions are known to occur and may have a role in the development of both benign hyperplasia and carcinoma of the prostate. To date, the expression of FGFs and their receptors is not fully understood, but there does appear to be a major difference between benign and malignant prostate in the activity of the FGF system. Splice variants occur in the FGFrs. It is likely that subtle changes occur in the FGF system during malignant progression. This has been demonstrated elegantly in a mouse prostate cancer model. During progression from the benign to the malignant phenotype, the prostate epithelial cells display a switch of expression of FGFr splice variants, conferring a switch of high-affinity binding from FGF-7 to FGF-2. FGF-2 was also concomitantly up-regulated, along with FGF-3 and FGF-5. Further evidence supporting a role for FGFs in the development of malignancy is that transformation of BHK-21 (baby hamster kidney) cells with plasmids carrying the bFGF coding sequence results in cells that exhibit the transformed phenotype. The prostatic cancer cell lines DU145 and PC-3 produce active FGF-2 and express large amounts of FGF-2. However, only the DU145 cell line and not the PC-3 cell line has been shown to respond to exogenous FGF-2.

The interaction between the androgen receptor and growth factor systems is important. It is known that certain growth factors, including FGF-7/KGF, IGFs and EGF, may activate androgen-dependent gene expression in the absence of androgen, which may represent a mechanism for the development of hormone insensitivity in prostate tumours.

Insulin-like growth factors

Insulin-like growth factor I (IGF-I) is a 70-amino acid polypeptide with functional homology to insulin. The mitogenic effect of IGF-I is due to its ability to facilitate the transfer of cells from the G1 phase to the S phase in the cell cycle. IGF-I and the closely related IGF-II are present in biological fluids and tissue extracts and are usually bound to an IGF-binding protein. There are two types of receptors for the IGFs. The type 1 receptor is a tyrosine kinase and binds both IGF-I and IGF-II. The type 2 receptor is structurally distinct and binds primarily IGF-II. The majority of the mitogenic effects of the IGFs appear to be mediated via the type 1 IGF receptor.

The growth of normal prostatic epithelial cells in culture is dependent on the presence of IGF-I and II. The response is most marked with IGF-I. The type 1 IGF receptor has been identified in normal, benign and malignant prostatic tissues. It is preferentially expressed in the basal cells. Production of IGF-II has been demonstrated by prostatic fibroblasts; IGF-I has not been identified as being produced by either prostatic fibroblasts or epithelial cells. However, IGF-1 mRNA has been identified in stromal cells from benign prostatic hyperplasia specimens. The mechanism of IGF-II-mediated stimulation of prostatic epithelial cells in benign prostatic hyperplasia appears to be similar to that in normal prostate, although the expression of IGF-II mRNA is ten-fold higher in fibroblasts from benign prostatic hyperplasia tissues. This led to the hypothesis that such cells may be 'reverting to a fetal-like state', in which IGF-II expression is normally high, causing stimulation of proliferation and the development of benign prostatic hyperplasia.

Transforming growth factor beta

TGF-β_1 is the predominant species in the TGF-β superfamily, which includes several modulators of growth, differentiation and morphogenesis (including bone morphogenetic proteins). TGF-β_1 is classically regarded as a stimulator for mesenchyme cells and an inhibitor for epithelial cells. Five isoforms of TGF-β have so far been identified, of which only the first three occur in mammals. TGF-β_1 is a homodimer of two 112-amino acid subunits linked by disulphide bonds. Cellular receptors for TGF-β_1 have been identified in the rat ventral prostate, where they are negatively regulated by androgens and involved in the mechanism of castration-induced prostatic cell death. Receptors for TGF-β_1 have been identified in the human prostate cancer cell lines DU145 and PC-3. TGF-β_1 has been shown to have an inhibitory effect on human prostatic fibroblasts and epithelial cells in culture. It has been suggested that TGF-β_1 causes inhibition of proliferation by preventing phosphorylation of the protein product of the retinoblastoma gene (pRb) by up-regulation of p15, which is a cyclin-dependent kinase inhibitor, and by stabilisation of the p27 protein.

Tumour suppressor genes

Evidence for the existence of tumour suppressor genes has come from several sources, although the significance of the observations was not appreciated at the time. Experiments dating back to the 1960s involving the fusion of normal and transformed cells had shown that normal genes can suppress transformation and malignancy in cell lines.

The second line of evidence came from an analysis of the inheritance of rare hereditary childhood cancers. Based on retinoblastoma, Knudson proposed a two-hit inactivation process in which both copies of a critical gene had to be inactivated for the disease to be manifest (see Figure 16.2). That these hereditary cancers are often associated with predisposition to a wide range of sporadic tumours of other tissues led to the further suggestion that somatic mutation or loss of these same genes was probably involved in the genesis of a wide range of cancers, including bladder cancer.

This also provided a possible explanation for the observation of non-random chromosome deletions seen in sporadic tumours. This concept in turn led to the identification of the p53 gene as a tumour suppressor gene.

Cytogenetic studies have shown that frequent non-random chromosome alterations occur in cancer. For instance, in bladder cancer, these alterations involve chromosomes 1p, 3p, 9p, 10q, 11, 13q, 17p and 18q. Loss of one copy of chromosome 9p was found as an early event in low-stage, low-grade tumours, unlike other chromosome losses that appeared more prevalent in advanced tumours. The high frequency of chromosome 9p losses in bladder cancer is not seen in other tumour types, and suggests the possible location of a tumour suppressor gene specific to bladder cancer.

The p53 tumour suppressor gene

The human p53 gene, located on the short arm of chromosome 17, encodes a nuclear phosphoprotein that binds to specific DNA sequences in the human genome and appears to play a key role in the control of DNA replication and hence cellular proliferation. Non-random chromosome 17 losses involving the p53 locus are commonly found in human tumours, including bladder cancer, and loss of one copy of the p53 gene has been found to be accompanied frequently by mutation of the remaining allele. Transfection studies have shown that the wild-type protein is able to suppress cell proliferation and transformation. It thus acts in such circumstances as a tumour suppressor gene, which can contribute to tumour formation by deletions or loss of function mutations. Germ-line mutations of the p53 gene have been found in certain inherited predispositions to cancer (e.g. Li–Fraumeni syndrome, in which there is clustering of soft tissue and bone sarcomas at any age, and cancers under the age of 45 in breast, brain, adrenal cortex and lung) and somatic cell mutations have frequently been detected in a wide range of common sporadic tumours, including breast, colon, brain and lung tumours as well as bladder cancer. These mutations are predominantly of the point mis-sense type and occur at many different locations within four highly conserved regions of the gene (codons 117–142,

171–181, 234–258 and 270–286) located in exons 4 to 9 of the p53 gene.

The p53 protein has three parts: a central DNA-binding domain in which mutations are usually of the mis-sense type, a transcription domain (N terminus) and a regulatory domain (C terminus) in which mutations result in non-sense or stop codons. The protein mdm2 binds near the N terminus of the protein. One of the genes activated by p53 is the p21 protein (WAF1), which inhibits the activity of cyclin-dependent kinases and which also binds to PCNA. Other genes include gadd45 and the protein bax (which promotes apoptosis).

The p53 protein has a short half-life, measured in the order of minutes, and is normally present at low levels not detectable by immunohistochemistry. One of the remarkable features of the p53 gene is that a broad spectrum of mutations can lead to an altered conformation and inactivation of the protein product, with an increased cellular half-life, resulting in accumulation in the cell to levels that are readily detectable by immunohistochemical staining. Although this initially led to suggestions that positive detection of p53 by immunohistochemistry was synonymous with the detection of mutations, this is now realised not to be the case. Moreover, some mutations do not result in accumulation of the altered protein product, and these have to be screened for by alternative complementary methods such as single strand conformation polymorphism assays to obtain a more complete picture. However, even combined, these techniques are at best a way of trawling for mutations rather than a way of systematically screening for all possible mutations. The definitive method of establishing the presence of a mutation in a sample is by DNA sequencing procedures.

Inactivation of normal p53 in tumours

Some proteins have been shown to bind to p53 and inactivate it. For instance, in sarcomas, it has been shown that p53 mutations are rare, but there is increased expression of a protein called mdm-2 which, like the large T antigen of the SV40 virus, binds to p53, inactivates and stabilises it. This confirms the frequent involvement of the p53 pathway in many human tumours.

p53 and G1 arrest

Irradiation of cells has been shown to result in marked up-regulation of the wild-type p53 protein. It may be that the primary event is DNA repair following radiotherapy which then activates p53. However, up-regulation of p53 switches on downstream genes such as *p21* which is a potent inhibitor of cell division, and places them into G1 arrest, which allows completion of DNA repair if this is possible.

p53 and apoptosis

Some authors believe that increased levels of p53 can, if DNA damage is too severe to repair during G1 arrest, force the cell into apoptosis. There is no doubt that with severe DNA damage there is an initial attempt at DNA repair followed by up-regulation of p53, stimulation of p21 and cell cycle arrest. With more severe DNA damage or with less severe damage in certain types of cells (e.g. thymocytes), this process may be followed by apoptosis, but currently it is controversial as to whether p53 is directly responsible for apoptosis in such circumstances. Certainly, p53 can up-regulate *bax* (a promoter of apoptosis) but, equally certainly in some cells, apoptosis can occur without recourse to the p53–bax pathway.

mdm2 oncogene

The *mdm2* gene (murine double minute 2) is located on chromosome 12q13-14 and encodes a 90-kDa nuclear protein. The mdm2 protein may act as an oncoprotein when over-expressed, by binding to the 'guardian of the genome', wild-type p53 protein, and abrogating its functions.

Retinoblastoma gene

The *Rb1* gene encodes a 105–115 kDa nuclear phosphoprotein that binds to DNA and appears to be involved in growth regulation in a wide variety of cell types. There are related p107 and p130 proteins whose function in humans has not been elucidated but which may have overlapping actions. The *Rb1* gene product binds to the transforming proteins of several DNA tumour viruses, including adenovirus E1A, SV40 large T antigen, and human papilloma virus E7 proteins. Abnormalities in the *Rb* gene were first reported in patients with inherited retinoblastoma who had one abnormal copy of the gene in all retinal cells; it is

thought that subsequent 'spontaneous' alterations in the remaining copy of the *Rb* gene cause tumour formation.

The Rb protein is central to the function of the cell cycle. It is inactive when phosphorylated or when bound to inactivating proteins. It is the target of cyclin-dependent kinases and cyclin D. When it is activated, it stimulates the E2F family of transcription factors (myc and jun are among them); it is a negative regulator of the cell cycle. Disruption of this pathway is central to many tumours. The cyclin-dependent kinase inhibitor p16 is particularly linked to *Rb*, so when p16 is up-regulated and the activity of cdk2 is inhibited, the Rb protein is not phosphorylated so it binds to DNA and inhibits transcription and the E2F family of transcription factors is switched off.

A wider role for the *Rb1* gene was suggested by the observation that those who inherit the mutant allele have a higher incidence of a wide range of non-ocular second tumours, particularly osteosarcomas but also lung, melanoma and bladder cancer.

Initial studies with the *Rb1* cDNA probe, based mainly on tumour cell lines, reported frequent structural abnormalities of the gene and absence of *Rb1* mRNA. Subsequent extensions of these studies with polyclonal antisera indicated that absence or abnormal forms of the Rb protein are almost universal in small cell lung cancer cell lines and present in one-third of bladder carcinoma cell lines, whilst being infrequent in colonic, breast and melanoma cell lines. Studies on primary bladder tumours have shown that loss of heterozygosity for *Rb1*-linked markers is associated with the development of invasive lesions. The overall frequency of *Rb1* allelic loss in bladder cancer was 3/63 (5%) for superficial (pTa/pT1) and 30/58 (52%) for invasive (T2–T4) tumours. Major rearrangements of the remaining *Rb1* gene were detected in only a small proportion of these cases, suggesting that generally more subtle small deletions or point mutations are involved, which have yet to be characterised. Altered Rb protein expression is associated with a poor outcome in several tumour types, including bladder.

Von Hippel–Lindau disease

This is inherited as a dominant abnormality and consists of retinal cysts, cerebellar haemangioblastomas, pancreatic cysts, phaeochromocytomas, renal cysts and renal cancer. The *VHL* gene is situated on chromosome 3 and also affects many sporadic renal cancers. It encodes a small protein (213 aa) with 3 exons and, in the human gene, there are 8 pentapeptide repeats in exon 1. Most mutations in *VHL* are found at the carboxy-terminus of exon 1 and at the beginning of exon 3. Similar mutations are found in sporadic tumours, but in addition mutations are found in exon 2, which is a rare event in von Hippel–Lindau disease. The VHL protein binds to the elongation factors elongin B and C, which help in the synthesis of mRNA. It is thought that the VHL/elongin B and C complex moves from the nucleus into the cytoplasm as a response to cell–cell contacts. VHL also up-regulates the peptide VEGF (see below), a feature that may be responsible for angiogenesis in renal cancer.

Degradation of extracellular matrix barriers

Metastasis requires cancer cells to penetrate extracellular matrix barriers. This involves the proteolytic degradation of extracellular matrix components. Metalloproteinases (MMPs) are a family of zinc-dependent endopeptidases (gelatinases) known to degrade extracellular matrix components. Their activity is inhibited by tissue inhibitors of metalloproteinases (TIMPs). High levels of TIMP-2 immunoreactivity detected both in tumour cells and in stroma have been reported to be associated with cancer-specific death. This is somewhat surprising given that TIMPs inhibit the degradation of extracellular matrix. However, recent studies have shown that under certain circumstances, TIMP-2 can also activate MMP-2. Other enzymes include the plasminogen activators. These enzymes may be expressed by host stroma around a tumour as an indicator merely of tissue remodelling. Thus, they have not shown consistent usefulness as prognostic markers.

Angiogenesis

This is the process of new blood vessel formation that is found in a number of diseases including cancer, diabetic retinopathy and the inflammatory arthritides. The initiation of angiogenesis in tumours is dependent on the co-ordinated expression of several factors (Table 16.7).

Angiogenesis requires dilatation of vessels, breakdown of perivascular stroma, migration and proliferation of endothelial cells, and canalisation of endothelial buds. Potent inhibitors of angiogenesis include angiostatin (which, paradoxically, is secreted by some primary tumours) and thrombospondin (which is involved in the binding of macrophages to apoptotic cells and which is also up-regulated by normal *p53*). A potent stimulus to angiogenesis is hypoxia, which up-regulates the expression of vascular endothelial growth factor (VEGF).

Vascular endothelial growth factor is a specific mitogen for endothelial cells. It exists in four forms (121, 165, 189 and 206 amino acid peptides) and is secreted by a number of cell types. VEGFr is found on endothelial cells. There are two forms of the VEGFr (Flt-1 and Flk-1), which is a tyrosine kinase.

Altered cell adhesion

Cell adhesion molecules

Decreased intercellular adhesiveness favours the detachment of tumour cells and this may play a role in regression to metastatic disease. At least four families of cell adhesion molecules are thought to be involved in cell–cell adhesion (cadherins, selectins, immunoglobulins and integrins). The most widely

Table 16.7 Peptides associated with angiogenesis

Vascular endothelial growth factor
Fibroblast growth factors
Platelet-derived growth factor
Tumour necrosis factor α
Angiogenin
Epidermal growth factor
Transforming growth factor alpha and beta
Platelet-derived endothelial cell growth factor or thymidine phosphorylase

studied have been E-cadherin, a cell-surface glycoprotein restricted to epithelial tissue and involved in calcium-dependent homotypic cell–cell adhesion, and vascular cell adhesion molecules, E-selectin, vascular cell adhesion molecule-1 (VCAM-1) and intercellular adhesion molecule-1 (ICAM-1). The regulation of the expression of E-cadherin on tumour cells is unclear. Post-translational modification of the protein product may affect function. It is known that three molecules (α, β and γ catenins) form bridges between the cytoplasmic tail of E-cadherin and the cytoskeleton, which may be necessary for E-cadherin to function normally.

Genes associated with chemoresistance

Chemotherapy with epirubicin or mitomycin C is increasingly used for recurrent superficial papillary tumours. In muscle-invasive disease, adjuvant and neoadjuvant chemotherapy regimes are currently being tested in clinical trials. Molecular mechanisms that mediate cellular drug resistance may play a role in the differential responsiveness of individual bladder tumours to chemotherapy. Transcript levels of the multidrug resistance (*mdr*1) gene have been found to vary 34-fold in high-grade muscle-invasive bladder tumours. In addition, renal cell carcinomas have very high levels of this gene, which may explain why it is chemoresistant.

Further reading

Alberts B, Bray D, Lewis J, Raff M, Roberts K, Watson JD. Cancer. In: Molecular Biology of the Cell. Chapter 24. Third Edition. Levittown, PA: Garland Publishing, 1998

Oliver RTD, Coptcoat MJ (eds). Bladder Cancer. Cancer Surveys. Volume 31. New York: Cold Spring Harbor Laboratory Press, 1998

The molecular genetics of renal cell carcinoma

17

S. C. Clifford and E. R. Maher

The epidemiology and pathology of renal cell carcinoma

Renal cell carcinoma is an adenocarcinoma that arises from the proximal tubular cells of the kidney, and represents between 2% and 3% of adult malignancies. It accounts for approximately 24 000 new cases and 10 000 deaths annually in the USA, with the highest prevalence observed in the 50–60-year age group, and a male : female ratio of about 2 : 1. Cigarette smoking has been identified as a positive risk factor for renal cell carcinoma development [1]. Whereas the majority of renal cell carcinomas (approximately 98%) are sporadic in nature, a significant hereditary component of the disease exists in approximately 2% of cases.

Renal cell carcinoma may be considered according to histopathological criteria. Among sporadic cases, most (78%) are classified as clear cell tumours. Non-clear cell tumours are predominantly classed as chromophilic (12%) or chromophobic (5%), and, less frequently, ductus Bellini or oncocytic [2]. An alternative but related classification is based on tumour structure rather than cell type, and divides renal cell carcinoma into papillary and non-papillary tumours [3]. Generally, the papillary tumours correspond to the chromophilic group and non-papillary tumours have a clear cell appearance.

Renal cell carcinoma as a genetic disease

There are many similarities between the processes and genes involved in normal development and tumorigenesis. Normal development requires precise control of gene expression such that the balance between growth-promoting and growth-suppressing influences is carefully co-ordinated. Thus, growth, differentiation and division of somatic cells are highly regulated, and cancer cells represent variants that have lost their usual growth and differentiation control. The conversion of cells into the neoplastic state involves three key types of change: firstly, immortalisation, or the acquirement of the ability to grow indefinitely; secondly, transformation, the failure to observe the normal constraints of growth; and thirdly, metastasis, in which the cancer cell gains the ability to invade normal tissue. Until recently, little was known of the molecular and genetic basis underlying these events. However, research has now highlighted two broad classes of genes, oncogenes and tumour suppressor genes, alterations in which contribute to the transformation of normal cells into tumour cells. A further class of cancer genes, those involved in DNA repair, has also been implicated in some tumour types, but appears not to have a major role in renal cell carcinoma [4].

Oncogenes
The normal cellular counterparts of oncogenes are called proto-oncogenes, which are involved in the normal positive regulation of cellular functions such as

growth control. The different types of oncogenes described have been classed into functional groups such as transmembrane receptors, growth factors and transcription factors, and over 100 have been identified to date. The generation of an oncogene represents a gain of function in which a proto-oncogene is activated aberrantly, by mechanisms including constitutive activation by gene mutation (e.g. c-Ha-*ras*), gene amplification (e.g. c-*erbB*-2), gene insertion (e.g. *int-2*) or by gene rearrangements such as translocations (e.g. *bcr-abl*), and frequently leads to gene over-expression either in the usual tissue or in a cell type in which it is not normally expressed [4].

Tumour suppressor genes

In normal cells, tumour suppressor genes are involved in the negative control of growth and usually impose a constraint on cell growth or the cell cycle. The loss of such constraints, therefore, causes abnormal growth control and the potential for tumorigenicity. Such genes have been detected in the form of genomic deletions of (part of) the gene or other inactivating mutations, and approximately ten different genes of varying intracellular function have thus far been identified, including the *p53*, Retinoblastoma (*RB*) and von Hippel–Lindau disease (*VHL*) genes [4].

Renal cell carcinoma may therefore be considered as a genetic disease, and numerous genes have been identified to date that are expressed aberrantly in this disease, many of which play a key role in normal renal development. This chapter reviews the more important changes described thus far, and aims to provide an insight into the broad range of genetic changes involved in the transformation of the normal proximal tubule cell into the neoplastic state, and the further development and progression of renal cell carcinoma.

The role of inherited disease in the identification of genes altered in sporadic renal cell carcinoma development

Only 2% of renal cell carcinoma cases are familial, but molecular genetic investigations of inherited forms of the disease have provided novel insights into the pathogenesis of sporadic and familial renal cell carcinoma. The mean age at onset is younger in familial than in sporadic cases [5, 6]. Familial renal cell carcinoma may be classified by whether (i) renal cell carcinoma is the only feature, or (ii) there are additional features as in von Hippel–Lindau disease.

Familial clear cell renal cell carcinoma and the von Hippel–Lindau disease tumour suppressor gene

The most common cause of inherited renal cell carcinoma is von Hippel–Lindau disease, a dominantly inherited familial cancer syndrome characterised by a high risk of renal cell carcinoma (>70% by the age of 60 years), retinal and cerebellar haemangioblastomas, phaeochromocytomas and renal pancreatic and epididymal cysts [7–9]. Pancreatic islet cell tumours and endolymphatic sac tumours are rare but significant complications. Renal cell carcinoma is the most common cause of death in von Hippel–Lindau disease, and all patients and at-risk relatives should receive routine annual renal imaging from the age of 15 years to ensure the early detection of renal tumours. Small (<3 cm) tumours detected presymptomatically may be carefully monitored [10], but larger tumours should be removed to prevent metastatic spread. The combination of early-onset renal cell carcinoma (the mean age of onset in von Hippel–Lindau patients is in the fifth decade, but renal cell carcinoma has been reported in a teenager with von Hippel–Lindau disease) and often multiple tumours (>50% patients have bilateral or multicentric tumours) in von Hippel–Lindau disease has resulted in the adoption of a nephron-sparing approach to the surgical management of renal cell carcinoma in von Hippel–Lindau disease in many centres [11, 12]. Patients and at-risk relatives also require surveillance for extrarenal complications [12]. The gene for von Hippel–Lindau disease has been localised to the distal region of the short arm of chromosome 3 (3p25–26), and was isolated in 1993 [13]. Most families have different mutations in the *VHL* gene, but DNA predictive testing (by direct mutation analysis or linked DNA markers) is possible in the majority of families, so that annual screening can be discontinued in relatives who are shown not to be gene carriers. In addition to identifying gene carriers, the identification of a *VHL* gene mutation may also provide a guide to the likely phenotype. Germ-line deletions or mutations predicted to cause a truncated protein product are associated with a low risk of phaeochromocytoma, whereas specific amino acid substitutions can cause a high risk of this condition. Most mis-sense mutations are associated with a high risk of renal cell carcinoma, but some are associated with a low risk of renal cell carcinoma and a high risk of phaeochromocytoma [14–18].

The *VHL* gene appears to function as a classic tumour suppressor gene, so that inactivation of both alleles is required to initiate tumorigenesis [19]. Thus, in von Hippel–Lindau patients, inactivation of one allele by a germ-line mutation is followed by inactivation (usually loss) of the second allele [20, 21]. Importantly, it appears that inactivation of both *VHL* alleles also occurs in the majority of sporadic clear cell renal carcinomas, so establishing that somatic inactivation of the *VHL* gene is a critical event in the pathogenesis of the most common form of non-familial renal cell carcinoma [22–25]. Somatic *VHL* gene mutations can

be identified in approximately 50% of clear cell tumours [22, 24]. A further 15% of tumours have *VHL* gene hypermethylation and silencing of *VHL* mRNA expression [25, 26]. However, *VHL* inactivation does not appear to be a feature of non-clear cell renal carcinoma. Chromosome 3p loss appears to be an early event in tumorigenesis, compatible with a role of *VHL* inactivation in tumour initiation [27]. The introduction of wild-type VHL protein into a *VHL*-deficient renal cell carcinoma cell line has been reported to suppress tumorigenicity of the renal carcinoma cells both in vitro and in a nude mice assay in vivo [28, 29], and recent studies suggest that the wild-type VHL protein may suppress the expression of proto-oncogenes and growth factors such as vascular endothelial growth factor [30, 31]. Indeed, investigators have recently demonstrated that the wild-type VHL protein can act to promote RNA polymerase II pausing during gene transcription by interaction with the elongin (SIII) complex and hence down-regulate the rate of transcriptional elongation (Figure 17.1) [32–34]. Therefore, molecular investigations of von Hippel–Lindau disease have defined a previously

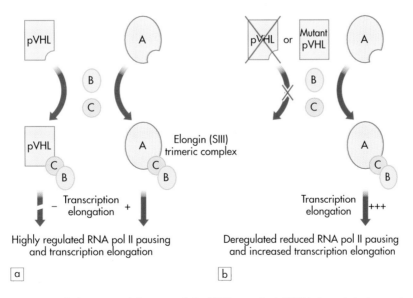

Figure 17.1 *Schematic representation of the proposed function of the VHL protein (pVHL) through its interaction with the elongin (SIII) complex (after Science 1995; 269: 1400). The elongin trimeric complex promotes transcriptional elongation via suppression of RNA polymerase II pausing during gene transcription. (a) In a normal cell, pVHL competes with elongin A for the binding of the elongin B and C subunits, and can so prevent assembly of the functional elongin complex (A + B + C) and suppress transcriptional elongation. The transcription of mRNA from target genes is thus highly regulated through this control of RNA polymerase II (pol II) pausing. (b) In a cancer cell, pVHL is absent or inactivated and elongin A binds to the B and C subunits in a deregulated fashion. The elongin complex (A + B + C) reduces pol II pausing and increases the transcription of target genes.*

undescribed mechanism of tumour suppressor gene function and may eventually lead to novel therapeutic approaches to von Hippel–Lindau disease and renal cell carcinoma.

Familial clear cell renal carcinoma with no additional features of von Hippel–Lindau disease occurs, but is uncommon. Although VHL gene mutations have been identified in some cases of familial phaeochromocytoma [35, 36], to date, germ-line VHL gene mutations have not been reported in familial clear cell renal carcinoma kindreds. In rare cases, inherited predisposition to clear cell renal carcinoma has been associated with balanced translocations involving the short arm of chromosome 3 [37, 38]. In these cases, the translocation breakpoints were centromeric (3p14) to the VHL locus (3p25), suggesting a possible renal cell carcinoma susceptibility gene at this breakpoint in proximal 3p. However, tumours from the t(3;8) family demonstrate somatic VHL gene mutations, suggesting that renal cell carcinoma susceptibility may result in the translocated chromosome being unstable and easily lost from cells in which a somatic VHL gene mutation has occurred. Thus, loss of the translocation chromosome occurs as a 'second-hit', resulting in the absence of functioning VHL protein within the cell containing a somatic VHL mutation, and a renal cell carcinoma is initiated [39]. These findings further implicate VHL gene inactivation in the pathogenesis of clear cell renal carcinoma. Recently, the FHIT putative tumour suppressor gene was isolated from the region close to the t(3;8) translocation breakpoint on 3p, but it is not yet known if inactivation of this gene has a role in the pathogenesis of sporadic renal cell carcinoma [40].

Familial non-clear cell renal carcinoma

Zbar et al. [41, 42] have described kindreds with dominantly inherited papillary non-clear cell renal carcinoma. Tumours were frequently bilateral and multiple, papillary tumours can be slow growing, and screening of at-risk relatives often revealed evidence of asymptomatic tumours [42]. Linkage to the VHL gene was excluded in families suitable for genetic linkage analysis [42]. Somatic VHL gene mutations have not been identified in sporadic non-clear cell renal carcinoma, and this further supports the concept that

clear cell and non-clear cell renal carcinomas have a different genetic basis [22–24]. The most frequent cytogenetic abnormality in non-clear cell renal carcinoma is trisomy 7, but chromosome 3 deletions (which occur in most clear cell tumours) are uncommon [41]. Molecular genetic analysis of sporadic renal cell carcinoma has indicated that, compared to clear cell tumours, deletions of the long arms of chromosomes 11 and 21 are common in papillary renal cell carcinoma [27]. A specific chromosomal translocation between chromosomes X and 1 (t(X;1)(p11;q21)) has been described for a subgroup of human papillary renal cell carcinoma [43], and a fusion gene that is created at the translocation breakpoint has recently been identified [44], although its role in the pathogenesis remains to be elucidated.

The Eker rat model of familial papillary renal cancer is caused by an inactivating mutation in the rat TSC2 gene [45, 46]. In humans, inherited mutations in the TSC2 gene cause tuberous sclerosis [47]. The most frequent renal complications of tuberous sclerosis are angiomyolipomas and renal cysts and, in addition, an increased incidence of renal cell carcinoma has been reported, but the absolute risk appears to be small. The TSC2 gene maps to the tip of the short arm of human chromosome 16 and encodes a protein (tuberin) that contains an area of sequence homology with the GTPase-activating protein rap1GAP [48]. Tuberous sclerosis can also be caused by mutations in the TSC1 gene, which maps to chromosome 9q34, but this gene has not yet been identified. There are no obvious differences between the clinical features of patients with TSC1 and TSC2 mutations, except that in some families large deletions of the TSC2 gene extend into the adjacent gene for adult polycystic kidney disease (PKD1) and are associated with the presence of severe and early-onset polycystic kidneys [49]. Both TSC1 and TSC2 appear to act as tumour suppressor genes, and loss of the wild-type allele has been detected in angiomyolipomas and other tuberous sclerosis neoplasms [50]. However, somatic TSC2 mutations or allele loss have not yet been reported in sporadic non-clear cell renal carcinoma.

Urothelial tumours, including carcinoma of the renal pelvis, may occur in hereditary non-polyposis colon cancer syndrome, a dominantly inherited disorder characterised by a susceptibility to early-onset and multiple colorectal cancer and, in some families, extraintestinal tumours, principally uterine and ovarian cancers. Hereditary non-polyposis colon cancer is frequently caused by inherited mutations in two DNA-mismatch repair genes (MSH2 and MLH1) and tumours from patients with this cancer usually show evidence of DNA replication errors [51]. However, mutations in these genes do not appear to have a major role in the pathogenesis of sporadic renal cell carcinoma [27].

Genetic alterations in the tumorigenesis of sporadic renal cell carcinoma

In addition to those genetic alterations specifically implicated in the development of sporadic renal cell carcinoma by their role in the tumorigenesis of inherited renal cell carcinoma, changes to a multitude of other genes have been investigated in this disease. These genes may have been implicated in renal cell carcinoma either by cytogenetic or molecular genetic evidence, or because of known roles in the pathogenesis of other tumour types and familial syndromes. These are classified into the two broad categories of (i) tumour suppressor genes and (ii) oncogenes.

Tumour suppressor genes in renal cell carcinoma

The p53 and retinoblastoma (RB) tumour suppressor genes

The p53 tumour suppressor gene at chromosome 17p13.1 encodes a 393-amino acid protein that plays a specific role in the maintenance of DNA integrity and cell cyle control. Among other functions, endogenously low p53 protein levels are increased in response to DNA damage and, dependent upon the level of DNA damage, can either block the damaged cell from entering S phase (G1 arrest) or induce programmed cell death (apoptosis). p53-induced G1 arrest is mediated, at least partially, by its ability to induce the expression of p21, an inhibitor of cyclin-dependent kinases. A substantial body of evidence has accumulated in recent years to suggest that loss of normal p53 function is associated with cell transformation in vitro and neoplastic development in vivo. The major implicating evidence of a role for p53 in tumorigenesis includes (i) the ability of the wild-type p53 gene to suppress tumorigenicity in vitro in cells either carrying defective p53 or transformed by cellular oncogenes; (ii) transgenic mice deficient for p53 are significantly more prone to tumour development; (iii) germ-line p53 mutations are associated with the Li–Fraumeni hereditary cancer syndrome; and (iv) mis-sense p53 mutations, the most commonly detected alteration of the p53 gene, and/or allelic losses occur frequently in diverse human cancers. Indeed, alterations to the p53 gene have been demonstrated to be the most common change identified in human cancer, specifically detected in most common carcinomas including lung (40–80% of tumours), gastric (30–60%), breast (10–40%), colorectal (40–70%) and bladder (30–60%) [52].

Loss of heterozygosity studies can be used to detect allelic loss in tumour samples, and those performed at the p53 locus in renal cell carcinoma [53, 54] have demonstrated a good accordance between the rates of loss detected (17–21%). However, using direct genetic analysis including direct DNA sequencing, p53 mutation detection rates in renal cell carcinoma have been consistently low (0–10%) [54–58], with those few mutations detected showing no overall association with any histopathological criteria. Many p53 mis-sense mutations induce changes that dramatically prolong the protein half-life, which can be readily detected. Detection of p53 protein levels in renal cell carcinoma by immunohistochemistry has, however, yielded ambiguous results, with p53 positivity rates ranging between 4% and 87%, dependent upon the study and the antibody used [59–63]. Whereas no study has reported any positive correlations between p53 protein staining and any particular histological renal cell carcinoma subtype, Uhlman et al. [61] did report significant correlations between positive p53 staining and both high tumour stage/grade and the development of distant metastases. It must be noted, however, that in addition to genetic mutation, the p53 protein may also be stabilised by factors such as the binding of cellular oncoproteins (e.g. MDM2) or

DNA damage [52], and therefore protein over-expression is not always indicative of gene mutation, and results must be interpreted with caution. Direct DNA analysis therefore remains the optimal method of *p53* mutation detection and, on the basis of the accumulated evidence, *p53* mutation is uncommon in renal cell carcinoma and does not appear to have a major role in its pathogenesis.

In the absence of *p53* mutations in renal cell carcinoma, the inhibition of apoptotic cell death in these tumours may occur by alternative mechanisms, and one such pathway may involve the over-expression of the *bcl-2* oncoprotein. *bcl-2* and *p53* play reciprocal roles in the mediation of cell death, with *bcl-2* appearing to play a pivotal role in cell survival by the inhibition of apoptotic cell death, including that mediated by *p53* [64]. *bcl-2* has also been suggested to play a key role in renal development and morphogenesis [65], and inverse correlations between the detection of *p53* mutation and *bcl-2* over-expression have been observed in breast cancer and glioma [59]. In a study of 25 renal cell carcinoma samples, Tomita *et al.* [59] detected positive *bcl-2* staining by immunohistochemistry in 68% of cases, whereas *p53* mutation was undetectable in any sample, although no histopathological comparisons were made and amplification of either gene was not observed. A more extensive immunohistochemical study of different renal cell carcinoma histopathological subtypes was reported by Paraf *et al.* [65], who compared *bcl-2* expression in 37 renal cell carcinomas with 26 adjacent normal tissue controls. While the majority of clear cell carcinomas (77%) were negative or contained sparsely distributed positive cells (15%), all papillary carcinomas were consistently positive for *bcl-2*. No particular correlations were observed with tumour grade. These results demonstrate that *bcl-2* over-expression in the absence of *p53* mutation is common in renal cell carcinoma samples, but suggest that this phenomenon may be specific to the papillary subtype of renal cell carcinoma, and shows no apparent correlation with tumour grade. Thus, *bcl-2* over-expression rather than *p53* mutation may play a specific role in the prevention of apoptosis during papillary development.

Retinoblastoma is a childhood tumour of the retina that can have both a sporadic and a hereditary pathogenesis. The gene responsible for the disease, the retinoblastoma (*RB*) tumour suppressor gene, has been localised to chromosome band 13q14, a region frequently deleted in both the sporadic and hereditary forms of the disease. The *RB* gene encodes a nuclear phosphoprotein (pRB) whose normal cellular functions are primarily centred around its ability to regulate the cell cycle through induction of G1 arrest, whereby its non-phosphorylated form can block progression through to S phase, and this block is then released upon the phosphorylation of pRB by cyclin-dependent kinase complexes. Futher functions include the ability to regulate transcription through interaction with transcription factors and repression of RNA polymerase I-specific transcription. Retinoblastoma arises when both alleles of the gene are inactivated. Deletions at the *RB* locus are observed in almost half of all retinoblastoma cases, with altered or absent transcripts found in other cases – both resulting in pRB protein loss. In addition to its role in retinoblastoma disease, *RB* loss has also been detected in other tumours, including small cell lung cancer and osteosarcomas [66–68].

No mutational analyses of the *RB* gene have been reported in renal cell carcinoma. However, studies by Suzuki *et al.* [69], showing no loss of heterozygosity at the *RB* locus in 15 informative renal cell carcinomas, and by Walther *et al.* [70], demonstrating no loss of pRB protein staining by immunohistochemistry in 30 tumours, suggest that alterations to the *RB* gene are not central to the development of renal cell carcinoma.

Given their roles in the development of many common neoplasia, the lack of involvement of the *p53* and *RB* genes in renal cell carcinoma development suggests that the molecular genetic pathways leading to the genesis of this disease differ considerably from many of the other common types of adult carcinoma.

Alterations to the short arm of chromosome 3 are central to renal cell carcinoma development

Allelotyping by loss of heterozygosity analysis using highly polymorphic markers is the technique most commonly used to map the positions of tumour suppressor genes across the genome by defining regions of allelic loss in tumour samples. Deletions of the short arm of chromosome 3 are the most common genetic aberration observed in renal cell carcinoma, with 3p loss of heterozygosity reported to occur in 45–90% of sporadic and hereditary renal cell carcinomas, although these changes are specifically associated with non-papillary disease and are not usually observed in papillary tumours [13, 71–75]. Furthermore, 3p allele loss is an early event that does not correlate with stage or grade. Several regions of 3p have been implicated in the development of renal cell carcinoma, suggesting the involvement of multiple tumour suppressor loci on this chromosome arm. The key regions most commonly implicated are (i) the von Hippel–Lindau disease gene locus at 3p25–26 (see above); (ii) 3p21, a common region of deletion in renal cell carcinoma [76, 77]; and (iii) 3p12–14, a common region of deletion overlap [78, 79], which includes the breakpoint of the familial t(3;8) constitutional translocation involved in hereditary bilateral renal cell carcinoma development (Figure 17.2). While the gene responsible for von Hippel–Lindau disease has been cloned and mutations detected in both familial and sporadic disease, thus defining a role in renal cell carcinoma development, no mutated genes have yet been isolated from either of the other candidate regions at 3p12–14 and 3p21.

Using a cohort of 44 sporadic renal cell carcinoma cases and multiple polymorphic markers clustered within the three candidate regions on 3p, van den Berg et al. [77] reported that when 3p deletions were detected, the 3p21 region was consistently included (loss of heterozygosity in 77% of informative cases), suggesting that this region may contain the most commonly altered tumour suppressor gene involved in renal cell carcinoma development. Loss of heterozygosity at the VHL locus was detected in 68%, and at the 3p14 region in 49% of cases. In a number of tumours in which two or three regions of loss of heterozygosity were detected separated by regions of retention of heterozygosity, 3p21 deletions were always detected in combination with loss of heterozygosity at the 3p14, VHL or both, further suggesting the involvement of multiple tumour suppressor loci on 3p in renal cell carcinoma development, with a primary role for the 3p21 region. As discussed previously, the FHIT putative tumour suppressor gene

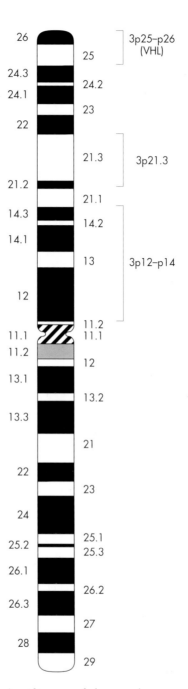

Figure 17.2 An idiogram of human chromosome 3 showing the three independent candidate regions implicated to harbour tumour suppressor genes involved in the tumorigenesis of renal cell carcinoma.

was recently isolated from the region close to the 3;8 translocation breakpoint, but so far there is little evidence that this gene has a significant role in renal cell carcinoma [40].

The involvement of alterations to tumour suppressor genes contained in these regions of 3p in renal cell carcinoma development is further supported by results from gene transfer experiments, which demonstrate the ability of these regions to suppress tumorigenicity. Firstly, Sanchez et al. [80] showed that transfer of the 3p14-q11 region into a highly malignant renal carcinoma cell line reduced their tumorigenicity in nude mice. No equivalent suppression was reported upon introduction of a 3p12-q24 fragment, thus functionally defining a tumour suppressor locus between 3p12 and 3p14. Seconly, Killary et al. [81] introduced a 2 Mb fragment of 3p21 into a mouse fibrosarcoma cell line, which dramatically reduced its tumorigenicity. Finally, the introduction of a wild-type VHL gene into renal carcinoma cell lines with either an altered or no VHL gene dramatically reduced the tumorigenicity of these cell lines [28, 29].

Mapping other putative renal cell carcinoma tumour suppressor genes by loss of heterozygosity analyses
Cytogenetic evidence suggests that, in addition to the loss of chromosome 3p, several other chromosomes are lost or rearranged in clear cell renal carcinoma and may be necessary for its development. Furthermore, since chromosome 3p loss is infrequent in papillary renal cell carcinoma, alternative genetic events are implicated in the development of this particular disease subtype. This section reviews several of the more recent molecular studies that have investigated such changes, and that have highlighted regions of the genome that may harbour genes involved in the development of renal cell carcinoma.

Using 70 polymorphic markers positioned across the entire genome, Thrash-Bingham et al. [75] analysed loss of heterozygosity in 28 renal cell carcinoma samples (22 non-papillary, 6 papillary). Consistent with previous findings, 3p loss was the most common aberration detected in non-papillary tumours (41%), and was not observed in any papillary renal cell carcinoma. Additionally, allelic losses on 6q (18%), 8p (18%), 9p (21%), 9q (15%) and 14q (21%) were also observed in both subtypes. These molecular data show good agreement with previous cytogenetic studies, which have shown loss of chromosomes 6p, 8p, 9pq and 14q in 14%, 22%, 14% and 30–50% of renal tumours, respectively [82]. Loss of heterozygosity for 21q was detected in 33% of papillary tumours, sug-

gesting the involvement of a tumour suppressor gene on this chromosome in papillary renal cell carcinoma. An extenstion of this study [27] revealed no correlation between disease stage and loss of heterozygosity of any particular chromosome. It is highly significant that 3p loss was never the sole aberration observed in any tumour, and usually occurred in association with losses on 6q, 8p, 9pq and/or 14q. These data suggest that alterations to genes on 3p are necessary, but not sufficient, for the development and/or progression of non-papillary renal cell carcinoma and that other tumour suppressor genes on these chromosomes are involved in the tumorigenesis of renal cell carcinoma.

Of the changes described, loss of chromosome 14q may be of particular interest because, in a study of 30 non-papillary renal cell carcinoma samples [83], 3p and 14q deletions were found in 90% and 37% of patients, respectively. However, while 3p loss showed no correlation with tumour stage or histological grade, the deletion of 14q significantly correlated with higher stage, histological grade, and patient outcome, suggesting that it may be a promising prognostic marker. These data are consistent with observations by Thrash-Bingham et al. [75] that loss of 14q is associated with an elevated level of overall allele loss compared to tumours with 14q retention, suggesting that 14q loss may be associated with aggressive disease and that a gene on 14q may be involved in the control of genomic stability.

In a study of loss of heterozygosity on chromosome 3p, 5q, 6q, 10q, 11q, 17p and 19p in Japanese populations, as well as observing chromosomes 3 loss of heterozygosity in 90% of cases, Morita et al. [72] observed frequent losses on chromosomes 5q (33%), 6q (39%) and 10q (41%), which seem apparently specific to this geographical population. Loss of chromosome 5q showed a significant correlation with increasing tumour grade. Moch et al. [84] analysed 41 clear cell stage 3 renal cell carcinomas using the technique of comparative genomic hybridisation. In addition to losses at 3p (54% of tumours), the most prevalent losses were observed at 9p and 13q (24% each). DNA gains were also observed, most often involving chromosomes 5q (17%) and 7 (15%), suggesting that these regions may harbour genes amplified in clear cell renal carcinoma development.

Schwerdtle et al. [85] analysed loss of heterozygosity in 50 renal cell carcinomas using a panel of non-3p chromosomal markers (1p, 2p, 6p, 7q, 10p, 11p, 13q, 14q, 17p, 21q, 22q) [31]. 14q loss of heterozygosity was detected at a high incidence in all subtypes (42–64%), but was the only loss that was detected frequently (>30%) in clear cell renal carcinoma. Losses at 2p (40%) and 17p (46%) were prevalent in chromophilic tumours. Chromophobe-specific losses were identified at high frequency (73–91%) at 1p, 2p, 6p, 10p, 13q, 17p and 21q. These data provide substantial evidence to define the chromophobe subtype of renal cell carcinoma as a distinct genetic entity. Finally, a study of papillary renal cell carcinoma by Corless et al. [86] confirmed previous cytogenic observations by demonstrating increased copy numbers of chromosomes 7 and 17 in 100% and 81% of cases, respectively.

This group of studies highlights the wide range of chromosomal alterations detected in renal cell carcinoma samples and are summarised in Table 17.1. Specific alterations have been detected that suggest that different genetic pathways lead to the development of each renal cell carcinoma subtype. More importantly, these data support a multistage, multi-event model for the tumorigenesis of renal cell carcinoma. Firstly, the frequent detection of multiple allelic losses in individual tumours in the studies described and, in particular, results showing that chromosome 3p loss is always accompanied by other chromosomal losses [27] indicate that the accumulation of multiple genetic aberrations is necessary for renal cell carcinoma development. Secondly, data suggest that different alterations play different roles in renal cell carcinoma tumorigenesis; for instance, whereas most of the alterations detected show no particular associations with tumour stage or grade (e.g. 3p loss), suggesting an early role in tumorigenesis, results for some allelic losses (e.g. 14q and 5q) suggest that these may be late-stage events in renal cell carcinoma development.

The role of p16/CDKN2/MTS1 in renal cell carcinoma
In the light of the common loss of the 9p21 region of chromosome 9 observed in renal cell carcinoma [27, 87], the role of p16/CDKN2/MTS1, a candidate tumour suppressor gene recently isolated from 9p21 [88, 89] and found to be deleted in many tumour cell lines including renal cell carcinoma lines [88], has recently been examined as a candidate tumour suppressor locus in renal cell carcinoma. In a study of primary renal cell tumours by Cairns et al. [87], apart from a homozygous deletion of 9p21–22 in one tumour sample, no further evidence of p16 gene rearrangement, homozygous deletion or point mutation was found in a further 11 cases. Thus, p16 inactivation appears to be infrequent in primary renal cell tumours, and a higher frequency of p16 mutation in cell lines than in primary tumours has been observed for other cancers.

Oncogenes in renal cell carcinoma

The ras gene family and the mitogen-activated protein kinase pathway
The ras family of proto-oncogenes encode small monomeric GTP-binding proteins involved in signal transduction across the cell membrane. Ras proteins have GTPase activity that is functionally important – GDP-bound ras protein is inactive, whereas GTP-bound ras is active and acts upon its target molecule. Following induction, wild-type ras is returned to the inactive condition by the hydrolysis of bound GTP to GDP by GTPase activity. Ras activation is an obligatory step in the signal transduction cascade initiated by the activation of certain tyrosine kinase growth factor receptors (e.g. epidermal growth factor receptor and platelet-derived growth factor). This important signal cascade passes to mitogen-activated protein kinase (a serine/threonine kinase) and terminates with the nuclear phosphorylation of nuclear transcription factors including c-fos and c-jun. The oncogenic variants of ras are constitutively activated by point mutation, with the majority of mutations occurring at specific codons, notably 12, 13 (GTP-binding domain) and 61 (GTP hydrolysis). Different oncogenic Ras proteins have been shown to be constitutively active, with a consistently reduced ability to hydrolyse GTP. Transfection of mutated ras genes into the appropriate recipient cells confers neoplastic properties, and ras gene mutations have been detected in approximately 50% of all colorectal carcinomas and adenomas [90–92].

Table 17.1 Summary of genetic alterations detected in sporadic renal cell carcinoma samples in the investigations reviewed in this chapter, their incidences, relationships to histopathological data and potential roles in renal cell carcinoma development. See individual sections for references and further information

Gene	Alteration (tumour vs. normal kidney)	Incidence (%)	Associations with tumour development		Tumour type (clear cell, papillary, chromophobic, chromophilic)
			Stage/grade	Early/late event	
Oncogenes					
VEGF	↑ mRNA/protein levels	45–95	no association	early	all
c-met	↑ protein levels	87	no association	early	all
PLGF	↑ mRNA levels	91	no association	early	all
bcl-2	↑ protein levels	100	no association	early	all
c-erbB-2	↓ mRNA levels	93	no association	early	papillary only
MAPK pathway	constitutive activation	48–55	↑ in high grade	early	clear cell only
EGFR	↑ mRNA/protein levels	21–73	↑ in high grade	late	all
TGF-α	↑ mRNA levels	60–100	↑ in high grade	late	all
bFGF	↑ tumour mRNA levels	47–67		late	all
	↑ serum protein levels	35–53	↑ in high grade	late	all
c-myc	↑ mRNA/protein levels	43–73	↑ in high grade	late	not investigated
c-fos	↓ mRNA levels	73	↓ in high grade	late	all
IR	↑ protein levels	100	not investigated	unknown	not investigated
IGF-1R	↑ protein levels	54–100	not investigated	unknown	not investigated
ras family	point mutation	not detected			all
Tumour suppressor genes					
VHL	mutation, methylation, LOH	50, 15, 77	no association	early	clear cell only
p53	mutation, LOH	<10, 17–21	no association	early	all
RB	↓ protein levels, LOH	not detected			all
p16	mutation	not detected			all
Other chromosome genes					
1p	LOH	89	not investigated	unknown	chromophobic only
2p	LOH	40–91	not investigated	unknown	chromophilic and chromophobic only
3p	LOH	41–90	no association	early	clear cell only
3p21	LOH	77	no association	early	clear cell only
3p12-14	LOH	49	no association	early	clear cell only
5q	DNA gains	17	not investigated	unknown	only clear cell investigated
5q	LOH	33	in high grade	late	all (Japanese populations)
6p	LOH	90	not investigated	unknown	chromophobic only
6q	LOH	39	no association	early	all (Japanese populations)
6q	LOH	14–18	no association	early	all
7	trisomy	81	not investigated	unknown	papillary only
7	DNA gains	15	not investigated	unknown	only clear cell investigated
8p	LOH	18–22	no association	early	all
9pq	LOH	14–24	no association	early	all
10p	LOH	91	not investigated	unknown	chromophobic only
10q	LOH	41	no association	early	all (Japanese populations)
13q	LOH	86	not investigated	unknown	chromophobic only
13q	LOH	24	not investigated	unknown	only clear cell investigated
14q	LOH	21–64	in high grade	late	all
17	trisomy	100	not investigated	unknown	papillary only
17p	LOH	46	not investigated	unknown	chromophilic only
17p	LOH	73	not investigated	unknown	chromophobic only
21q	LOH	33	no association	early	papillary only
21q	LOH	90	not investigated	unknown	chromophobic only

OH, loss of heterozygosity.

The incidence of point mutations in the *ras* family of genes has now been extensively investigated in all histological subtypes of renal cell carcinoma. No mutations in any of the *ras* family members (c-Ha-*ras*, c-Ki-*ras* and N-*ras*) have been reported in any of the five studies reviewed [69, 93–96], implying that mutations of the *ras* family of proto-oncogenes do not play a role in the tumorigenesis of renal cell carcinoma. Therefore, attention has recently shifted onto the mitogen-activated protein kinases as the possible focus of alterations to the ras-related signal transduction cascade in this disease. Two mitogen-activated protein kinases have been identified to date (ERK1 and ERK2), which are rapidly phosphorylated and activated as a result of the sequential activation of a dual specificity kinase known as mitogen-activated protein kinase-kinase, in response to many growth factors, hormones and neurotransmitters that influence cell proliferation and differentiation. In addition to ras activation, phosphorylation of the *raf*-1 proto-oncogene is also involved as an upstream event in the mitogen-activated protein kinase/ras cascade [96]. Strong evidence of a role for constitutive mitogen-activated protein kinase activation in carcinogenesis was provided by Mansour *et al.* [97], who demonstrated that a constitutively active mitogen-activated protein kinase-kinase mutant could transform NIH3T3 cells. In a study of 25 renal cell carcinomas and corresponding normal kidney biopsies, Oka *et al.* [96] demonstrated constitutive mitogen-activated protein kinase activation in 48% of tumours, over-expression and phosphorylation of mitogen-activated protein kinase-kinase in 52% and 50% of tumours respectively, and *raf*-1 phosphorylation in 55% of tumours. No *ras* mutations were detected in any sample, and mitogen-activated protein kinase-kinase over-expression was significantly correlated with mitogen-activated protein kinase activation, which in turn correlated significantly with *raf*-1 and mitogen-activated protein kinase-kinase activation. A significantly higher incidence of mitogen-activated protein kinase activation was observed in grade 2 and 3 tumours than in grade 1 cases. No associations were observed between this activation and renal cell carcinoma histopathological subtype.

Constitutive activation of the mitogen-activated protein kinase cascade would therefore appear to play an important role in the tumorigenesis of renal cell carcinoma, and would seem to be particularly associated with the development of late-stage tumours with increased malignant potential. In view of the low incidence of *ras* mutations in renal cell carcinoma samples, the underlying cause of mitogen-activated protein kinase activation in this disease remains open to speculation, although other oncogenes involved in the mitogen-activated protein kinase cascade have been shown to participate in the carcinogenesis of renal cell carcinoma. Of these, the *EGFR* gene and its transforming growth factor alpha ligand are of particular note, given that they are also over-expressed in high-grade tumours, suggesting a possible correlation between these different events observed in renal cell carcinoma development.

The erbB family

The epidermal growth factor receptor (*EGFR*/c-*erb*B) gene encodes a 170-kDa membrane-bound glycoprotein with intracellular tyrosine kinase activity and an extracellular binding site for substrates including epidermal growth factor and transforming growth factor alpha [98]. The c-*erb*B2 (*HER2/neu*) gene product is also a receptor-like glycoprotein (185 kDa in size) with a cytoplasmic tyrosine kinase domain that shares 50% sequence homology with EGFR [99], although, in contrast to EGFR, a ligand for c-*erb*B2 has not yet been identified. Recent work has demonstrated the formation of heterodimers between c-*erb*B2 and EGFR that appear to facilitate by transactivation the enhanced intracellular transduction of growth signals from EGFR [100]. The chromosomal locations of these proto-oncogenes are at 7p12–13 (*EGFR*) and 17q11.2–12 (c-*erb*B2) [101]. Amplification and/or over-expression of the *EGFR* gene have been reported in a number of human malignancies including glioblastomas, thyroid, oesophageal and breast cancers [102–106], and of the c-*erb*B2 gene in tumours including thyroid [102], ovarian [107] and, most notably, breast cancer, in which a strong correlation has been observed between high-level amplification of the c-*erb*B2 gene and poor prognosis [108]. Both genes are transforming when over-expressed in fibroblasts, although studies have suggested that c-*erb*B2 may be the more potent in this respect [109, 110].

Several studies have investigated the expression of these two members of the c-erbB family in renal cell carcinoma. Studies performed at the mRNA level have demonstrated lower expression levels of the c-erbB2 gene in renal cell carcinoma compared with paired normal kidney tissue [111, 112]. Rotter et al. [112] found a reduction in c-erbB2 mRNA levels in clear cell renal carcinoma compared with normal tissue but not in papillary, chromophobic and chromophilic subtypes, suggesting that these changes may be specific to clear cell renal carcinoma. Neither study observed any associations between c-erbB2 mRNA levels and tumour stage, or evidence of c-erbB2 gene amplification by Southern blot hybridisation in any tumour.

A good general agreement exists between the various studies examining EGFR expression in renal cell carcinoma. Studies at the mRNA level have consistently demonstrated higher EGFR expression in this disease compared to surrounding normal kidney tissue [113–115]. While no correlations have been observed between EGFR mRNA levels and tumour stage or grade [114, 115], three different immunohistochemistry studies have all demonstrated good correlations between strong EGFR staining intensity and high-grade tumours [116–118], with EGFR positivity in primary tumours reportedly associated with metastatic disease [117]. Protein-binding studies have also demonstrated a higher EGFR-binding capacity in renal cell carcinoma than in normal kidney samples [115–119]. A low incidence of EGFR gene amplification, ranging between 0% and 27%, has been reported in three different studies [114, 116, 118], suggesting this as a potential cause of EGFR over-expression in only a small subset of renal cell tumours. Few studies have investigated the pattern of EGFR expression between different renal cell carcinoma histopathological subtypes; however, Uhlman et al. [117] reported significantly lower EGFR positivity in papillary than in non-papillary renal cell carcinoma by immunohistochemistry.

Taken together, reports in the literature indicate that c-erbB2 expression is reduced as an early-stage event in the tumorigenesis of clear cell renal carcinoma on the basis of the lack of association observed with tumour stage or grade. Conversely, EGFR over-expression is associated with the development of late-stage/grade clear cell tumours, which suggests that an inverse relationship may exist between the expression of these two members of the c-erbB gene family during the development of renal cell carcinoma.

Vascular endothelial growth factor

The VEGF gene was recently assigned to human chromosome 6p12-p21 [120], and four differentially spliced vascular endothelial growth factor isoforms have been described, the larger two of which are cell associated (VEGF$_{189}$ and VEGF$_{206}$), while the smaller two are secreted proteins (VEGF$_{121}$ and VEGF$_{165}$) [121, 122]. Vascular endothelial growth factor is an endothelial cell-specific mitogen that induces angiogenesis and vascular permeability in vivo [123–125], and has previously been reported to be up-regulated in neoplasia, including von Hippel–Lindau disease-associated hereditary and sporadic haemangioblastomas [126] and in glioblastoma cells of highly vascularised lesions [127]. Over-expression of VEGF$_{121}$ by transfection into breast carcinoma cells has been shown to confer a growth advantage in vivo but not in vitro, forming more vascular tumours than those formed by the untransfected cells, thus suggesting that the growth advantage induced by vascular endothelial growth factor arises from increased tumour vascularisation [128].

Various studies have now demonstrated VEGF mRNA levels to be commonly up-regulated in renal cell carcinoma. Takahashi et al. [129] reported the over-expression of VEGF mRNA (3 to 13-fold) in 96% of hypervascular renal cell carcinomas analysed, compared with surrounding normal tissue. Interestingly, two tumours classified as 'hypovascular' had VEGF mRNA levels equivalent to or less than those in matched normal kidney. In a study of 20 renal cell carcinomas by Northern blot, Sato et al. [130] similarly reported VEGF over-expression (more than three-fold higher than normal renal tissues) in 60% of renal cell carcinomas. By in-situ hybridisation, high levels of VEGF mRNA were reported in 91% of renal cell carcinomas compared with surrounding normal tissue, with concomitantly strong staining for the VEGF protein observed in the same samples by immunohistochemistry [131]. Accentuated VEGF expression was observed adjacent to areas of tumour necrosis, suggesting a role for VEGF in response to tumour hypoxia in renal cell carcinoma. None of these studies found any consistent correlation between *VEGF* mRNA over-expression and tumour stage, grade or histological subtype. At the protein level, Mattern and Volm [132] reported that 45% of renal cell carcinomas (n = 20) were positive for VEGF protein by immunohistochemistry, although no normal tissue or clinicopathological comparisons were reported.

The available evidence indicates that *VEGF* over-expression is characteristic of all renal cell carcinoma subtypes, and is implicated both as an early event (on the basis of no tumour stage or grade correlation) in renal cell carcinoma tumorigenesis and in having a role in angiogenesis and the characteristically high degree of vascularisation observed in renal cell carcinoma. Enhanced *VEGF* mRNA levels have been demonstrated in response to a number of upstream events, including stimulation with platelet-derived growth factor, epidermal growth factor and tumour-promoting agents, induction of hypoxia and oncogene activation [130], many of which are characteristic of renal cell tumours and may go some way to explaining the high levels of *VEGF* expression observed in renal cell carcinoma. *VEGF* expression in sporadic renal cell carcinoma may also be influenced by the von Hippel–Lindau disease protein. Siemeister *et al.* [30] recently demonstrated de-regulated (increased) *VEGF* expression in renal cell carcinoma cells lacking endogenous wild-type *VHL*, which was reverted by the introduction of wild-type but not mutant *VHL*, and Iliopoulos *et al.* [31] have demonstrated that the effect of *pVHL* on *VEGF* mRNA abundance primarily acts at the level of mRNA stabilisation.

Basic fibroblast growth factor

Basic fibroblast growth factor (bFGF) is a 15–16 kDa protein that has been demonstrated to trigger the proliferation and differentiation of endothelial cells and capillaries, and has additionally been reported to play an important role in the regulation of epithelial cell growth [133–135]. The potential importance of bFGF in tumour development is supported by the discovery of the *hst*-1 and *int*-2 oncogenes, which are structurally related to the fibroblast growth factor family [136]. This notion is lent further weight by the tumour-based observations that mRNA expression is higher in gastric carcinoma than in normal gastric mucosa [137], and that *bFGF* transcript levels are higher in schwannoma samples than in benign meningioma samples [138].

Studies performed on renal cell carcinoma samples would suggest that serum bFGF levels are elevated in renal cell carcinoma patients, although findings at the tumour mRNA level are rather more equivocal. Three studies of serum bFGF levels in renal cell carcinoma patients have produced consistent findings of increased levels (between 35% and 53%), which were highest in advanced cases [139–141]. Fujimoto *et al.* [139] indicated that the increased serum bFGF levels measured specifically arose from renal cell carcinoma tumours by sampling from the renal veins of the affected and non-affected kidneys, both before and after resection. At the tumour mRNA level, two studies have independently reported elevated *bFGF* mRNA levels in renal cell carcinoma compared to corresponding normal kidney tissue in between 47% and 67% of renal cell carcinomas [142, 143], although the level of elevation observed was often small (about two-fold). However, a study of 29 renal cell carcinomas by Takahashi *et al.* [129] reported no difference between *bFGF* expression in tumour and normal tissue. None of the tumour or serum-based studies reviewed has reported any correlation between bFGF levels and histological renal cell carcinoma subtype.

The disagreement between the reported findings of bFGF serum and tumour mRNA levels are consistent with the findings of Kandel *et al.* [144], who demonstrated in a transgenic mouse model that a switch from cell-associated to exported bFGF, despite no change in mRNA levels, correlates with tumorigenesis and neovascularisation *in vivo*, which suggests that increased bFGF serum levels may be involved in the development and neovascularisation/angiogenesis of renal cell carcinoma, showing particular association with late-stage, metastatic disease.

The c-myc and c-fos nuclear oncoproteins

The products of the *c-myc* and *c-fos* proto-oncogenes are highly conserved nuclear phosphoprotein transcription factors whose expression is closely linked to cellular proliferation and with pathways of differentiation. Constitutive over-expression of the c-*myc* gene can partially relieve cells from growth factor dependence, block differentiation and provide one step towards malignancy in cultured cells [145]. Transfection of the c-*fos* proto-oncogene has similarly been demonstrated to be sufficient to induce the malignant conversion of tumour cell lines [e.g. 146]. Increased expression of both c-*myc* and c-*fos* has been reported for a wide spectrum of human malignancies [147].

In renal cell carcinoma, c-*myc* mRNA expression has been shown to be greater than that of normal kidney in between 43% and 73% of cases, while no evidence of c-*myc* gene amplification in renal cell carcinoma tumours has been found [111, 148]. Weidner *et al.* [111] reported a good association between c-*myc* over-expression and increasing tumour grade, but Yao *et al.* [148] did not report any such association. Neither study attempted any correlations between c-*myc* expression and histological subtype. Two studies of c-*myc* protein expression in renal cell carcinoma show good accordance with the mRNA findings. By immunohistochemistry, Kinouchi *et al.* [149] showed a good relationship between strong nuclear staining and increasing tumour grade in a panel of 41 renal cell carcinomas. Lanigan *et al.* [150] also reported a strong correlation between high levels of c-*myc* expression and both tumour stage and grade in a cohort of 95 tumours, although no correlations with renal cell carcinoma subtype were observed. In contrast to c-*myc*, the c-*fos* proto-oncogene has not been as widely studied, but there appears to be little association between c-*fos* expression and renal cell carcinoma. In two notable studies, Weidner *et al.* [111] reported decreased c-*fos* mRNA levels in 73% of cases, showing a good correlation between the level of decrease and increasing tumour grade. The study by Yao *et al.* [148] reported no differential c-*fos* expression between normal kidney and renal cell carcinoma samples in 15 pairs of samples, although a wide level of variation in expression was observed between individuals. No attempts were made at correlations with renal cell carcinoma subtype in either study.

In summary, expression of the c-*myc* proto-oncogene is elevated in renal cell carcinoma samples compared to parallel normal kidney samples, showing a good correlation between high expression levels and increasing tumour grade, thus suggesting a late-stage involvement in renal cell carcinoma development. Consistent with studies in other tumour types [151], gene amplification would not appear to be a contributing mechanism to c-*myc* over-expression in renal cell carcinoma development.

Transforming growth factor-alpha

Transforming growth factor alpha (TGF-α) is a 50-amino acid polypeptide growth factor that stimulates cell growth by binding to and activating the epidermal growth factor receptor (EGFR). It is expressed in the kidney, can stimulate angiogenesis and may therefore play a role in tissue vascularisation, and has been demonstrated to cause the transformation of certain cell lines, although its precise biological role and function remain unclear [152]. Transforming growth factor alpha has been investigated in renal cell carcinoma by a number of groups [113, 116, 152–154] and the consensus view is that *TGF-α* mRNA levels are elevated in the majority of renal cell carcinoma samples, but that this over-expression does not result from gene amplification. These data suggest the *TGF-α* mRNA levels may be increased in a tumour grade-dependent fashion, but are also increased relative to normal kidney in most low-grade samples. Thus, despite this association with tumour development, the patient numbers involved in these studies have not yet allowed definitive correlations with stage and grade of tumour development to be made. Previous studies would suggest that the elevated *TGF-α* mRNA levels observed may be associated with angiogenesis and renal cell carcinoma hypervascularity. Inconsistent results have been reported at the protein level, and further studies are therefore necessary to clarify the role or association of *TGF-α* protein levels with renal cell carcinoma development.

Other proto-oncogenes aberrantly expressed in renal cell carcinoma

In this final section, three proto-oncogenes are discussed that, although less extensively investigated in renal cell carcinoma samples than others reviewed in this chapter, have been associated with patterns of expression in renal cell carcinoma that suggest potential roles in its tumorigenesis and development, although further experimentation at both the basic functional and tumour pathology levels is required to elucidate more clearly their roles in renal cell carcinoma tumorigenesis.

Placenta growth factor

Placenta growth factor (PLGF) was recently isolated from human placenta and choriocarcinoma, and shares 53% amino-acid homology with vascular endothelial growth factor in the 94-amino acid cysteine-rich domain that contains the platelet-derived growth factor-like domain of vascular endothelial growth factor. On the basis of these similarities to vascular endothelial growth factor, and in particular the observation that PLGF can stimulate the growth of endothelial cells in vitro, PLGF has been hypothesised to play a potential role in angiogenesis and neovascularisation [155, 156]. Takahashi et al. [129] detected variable levels of PLGF mRNA in 91% (n = 23) of renal cell carcinomas despite it being undetectable in all corresponding normal kidney samples. Elevated PLGF expression showed no correlation with stage, grade or subtype, and may therefore be an early event in renal cell carcinoma development and have a role in renal cell carcinoma angiogenesis.

The c-met proto-oncogene

Hepatocyte growth factor is a 97 kDa peptide growth factor that, together with its high-affinity membrane receptor (the c-met proto-oncogene product), appears to play an important role in the early development of the metanephros and branching tubulogenesis of the developing kidney [157, 158]. It exerts powerful mitogenic effects on epithelial cells including renal proximal tubule cells [159], having been shown in mice to prevent the onset of renal dysfunction and to stimulate DNA synthesis of renal tubular cells (renal regeneration) following injury [160]. c-met has been shown to be over-expressed in tumours, including hepatocellular and prostate carcinomas [161, 162], and, furthermore, met over-expression in fibroblast cells has been demonstrated to lead directly to cell transformation and tumorigenicity [163]. Using immunohistochemistry techniques, Natali et al. [164] demonstrated that, in normal kidneys, weak staining for the c-met protein

was restricted to the distal tubules, whereas increased expression at various levels was found in 87% (n = 50) of renal cell carcinomas, showing no correlation with any histopathological feature. Results from this study therefore suggest that over-expression of c-met proto-oncogene may be involved as an early event in the development of renal cell carcinoma.

Insulin and insulin-like growth factor-1 receptors

Both insulin and insulin-like growth factor-1 can promote growth in normal tissues [165], and over-expression of insulin receptors in fibroblast and ovary cells has been shown to lead to a ligand-mediated transformed phenotype [166]. The insulin (IR) and insulin-like growth factor-1 (IGFR) receptors both have intrinsic tyrosine kinase activity located in the cytoplasmic part of the β-subunit, and it is this region in which the two receptors show their highest level of sequence homology (approximately 80%) [167]. There is evidence to suggest that insulin, IGF-1 and their receptors may be increased in breast [168] and gastrointestinal [169] tumour biopsies, and the observation that many renal cell carcinomas contain increased levels of glycogen, phospholipids and triglycerides suggests an involvement of insulin pathways in renal cell carcinoma development. Analysing IGF-1 binding in 13 renal cell carcinomas (grade 2 or higher) and paired normal kidney samples, Pekonen et al. [170] demonstrated increased IGF-1 membrane binding in seven renal cell carcinomas relative to normal kidney, with reduced levels found in the remaining six samples. Notably, the highest levels of IGF-1 binding were observed in five renal cancers. In a study of high-stage and grade (≥ T3, G2) renal cell carcinomas from eight patients, Kellerer et al. [171] demonstrated increased levels of insulin-binding (three- to four-fold) and IGF-1-binding (two-fold) sites in renal cell carcinoma compared to adjacent normal kidney in all eight tumours. Both types of receptor also possessed increased specific tyrosine kinase and autophosphorylation activity compared to normal kidney, which could not be attributed to altered expression levels of the receptors of their isoforms. Although no histological subtype or mRNA expression data were given in either study, taken together these data suggest that both receptor systems may be expressed at increased levels in renal tumours and may therefore contribute to the growth, proliferation and/or metabolism of renal cell carcinoma.

Summary and discussion

Molecular genetic techniques have provided a powerful research tool that has allowed the elucidation of a broad spectrum of genetic changes to oncogenes and tumour suppressor genes which are involved in the development and progression of renal cell carcinoma. The genetic alterations detected in renal cell carcinoma and reviewed in this chapter are summarised in Table 17.1. This review highlights the distinctive pathogenesis of renal cell tumours compared to other major tumour types, most notably through the lack of p53/RB/ras mutations coupled with the involvement of multiple tumour suppressor genes on the short arm of chromosome 3. Furthermore, the distinct genetic events in the genesis of the different histopathological renal cell carcinoma subtypes are clearly apparent, and correlations with disease stage and grade provide indications of the roles of particular alterations in renal cell carcinoma tumorigenesis. The nature of the genetic alterations observed allows some correlation between over-expression of a number of different angiogenic growth factors (e.g. VEGF, PLGF, bFGF) and the frequently observed highly vascular nature of renal cell carcinoma.

Further elucidation of the oncogenetic processes involved in renal cell carcinoma development is anticipated over the coming years. Loss of heterozygosity studies have now identified a number of regions of chromosomal loss specific to each subtype of renal cell carcinoma, and the identification and further analysis of the putative tumour suppressor genes lying within these regions are of prime importance. The discovery and analysis of cancer genes have frequently entailed a reductionist approach to the identification of individual genes in renal cell carcinoma. Further investigations will be driven to understanding the complex interrelationships between the different genes involved in renal cell carcinoma development, their upstream modifiers and downstream effects (e.g. between growth factors, their receptors, signal trans-

duction pathways and transcription factors). Meanwhile, the identification of the molecular basis of von Hippel–Lindau disease has improved the support of von Hippel–Lindau families.

References

1. Fleischmann J, Huntley NH. Renal tumours. In: Krane RJ, Siroky MB, Fitzpatrick JM (eds) Clinical urology. Philadelphia: JP Lippincott, 1994: 359–73
2. Thoenes W, Storkel S, Rumpelt HJ. Histopathology and classification of renal cell tumours (adenomas, oncocytomas and carcinomas). The basic cytological and histopathological elements and their use for diagnostics. Path Res Pract 1986; 181: 125–143
3. Kovacs G, Wilkens L, Papp T, De Riese W. Differentiation between papillary and nonpapillary renal cell carcinomas by DNA analysis. J Natl Cancer Inst 1989; 81: 527–30
4. Lewin B. Oncogenes: gene expression and cancer. In: Lewin B (ed) Genes V. Oxford: Oxford University Press, 1994: 1181–229
5. Maher ER, Yates JRW. Familial renal cell carcinoma: clinical and molecular genetic aspects. Br J Cancer 1991; 63: 176–9
6. Maher ER, Yates JRW, Ferguson-Smith MA. Statistical analysis of the two stage mutation model in von Hippel–Lindau disease and in sporadic cerebellar haemangioblastoma and renal cell carcinoma. J Med Genet 190; 27: 311–14
7. Maher ER, Yates JRW, Harries R, et al. Clinical features and natural history of von Hippel–Lindau disease. Quart J Med 1990; 77: 1151–63
8. Maher ER. Von Hippel–Lindau disease. Eur J Cancer 1994; 30A: 1987–90
9. Choyke PL, Glenn GM, Walther MM, Patronas NJ, Linehan WM, Zbar B. von Hippel–Lindau disease: genetic, clinical, and imaging features. Radiology 1995; 194: 629–42
10. Choyke PL, Glenn GM, Walther MCM, et al. The natural history of renal lesions in von Hippel–Lindau disease: a serial CT study in 28 patients. Am J Radiol 1992; 159: 1229–34
11. Steinbach F, Novick AC, Zincke H, et al. Treatment of renal cell carcinoma in von Hippel–Lindau disease: a multicenter study. J Urol 1995; 153: 1812–16
12. Walther MM, Choyke PL, Weiss G, et al. Parenchymal sparing surgery in patients with hereditary renal cell carcinoma. J Urol 1995; 153: 913–16

13. Latif F, Tory K, Gnarra J, et al. Isolation of the von Hippel–Lindau disease tumour suppressor gene. Science 1993; 260: 1317–20

14. Crossey PA, Richards FM, Foster K, et al. Identification of intragenic mutations in the von Hippel–Lindau disease tumour suppressor gene and correlation with disease phenotype. Hum Mol Genet 1994; 3: 1303–8

15. Chen F, Kishida T, Yao M, et al. Germ line mutations in the von Hippel–Lindau disease tumor suppressor gene: correlations with phenotype. Human Mutation 1995; 5: 66–75

16. Brauch H, Kishida T, Glavac D, et al. von Hippel–Lindau disease with pheochromocytoma in the Black Forest region of Germany: evidence for a founder effect. Hum Genet 1995; 95: 551–6

17. Maher ER, Webster AR, Richards FM, et al. Phenotypic expression in von Hippel–Lindau disease: correlations with germline VHL gene mutations. J Med Genet 1996; 33: 328–32

18. Zbar B, Kishida T, Chen F, et al. Germline mutations in the von Hippel–Lindau disease (VHL) gene in families from North America, Europe and Japan. Human Mutation 1996; 8: 348–57

19. Knudson AG. Hereditary cancer, oncogenes and antioncogenes. Cancer Res 1985; 45: 1437–43

20. Tory K, Brauch H, Linehan M, et al. Specific genetic change in tumors associted with von Hippel–Lindau disease. J Natl Cancer Inst 1989; 81: 1097–101

21. Crossey PA, Foster K, Richards FM, et al. Molecular genetic investigation of the mechanism of tumourigenesis in von Hippel–Lindau disease: analysis of allele loss in VHL tumours. Human Genetics 1994; 93: 53–8

22. Foster K, Prowse A, Van den Berg A, et al. Somatic mutations of the von Hippel–Lindau disease tumour suppressor gene in nonfamilial clear cell renal carcinoma. Hum Mol Genet 1994; 3: 2169–73

23. Chen F, Duh FM, Lubensky I, et al. Mutations of the VHL tumour suppressor gene in renal carcinoma. Nature Genet 1994; 7: 85–90

24. Shuin T, Kondo K, Torigoe S, et al. Frequent somatic mutations and loss of heterozygosity of the von Hippel–Lindau tumor suppressor gene in primary human renal cell carcinomas. Cancer Res 1994; 54: 2852–5

25. Herman JG, Latif F, Weng YK, et al. Silencing of the VHL tumor suppressor gene by DNA methylation in renal carcinomas. Proc Natl Acad Sci USA 1994; 91: 9700–4

26. Clifford SC, Prowse AH, Affara NA, et al. Mutation and methylation of the von Hippel–Lindau tumour suppressor gene and allelic loss on chromosome 3p: evidence for a VHL-independent pathway in clear cell renal carcinogenesis. Genes Chrom Cancer 1998; 22: 200–09

27. Thrash-Bingham CA, Salazar H, Freed JJ, Greenberg RE, Tartof KD. Genomic alterations and instabilities in renal cell carcinomas and their relationship to tumor pathology. Cancer Res 1995; 55: 6189–95

28. Iliopoulos O, Kibel A, Gray S, Kaelin WG Jr. Tumour suppression by the human von Hippel–Lindau gene product. Nature Med 1995; 1: 822–6

29. Chen F, Kishida T, Duh FM, et al. Suppression of growth of renal carcinoma cells by the von Hippel–Lindau tumour suppressor gene. Cancer Res 1995; 55: 4804–7

30. Siemeister G, Weindel K, Mohrs K, Barleton B, Martiny-Baron G, Marme D. Reversion of deregulated expression of vascular endothelial growth factor in human renal carcinoma cells by von Hippel–Lindau tumour suppressor protein. Cancer Res 1996; 56: 2299–301

31. Iliopoulos O, Levy AP, Jiang C, Kaelin WG Jr, Goldberg MA. Negative regulation of hypoxia-inducible genes by the von Hippel–Lindau protein. Proc Natl Acad Sci USA 1996; 93: 10595–99

32. Duan DR, Pause A, Burgess WH, et al. Inhibition of transcription elongation by the VHL tumor suppressor protein. Science 1995; 269: 1402–6

33. Aso T, Lane WS, Conaway JW, Conaway RC. Elongin (SIII): a multisubunit regulator of elongation by RNA polymerase II. Science 1995; 269: 1439–43

34. Kibel A, Iliopoulos O, DeCaprio JA, Kaelin WG. Binding of the von Hippel–Lindau tumor suppressor protein to Elongin B and C. Science 1995; 269: 1444–6

35. Crossey PA, Eng C, Ginalska-Malinowska M, et al. Molecular genetic diagnosis of von Hippel–Lindau disease in familial phaeochromocytoma. J Med Genet 1995; 32: 885–6

36. Neumann HPH, Eng C, Mulligan L, et al. Consequences of direct genetic testing for germline mutations in the clinical management of families with multiple endocrine neoplasia type 2. JAMA 1995; 274: 1149–51

37. Cohen AJ, Li FP, Berg S, et al. Hereditary renal cell carcinoma associated with a chromosomal translocation. N Engl J Med 1979; 301: 592–5

38. Kovacs G, Brusa P, De Riese W. Tissue-specific expression of a constitutional 3;6 translocation: development of multiple bilateral renal-cell carcinomas. Int J Cancer 1989; 43: 422–7

39. Schmidt L, Li F, Bron RS, et al. Mechanism of tumorigenesis of renal carcinomas associated with the constitutional 3;8 translocation. Cancer J Sci Am 1995; 1: 191–5

40. Ohta M, Inoue H, Cotticelli MG, et al. The FHIT gene, spanning the chromosome 3p14.2 fragile site and renal carcinoma-associated t(3;8) breakpoint, is abnormal in digestive tract cancers. Cell 1996; 84: 587–97

41. Zbar B, Glenn G, Lubensky I, et al. Hereditary papillary renal cell carcinoma: clinical studies in 10 families. J Urol 1995; 153: 907–12

42. Zbar B, Tory K, Merino M, et al. Hereditary papillary renal cell carcinoma. J Urol 1994; 151: 561–6

43. Suijkerbuijk RF, Meloni AM, Sinke RJ, et al. Identification of a yeast artificial chromosome that spans the human papillary renal cell carcinoma-associated t(X;1) breakpoint in Xp11.2. Cancer Genet Cytogenet 1993; 71: 164–9

44. Sidhar SK, Clark J, Gill S, et al. The t(x-l)(p11.2-q21.2) translocation in papillary renal-cell carcinoma fuses a novel gene PRCC to the TFE3 transcription factor gene. Hum Mol Genet 1996; 5: 1333–8

45. Yeung RS, Xiao GH, Jin F, Lee WC, Testa JR, Knudson AG. Predisposition to renal carcinoma in the Eker rat is determined by germ-line mutation of the tuberous sclerosis 2 (TSC2) gene. Proc Nat Acad Sci USA 1994; 91: 11413–16

46. Kobayashi T, Hirayama Y, Kobayashi E, Kubo Y, Hino O. A germline insertion in the tuberous sclerosis (TSC2) gene gives rise to the Eker rat model of dominantly inherited cancer. Nature Genet 1995; 9: 70–4

47. The European Chromosome 16 Tuberous Sclerosis Consortium. Identification and characterization of the tuberous sclerosis gene on chromosome 16. Cell 1993; 75: 1305–15

48. Sampson JR, Harris PC. The molecular genetics of tuberous sclerosis. Hum Mol Genet 1994; 3: 1477–80

49. Brook-Carter PT, Peral B, Ward CJ, et al. Deletion of the TSC2 and PKD1 genes associated with severe infantile polycystic kidney disease – a contiguous gene syndrome. Nature Genet 1994; 8: 328–32

50. Green AJ, Smith M, Yates JR. Loss of heterozygosity on chromosome 16p13.3 in hamartomas from tuberous sclerosis patients. Nature Genet 1994; 6: 193–6

51. Aaltonen LA, Peltomaki P, Leach FS, et al. Clues to the pathogenesis of familial colorectal cancer. Science 1993; 260: 810–12

52. Chang F, Syrjanen S, Syrjanen K. Implications of the p53 tumour-suppressor gene in clinical oncology. J Clin Oncol 1995; 13: 1009–22

53. Ogawa O, Habuchi T, Kakehi Y, Koshiba M, Sugiyama T, Yoshida O. Allelic losses at chromosome-17p in human renal-cell carcinoma are inversely related to allelic losses at chromosome-3p. Cancer Res 1992; 52: 1881–5

54. Uchida T, Wada C, Shitara T, Egawa S, Mashimo S, Koshiba K. Infrequent involvement of p53 mutations and loss of heterozygosity of 17p in the tumorigenesis of renal-cell carcinoma. J Urol 1993; 150: 1298–301

55. Suzuki Y, Tamura G, Satodate R, Fujioka T. Infrequent mutation of p53 gene in human renal-cell carcinoma detected by polymerase chain-reaction single-strand conformation polymorphism analysis. Jap J Cancer Res 1992; 83: 233–5

56. Torigoe S, Shuin T, Kubota Y, Horikoshi T, Danenberg K, Danenberg PV. p53 gene mutation in primary human renal-cell carcinoma. Oncol Res 1992; 4: 467–72

57. Suzuki Y, Tamura G. Mutations of the p53 gene in carcinomas of the urinary system. Acta Path Jap 1993; 43: 745–50

58. Uchida T, Wada LC, Wang CX, Egawa S, Ohtani H, Koshida K. Genomic instability of microsatellite repeats and mutations of H-, K-, and N-ras, and p53 genes in renal-cell carcinoma. Cancer Res 1994; 54: 3682–5

59. Tomita Y, Bilim V, Kawasaki T, et al. Frequent expression of bcl-2 in renal-cell carcinomas carrying wild-type p53. Int J Cancer 1996; 66: 322–5

60. Bot FJ, Godschalk JCJ, Krishnadath KK, Vanderkwast THM, Bosman FT. Prognostic factors in renal-cell carcinoma – immunohistochemical detection of p53 protein versus clinicopathological parameters. Int J Cancer 1994; 57: 634–7

61. Uhlman DL, Nguyen PL, Manivel JC, et al. Association of immunohistochemical staining for p53 with metastatic progression and poor survival in patients with renal-cell carcinoma. J Nat Canc Inst 1994; 86: 1470–5

62. Kamel D, Turpeenniemihujanen T, Vahakangas K, Paakko P, Soini Y. Proliferating cell nuclear antigen but not p53 or human papillomavirus DNA correlates with advanced clinical stage in renal-cell carcinoma. Histopathology 1994; 25: 339–47

63. Lai R, Eldabbagh L, Mourad WA. Mutant p53 expression in kidney-tubules adjacent to renal-cell carcinoma – evidence of a precursor lesion. Mod Pathol 1996; 9: 690–5

64. Williams GT, Smith CA. Molecular regulation of apoptosis – genetic-controls on cell-death. Cell 1993; 74: 777–9

65. Paraf F, Gogusev J, Chretien Y, Droz D. Expression of

bcl-2 oncoprotein in renal-cell tumors. J Pathol 1995; 177: 247–52

66. Kouzarides K. Functions of pRb and p53: what's the connection? Trends Cell Biol 1995; 5: 448–50

67. Marshall CJ. Tumor suppressor genes. Cell 1991; 64: 313–26

68. Cavenee WK, Dryja TP, Phillips RA, et al. Expression of recessive alleles by chromosomal mechanisms in retinoblastoma. Nature 1983; 305: 779–84

69. Suzuki Y, Tamura G, Maesawa C, Fujioka T, Kubo T, Satodate R. Analysis of genetic alterations in renal-cell carcinoma using the polymerase chain-reaction. Vir Archiv Int J Pathol 1994; 424: 453–7

70. Walther MM, Gnarra JR, Elwood L, et al. Loss of heterozygosity occurs centromeric to Rb without associated abnormalities in the retinoblastoma gene in tumors from patients with metastatic renal-cell carcinoma. J Urol 1995; 153: 2050–4

71. Presti JC, Rao PH, Chen Q, et al. Histopathological, cytogenetic, and molecular characterization of renal cortical tumors. Cancer Res 1991; 51: 1544–52

72. Morita R, Ishikawa J, Tsutsumi M, et al. Allelotype of renal-cell carcinoma. Cancer Res 1991; 51: 820–3

73. Zbar B, Brauch H, Talmadge C, Linehan M. Loss of alleles of loci on the short arm of chromosome-3 in renal-cell carcinoma. Nature 1987; 327: 721–4

74. Kovacs G, Frisch S. Clonal chromosome abnormalities in tumor cells from patients with sporadic renal-cell carcinomas. Cancer Res 1989; 49: 651–9

75. Thrash-Bingham CA, Greenberg RE, Howard S, et al. Comprehensive allelotyping of human renal-cell carcinomas using microsatellite DNA probes. Proc Natl Acad Sci USA 1995; 92: 2854–8

76. Van der Hout AH, Vandervlies P, Wijmenga C, Li FP, Oosterhuis JW, Buys CHCM. The region of common allelic losses in sporadic renal-cell carcinoma is bordered by the loci-D3S2 and THRB. Genomics 1991; 11: 537–42

77. Van den Berg A, Hulsbeek MMF, Dejong D, et al. Major role for a 3p21 region and lack of involvement of the t(3–8) breakpoint region in the development of renal-cell carcinoma suggested by loss of heterozygosity analysis. Gen Chrom Cancer 1996; 15: 64–72

78. Lubinski J, Hadaczek P, Podolski J, et al. Common regions of deletion in chromosome regions 3p12 and 3p14.2 in primary clear-cell renal carcinomas. Cancer Res 1994; 54: 3710–13

79. Yamakawa K, Morita R, Takahashi E, Hori T, Ishikawa J, Nakamura Y. A detailed deletion mapping of the short arm of chromosome-3 in sporadic renal-cell carcinoma. Cancer Res 1991; 51: 4707–11

80. Sanchez Y, Elnaggar A, Pathak S, Killary AM. A tumor-suppressor locus within 3p14-p12 mediates rapid cell death of renal-cell carcinoma in-vivo. Proc Natl Acad Sci USA 1994; 91: 3383–7

81. Killary AM, Wolf ME, Giambernardi TA, Naylor SL. Definition of a tumor suppressor locus within human chromosome-3p21-p22. Proc Natl Acad Sci USA 1992; 89: 10877–81

82. Kovacs G. Molecular cytogenetics of renal-cell tumors. Adv Cancer Res 1993; 62: 89–124

83. Wu Sq, Hafez GR, Xing WR, Newton M, Chen XR, Messing E. The correlation between the loss of chromosome 14q with histologic tumor grade, pathological stage, and outcome of patients with nonpapillary renal-cell carcinoma. Cancer 1996; 77: 1154–60

84. Moch H, Presti JC, Sauter G, et al. Genetic aberrations detected by comparative genomic hybridization are associated with clinical outcome in renal-cell carcinoma. Cancer Res 1996; 56: 27–30

85. Schwerdtle RF, Storkel S, Neuhaus C, et al. Allelic losses at chromosomes 1p, 2p, 6p, 10p, 13q, 17p and 21q significantly correlate with the chromophobe subtype of renal-cell carcinoma. Cancer Res 1996; 56: 2927–30

86. Corless CL, Aburatani H, Fletcher JA, Housman DE, Amin MB, Weinberg DS. Papillary renal-cell carcinoma – quantitation of chromosome-7 and chromosome-17 by FISH, analysis of chromosome 3p for LOH, and DNA-ploidy. Diag Mol Pathol 1996; 5: 53–64

87. Cairns P, Tokino K, Eby Y, Sidransky D. Localization of tumor-suppressor loci on chromosome-9 in primary human renal-cell carcinomas. Cancer Res 1995; 55: 224–7

88. Kamb A, Gruis NA, Weaverfeldhaus J, et al. A cell-cyle regulator potentially involved in genesis of many tumor types. Science 1994; 264: 436–40

89. Nobori T, Miura K, Wu DJ, Lois A, Takabayashi K, Carson DA. Deletions of the cyclin-dependent kinase-4 inhibitor gene in multiple human cancers. Nature 1994; 368: 753–6

90. Barbacid M. Ras genes. Ann Rev Biochem 1987; 56: 779–827

91. Lowy DR, Willumsen BM. Function and regulation of ras. Ann Rev Biochem 1993; 62: 851–91

92. Fearon ER, Vogelstein B. A genetic model for colorectal tumorigenesis. Cell 1991; 61: 759–67

93. Nanus DM, Mentle IR, Motzer RJ, Bander NH, Albino

AP. Infrequent ras oncogene point mutations in renal-cell carcinoma. J Urol 1990; 143: 175–8

94. Rochlitz CF, Willroth G, Herrmann R, Peter S. Polymerase chain-reaction (PCR) to determine oncogenes in renal-cell carcinoma. Aktuelle Urologie 1992; 23: 58–63

95. Uchida T, Wada LC, Wang CX, Egawa S, Ohtani H, Koshiba K. Genomic instability of microsatellite repeats and mutations of H-, K-, and N-ras, and p53 genes in renal-cell carcinoma. Cancer Research 1994; 54: 3682–5

96. Oka H, Chatani Y, Hoshino R, et al. Constitutive activation of mitogen-activated protein (MAP) kinases in human renal-cell carcinoma. Cancer Research 1995; 55: 4182–7

97. Mansour SJ, Matten WT, Hermann AS, et al. Transformation of mammalian cells by constitutively active MAP kinase kinase. Science 1994; 265: 966–70

98. Carpenter G. Receptors for epidermal growth factor and other polypeptide mitogens. Ann Rev Biochem 1987; 56: 881–914

99. Yamamoto T, Ikawa S, Akiyama T, et al. Similarity of protein encoded by the human c-erbB2 gene to epidermal growth factor receptor. Nature 1986; 319: 230–4

100. Dougall WC, Qian XL, Peterson NC, Miller MJ, Samanta A, Greene MI. The neu-oncogene – signal transduction pathways, transformation mechanisms and evolving therapies. Oncogene 1994; 9: 2109–23

101. Tenth International Workshop on Human Gene Mapping. New Haven. Cytogenet Cell Genet 1989; 51: 166–337

102. Aasland R, Lillehaug JR, Male R, Josendal O, Varhaug JE, Kleppe K. Expression of oncogenes in thyroid tumors – coexpression of c-erbB2/neu and c-erbB. Br J Cancer 1988; 57: 358–63

103. Lu SH, Hsieh LL, Luo FC, Weinstein IB. Amplification of the EGF receptor and c-myc genes in human esophageal cancers. Int J Cancer 1988; 42: 502–5

104. Libermann TA, Nusbaum HR, Razon N, et al. Amplification, enhanced expression and possible rearrangement of EGF receptor gene in primary human brain tumors of glial origin. Nature 1985; 313: 144–7

105. Berger MS, Greenfield C, Gullick WJ, et al. Evaluation of epidermal growth-factor receptors in bladder tumors. Br J Cancer 1987; 56: 533–7

106. Ro J, North SM, Gallick GE, Hortobagyi GN, Gutterman JU, Blick M. Amplified and overexpressed epidermal growth-factor receptor gene in uncultured primary human breast carcinoma. Cancer Res 1988; 48: 161–4

107. Berchuck A, Kamel A, Whitaker R, et al. Overexpression of her-2/neu is associated with poor survival in advanced epithelial ovarian cancer. Cancer Res 1990; 50: 4087–91

108. Slamon DJ, Clark GM, Wong, SG, Levin WJ, Ullrich A, McGuire WL. Human breast cancer – correlation of relapse and survival with amplification of the her-2 neu oncogene. Science 1987; 235: 177–82

109. Hudziak RM, Schlessinger J, Ullrich A. Increased expression of the putative growth-factor receptor p185her2 causes transformation and tumorigenesis of NIH-3T3 cells. Proc Natl Acad Sci USA 1987; 84: 7159–63

110. DiFiore PP, Pierce JH, Kraus MH, Segatto O, King CR, Aaronson SA. erbB-2 is a potent oncogene when overexpressed in NIH/3T3 cells. Science 1987; 237: 178–82

111. Weidner U, Peter S, Strohmeyer T, Hussnatter R, Ackermann R, Sies H. Inverse relationship of epidermal growth-factor receptor and her2/neu gene expression in human renal-cell carcinoma. Cancer Res 1990; 50: 4504–9

112. Rotter M, Block T, Busch R, Thanner S, Hofler H. Expression of her-2/neu in renal-cell carcinoma – correlation with histologic subtypes and differentiation. Int J Cancer 1992; 52: 213–17

113. Mydlo JH, Michaeli J, Cordoncardo G, Goldenberg AS, Heston WDW, Fair WR. Expression of transforming growth factor-alpha and epidermal growth-factor receptor messenger-RNA in neoplastic and non-neoplastic human kidney tissue. Cancer Res 1989; 49: 3407–11

114. Ishikawa J, Maeda S, Umezu K, Sugiyama T, Kamidono S. Amplification and overexpression of the epidermal growth-factor receptor gene in human renal-cell carcinoma. Int J Cancer 1990; 45: 1018–21

115. Ljundberg B, Gafvels M, Damber JE. Epidermal growth-factor receptor gene expression and binding capacity in renal-cell carcinoma, in relation to tumor stage, grade and DNA-ploidy. Urol Res 1994; 22: 305–8

116. Lager DJ, Slagel DD, Palechek PL. The expression of epidermal growth-factor receptor and transforming growth-factor-alpha in renal-cell carcinoma. Mod Pathol 1994; 7: 544–8

117. Uhlman DL, Nguyen P, Manivel JC, et al. Epidermal growth-factor receptor and transforming growth-

factor-alpha expression in papillary and non-papillary renal-cell carcinoma – correlation with metastatic behavior and prognosis. Clin Cancer Res 1995; 1: 913–20

118. Stumm G, Eberwein S, Rostockwolf S, et al. Concomitant overexpression of the EGFR and erbB-2 genes in renal-cell carcinoma (RCC) is correlated with dedifferentiation and metastasis. Int J Cancer 1996; 69: 17–22

119. Pekonen F, Partanen S, Rutanen EM. Binding of epidermal growth-factor and insulin-like growth-factor-1 in renal-carcinoma and adjacent normal kidney tissue. Int J Cancer 1989; 43: 1029–33

120. Mattei MG, Borg JP, Rosnet O, Marme D, Bimbaum D. Assignment of vascular endothelial growth-factor (VEGF) and placenta growth-factor (PIGF) genes to human-chromosome 6p12-p21 and 14q24-q31 regions, respectively. Genomics 1996; 32: 168–9

121. Ferrara N, Houck KA, Jakeman LB, Winer J, Leung DW. The vascular endothelial growth-factor family of polypeptides. J Cell Biochem 1991; 47: 211–18

122. Breier G, Albrecht U, Sterrer S, Risau W. Expression of vascular endothelial growth-factor during embryonic angiogenesis and endothelial-cell differentiation. Development 1992; 114: 521–32

123. Leung DW, Cachianes G, Kuang WJ, Goeddel DV, Ferrara N. Vascular endothelial growth-factor is a secreted angiogenic mitogen. Science 1989; 246: 1306–9

124. Keck PJ, Hauser SD, Krivi G, et al. Vascular-permeability factor, an endothelial-cell mitogen related to PDGF. Science 1989; 246: 1309–12

125. Connolly DT, Heuvelman DM, Nelson R, et al. Tumor vascular-permeability factor stimulates endothelial-cell growth and angiogenesis. J Clin Invest 1989; 84: 1470–8

126. Wizigmann-Voos S, Breier G, Risau W, Plate KH. Up-regulation of vascular endothelial growth-factor and its receptors in von Hippel–Lindau disease-associated and sporadic hemangioblastomas. Cancer Res 1995; 55: 1358–64

127. Plate KH, Breier G, Weich HA, Risau W. Vascular endothelial growth-factor is a potential tumor angiogenesis factor in human gliomas in vivo. Nature 1992; 359: 845–8

128. Zhang HT, Craft P, Scott PAE, et al. Enhancement of tumor growth and vascular density by transfection of vascular endothelial-cell growth-factor into MCF-7 human breast carcinoma cells. J Natl Cancer Inst 1995; 87: 213–19

129. Takahashi A, Sasaki H, Kim SJ, et al. Markedly increased amounts of messenger-RNAs for vascular endothelial growth-factor and placenta growth-factor in renal-cell carcinoma associated with angiogenesis. Cancer Res 1994; 54: 4233–7

130. Sato K, Terada K, Sugiyama T, et al. Frequent overexpression of vascular endothelial growth-factor gene in human renal-cell carcinoma. Tohoku J Exp Med 1994; 173: 355–60

131. Brown LF, Berse B, Jackman RW, et al. Increased expression of vascular-permeability factor (vascular endothelial growth-factor) and its receptors in kidney and bladder carcinomas. Am J Pathol 1993; 143: 1255–62

132. Mattern J, Volm M. Microvessel density and vascular endothelial growth-factor expression in human tumors of different localization. Oncol Reps 1996; 3: 465–8

133. Gospodarowicz D, Neufeld G, Schweigerer L. Fibroblast growth-factor. Mol Cell Endocrinol 1986; 46: 187–204

134. Crabb JW, Armes LG, Johnson CM, McKeehan WL. Characterization of multiple forms of prostatropin (prostate epithelial-cell growth-factor) from bovine brain. Biochem Biophys Res Comm 1986; 136: 1155–61

135. Takahashi K, Suzuki K, Kawahara S, Ono T. Growth stimulation of human breast epithelial cells by basic fibroblast growth-factor in serum-free medium. Int J Cancer 1989; 43: 870–4

136. Yoshida T, Miyagawa K, Odagiri H, et al. Genomic sequence of hst, a transforming gene encoding a protein homologous to fibroblast growth-factors and the int-2-encoded protein. Proc Natl Acad Sci USA 1987; 84: 7305–9

137. Tanimoto H, Yoshida K, Yokozaki H, et al. Expression of basic fibroblast growth-factor in human genetic carcinomas. Virchows Archiv 1991; 61: 263–7

138. Murphy PR, Myal Y, Sato Y, Sato R, West M, Friesen HG. Elevated expression of basic fibroblast growth-factor messenger ribonucleic-acid in acoustic neuromas. Mol Endocrinol 1989; 3: 225–31

139. Fujimoto K, Ichimori Y, Yamaguchi H, et al. Basic fibroblast growth-factor as a candidate tumor-marker for renal-cell carcinoma. Jap J Cancer Res 1995; 86: 182–6

140. Duensing S, Grosse J, Atzpodien J. Increased serum levels of basic fibroblast growth-factor (bFGF) are associated with progressive lung metastases in

advanced renal-cell carcinoma patients. Anticancer Res 1995; 15: 2331–3

141. Fujimoto K, Ichimori Y, Kakizoe T, et al. Increased serum levels of basic fibroblast growth-factor in patients with renal-cell carcinoma. Biochem Biophys Res Comm 1991; 180: 386–92

142. Emoto N, Isozaki O, Ohmura E, et al. Basic fibroblast growth-factor (FGF-2) in renal-cell carcinoma, which is indistinguishable from that in normal kidney, is involved in renal-cell carcinoma growth. J Urol 1994; 152: 1626–31

143. Eguchi J, Nomata K, Kanta S, et al. Gene expression and immunohistochemical localization of basic fibroblast growth-factor in renal-cell carcinoma. Biochem Biophys Res Comm 1992; 183: 937–44

144. Kandel J, Bossywetzel E, Radvanyi F, Klagsbrun M, Folkman J, Hanahan D. Neovascularization is associated with a switch to the export of bFGF in the multistep development of fibrosarcoma. Cell 1991; 66: 1095–104

145. Spencer CA, Groudine M. Control of c-myc regulation in normal and neoplastic cells. Adv Cancer Res 1991; 56: 1–48

146. Greenhalgh DA, Yuspa SH. Malignant conversion of murine squamous papilloma cell-lines by transfection with the fos oncogene. Mol Carcinogen 1988; 1: 134–43

147. Slamon DJ, Dekernion JB, Verma IM, Cline MJ. Expression of cellular oncogenes in human malignancies. Science 1984; 224: 256–62

148. Yao M, Shuin T, Misaki H, Kubota Y. Enhanced expression of c-myc and epidermal growth-factor receptor (c-erbB-1) genes in primary human renal cancer. Cancer Res 1988; 48: 6753–7

149. Kinouchi T, Saiki S, Naoe T, et al. Correlation of c-myc expression with nuclear pleomorphism in human renal-cell carcinoma. Cancer Res 1989; 49: 3627–30

150. Lanigan D, Mclean PA, Murphy DM, Donovan MG, Curran B, Leader M. c-myc expression in renal carcinoma – correlation with clinical parameters. Br J Urol 1993; 72: 143–7

151. Erisman MD, Rothberg PG, Diehl RE, Morse CC, Spandorfer JM, Astrin SM. Deregulation of c-myc gene expression in human-colon carcinoma is not accompanied by amplification or rearrangement of the gene. Mol Cell Biol 1985; 5: 1969–76

152. Hise MK, Jacobs SC, Papadimitriou JC, Drachenberg CI. Transforming growth-factor-alpha expression in human renal-cell carcinoma. Urology 1996; 47: 29–33

153. Petrides PE, Bock S, Bovens J, Hofmann R, Jakse G. Modulation of pro-epidermal growth-factor, pro-transforming growth factor-alpha and epidermal growth-factor receptor gene expression in human renal carcinomas. Cancer Res 1990; 50: 3934–9

154. Gomella LG, Sargent ER, Wade TP, Angland P, Linehan WM, Kasid A. Expression of transforming growth factor-alpha in normal human adult kidney and enhanced expression of transforming growth factor-alpha and factor-beta-1 in renal-cell carcinoma. Cancer Res 1989; 49: 6972–5

155. Maglione D, Guerriero V, Viglietto G, Dellibovi P, Persico MG. Isolation of a human placenta cDNA coding for a protein related to the vascular-permeability factor. Proc Natl Acad Sci USA 1991; 88: 9267–71

156. Maglione D, Guerriero V, Viglietto G, et al. Alternative messenger RNAs coding for the angiogenic factor, placenta growth-factor (P1GF), are transcribed from a single gene of chromosome-14. Oncogene 1993; 8: 925–31

157. Cantley LG, Barros EJG, Gandhi M, Rauchman M, Nigam SK. Regulation of mitogenesis, motogenesis, and tubulogenesis by hepatocyte growth-factor in renal collecting duct cells. Am J Physiol 1994; 267: 271–80

158. Woolf AS, Kolatsijoannou M, Hardman P, et al. Roles of hepatocyte growth factor/scatter factor and the met receptor in the early development of the metanephros. J Cell Biol 1995; 128: 171–84

159. Harris RC, Burns KD, Alattar M, Homma T, Nakamura T. Hepatocyte growth-factor stimulates phosphoinositide hydrolysis and mitogenesis in cultured renal epithelial cells. Life Sciences 1993; 52: 1091–100

160. Kawaida K, Matsumoto K, Shimazu H, Nakamura T. Hepatocyte growth-factor prevents acute renal failure and accelerates renal regeneration in mice. Proc Natl Acad Sci USA 1994; 91: 4357–61

161. Suzuki K, Hayashi N, Yamada Y, et al. Expression of the c-met protooncogene in human hepatocellular carcinoma. Hepatology 1994; 20: 1231–6

162. Pisters LL, Troncoso P, Zhau HE, Li W, Voneschenbach AC, Chung LWK. C-met protooncogene expression in benign and malignant human prostate tissues. J Urol 1995; 154: 293–8

163. Iyer A, Kmiecik TE, Park M, et al. Structure, tissue-specific expression, and transforming activity of the mouse met protooncogene. Cell Growth Diff 1990; 1: 87–95

164. Natali PG, Prat M, Nicotra MR, et al. Overexpression

of the met/HGF receptor in renal-cell carcinomas. Int J Cancer 1996; 69: 212–17

165. Petrides PE, Bolen P. The mitogeneic property of insulin: an intrinsic property of the molecule. Biochem Biophys Res Comm 1980; 95: 1138–44

166. Giorgino F, Belfiore A, Milazzo G, *et al*. Overexpression of insulin-receptors in fibroblast and ovary cells induces a ligand-mediated transformed phenotype. Mol Endocrinol 1991; 5: 452–9

167. Duronio V, Jacobs S. Comparison of insulin and IGF-1 receptors. In: Venter CJ, Harrison LC (eds) Receptor biochemistry and methodology. New York: AR Liss, 1988: 3–18

168. Milazzo G, Giorgino F, Damante G, *et al*. Insulin-receptor expression and function in human breast-cancer cell-lines. Cancer Res 1992; 52: 3924–30

169. Chung CK, Antoniades HN. Expression of c-sis/platelet-derived growth factor-β, insulin-like growth factor-1, and transforming growth factor-alpha messenger-RNAs and their respective receptor messenger-RNAs in primary human gastric carcinomas – in vivo studies with in situ hybridization and immunocytochemistry. Cancer Res 1992; 52: 3453–9

170. Pekonen F, Partanen S, Rutanen EM. Binding of epidermal growth-factor and insulin-like growth-factor-1 in renal carcinoma and adjacent normal kidney tissue. Int J Cancer 1989; 43: 1029–33

171. Kellerer M, Corleta HVE, Muhlhofer A, *et al*. Insulin and insulin-like growth-factor-1 receptor tyrosine-kinase activities in human renal carcinoma. Int J Cancer 1995; 62: 501–7

Transitional cell carcinoma of the bladder

18

T. R. L. Griffiths and D. E. Neal

Introduction

Each year in England and Wales, around 8500 men and 3000 women develop cancer of the bladder; it is the fourth most common cancer after lung, colorectal and prostate/breast cancer [1]. In the developed world, transitional cell carcinoma (rather than squamous carcinoma or adenocarcinoma) is responsible for most bladder carcinoma. About 25% of newly diagnosed cancers are muscle invasive (T2–T4); the remainder are superficial (70%), classified as limited to the mucosa (pTa), lamina propria (pT1) or being in-situ changes (Tis – 5%).

Aetiology

The aetiology of bladder cancer is heavily dependent on chemical exposure from smoking and occupation, although genetic polymorphisms for certain enzymes involved in detoxification affect susceptibility. These enzymes include N-acetyl transferase, one of the cytochrome P450s (CYP 2D6) and glutathione transferase M1. Squamous metaplasia induced by stones, strictures and infection by *Schistosoma haematobium* is a risk factor in the development of squamous carcinoma.

Industrial chemicals (Tables 18.1 and 18.2)
Occupational exposure to chemicals is thought to precipitate up to one-third of bladder cancers. Most carcinogens have a latent period of 15 to 20 years between exposure and the development of tumours; this means that occupational exposure could result in tumour formation at an earlier age than in those patients not exposed to industrial carcinogens. In 1938, Heupner produced the first experimental evidence showing that the aromatic amine β-naphthylamine could induce bladder cancer in dogs. Following this and other reports, a full epidemiological survey headed by Case was performed; this showed that exposure to α-naphthylamine, β-naphthylamine or benzidine, rather than to aniline itself, was the main factor associated with the development of bladder cancer.

Smoking
Lilienfield first identified the association between smoking and bladder cancer. Since then, most studies have indicated a direct relationship between the

Table 18.1 Compounds associated with bladder cancer

2-Naphthylamine
4-Aminobiphenyl
Benzidine
Chlornaphazine
4-Chloro-*o*-toluidine
o-Toluidine
4,4′-Methylene *bis* (2-choloranliline)
Methylene dianiline
Benzidine-derived azo dyes

Table 18.2 Occupations associated with bladder cancer

Textile workers
Dye workers
Tyre rubber and cable workers
Petrol workers
Leather workers
Shoe manufacturers and cleaners
Painters
Hairdressers
Lorry drivers
Drill press operators
Chemical workers
Rodent exterminators and sewage workers

incidence of bladder cancer and the prevalence of smoking among any particular patient cohort. Indeed, a third of all bladder cancers may be related to cigarette smoking. It is of interest that nitrosamines and 2-naphthylamine have been found in cigarette smoke and may be the causative agents.

Drugs

In the 1950s and 1960s, analgesic abuse was rife in Australia and New Zealand, and both upper tract and bladder transitional cell carcinomas were linked to phenacetin administration. Being an aniline derivative, the carcinogenicity of phenacetin may be related to orthohydroxyamine metabolites. Subsequently, cyclophosphamide was shown to induce bladder cancer. In comparison to other carcinogenic agents, the latency period was relatively short.

Pelvic irradiation

Patients who are treated with pelvic radiotherapy for cervical carcinoma have an increased risk of developing bladder cancer. One retrospective study in which patients were followed up for 25 years identified the risk as 57-fold higher than that of the general female population.

Genetic polymorphisms

Drug- and carcinogen-metabolising enzymes have evolved as multigene families of proteins to combat the potential toxic effects of environmental chemicals. The predominant role of these proteins is the metabolism of lipophilic chemicals to products that are more water soluble and can be excreted. The activity of these enzyme systems is to a degree controlled by genetic polymorphism. Metabolic activation occurs in the liver and involves N-oxidation by cytochrome P4501A2 (CYP1A2), while detoxification involves N-acetylation by N-acetyltransferase (NAT)2 [2]. The toxic or mutagenic effects of chemical intermediates generated by the P450 system can also be inactivated by their conjugation with glutathione. This reaction is predominantly catalysed by the glutathione S-transferases (GST). Genotyping studies have suggested that GST M1 may play an important role in the detoxification of bladder carcinogens, because individuals with the GST M1 deletion are at higher risk for bladder cancer [3]. GST P1 represents approximately 90% of the glutathione S-transferases in bladder cytosol, and the levels of this enzyme in the bladder are expressed in a polymorphic manner.

Pathology

The calyces, renal pelvis, ureter, bladder and urethra as far as the navicular fossa are lined by transitional cell epithelium. Tumours of the bladder are about 50 times as common as those of the ureter or renal pelvis. Most are trainsitional cell carcinomas (70% pure transitional cell carcinomas; 20% transitional cell carcinomas with squamous or glandular portions). The remainder present with rare tumours including pure squamous cell carcinoma, adenocarcinoma, sarcoma and undifferentiated tumours. Adenocarcinomas of the rectum, uterus, breast, ovary and prostate may metastasise to the bladder, and, very rarely, adenocarcinoma may arise in a urachal remnant.

Premalignant conditions

Bladder leucoplakia is a premalignant condition, especially when associated with chronic infection. Squamous metaplasia seen in exstrophy, chronic bladder inflammation and schistosomiasis is premalignant. In contrast, metaplasia of the trigone, as seen in women with trigonitis, is not premalignant.

Histologically, dysplasia is a flat, non-invasive, urothelial lesion recognised at low magnifications by lack of cytoplasmic clearing and the presence of nuclear clustering. Urothelial dysplasia has been detected in 20–86% of bladder cancer patients, depending on the amount of tissue available and the thoroughness of the examination. Dysplastic changes are more commonly detected in muscle-invasive and high-grade tumours (Figure 18.1). Investigators supporting dysplasia as a premalignant condition cite the frequent co-existence of dysplastic and neoplastic lesions, the frequency of tumour recurrence and progression among bladder cancer patients with dysplasia, and experimental studies that document a progression of morphological changes from normal through dysplasia to invasive cancer. Sceptics point out that it is not clear whether dysplasia develops before or concomitantly with clinically manifest bladder cancer. Furthermore, in clinical studies showing progression, dysplasia is often confused with carcinoma in situ.

Clinical features

The natural history of bladder cancer can be classified as follows:

no further recurrence;
local recurrence, which can occur on a single occasion or on multiple occasions; it can involve single or multiple tumour recurrences, but recurrent tumours are usually of the same stage and grade as the primary tumour;
local progression – an increase in local stage with time; the appearance of distant metastases (which usually presages death).

Prediction of these events depends strongly on the presenting stage and grade of the primary tumour.

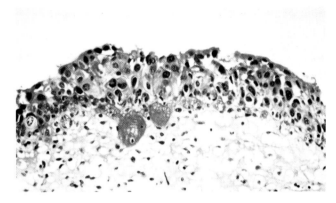

Figure 18.1 *Section taken from a patient with primary carcinoma in situ of the urinary bladder showing abnormal atypical cells throughout the width of the urothelium.*

The addition of molecular markers may well improve the prediction of tumour behaviour in the future.

Tumour stage

The TNM staging system provides the basis for assessing the future behaviour of a newly diagnosed tumour (Table 18.3) [4]. In superficial tumours (pTa and pT1), good data on the pT category should be obtained from histological examination of resection biopsies, although, if deep muscle is not included, accurate staging will be impossible (approximately 5% of cases). On examination under anaesthesia, a soft, palpable mass may be present before resection in large Ta or T1 tumours.

On the basis of resection biopsies, the pathologist can only state that muscle invasion is present or absent. Careful examination under anaesthesia can determine the clinical stage and tumour size, but will understage 40–50% of T2 and T3a tumours.

Tumour grade

Considerable disagreement has been shown in the interpretation of histological grade between pathologists [5]. There are several grading systems in use, but there is no evidence that any one system is better than another; it is more important that the pathologist is familiar with one system.

Tumour size

Tumours more than 5 cm in diameter have a worse prognosis than smaller tumours. Superficial tumours

Table 18.3 TNM classification of bladder cancer

Tis	Pre-invasive carcinoma (carcinoma in situ)
Ta	Papillary non-invasive carcinoma showing no lamina propria invasion
T1	Tumour invading beyond the lamina propria but confined within the submucosal tissue
T2	Tumour invading the superficial muscle
T3a	Tumour invading the deep muscle
T3b	Tumour invading through the bladder wall
T4a	Tumour infiltrating the prostate in men and the uterus or vagina in women
T4b	Tumour fixed to the pelvic wall and/or abdominal wall
N1	Single ipsilateral regional lymph node involvement
N2	Contralateral or bilateral or multiple regional lymph node involvement
N3	Fixed regional lymph nodes as a fixed mass separated from the tumour within the bladder
N4	Juxtaregional lymph node involvement
M1	Distant metastases

less than 2 cm in size have a significantly lower risk of recurrence. A simple system has been proposed of stratifying risks of recurrence on the basis of size, multifocality and recurrence at three months (Table 18.4) [6, 7].

Abnormalities of urothelium distant from the primary lesion

Urine cytology may detect carcinoma in situ that has not been found by random mucosal biopsies because surface urothelial cells are not adherent in carcinoma in situ. In patients with marked irritative symptoms such as bladder pain, urethral irritation and dysuria, but no abnormal clinical findings, the cytological examination of several specimens of urine is recommended. A biopsy of abnormal mucosa should be performed.

Prognostic factors and natural history
(Tables 18.5 and 18.6)

Bladder cancer can be classified into superficial and muscle-invasive tumours, but urologists now prefer to separate pT1 and pTa tumours. Of patients presenting with transitional cell carcinomas, 70% have superficial tumours (50% pTa and 20% pT1) not invading detrusor muscle, and 25% have muscle-invasive tumours. The latter account for the majority of deaths from bladder cancer and such patients have an overall

Table 18.4 Prognostic groups, their relationship to risks of recurrence and recommended management plans for Ta and T1 (G1 and G2) tumours

Prognostic groups	Cystoscopic findings	Management plan
Group 1	Solitary tumour at presentation; no tumour recurrence at three months (20% risk of recurrence at one year)	Followed up safely by annual flexible cytoscopy
Group 2	Solitary tumour at presentation; tumour recurrence at three months; multiple tumours at presentation; no tumour recurrence at three months (40% risk of recurrence at one year)	Followed up three-monthly by flexible cytoscopy for the first year, then annually if no recurrence
Group 3	Multiple tumours at presentation; tumour recurrence at three months (90% risk of recurrence at one to two years)	Three-monthly rigid cystoscopic assessment under general anaesthesia

Table 18.5 Risk of recurrence in superficial tumours [25]

	Number	Recurrence rate (+ve cystoscopies per 100 patient months)
Tumour status		
Primary	190	5.2
Recurrent	118	10.4
Number of prior recurrences per year		
Primary tumours (none)	190	5.2
≤1	38	5.6
1–2	28	12.7
>2	42	12.8
Number of tumours		
1	161	4.8
2–3	71	7.8
>3	68	12.3
Diameter of largest (cm)		
<2	201	6.4
>3	95	7.9
Grade		
1	241	6.4
2–3	60	8.9

Table 18.6 Risk of progression

	Percentage risk
Ta	10
T1	24
T1 (recurrent)	56
Solitary versus multiple	
Ta single	5
Ta multiple	20
T1 single	33
T1 multiple	46
Grade	
pTa grade 1	None
pTa grade 2	6
pTa grade 3	25
pT1 grade 2	25
pT1 grade 3	50

survival of 50% at five years. Of newly diagnosed superficial bladder tumours, approximately 30% are multifocal at presentation, 60–70% will recur, and 10–20% will undergo stage progression to muscle-invasive or metastatic disease [8]. Of newly diagnosed muscle-invasive tumours, 50% have occult metastases that manifest themselves within 12 months. Few patients with metastatic disease survive more than two years.

Superficial tumours

Ta disease

After five to ten years of follow-up, 50% of patients have no recurrence; 20% have only one recurrence; and 30% have more than one recurrence. Recurrence at three months' follow-up is highly predictive of further recurrence (90% continue to recur) [9]. Small papillary tumours have a significantly lower risk of recurrence (30%) compared with multifocal or large sessile tumours (80%; see Table 18.3).

Among patients with Ta tumours who develop recurrence, about 15% progress. The survival of patients with Ta G1/G2 disease is similar to that of an age-matched and sex-matched control population.

T1 disease

About 20% of patients with T1 disease will die from bladder cancer within five years [10]. The presence of carcinoma in situ near the site of the initial tumour is associated with a greater risk of tumour progression. The survival of patients with early T1 recurrence at the site of the initial T1 tumour is poor, being similar to that of patients with muscle-invasive cancer, which may indicate that some of these tumours are under-staged.

Grade

Despite inaccuracies in grading, most authors report that tumour grade has a pronounced influence on progression, and the poor prognosis of T1 Grade 3 tumours is well described (50% progression rate if accompanied by carcinoma in situ) [11, 12].

Morphometric measurements correlate well with tumour grade. Flow-cytometric DNA analysis correlates in general with grade, recurrence rate, risk of progression and survival, and represents an objective method that may be used to improve the reproducibility of tumour characterisation. However, it is unclear whether such objective assessments improve prediction over conventional grading.

Carcinoma in situ

Carcinoma in situ is usually classified as primary and secondary. In primary carcinoma in situ, there is no history of previous or concurrent tumour. The term concomitant carcinoma in situ is used when a tumour is present at the same time.

Primary carcinoma in situ

Patients presenting with bladder pain and dysuria and positive cytology have primary carcinoma in situ, which is a serious risk to life, around 50% of patients dying of metastatic bladder cancer within a year or two if aggressive treatment with intravesical therapy is not instituted [13].

Secondary carcinoma in situ

This can be demonstrated by carrying out random or preselected site biopsies in patients with bladder cancer. However, most authors have found that random biopsies of apparently normal urothelium do not add prognostic information.

Concomitant carcinoma in situ

Concomitant carcinoma in situ can be demonstrated in around 40% of patients. Its presence is highly predictive of recurrent disease [14]. It also predicts the progression of superficial bladder cancer. Fifty per cent of those with carcinoma in situ or severe dysplasia progress to muscle invasion. There is a good case to be made for carrying out near and far biopsies of urothelium at initial tumour presentation to detect unsuspected carcinoma in situ, though such changes are uncommon if the mucosa appears normal.

Failure of carcinoma in situ to respond to intravesical treatment should lead to the consideration of early cystectomy.

Muscle-invasive disease

Tumour stage at presentation is the most useful prognostic indicator associated with outcome. The presence of lymph node metastases is clearly related to tumour stage, a gradually increasing proportion of lymph node metastases being found with increasing stage. In most series, few patients (about 10%) with even N1 disease survive following radical cystectomy, although some authors have reported 20% survival rates following extensive pelvic lymphadenectomy.

Over 50% of patients with muscle-invasive disease have occult systemic or nodal metastatic disease at presentation; its presence is strongly related to initial tumour stage, being most frequent in T4 disease. Other non-specific features of poor prognostic import include systemic signs such as anaemia, renal failure and performance status. The presence of upper tract dilatation in muscle-invasive disease is associated with increased risks of lymph node metastases, systemic spread and a worse clinical outcome.

Molecular studies and bladder cancer

For patients with a superficial bladder tumour, the difficulty lies in identifying those who will progress to muscle invasion or metastatic disease. None of the established prognostic factors is sufficiently sensitive or specific to identify precisely those in whom early radical therapy would be beneficial. For muscle-invasive tumours, criteria are needed to distinguish tumours likely to respond to local therapy and those likely to metastasise. Genetic changes that identify different subsets of tumours may provide the key. Several of these factors have been studied in bladder cancer.

Oncogenes and growth factors

These are dealt with in greater detail in Chapter 16.

ras oncogenes

The detection of an activated H-ras gene in the bladder tumour cell line EJ/T24 prompted researchers to look for ras mutations in human tumours. Using a combination of NIIH-3T3 transfection assays, single strand conformation polymorphism, restriction fragment length polymorphism analysis and direct sequencing and polymerase chain reation-based direct DNA sequencing, mutations for H-ras have been found in between 10% and 20% of tumours. H-ras mutations are found with equal frequency in both well-differentiated superficial tumours and poorly differentiated muscle-invasive tumours, which suggests that this is an early event in the development of bladder cancer.

c-myc oncogene

The *c-myc* gene maps to chromosome 8q24 and encodes a nuclear phosphoprotein of about 60 kDa that is involved in transcriptional regulation. Its function has been linked to growth regulation, cell differentiation and apoptosis. Two studies showed a higher level of *c-myc* in superficial than in muscle-invasive tumours assessed by flow cytometry and immunohistochemistry. Other studies have shown an association with increased *c-myc* transcript levels and poor grade.

mdm-2 oncogene

High levels of *mdm-2* in bladder cancer are associated with low-stage, low-grade tumours and p53 protein accumulation. In keeping with studies of other oncogenes in bladder cancer, gene amplification assessed by Southern blotting is a rare cause of oncoprotein over-expression: *mdm-2* gene amplification was only detected in one of 26 tumours with high *mdm-2* immunoreactivity. In another study, *mdm-2* gene amplification was detected in two of 50 bladder tumours (4%) that were high-grade, muscle-invasive tumours, neither of which harboured *p53* gene mutations.

Epidermal growth factor receptor family

Epidermal growth factor receptor

In 1984, epidermal growth factor was reported to stimulate the proliferation of transitional cell malignant cell lines. In the same year, the immunohistochemical detection of epidermal growth factor receptor was described. Epidermal growth factor is a 53-amino acid peptide of 6000 Da, originally extracted from murine submaxillary gland extracts. High levels of this growth factor have been found in milk, urine and prostatic secretion. These initial studies provided the impetus to investigate epidermal growth factor receptor levels in bladder cancer. Epidermal growth factor levels are consistently reduced in the urine of patients with bladder tumours of increasing stage, the levels rising again following

tumour ablation [15]. In bladder cancer, tissue transforming growth factor alpha levels assessed using a standard radio-immunoassay have been found to correlate with epidermal growth factor receptor assessed by immunohistochemistry. In these specimens, epidermal growth factor was barely detectable. This finding suggests that transforming growth factor alpha is the more important ligand for epidermal growth factor receptor in tissues, where it acts in an autocrine/paracrine mode.

Epidermal growth factor receptor status has prognostic value in bladder cancer (Figure 18.2). A prospective study found that receptor positivity was associted with a poor prognosis (Figure 18.3) [16]. Mechanisms underlying epidermal growth factor

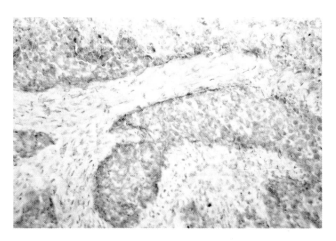

Figure 18.2 *An invasive bladder cancer showing over-expression for the epidermal growth factor receptor.*

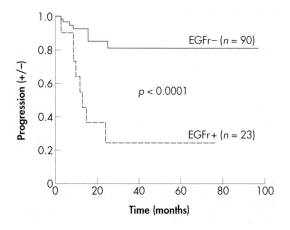

Figure 18.3 *A graph showing time to progression against epidermal growth factor receptor (EGFr) status for 90 patients who were receptor negative and 23 patients who were receptor positive.*

receptor over-expression in bladder cancer are not clear, although gene amplification is not the principal mechanism. Furthermore, despite the absence of altered gene copy numbers or chromosomal translocations, elevated levels of epidermal growth factor receptor messenger RNA have been detected in tumours compared with normal urothelium.

c-erb-B2

The finding that, in breast cancer, amplification and over-expression of c-erb-B2 were associated with a poor clinical outcome prompted studies in transitional cell carcinoma. In a study of 141 bladder tumour specimens, gene amplification for c-erbB2, assessed using fluorescence in-situ hybridisation, was detected in only 7% of cases and was associated with c-erb-B2 over-expression[17]. However, over-expression without gene amplification was detected in 51 tumours.

Fibroblast growth factors

Both int2 and hst are located on chromosome band 11q13, which was found to be amplified in 7% of bladder tumors. Gene amplification at the 11q13 locus involving int2 and hst co-amplification has also been reported in 21% of bladder tumours. A fibroblast growth factor-like factor has previously been reported in raised amounts in the urine of patients with bladder cancer.

Tumour suppressor genes

Loss of heterozygosity studies

Karyotyping is time consuming, and reliable results can only be achieved by analysing cells stimulated into mitosis. Fluorescence in-situ hybridisation enabled the rapid characterisation of minor genetic aberrations in the interphase nuclei of individual cells. However, polymerase chain reaction methods, based on the amplification of the area of interest in the genome, are the most sensitive indicators of chromosomal aberrations. The systematic study of all chromosome arms in a particular type of tumour has been termed an allelotype, and aims to identify the common sites of deletion in that tumour. In bladder cancer, loss of heterozygosity has been commonly detected on chromosomes 9p, 9q, 17p, 13p, 4p, 8p and 3p.

Chromosome 4, 8 and 9 deletions

Loss of heterozygosity of chromosome 9 has been detected in at least 60% of bladder tumours of all grades and stages. It is of particular interest because it is the only genetic alteration found in low-grade pTa bladder tumours and therefore represents a candidate for an initiating event in bladder cancer. The 9p21 region is mutated in a wide variety of tumour cell lines [18]. Lesions of chromosome 9 appear to involve proximal 9q extending to proximal 9p and lie between 9p12 and 9q34.1. Further study has shown that the common site of deletion on 9p is between the α-interferon gene and D9S171, and on 9q it is in the region of 9q34.1–2. Lesions of 9p are particularly found in pTa tumours (70% of cases), whereas pT1 tumours tend to have both regions affected, suggesting that there may be two tumour suppressor genes involved. The search for a putative tumour suppressor gene initially suggested that it might be p16. However, early enthusiasm was restrained following reports suggesting that although p16 gene alterations were commonly detected in cell lines, they were infrequent in many primary tumours [19].

In one study, loss of heterozygosity for chromosome 9 was reported to be less common in carcinoma in situ compared with papillary or muscle-invasive transitional cell carcinoma. Using a larger number of microsatellite markers directed within the critical region of chromosome 9p, these findings were recently disputed; loss of heterozygosity on chromosome 9 was detected in the majority of carcinoma in situ lesions, with both arms being deleted with a similar frequency.

Other studies have found that alterations in chromosome 8 (between 8p21 and 8q11.2) are also associated with high-grade disease. In addition, 22% of tumours have losses of chromosome 4 in the region of 4p (D4S43 and D4S127). D4S174 was also deleted in 7/23 (30%) of tumours with deletions in 4.

Deletions of chromosome 13q and the retinoblastoma gene

Loss of the Rb1 locus on chromosome 13q is a common finding in sporadic cases of muscle invasive bladder cancer, being detected in 29% of cases, most of which were muscle invasive. Whether positive immunostaining for the Rb protein reflects normal levels of protein is still under debate, though it would be expected that loss of Rb immunoreactivity would be associated with chromosome 13q deletions. There is a general consensus that altered *Rb* expression is associated with high-stage tumours [20].

Deletions of chromosome 17p and the p53 *gene*
Estimates of the frequency of 17p loss of heterozygosity in bladder cancer vary and probably reflect the stage and grade profiles of the tumours studied. Chromosome 17p deletions are more commonly detected in tumours of high stage and poor histological grade. In muscle-invasive tumours, detection of loss of heterozygosity of 17p has varied between 57% and 70%. In superficial tumours (pTa and pT1), loss of heterozygosity of 17p is found in about 30%, being more common in pT1 grade 3 tumours. One of the underlying molecular mechanisms distinguishing low-grade from high-grade tumours involves *p53*. Genetic alterations of *p53* are found in 66% of muscle-invasive tumours and in 33% of pT1 tumours examined by direct polymerase chain reaction-based DNA sequencing of exons 5 to 9. In the largest series to date, *p53* gene mutation was only detected in one of 36 pTa tumours (3%). The high frequency of *p53* gene mutations in carcinoma in situ may explain the high propensity for patients with these tumours to progress to muscle-invasive or metastatic disease.

In one study, the frequency of *p53* mutations was similar in smokers and non-smokers. In another study, A:T–G:C transitions were associated with smoking. However G:C–T:A transversions, mutations known to be produced by benzo-(α)-pyrene, a constituent of cigarette smoke, did not predominate. This indicates that other carcinogenic components of cigarette smoke may be involved.

Many *p53* gene mis-sense mutations result in the production of a mutant p53 protein in a denatured conformation. A pathophysiological effect of the denatured conformation is to prolong the half-life of the p53 molecule by a factor of 10 to 20, enabling detection by immunohistochemical methods. Consequently, immunohistochemical detection of p53 protein was initially suggested as being synonymous with the presence of mutations. However, it is now clear that whilst most very strongly stained invasive tumours contain mutations, less intense but nonetheless increased levels of staining are associated with increased levels, or at least stabilised forms, of the wild-type molecule.

Two reports have shown that more than 20% staining of tumour cell nuclei for *p53* using the antibody 1801 was an independent predictor of progression in patients with pT1 transitional cell carcinoma [21, 22]. However, the prognostic value of *p53* immunoreactivity in bladder cancer is far from clear cut.

Apoptosis

Only one study has assessed the prognostic value of apoptosis in bladder cancer. bcl-2 immunoreactivity was significantly elevated in poorly differentiated tumours, pointing to a critical role of this protein in bladder cancer progression. However, in this study, the proliferation index, determined using Ki67 antigen, had more prognostic value than the apoptotic index, assessed by end-labelling of DNA fragments.

Degradation of extracellular matrix barriers

High levels of matrix metallo-proteinases (MMPs) and tissue inhibitors of MMPs (TIMPs) detected both in tumour cells and in stroma have been reported to be associated with cancer-specific death in patients with tumours staged ≥ pT1. This is somewhat surprising given that TIMPs inhibit the degradation of extracellular matrix. However, recent studies have shown that under certain circumstances, TIMP-2 can also activate MMP-2. The pattern of expression of such enzymes is specific to particular tumour types and the activity may reflect the host stromal responses to tissue remodelling rather than over-expression by the tumour cells.

Angiogenesis

A recent study assessed microvessel density by immunohistochemical methods using HPCA-1, a mouse monoclonal antibody directed against the endothelial cell antigen, CD34, in 164 patients with muscle-invasive transitional cell carcinoma who had undergone radical cystectomy. It was found that tumour angiogenesis can contribute independent prognostic information in terms of tumour recurrence ($p<0.001$) and overall survival ($p<0.001$) [23]. The Oxford Molecular group has detected elevated levels of basic fibroblast growth factor in the urine of patients with bladder cancer. However, elevated levels were also found in the urine of symptomatic patients with benign prostatic hypertrophy. It is therefore of limited use in surveillance, although it is a potential therapeutic target.

Cell adhesion molecules

In normal urothelial cells, E-cadherin is homogenously expressed at cell–cell borders. Loss of expression of E-cadherin on cell membranes has been reported in patients with high-grade muscle-invasive bladder tumours [24]. Abnormal expression of E-cadherin in superficial tumours is associated with reduced recurrence-free survival and higher progression rates and also reduced survival in patients with muscle-invasive tumours.

Soluble cell adhesion molecules

A 80-kDa, soluble form of E-cadherin (sE-cadherin) has been detected in the urine of healthy individuals and patients with bladder cancer. It has been found that, in superficial transitional cell carcinoma, elevated levels correlate with multifocal tumours at presentation and tumour recurrence at three months.

Genes associated with chemoresistance

Adjuvant intravesical chemotherapy with epirubicin or mitomycin C is increasingly used as prophylaxis against recurrent superficial papillary tumours. In muscle-invasive disease, adjuvant and neo-adjuvant systemic chemotherapy regimes are currently being tested in clinical trials. Molecular mechanisms that mediate cellular drug resistance may play a role in the differential responsiveness of individual bladder tumours to chemotherapy. Transcript levels of the multidrug resistance (mdr1) gene have been found to vary 34-fold in high-grade muscle-invasive bladder tumours, which may be a significant determinant of chemotherapeutic outcome. High-grade transitional cell carcinoma was significantly associated with elevated transcript levels.

Other markers

Levels of urinary total beta human chorionic gonadotrophin are elevated in patients with muscle-invasive bladder cancer and are associated with subsequent metastatic spread and reduced survival ($p<0.01$). Furthermore, whereas human chorionic gonadotrophin beta 7 (hCGβ7) mRNA has been found in normal urothelium and Ta tumours, the β7, β5, β8, β3 mRNA forms of human chorionic gonadotrophin have all been detected in 45% of T1 and 95% of muscle-invasive tumours.

Leucocytosis in association with transitional cell carcinoma has been reported to reflect aggressive biological activity. There is good evidence that elevated levels of granulocyte colony stimulating factor in serum are derived from secretion by bladder tumour cells and may be responsible for leucocytosis. Granulocyte colony stimulating factor has been shown to stimulate the growth of some tumour cell lines by activating granulocyte colony stimulating factor receptors.

The molecular basis of tumour recurrence and progression

Intense debate surrounds the molecular basis of synchronous and metachronous bladder cancer. Patients with bladder cancer often present with metachronous tumours, presenting at different times and different places in the bladder. Some investigators attribute this observation to a 'field defect' such as dysplasia or carcinoma in situ in the bladder that allows the individual transformation of epithelial cells at a number of sites. In contrast, recent reports based on molecular biological studies have added a new dimension suggesting a common clonal origin for concomitant urothelial tumours, at least in some cases. Cells of adult tissues in females have either one of the two X chromosomes randomly inactivated by methylation. Therefore, if cells are individually transformed, multiple tumours would be heterogeneous with respect to which X chromosome remained active. For each of four female patients with multiple tumours, it was found that all the tumours from a given individual had inactivation of the same X chromosome. Lunec reported identical *p*53 mutations and c-erbB-2 gene amplification in a case of concomitant transitional carcinomas of the renal pelvis and urinary bladder. Lateral intra-epithelial spread of transformed cells from the origin of a bladder carcinoma and dispersal of tumour cells are possible mechanisms underlying multifocal disease. In support of these theories, a single instillation of intravesical mitomycin C or epirubicin immediately following transurethral resection increases tumour-free rates.

References

1. OPCS. (1988). Cancer statistics registration: OPCS – A publication of the government statistical service.

2. Kadlubar FF, Badawi A.F. Genetic susceptibility and carcinogen-DNA adduct formation in human urinary bladder carcinogenesis. Toxicol Lett 1995; 82: 627–32

3. Daly AK, Thomas DJ, Cooper J, et al. Homozygous deletion of gene for glutathione S-transferase M1 gene in bladder cancer. BMJ 1993; 307: 481–82

4. The TNM classification of tumours. Union Internationale Contre le Cancer, 1992.

5. Ooms EC, Anderson WA, Alons CL, Boon ME, Veldhuizen RW. Analysis of the performance of pathologists in the grading of bladder tumors. Hum Pathol 1983; 14: 140–3

6. Parmar MK, Freedman LS, Hargreave TB, Tolley DA. Prognostic factors for recurrence and follow-up policies in the treatment of superficial bladder cancer: report from the British Medical Research Council Subgroup on Superficial Bladder Cancer (Urological Cancer Working Party). J Urol 1989; 142: 284–8

7. Hall RR, Parmar MK, Richards AB, Smith PH. Proposal for changes in cystoscopic follow up of patients with bladder cancer and adjuvant intravesical chemotherapy. BMJ 1994; 308: 257–60

8. Lutzeyer W, Rubben H, Dahm H. Prognostic parameters in superficial bladder cancer: an analysis of 315 cases. J Urol 1982; 127: 250–2

9. Fitzpatrick JM, West AB, Butler MR, et al. Superficial bladder tumors (stage pTa, grades 1 and 2): the importance of recurrence pattern following initial resection. J Urol 1986; 135: 920–2

10. Anderstrøm C, Johansson S, Nilsson S. The significance of lamina propria invasion on the prognosis of patients with bladder cancer. J Urol 1980; 124: 23–6

11. Heney NM, Ahmed S, Flanagan MJ, et al. Superficial bladder cancer: progression and recurrence. J Urol 1983; 130: 1083–6

12. Jakse G, Loidl W, Sieber G, Hofstadter F. Stage T1 grade G3 transitional cell carcinoma of the bladder: an unfavourable tumor? J Urol 1987; 137: 39–43

13. Utz DC, Farrow GM. The management of carcinoma in situ of the urinary bladder: the case for surgical management. Urol Clin N Am 1981; 7: 160–4

14. Wolf H, Olsen PR, Fischer A, Højgaard. Urothelial atypia concomitant with primary bladder tumour. Incidence in a consecutive series of 500 unselected patients. Scand J Urol Nephrol 1987; 21: 33–8

15. Kristensen JK, Lose J, Lund F, Nexo E. Epidermal growth factor in urine from patients with urinary bladder tumours. Eur Urol 1988; 14: 313–4

16. Mellon K, Wright C, Kelly P, Horne CH, Neal DE. Long-term outcome related to epidermal growth factor receptor status in bladder cancer. J Urol 1995; 153: 919–25

17. Sauter G, Moch D, Moore P. Heterogeneity of erbB-2 gene amplification in bladder cancer. Cancer Res 1993; 53: 2199–203

18. Knowles MA, Elder PA, Williamson M, et al. Allelotype of human bladder cancer. Cancer Res 1994; 54: 531–8

19. Cairns P, Tokino K, Eby Y, Sidransky D. Homozygous deletions of 9p21 in primary human bladder tumours detected by comparative multiplex polymerase chain reaction. Cancer Res 1994; 54: 1422–4

20. Cordon-Cardo C, Wartinger D, Petrylak D, et al. Altered expression of the retinoblastoma gene product: prognostic indicator in bladder cancer [see comments]. J Natl Cancer Inst 1992; 84: 1251–6

21. Sarkis A.S, Bajorin DF, Reuter VE, et al. Prognostic value of p53 nuclear overexpression in patients with invasive bladder cancer treated with neoadjuvant MVAC. J Clin Oncol 1995; 13: 1384–90

22. Serth J, Kuczyk MA, Bokemeyer C, et al. p53 immunohistochemistry as an independent prognostic factor for superficial transitional cell carcinoma of the bladder. Br J Cancer 1995; 71: 201–5

23. Dickinson AJ, Fox SB, Persad RA, et al. Quantification of angiogenesis as an independent predictor of prognosis in invasive bladder carcinomas. Br J Urol 1994; 74: 762–6

24. Bringuier PP, Umbas R, Schaafsma HE, et al. Decreased E-cadherin immunoreactivity correlates with poor survival in patients with bladder tumors. Cancer Res 1993; 53: 3241–5

25. Dalesio O, Schulman CC, Sylvester R, et al. Prognostic factors in superficial bladder tumors. A study of the European Organization for Research on Treatment of Cancer: Genitourinary Tract Cancer Cooperative Group. J Urol 1983; 129: 730–3

Prostate cancer

19

F. C. Hamdy, M. I. Johnson and C. N. Robson

As the eyes grow dim, the trunk bends, the cartilages ossify, and the arteries change in their coats, so the prostate is supposed to grow large and hard ...

James Miller, 1864

Introduction

Prostate cancer is the second most common malignancy in males in the European Union, with approximately 95 000 new cases registered, and 35 000 men dying from the disease every year [1]. In the USA, it is the most common malignancy in males, with an estimated 209 900 cases diagnosed in 1997 [2]. In England and Wales, there were 10 837 new cases of prostate cancer registered in 1987, rising to 13 481 in 1990 [3]. Public awareness about the disease is clearly on the increase, partly because of media interest and growing general interest in men's health issues.

Evidence of carcinoma has been found in postmortem studies in approximately 30% of men aged 50 years and in 70% of men over the age of 80 years [4, 5], but only a small proportion of these tumours progress to become clinically significant. With well-conducted screening programmes, it is now possible to detect small-volume tumours amenable to cure. However, clinicians are still unable to predict which tumour is likely to progress and which will remain quiescent.

Aetiology

Prostate cancer results from a complex and yet unclear interaction between ageing, genetic factors, hormones, growth factors and the environment, and there is an increasing body of evidence incriminating dietary fat [4–7].

Prostate cancer can be sporadic, familial, with clustering of disease within families due to exposure to common risk factors, or hereditary, with typical characteristics of early age onset and an autosomal dominant inheritance pattern. The hereditary form is likely to be triggered by a single gene present in family members that is yet to be discovered and possibly located in chromosome 1 [8]. It has been estimated that men who have three first-degree relatives with the disease have a 10.9-fold increase in risk of developing prostate cancer [9]. An increased risk of prostate cancer has also been associated with familial breast cancer [7]. It is generally accepted that prostate cancer is not divided into latent and clinically significant tumour, but that its very long natural history, coupled with cumulative genetic and biological changes, eventually leads to progressive disease. It is the length of this natural history that allows more men to die *with* the disease than *from* it.

Pathology

Adenocarcinoma arising from the prostatic epithelium accounts for about 95% of prostatic malignancies and is usually composed of small glandular acini that infiltrate in an irregular, haphazard manner [10]. The critical feature in prostatic adenocarcinoma is absence of the basal cell layer (Figure 19.1), which may be detected immunohistochemically by using monoclonal antibodies against high molecular weight cytokeratin. Perineural and microvascular invasion may be seen, the latter correlating with histological grade.

Prostatic adenocarcinoma originates in the peripheral zone in approximately 75% of cases, with the

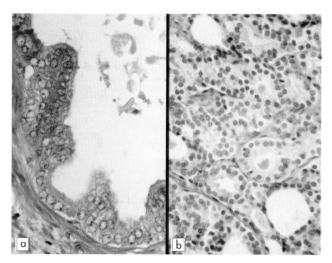

Figure 19.1 *(a) A photomicrograph of the prostate demonstrating high-grade prostatic intraepithelial neoplasia with dysplastic changes, nuclear enlargement, hyperchromatism, prominent nuclei, cellular crowding, overlapping nuclei and epithelial hyperplasia. (H & E staining; magnification approximately × 400.) (b) A photomicrograph of the prostate demonstrating adenocarcinoma with small glandular acini infiltrating in an irregular haphazard manner. The acini are composed of a single layer of cells showing nuclear enlargement with prominent nucleoli. The critical diagnostic feature in prostatic adenocarcinoma is absence of the basal layer. (H & E staining; magnification approximately × 400.)*

rest originating in the transition zone [11]. The tumours arising from these separate zones have different pathological features and clinical behaviour. Transition zone tumours arise in or near foci of benign prostatic hyperplasia and are usually smaller

and better differentiated (Gleason pattern 1 and 2). Peripheral zone cancers are often less well differentiated (Gleason pattern 2, 3 or 4), larger in volume than transition zone tumours, and are frequently associated with greater stromal fibrosis, extracapsular extension, seminal vesicle invasion and lymph node metastases [12].

Histological grading

There are numerous grading systems, but the accepted standard is that developed by Gleason [13]. The system is based on the degree of architectural differentiation, and individual cell cytology does not play a role. The system identifies five patterns that are often seen in prostatic adenocarcinoma and, to accommodate this, a primary and a secondary pattern are assigned and the Gleason score is given as their sum, ranging from 2 to 10, with the dominant pattern recorded first, e.g. 3 + 4 = 7 (Figure 19.2). The Gleason score correlates strongly with crude survival, tumour-free survival and cause-specific survival, and is a significant predictor of time to recurrence following radical prostatectomy [14].

Grading errors are common in needle biopsy specimens of the prostate, with underestimation of the grade in 40% of cases, and overestimation in 25% when compared with the whole specimen following prostatectomy. Grading errors occur more readily in biopsies containing small foci and low-

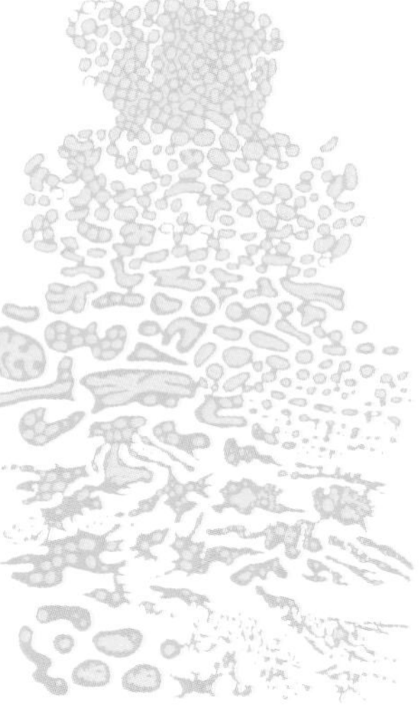

Grade	Margins	Gland pattern	Gland size	Gland distribution
1	Well defined	Single, separate, round	Medium	Closely packed
2	Less defined	Same as one but more variable	Medium	Spaced up to one gland apart
3	Poorly defined	Single, separate, irregular rounded masses of cribriform epithelium	Small medium or large	Spaced more than one gland apart, rarely packed
4	Ragged infiltrating	Fused glandular masses	Small	Fused ragged masses
5	Ragged infiltrating. Poorly defined	Almost absent, few tiny glands or signet ring cells	Small	Ragged anaplastic masses of epithelium

Figure 19.2 *The Gleason system of grading adenocarcinoma of the prostate.*

grade cancers, reflecting sampling error and tumour heterogeneity. Nevertheless, useful predictive information can be provided by Gleason grading needle biopsies [15].

Tumour staging

The TNM system, recently modified [16], is the most common classification used worldwide (Table 19.1). Clinical staging is limited by a number of factors, including clinical understaging with digital rectal examination and transurethral resection specimens, limited accuracy of imaging, and the wide pathological variation of tumours identified on needle biopsy (stage T1c). The inaccuracy of clinical staging is especially important when comparing non-surgical treatment methods (observation or radiotherapy) with pathologically staged disease following radical prostatectomy.

Prostate cancer commonly spreads to the pelvic lymph nodes, bones, especially the axial skeleton, and lung. Unlike most other malignancies, skeletal metastases from prostate cancer are osteoblastic in over 80% of cases and, despite the increase in bone formation, they lead to disturbance in the normal skeletal architecture and subsequent pathological fractures if left untreated.

Putative premalignant lesions of the prostate

Prostatic intraepithelial neoplasia

Prostatic intraepithelial neoplasia is believed to be the pre-invasive end of a morphological continuum of cellular proliferation affecting prostatic ducts, ductules and acini. It tends to be multifocal and occurs in the peripheral zone, as does prostate cancer. It is divided into two groups: low and high grade. The continuum from normal prostatic epithelium through low-grade and high-grade prostatic intraepithelial neoplasia to invasive cancer is characterised by increased epithelial dysplasia within the luminal secretory cell

Table 19.1 TNM classification of prostate cancer

Tumour	Tx	Primary tumour cannot be assessed
	T0	No evidence of primary tumour
	T1	Tumour clinically inapparent, not palpable nor visible by imaging
	T1a	Incidental finding following TURP in up to 5% of tissue
	T1b	Incidental finding following TURP in more than 5% of tissue
	T1c	Tumour identified by needle biopsy (e.g. because of elevated PSA)
	T2	Tumour confined to the prostate, palpable or visible by imaging
	T2a	Tumour involves one lobe
	T2b	Tumour involves both lobes
	T3	Locally advanced tumour
	T3a	Extracapsular extension
	T3b	Invasion of seminal vesicle
		Invasion into the prostatic apex or into (but not beyond) the prostatic capsule is not classified as T3, but as T2
	T4	Tumour is fixed or invades adjacent structures other than seminal vesicles; i.e. bladder neck, external sphincter, rectum, levator muscles, and/or pelvic wall
Nodes	Nx	Regional lymph nodes cannot be assessed
	N0	No regional lymph node metastases
	N1	Regional lymph node metastasis
Metastasis	Mx	Presence of distant metastases cannot be assessed
	M0	No distant metastases
	M1	Distant metastases present
	M1a	Non-regional lymph nodes
	M1b	Skeletal metastases
	M1c	Other sites

layer. The dysplastic changes with increasing grade of neoplasia include nuclear enlargement, hyperchromatism, prominent nucleoli, cellular crowding with overlapping nuclei and epithelial hyperplasia (see Figure 19.1). The basal cell layer remains intact, though there may be some disruption in high-grade prostatic intraepithelial neoplasia. There is strong clinical, histological and molecular evidence linking high-grade neoplasia with prostate cancer [24]. High-grade neoplasia is seen in up to 16% of needle biopsies in men over 50 years of age [25]. In malignant prostates, it is more frequent and of higher grade than in glands without cancer. The incidence of prostatic intraepithelial neoplasia increases with age, with low-grade neoplasia occurring in men in their third and fourth decades and high-grade neoplasia occurring in their fifth decade [17–19].

Atypical adenomatous hyperplasia

Atypical adenomatous hyperplasia is a small acinar proliferation that may be confused histologically with low-grade prostatic adenocarcinoma. It consists of crowded small glands with a predominantly lobular growth pattern. Basal cells are never seen in carcinoma, but are distributed in a patchy discontinuous manner in atypical adenomatous hyperplasia. Atypical adenomatous hyperplasia is characteristically found near the apex, in the transition zone and periurethral region, and is therefore most commonly seen in transurethral resection specimens. It has been suggested that it may be a precursor of low-grade transition zone cancer, though the data linking them together are inconclusive [20].

Prostate specific antigen

Prostate specific antigen is a serine protease and organ-specific glycoprotein (molecular weight 34 000) that originates in the cytoplasm of ductal cells of the prostate. It is responsible for liquefaction of seminal coagulation. The measurement of serum concentrations of prostate specific antigen is now well established as a useful investigation in the diagnosis and follow-up of patients with prostate cancer [21]. The greatest limitation of this antigen is that it is *tissue* and not *tumour* specific in the prostate. However, prostate specific antigen concentrations are the best overall predictor of bone scan findings and can be used as a screening test for prostate cancer [22, 23]. The antigen circulates in blood mainly bound to protease inhibitors, including alpha-1-antichymotrypsin (ACT) and alpha-2-macroglobulin (AMG); only a small fraction of the total prostate specific antigen exists in a free state. Whereas alpha-2-macroglobulin encapsulates all epitopes of the prostate specific antigen protein, alpha-1-antichymotrypsin leaves some exposed; therefore, immunoassay techniques have been developed to assess free prostate specific antigen and that bound to alpha-1-antichymotrypsin but not to alpha-2-macroglobulin [24]. Recent reports suggest that the free:total prostate specific antigen ratio in patients with benign prostatic hyperplasia is significantly higher than in prostate cancer, but its role is not yet fully established in diagnosing the disease. Several studies report various optimal cut-off levels, largely due to the different nature of the assays used [25]. A recent large study using the Hybritech assay (Hybritech Inc., USA) demonstrated a sensitivity of 90% in diagnosing prostate cancer in the total prostate specific antigen range of 2.6 to 4.0 ng/ml, whilst sparing approximately 18% of patients from having prostatic biopsies [26]. The use of free:total prostate specific antigen ratios in routine clinical practice remains to be determined [27].

Circulating prostate specific antigen-positive cells in prostate cancer

Clinically localised prostate cancers are frequently understaged in over 50% of cases, with resulting positive surgical margins, extracapsular extension and potential treatment failure. This has stimulated researchers to detect circulating micrometastases prior to the establishment of overt secondaries, to avoid unnecessary radical treatment. Metastasis does not rely on the random survival of cells released from the primary tumour, but on the selective growth of specialised subpopulations of highly metastatic cells endowed with properties that will allow them successfully to complete each step of the metastatic cascade [28, 29]. In recent years, new technology, including flow cytometry and the reverse transcription polymerase chain reaction, has given researchers the opportunity of detecting circulating tumour cells with high levels of sensitivity. In that sense, prostate cancer has a significant advantage over other malignancies, due to the specificity of prostate specific antigen as a reliable marker. However, it has to be emphasised again that prostate specific antigen is not tumour specific, a major drawback of all techniques attempting to detect circulating tumour cells. A prostate specific antigen-positive cell in the peripheral blood, therefore, does not necessarily mean a prostate tumour cell, but a cell expressing this antigen, which is likely to be of prostatic origin, in particular if the cell is found to express the gene constitutively, i.e. mRNA for prostate specific antigen. Based on these principles, analytical flow cytometry and reverse transcription polymerase chain reaction have been used in an attempt to detect and isolate circulating tumour cells from patients with prostate cancer. Studies have shown that although quantification of circulating prostate specific antigen-positive cells by flow cytometry was a better predictor of skeletal metastases than isotope bone scanning, the majority of these cells were not of prostatic origin, raising important questions regarding the role of non-prostatic, circulating, prostate specific antigen-positive cells in patients with prostate cancer [30, 31]. Reverse transcription polymerase chain reaction methods, on the other hand, are considerably more sensitive in detecting circulating prostate specific antigen-positive cells, relying on the identification of mRNA for the antigen, an unequivocal proof that the cells are of prostatic origin. A number of studies demonstrated the ability of reverse transcription polymerase chain reaction to detect circulating prostate cells in patients with apparently localised disease, undergoing radical prostatectomy, and some found a strong correlation between a positive polymerase chain reaction, capsular tumour penetration and positive surgical margins, suggesting the potential of this technique to be used for 'molecular staging' of prostate cancer [32]. Other workers used nested reverse transcription polymerase chain reaction to compare the sensitivity of prostate specific antigen with a more recently identified marker, prostate specific membrane antigen in the detection of circulating prostatic cells [33]. The authors of all these studies assume that circulating prostate specific antigen-positive cells are endowed with metastatic

propensity, despite the fact that the results only demonstrate the presence of cells of prostatic origin. Furthermore, the specificity of prostate specific antigen mRNA in identifying cells of prostatic origin has been questioned in a recent study [34]. The role of detecting circulating prostate specific antigen-positive cells in the circulation of patients with prostate cancer remains unclear [35].

Screening for early prostate cancer

Primum non nocere.

Hippocrates

There is an apparent consensus, based on the evidence, that there is no justification to introduce population screening for prostate cancer. The classic triad of screening tests consists of serum prostate specific antigen measurement, digital rectal examination and transrectal ultrasound of the prostate and biopsy, which detect up to 6% of a sreeened population as having prostate cancer. A number of groups is addressing this issue, particularly in Europe. These studies will utilise mortality from prostate cancer as their end-point in the screened compared with the unscreened population, indirectly revealing whether treating the disease early may improve survival [36]. However, methods of screening are changing rapidly, and when the results of these studies are available, it may well be that urologists will be detecting a different category of disease altogether compared with current screening modalities [37].

Clinical presentation

We found the patient complaining of excruciating pains in various parts of the body, which could be compared to nothing except the pains under which persons afflicted with carcinoma occasionally labour. He could void no urine without the assistance of a catheter. The prostate gland, examined by the rectum was found to be much enlarged and of a stony hardness. I continued to visit him in consultation for nearly a year, at the end of which time he suddenly lost the use of the muscles of his lower limbs and died a fortnight afterwards.

Sir Benjamin Brodie, 1842

Early prostate cancer is asymptomatic. The above description by Benjamin Brodie, over 150 years ago, illustrates all the relevant symptoms in advanced prostate cancer. Patients with symptomatic disease can present in a variety of ways, including with bladder outflow obstruction, irritative bladder symptoms secondary to trigonal involvement and haematuria. Metastatic disease may present with skeletal pain, spinal cord compression secondary to collapsed vertebrae and pathological fractures, or with general systemic manifestations, including weight loss, weakness and anorexia. With locally advanced disease, prostate cancer may manifest itself as renal failure secondary to bilateral ureteric orifices involvement.

Treatment

The more resources we have, and the more complex they are, the greater are the demands on our clinical skill. These resources are calls upon our judgement, and not substitutes for it.

Sir Francis Walsh

For the sake of simplicity, prostate cancer can be classified into early organ-confined and advanced disease when treatment is dicussed.

Organ-confined prostate cancer

Conventional 'curative' treatments of localised disease include surgery in the form of radical prostatectomy through the retropubic or perineal routes, or radiotherapy with its variations, including conformal approaches and radioactive seed implantation, otherwise known as brachytherapy. These treatments carry relatively low morbidity in experienced hands, and a high cure rate. Watchful waiting, on the other hand, remains a reasonable option in men with low-grade, small-volume tumours and a life expectancy less than 10 years. Evidence concerning the effectiveness of treatments is limited to observational studies with the full range of well-described limitations of such material, including differences in patient selection criteria, operative techniques, postoperative assessments, variable definitions and lengths of follow-up, and methods of data analysis. Survival following treatment for localised prostate cancer is good for all modes of treatment: 85–90% for radical prostatectomy, 65–90% for radiotherapy, and 70–90% for conservative management. Radical interventions are not recommended for men who are likely to have a life expectancy of less than 10 years. Studies indicate that selected groups of men may benefit from radical intervention, particularly those who are youngest and fittest and have high-grade tumours. However, problems with the accuracy of clinical staging using the classical triad of serum prostate specific antigen levels, digital rectal examination and transrectal ultrasound of the prostate mean that up to 50% of men with apparently localised tumours are found to have extracapsular disease and positive margins following radical prostatectomy. This major issue of treatment efficacy in early prostate cancer can be resolved only by well-conducted, randomised controlled trials, some of which are underway in the USA and Europe but will take more than a decade to yield any significant results.

Advanced prostate cancer

Locally advanced disease
External beam irradiation is widely accepted in treating locally advanced prostate cancer. There is evidence, however, that a large number of clinicians adopted the policy of no treatment in the absence of symptoms. This problem was addressed recently by the Medical Research Council trial of immediate versus deferred treatment, and the results suggest that there is a small but significant advantage in treating these patients early, albeit to delay or prevent the advent of serious morbidity and complications from progressive disease [38]. Downstaging of extracapsular disease has also been attempted in a number of studies, whereby androgen ablation is performed for three to six months prior to radical prostatectomy. Although the incidence of positive margins decreases in clinically T2 tumours, there is no apparent change in T3 disease, and disease-free survival is not affected [39, 40].

Metastatic disease

In 1940, Charles Huggins discovered the beneficial effects of androgen deprivation in patients with metastatic prostate cancer [41]. Since then, hormonal manipulation has remained the mainstay of treatment in advanced stages of the disease. It is still expected that about 80% of all patients with advanced prostate cancer will respond to androgen blockade. Patients will show both subjective and objective responses, manifested by considerable and rapid symptomatic improvement, particularly in metastatic skeletal pain, together with local and distant regression of the disease. This is complemented by normalisation of serum tumour markers. Relapse, however, is common at a mean interval of two years following the initiation of treatment. The disease is then hormone resistant and prognosis becomes extremely poor. Methods of hormonal manipulation include bilateral orchidectomy and oestrogen preparations that are rarely prescribed nowadays in view of the serious cardiovascular side-effects encountered with the recognised 3 mg daily dose, in order to achieve castrate levels. The use of the smaller dose of 1 mg daily remains controversial, as castrate levels are not reached in 30% of patients. Alternative therapy includes the use of analogues of the hypothalamic luteinising hormone-releasing hormone. These analogues occupy the receptors of luteinising hormone-releasing hormone in the pituitary, initially stimulating the release of luteinising hormone and then blocking the subsequent stimulation of the receptors by the endogenous pulsatile secretion of luteinising hormone. Finally, synthetic anti-androgens are also being used. They all act by competing with androgen receptors in hormone-sensitive prostatic cells, benign or malignant. In the late 1980s, total androgen blockade has been advocated to prevent the effect of the non-testicular circulating testosterone formation by the adrenals. After initial enthusiasm, recent studies have failed to show any survival advantage in patients treated with maximum androgen blockade [42, 43].

Novel therapies in prostate cancer

The development of new therapeutic approaches in prostate cancer will rely on continuing progress made in three specific areas: (1) imaging of the prostate and identification of cancerous lesions; (2) the delivery of different forms of energy to achieve safe and targetted tissue ablation; and (3) understanding the biology of prostate cancer from its early genetic alterations to the molecular changes responsible for tumour progression. Based on modern transurethral ultrasound technology, two distinct modes of energy delivery systems for tissue ablation have been revived in recent years: cryotherapy and high-intensity focused ultrasound.

Cryotherapy

The in-situ destruction of tumours by the application of low temperatures was first developed in the 1970s to treat localised prostate cancer with reasonable success. Cryoablation had a number of advantages over other forms of treatment, but suffered from many limitations: the equipment was cumbersome, probes were placed mostly transurethrally under digital rectal guidance, temperature control was poor, and damage to adjacent tissue was common. The ability of real-time transurethral ultrasound to guide cryoprobe placement and accurately monitor the freezing process, in addition to the development of urethral warming devices, encouraged clinicians to attempt again the destruction of prostate cancer by freezing. A number of studies on humans followed the animal work, and results are emerging slowly [44, 45].

High-intensity focused ultrasound

The technique consists of delivering ultrasonic energy with resultant heat and tissue destruction to a discrete point without damaging the intervening tissue. Much higher temperatures are generated at the focal point using this technique (approximately 98 °C) than with diffuse ultrasound hyperthermia (approximately 42 °C), leading to complete tumour necrosis. After evaluating the technique initially in animal models and in vitro using cell lines, its use was reported in the treatment of benign prostatic hyperplasia without significant side-effects as a minimally invasive therapeutic option in symptomatic patients. The relative safety of high-intensity focused ultrasound coupled with its documented ability to cause targeted tissue necrosis prompted researchers to extrapolate its application to the treatment of prostate cancer, as an alternative to surgery and radiotherapy [46, 47].

Gene therapy

Since the discovery of DNA and its structure by James Watson and Francis Crick in 1953, our knowledge of the molecular basis and human genetics in health and disease has made giant steps forward, bringing closer the 'double-helix' to the bedside of patients where every other conventional treatment may be failing. Advances in molecular biology, particularly in recombinant DNA technology, have paved the way to unlimited possibilities in predicting, controlling and preventing disease at its molecular origin.

The prostate is a prime target in the development of successful gene therapy for the following reasons: (1) prostate cancer is slow growing; (2) tumour burden can be significantly reduced by surgery; and (3) the prostate expresses unique antigens, including prostate specific antigen and prostate specific membrane antigen.

The most significant limitation of gene therapy is the difficulty associated with gene delivery to the relevant cells. Gene transfer can be achieved in vitro or in vivo. In-vitro methods can be chemical, through calcium-phosphate transfection, physical, through electroporation or microinjection, by fusion with liposomes, through receptor-mediated endocytosis, or using recombinant viruses. In-vivo methods include direct injection of DNA, naked, contained in liposomes, conjugated to a carrier (e.g. antibodies to a specific cell-surface protein) or by particle bombardment [48].

Gene-directed enzyme prodrug therapy is based on the potential use of prodrugs that are essentially inert but that can be converted in vivo to highly toxic active species with the aim of specifically destroying tumour cells. Activation can be the result of metabolism by an enzyme that is either unique to the target organ or present at much higher concentrations compared with other tissues. Tumour destruction involves two essential steps: (1) specific targeting of malignant cells with the gene encoding enzyme, which can also be under the control of a specfic promoter (e.g. prostate specific antigen or prostate specific membrane antigen in the prostate); and (2) administration of the prodrug, which will be activated into its toxic derivative by the appropriate enzyme *within* the target tissue concerned, with few or no systemic consequences [49].

Tumour vaccines represent a potentially new and different treatment modality. There are three basic approaches to construct cancer vaccines: (1) using whole tumour cells or non-purified cellular extract preparations in an attempt to include relevant tumour antigens that can stimulate protective immune responses; (2) using partially purified preparations enriched in the cellular fraction most likely to contain relevant tumour antigens; and (3) using preparations from highly purified tumour antigens. The development of these 'vaccines' depends on the expression of a family of genes reported to encode antigens recognised by autologous cytotoxic T lymphocytes. Such genes have now been identified in melanoma cells, (*MAGE-1, MAGE-3, BAGE, GAGE*) as well as in head and neck tumours, non-small lung cancers and bladder carcinomas. Recent work from Chen *et al.* [50] demonstrated the presence of two new genes (*PAGE* and *GAGE-7*) expressed in the LNCaP cell line that may be specific to prostate cancer and serve as a potential target for tumour immunisation.

Every technique mentioned above has specific advantages and disadvantages, the details of which are beyond the scope of this chapter. Experimental studies of gene therapy in prostate cancer are emerging in the literature at an increasing frequency.

Apoptosis-regulating genes in prostate cancer

Apoptosis

Hormone ablation in prostate cancer achieves its effect by the activation of apoptosis (programmed cell death) [51, 52], which is a distinct mode of cell death occurring in normal physiological conditions as well as in disease, including cancer [53]. Apoptosis is an active process characterised by distinct morphological changes in single cells, with compaction and margination of nuclear chromatin, cytoplasmic condensation and convolution of nuclear and cell outlines. Later changes involve nuclear fragmentation and budding of the cell, with the development of membrane-bound apoptotic bodies, which are removed by phagocytosis [53]. In contrast to necrosis, which is a passive process, there is no associated inflammation.

Numerous genes are involved in the control of apoptosis, including the proto-oncogene bcl-2 on chromosome 18 region 18q21 [54, 55] and the tumour suppressor gene p53 on chromosome 17 region 17p13 [56].

bcl-2

The bcl-2 gene was initially identified in B cell lymphomas [57]; the gene product acts by inhibiting apoptosis, but has no direct effect on cell proliferation [54]. A rapidly expanding group of genes showing homology to bcl-2 has been described, named the bcl-2 gene family, forming two functionally antagonistic groups controlling the balance between cell death and survival [55, 57]. Bax accelerates apoptotic cell death by forming heterodimers with bcl-2, leading to the suppression of apoptosis [58]. The molecular mechanisms by which the bcl-2 protein suppresses apoptosis remain unresolved. In the prostate, bcl-2 is normally expressed in basal epithelial cells, seminal vesicles and ejaculatory ducts [54].

In primary prostate cancer, bcl-2 is expressed in around 25% of cases [59]. bcl-2 over-expression is associated with increasing tumour stage and the development of hormone refractory disease [60, 61].

In high-grade prostatic intraepithelial neoplasia, the reported expression of bcl-2 has shown a wide variation, from 0% to 100% [59, 62, 63]. The largest study reported bcl-2 expression in 4/24 (17%) cases of this neoplasia [62].

p53

Inactivation of the tumour suppressor gene p53 is presently the most common mutation identified in human cancers [56]. Functional (wild-type) p53 protein has DNA-binding properties and forms a key part of the mechanism by which mammalian cells undergo growth arrest or apoptosis in response to DNA damage. Mutation of p53 may result in the loss of its normal function [64]. Mutations in the p53 gene commonly occur in the highly conserved exons 5, 6, 7 and 8. In most cases, one allele is completely deleted, with a mis-sense mutation in the remaining allele [65]. Mutant p53 protein has a prolonged half-life compared to the wild-type p53 protein, and its nuclear accumulation is detectable by immunohistochemistry.

In benign prostatic epithelium, p53 positivity is absent. In primary prostate cancer, p53 nuclear positivity is present in around 20% of cases [66–68]. p53 protein accumulation appears to be a late event, being associated with advanced stage, high Gleason tumour grade, hormonal resistance, poor-survival DNA aneuploidy and high cell proliferation rate [68–71]. A good correlation is seen between p53 immunoreactivity in prostate cancer and direct evidence of gene mutation using the polymerase chain reaction and single strand conformational polymorphism and direct sequencing [72]. p53 positivity is infrequent in high-grade prostatic intraepithelial neoplasia, the largest study showing strong nuclear staining in 14% [73].

Wild-type p53 may participate with bcl-2 and bax in a common pathway regulating cell death by decreasing the expression of bcl-2 while simultaneously increasing the expression of bax, resulting in apoptosis [74]. The combination of bcl-2 over-expression and p53 nuclear protein accumulation in human prostate cancer has been shown to correlate with the development of hormone refractory disease [61], and these are independent prognostic markers for post-radical prostatectomy recurrence [75].

Angiogenesis

Microvessel density

The ability of a tumour to grow and metastasise depends on tumour angiogenesis. The quantification of new microvessels within a tumour is commonly performed using antibodies against Factor VIII to identify endothelial cells. Increasing microvessel density correlates with increasing Gleason score and presence of metastases, and is an independent predictor of progression after radical prostatectomy for Gleason score 5 to 7 tumour [76, 77].

Vascular endothelial growth factor

Angiogenesis is controlled by a group of substances known as angiogenic factors. Vascular endothelial growth factor is a potent inducer of endothelial cell growth and is expressed in a variety of tumours. In prostate cancer, expression of this factor is increased compared to benign prostatic epithelium [78].

Growth factors

Growth factors may act as positive or negative effectors of various cellular processes, including proliferation, differentiation and cell death. Interaction occurs with specific membrane receptors, which results in the transmission of signals through an intracellular protein cascade and the activation or the repression of a number of target genes. Several growth factors have been associated with prostatic growth, including transforming growth factors alpha and beta, fibroblast growth factors, insulin-like growth factors, epidermal growth factor, nerve growth factor and various cytokines.

Growth factors act primarily over short distances in either an autocrine or paracrine manner. In addition, growth factors may act through an endocrine pathway, affecting target cells at distant sites. Many growth factors possess a mitogenic activity that is mediated through a membrane-bound receptor. Interaction occurs with an extracellular ligand-binding domain, leading to a change in receptor conformation that results in the activation of an intracellular tyrosine kinase domain. Tyrosine phosphorylation of specific intracellular proteins is responsible for the mitogenic signal. In many cases, the protein components of the intracellular cascade remain to be elucidated. Aberrant signalling may result from mutation in growth factors or their downstream effector proteins, leading to either loss of growth factor function, i.e. switching off the signalling pathway, or to uncontrolled expression or activation, i.e. a permanently switched on signalling pathway. Such changes are commonly associated with the malignant state and the aggressive phenotypes of cancer cells.

Transforming growth factor β-1

Transforming growth factor β-1 belongs to a superfamily of structurally related regulatory polypeptides, which includes activins/inhibins and bone morphogenetic proteins. It is a multifunctional cytokine that acts through type I and II receptor kinases to positively or negatively regulate the proliferation of various cell types. Generally, transforming growth factor β-1 functions as a mitogen for various mesenchymal cells and a potent growth inhibitor of lymphoid, endothelial and epithelial cells. Transforming growth factors β-1 and β-2 have been implicated in the development of prostatic disease. The β-1 form has been detected immunohistochemically in both human prostatic stromal and epithelial cells, and the β-2 mRNA has been identified in normal and malignant human prostate. The addition of transforming growth factor β-1 to cultured prostatic epithelial and stromal cells inhibits proliferation [79].

Bone morphogenetic proteins

The term bone morphogenetic protein (BMP) refers to an activity derived from bone that induces ectopic bone formation in vivo [80]. The proteins belong to the transforming growth factor β superfamily and, to date, 15 have been identified. Since their discovery in 1965, researchers have focused their attention on the identification of these proteins and, more recently, on understanding their role in normal human embryonic development. To date, very few efforts have been made to link bone morphogenetic protein activity with the development and progression of cancer. This is not surprising because the majority of bony secondaries result in osteolytic lesions, with increased bone resorption and osteoclastic activity, unlike prostatic secondaries which are mostly osteoblastic. Several studies have shown an association between bone morphogenetic protein expression and skeletal metastases in prostate cancer. BMP-6, in particular, is expressed in the majority of primary prostate cancers with established skeletal secondaries, and rarely in localised disease. Primary and secondary prostate cancer expresses BMP-6, which is found infrequently in skeletal metastases from other human malignancies. BMP-6 may have a role in the initiation of skeletal secondaries, and in the osteoblastic reaction commonly seen in these deposits [81].

Fibroblast growth factors

Members of the fibroblast growth factor (FGF) family of polypeptide growth factors have diverse physiological and pathological functions, including development, wound healing, angiogenesis and tumorigenesis [82]. In humans, the fibroblast growth factors comprise at least ten genes, and the receptor family comprises four members. Multiple ligands and receptors allow interaction between a single receptor and several ligands, and between different receptor monomers through heterodimerisation following activation by fibroblast growth factor [83].

Basic fibroblast growth factor (FGF-2) is secreted by prostatic fibroblasts in response to androgen and acts in an autocrine fashion to stimulate fibroblast cell growth [84]. Stromal-derived keratinocyte growth factor (KGF/ FGF-7) is up-regulated in hormone-resistant prostate cancer and has a role as a potential paracrine growth factor on epithelial cells [85]. It has a potent mitogenic action on epithelial cells and has been proposed to act as an androgen-regulated mediator of epithelial cell growth [86]. A similar paracrine action applies to FGF-8 (androgen-induced growth factor), which is secreted in response to androgens and can stimulate the growth of epithelial and fibroblast cells.

Insulin-like growth factors

The insulin-like growth factors IGF-1 and IGF-2 are important mitogens that mediate normal and neoplastic cell growth. The insulin-like growth factors bind to specific receptors, designated type I and II insulin-like growth factor receptors (IGFr). Type I IGFr is a transmembrane heterotetramer tyrosine kinase that primarily mediates the mitogenic actions of these growth factors. The insulin-like growth factors are two of the most abundant growth factors in bone [87], the preferential site for metastatic prostate cancer. Type I IGFr is expressed by prostate cancer cells, which could facilitate the development of bone metastases.

The insulin-like growth factors also have high affinity for a family of at least six insulin-like growth factor-binding proteins (IGFBPs), which act to regulate their bioavailability [88]. The levels of circulating insulin-like growth factor-binding proteins are regulated by endocrine factors and by specific proteases that cleave them to small, inactive peptides. They are believed to modulate the proliferative and mitogenic effects of the insulin-like growth factors as well as modulating cell growth independently of them. Although all insulin-like growth factor-binding proteins have high affinity for the insulin-like growth factors, IGFBP-3 is the major transporter of these factors in serum. A number of studies have suggested that insulin-like growth factor-binding proteins may be involved in the growth modulation of prostate malignancy. One study showed elevated IGFBP-2 and decreased IGFBP-3 in patients with prostate cancer [89].

Epidermal growth factor

Binding of epidermal growth factor to the extracellular domain of its receptor, EGFr, results in the activation of the receptor's cytoplasmic tyrosine kinase, phosphorylation of substrate proteins and stimulation of cell proliferation. Members of the epidermal growth factor family play a role in the modulation of prostatic growth. Withdrawal of androgen from the rodent prostate leads to reduced expression of epidermal growth factor, which is a potent mitogen for epithelial cells [90]. Thus, the continued presence of androgens within the prostate helps maintain epithelial cell proliferation mediated through the expression of epidermal growth factor.

Cell adhesion

Cell adhesion is of fundamental importance in establishing and maintaining tissue form and function. Several molecules, including cadherins, integrins, selectins and members of the immunoglobulin superfamily, are involved in the mechanisms by which a cell maintains contact with other cells and interacts with the extracellular matrix. Fibronectin, collagen, laminin and vitronectin are major components of this complex extracellular matrix which interact with their cognate receptors, most of which are integrins. Integrins function as heterodimeric membrane glycoproteins, the combination of alpha and beta subunits determining the ligand specificity. Differential expression of members of the large integrin family allows the cell to modulate its interaction with other cells and the extracellular matrix. Integrins are important components of cellular signal transduction, mediating cell–matrix interactions, whereas cadherins principally mediate intercellular interactions.

Cadherins are a large family of calcium-dependent morphoregulatory proteins. The best-studied proteins within this family are E-cadherin and N-cadherin. Membrane-associated cadherins require members of the catenin family of proteins to mediate their interaction with the cytoskeleton. Catenins probably act by oligomerising proteins to which they bind and/or attaching proteins to the actin cytoskeleton.

E-cadherin

The E-cadherin gene plays a critical role in embryogenesis and organogenesis through mediating epithelial cell–cell recognition and adhesion processes [91]. E-cadherin protein is frequently found to be reduced or absent in cancer cell lines. Experiments performed with the Dunning rat model for prostate cancer showed a correlation between a lack of E-cadherin and tumour invasion, demonstrated by the progession of a non-invasive, E-cadherin-positive tumour to an invasive, E-cadherin-negative tumour. Immunocytochemistry performed on human prostate cancer samples showed a general reduction of E-cadherin expression in high-grade tumours associated with aberrant staining. This aberrant E-cadherin staining is proving to be a powerful predictor of poor outcome, both in terms of disease progression and patient survival [92].

CD44

The CD44 gene is an integral transmembrane glycoprotein involved in specific cell–cell and cell–extracellular matrix interactions [93]. The gene is encoded by 20 exons, at least ten of which are differentially expressed due to alternative splicing of mRNA. CD44 is expressed on the plasma membrane of prostatic glandular cells. It is involved in cell adhesion because it acts as a receptor for the extracellular matrix components hyaluronic acid and osteopontin. CD44 is believed to play a major role in tumour metastases; alternative splice variants of the receptor differ in their capacity to enhance or decrease metastatic potential. In human prostate cancer, CD44 downregulation is correlated with high tumour grade, aneuploidy and distant metastases [94].

Proliferation

The hallmark of malignancy is uncontrolled growth. It is therefore logical to assume that measuring prolif-

erative activity within a tumour may indicate its invasive potential and capacity to progress. Several methods are available to assess proliferation, including the determination of S-phase fraction by flow cytometry, labelling of replicating DNA with bromodeoxyuridine and by immunohistochemistry using antibodies against proliferation-related antigens (Ki67 and MIB-1) [95, 96]. The use of these methods in clinical practice, however, remains to be determined.

Tumour ploidy and nuclear morphometry

Nuclear DNA content, otherwise known as ploidy, can be studied by flow cytometry and image or static cytometry. Tumours can be broadly classified as diploid, tetraploid or aneuploid, with accompanying variations in view of the well-documented heterogeneity of prostatic adenocarcinoma. Several reports have emerged in the last three decades correlating DNA ploidy with prognosis in prostate cancer. The results are conflicting, and only half the studies published confirm ploidy to be an independent prognostic marker [97]. A more modern and sensitive method of assessing ploidy has been developed recently, using fluorescent and non-fluorescent DNA in-situ hybridisation of interphase cells. These techniques visualise individual chromosomes by specific binding of a labelled probe to a particular DNA sequence, mostly localised at the centromere region. There is good correlation with flow cytometry, but fluorescent DNA in-situ hybridisation appears to be more sensitive [98]. If these methods are to have an impact on clinical practice, large studies analysing ploidy determination in biopsy specimens must be conducted.

Androgen regulation

Androgens are important male sex hormones, which, in addition to being essential for the growth and differentiation of all male sex accessory organs, are strongly associated with the development and progression of prostate cancer. Androgen action in prostate cancer is mediated through the androgen receptor, a ligand-dependent transcription factor that is a member of the steroid/thyroid hormone receptor gene superfamily. The mitogenic effects of androgens on prostatic growth appear to be mediated through the action of soluble peptide growth factors, acting in either an autocrine or paracrine manner. Various model systems for prostate cancer have shown FGF-7 and TGF-β1 to be paracrine mediators of androgen action and FGF-2 to be an androgen-mediated autocrine growth factor.

Androgen depletion prolongs the disease-free interval for prostate cancer patients, indicating that the cancer cells are androgen sensitive. However, this treatment is only palliative because androgen-independent clones of cancer cells expand and progress. This observation has been made in almost every case of prostate cancer. These androgen-independent cells acquire the ability to proliferate in the absence of androgen through genetic mutations. Mutations may result in changes in the function/expression of androgen receptor protein or growth factors and their receptors.

Androgen receptor

The androgen receptor can be structurally divided into three domains: a transcriptional activation domain, a DNA-binding domain, and a ligand-binding domain [99] (Figure 19.3). Cellular signalling occurs following androgen binding to the androgen receptor and translocation to the nucleus. This activated complex associates with androgen responsive elements contained in the DNA sequence of a number of target genes to affect their transcriptional activity. The possible presence in vivo of alternate androgen receptor isoforms, the extent of androgen receptor phosphorylation, the association with other proteins and the presence of polymorphic glutamine and glycine regions may provide additional levels of control for androgen receptor action.

Radioligand binding studies and immunohistochemistry have been used to detect androgen receptor protein expression. Both primary and metastatic prostate cancers have shown elevated levels of androgen receptors by ligand-binding assays when compared to non-malignant prostate tissue [100]. Immunohistochemistry supports elevated androgen receptor in prostate cancer, with strong nuclear staining, mostly of a heterogeneous nature, in hormone-relapsed and in primary and metastatic hormone-refractory prostate cancer [101].

Recent studies have suggested that a high frequency of amino acid substitutions occur in the androgen receptor protein (25–50%) for untreated advanced prostate cancer and in hormone-relapsed tumours from primary and metastatic sites. Functional analysis of these mutations has revealed alterations in ligand binding and transcriptional activation. Additionally, androgen receptor gene amplification has been identified in 30% of recurrent prostate tumours [102]. Examination of the corresponding primary tumour prior to the initiation of hormone therapy showed no evidence of amplification, suggesting amplification occurred during androgen deprivation, conferring a growth advantage on the prostate cancer cells. Variation in the length of a polyglutamine stretch in the N-terminal domain of the androgen receptor protein, causing an alteration in androgen receptor function, has been suggested as a contributory factor towards an increased lifetime risk for the development of prostate cancer.

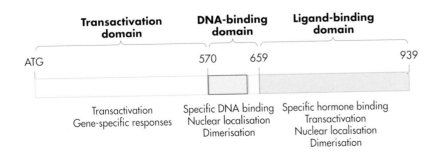

Figure **19.3** *Functional organisation of the androgen receptor.*

Genetic factors

Genetic alterations are important contributory events in neoplasia. Various genes have been identified that are associated with predisposition or progression for most of the common epithelial neoplasms, with the exception of prostate cancer. Most known oncogenes and suppressor genes have been screened for their importance in primary prostate cancer but no common mutations have been identified. *p53* mutations are rare in early prostate cancer but have been observed in almost 50% of advanced, metastatic disease [72]. Mutations in the retinoblastoma (*Rb*) gene and deletion or methylation of p16^{INK4a} (*CDKN2*), two genes intimately linked to cell cycle progression, have been described in a few prostate tumours and cell lines.

Allelic loss, defined by the absence of one of the two copies of an autosomal locus present in somatic cells, commonly occurs in prostate cancer. Loss of heterozygosity and comparative genomic hybridisation analyses have revealed frequent loss of genetic material from chromosome regions 7q, 8p, 10pq, 13q, 16q, 17p and 18q in primary and metastatic prostate cancer. More recently, specific gene loci have been identified as metastatic suppressors in prostate cancer. The introduction of the genes for KAI1 (chromosome 11p11.2), E-cadherin (chromosome 16q22) or CD44 (chromosome 11p13) into prostate cancer cells has been shown to suppress metastatic ability.

A number of studies revealed a familial clustering for prostate cancer. A risk factor of between two and three has been indicated for a relative of a prostate cancer patient acquiring the disease. This risk factor depends on the relationship within the family: a first-degree relative (brother, father) presents the highest risk. Additionally, the risk factor increases if two or more family members have the disease.

Hereditary prostate cancer, which can be separated from familial prostate cancer, has been reported to account for some 9% of all prostate cancers and for more than 40% of early-onset disease [103]. Recent work provides strong evidence for a major susceptibility locus for prostate cancer on chromosome 1 (1q24-25) [104].

Matrix metalloproteinases and their inhibitors

Tumour invasion and metastasis represent key events in the natural history of cancer. To complete the different steps involved in the metastatic cascade of events, a malignant cell has to overcome a number of natural barriers, including extracellular matrix and basement membranes. This can be partly achieved through excess production of proteolytic enzymes, either by the tumour cells themselves or through stimulation of surrounding stromal cells to secrete such enzymes [105]. The matrix metalloproteinases (MMPs) are extracellular zinc enzymes that mediate a number of tissue-remodelling processes, and have been heavily incriminated in cancer progression. A number of malignancies, including prostate cancer, have been shown to differentially express MMPs, which when highly expressed correlated strongly with aggressive disease [106–108]. More recently, a new membrane-type matrix metalloproteinase (MT-MMP) has been found to be specifcally expressed in fibroblastic cells of human carcinomas and in prostate cancer [109]. The matrix metalloproteinases are tightly regulated by their inhibitors, called tissue inhibitors of metalloproteinases (TIMPs), synthetic forms of which have been developed recently, and may represent a novel therapeutic approach in prostate cancer.

In-vitro and in-vivo models of prostate cancer

In order to investigate the biology of prostate cancer, numerous models have been developed over the years. The three most widely used cell lines are LNCaP, an androgen receptor-positive epithelial prostate cancer cell line originating from a metastatic lymph node; DU-145, an androgen receptor-positive epithelial prostate cancer line originating from metastatic bone secondaries; and PC-3, an androgen receptor-negative epithelial prostate cancer line originating from metastatic brain secondaries [110–112]. Animals used for in-vivo experiments include spontaneous models (canine, Lobund–Wistar), inducible cancer models (Noble and Lobund–Wistar rat), transplantable cancer models (Dunning R-3327 rat, Pollard rat, Shain rat and Noble rat), and xenograft nude mice models [113–116]. These models are extremely useful in studying a variety of factors thought to affect the development and progression of prostate cancer, but suffer from limitations in terms of reproducibility in humans.

References

1. Møller Jensen O, Estève J, Møller H, Renard H. Cancer in the European community and its member states. Eur J Cancer 1990; 26: 1167–256

2. Wingo PA, Landis S, Ries LA. An adjustment to the 1997 estimate of new prostate cancer cases. CA Cancer J Clin 1997; 47: 239–42

3. Office of Population Censuses and Surveys. Cancer Statistics. Registrations 1991 England and Wales. MB1 1996; No 20. HMSO: London

4. Pienta KJ. The epidemiology of prostate cancer: clues for chemoprevention. In Vivo 1994; 8: 419–22

5. Muir CS, Nectoux J, Statzsewski J. The epidemiology of prostatic cancer. Acta Oncol 1991; 30: 133–40

6. Whitmore WF. Localised prostate cancer: management and detection issues. Lancet 1994; 343: 1263–67

7. Pienta KJ, Esper PS. Risk factors for prostate cancer. Ann Int Med 1993; 118: 793–803

8. Smith JR, Freije D, Carpten JD, et al. Major susceptibility locus for prostate cancer on chromosome 1 suggested by a genome-wide search. Science 1996; 274: 1371–4

9. Bova GS, Beaty TH, Steinberg GD, et al. Hereditary prostate cancer: epidemiologic and clinical features. J Urol 1993; 150: 797–802

10. Ellis WJ, Lange PH. Prostate cancer. Endocrinol Metab Clin North Am 1994; 23: 809–24

11. McNeal JE, Redwine EA, Frieha FS, Stamey TA. Zonal distribution of prostatic adenocarcinoma: correlation with histologic pattern and direction of spread. Am J Surg Pathol 1988; 12: 897–906

12. Bostwick DG, Cooner WH, Denis L, Jones GW, Scardino PT, Murphy GP. The association of benign prostatic hyperplasia and cancer of the prostate. Cancer 1992; 70: 291–301

13. Gleason DF. Histologic grading of prostate cancer: a perspective. Hum Pathol 1992; 23: 273–9

14. Humphrey PA, Frazier HA, Vollmer RT, Paulson DF. Stratification of pathologic features in radical prostatectomy specimens that are predictive of elevated initial postoperative serum prostate-specific antigen levels. Cancer 1993; 71: 1821–7

15. Bostwick DG. Gleason grading of prostatic needle biopsies; correlation with grade in 316 matched prostatectomies. Am J Surg Pathol 1994; 18: 796–803

16. Hermanek P, Hutter RVP, Sobin LH, Wagner G, Wittekind Ch. TNM atlas. Fourth edition. UICC: Springer, 1997

17. Helpap B, Bonkhoff H, Cockett A, et al. Relationship between atypical adenomatous hyperplasia (AAH), prostatic intraepithelial neoplasia (PIN) and prostatic adenocarcinoma. Pathologica 1997; 89: 288–300

18. Sakr WA, Haas GP, Cassin BF, Pontes JE, Crissman JD. The frequency of carcinoma and intraepithelial neoplasia of the prostate in young male patients. J Urol 1993; 150: 379–85

19. Häggman MJ, Macoska JA, Wojna KJ, Oesterling JE. The relationship between prostatic intraepithelial neoplasia and prostate cancer: critical issues. J Urol 1997; 158: 12–22

20. Epstein JI, Armas OA. Atypical basal cell hyperplasia of the prostate. Am J Surg Pathol 1992; 16: 1205–14

21. Oesterling JE. Prostate specific antigen: a critical assessment of the most useful tumour marker for adenocarcinoma of the prostate. J Urol 1991; 145: 907–23

22. Chybowski FM, Larson Keller JJ, Beerstralh EH, Oesterling JE. Predicting radionuclide bone scan findings in patients with newly diagnosed, untreated prostate cancer: prostate specific antigen is superior to all other clinical parameters. J Urol 1991; 145: 313–18

23. Catalona WJ, Ritchie JP, Ahmann FB, et al. Comparison of digital rectal examination and serum prostate specific antigen in the early detection of prostate cancer: results of a multicentre clinical trial of 6,630 men. J Urol 1994; 151: 1283–90

24. Christensson A, Bjork T, Nilsson O, et al. Serum prostate specific antigen complexed to alpha-1-antichymotrypsin as an indicator of prostate cancer. J Urol 1993; 150: 100–5

25. Leung H, Lai L, Day J, Thomson J, Neal DE, Hamdy FC. Serum free PSA in the diagnosis of prostate cancer. Br J Urol 1997; 80: 256–9

26. Catalona WJ, Smith DS, Ornstein DK. Prostate cancer detection in men with serum PSA concentrations

of 2.6 to 4.0 ng/ml and benign prostate examination: enhancement of specificity with free PSA measurements. J Am Med Assoc 1997; 227: 1452–5

27. Woodrum DL, Brawer MK, Partin AW, Catalona WJ, Southwick PC. Interpretation of free prostate specific antigen clinical research studies for the detection of prostate cancer. J Urol 1998; 159: 5–12

28. Fidler IJ. Metastasis: quantitative analysis of distribution and fate of tumour emboli labelled with ^{125}I-5-iodo-2′-deoxyuridine. J Natl Cancer Inst 1970; 45: 773–82

29. Fidler IJ, Hart IR. Biological diversity in metastatic neoplasms: origins and implications. Science 1982; 217: 998–1003

30. Hamdy FC, Lawry J, Anderson JB, Parsons MA, Rees RC, Williams JL. Circulating prostate-specific antigen-positive cells correlate with metastatic prostate cancer. Br J Urol 1992; 69: 392–6

31. Fadlon EJ, Rees RC, Lawry J, McIntyre C, Sharrard M, Hamdy FC. Detection of circulating PSA-positive cells in patients with prostate cancer by flow cytometry and reverse transcription polymerase chain reaction. Br J Cancer 1996; 74: 400–5

32. Katz AE, Olsson CA, Raffo AJ, et al. Molecular staging of prostate cancer with the use of an enhanced reverse transcriptase-PCR assay. Urology 1994; 43: 765–74

33. Israeli RS, Miller WH, Su SL, et al. Sensitive nested reverse transcription polymerase chain reaction detection of circulating prostatic tumor cells: comparison of prostate-specific membrane antigen and prostate-specific antigen-based assays. Cancer Res 1994; 54: 6306–10

34. Smith MR, Biggar S, Hussain M. Prostate specific antigen messenger RNA is expressed in non-prostate cells: implications for the detection of micrometastases. Cancer Res 1995; 55: 2640–4

35. Gomella LG, Ganesh VR, Moreno JG. Reverse transcriptase polymerase chain reaction for prostate specific antigen in the management of prostate cancer. J Urol 1997; 158: 326–37

36. Schröder FH. Detection of prostate cancer. Br Med J 1995; 310: 140–1

37. Hamdy FC, Neal DE. Screening for prostate cancer: methods are changing rapidly. Br Med J 1995; 310: 1139–40

38. Adib RS, Anderson JB, Ashken MH, et al. Immediate versus deferred treatment for advanced prostatic cancer: initial results of the Medical Research Council trial. Br J Urol 1997; 79: 235–46

39. Abbas F, Scardino PT. Why neoadjuvant androgen deprivation prior to radical prostatectomy is unnecessary. Urol Clin North Am 1996; 23(4): 587–604

40. Witjes WP, Schulman CC, Debruyne FM. Preliminary results of a prospective randomized study comparing radical prostatectomy versus radical prostatectomy associated with neoadjuvant hormonal combination therapy in T2–T3 N0 M0 prostatic carcinoma. The European Study Group on Neoadjuvant Treatment of Prostate Cancer. Urology 1997; 49: (3A Suppl.): 65–9

41. Huggins C, Hodges CV. Studies on prostate cancer. The effect of castration, of oestrogen and of androgen injection on serum phosphatase in metastatic carcinoma of the prostate. Cancer Res 1941; 1: 293–7

42. Maximum androgen blockade in advanced prostate cancer: an overview of 22 randomised trials with 3283 deaths in 5710 patients. Prostate Cancer Trialists' Collaborative Group. Lancet 1995; 346: 265–9

43. Caubet JF, Tosteson TD, Dong EW, et al. Maximum androgen blockade in advanced prostate cancer: a meta-analysis of published randomized controlled trials using nonsteroidal antiandrogens. Urology 1997; 49: 71–8

44. Onik GM, Cohen JK, Reyes GD, Rubinsky B, Chang Z, Baust J. Transrectal ultrasound-guided percutaneous radical cryosurgical ablation of the prostate. Cancer 1993; 72: 1291–9

45. Wieder J, Schmidt JD, Casola E, vanSonnenberg E, Stainken BF, Parsons CL. Transrectal ultrasound-guided transperineal cryoablation in the treatment of prostatic carcinoma: preliminary results. J Urol 1995; 154: 435–41

46. Gelet A, Chapelon JY, Bouvier R, et al. Treatment of prostate cancer with transrectal focused ultrasound: early clinical experience. European Urol 1996; 29: 174–83

47. Madersbacher S, Pedevilla M, Vingers L, Susani M, Marberger M. Effect of high-intensity focused ultrasound on human prostate cancer in vivo. Cancer Res 1995; 55: 3346–51

48. Culver KW. Gene therapy. A handbook for physicians. New York: Liebert MA, 1994

49. Connors TA. The choice of prodrugs for gene directed enzyme prodrug therapy of cancer. Gene Therapy 1995; 2: 702–9

50. Chen ME, Sikes RA, Troncoso P, Lin S-H, von Eschenbach AC, Chung LWK. PAGE and GAGE-7 are novel genes expressed in the LNCaP prostatic

carcinogenesis model that share homology with melanoma associated antigens. J Urol 1996; 155: 642A

51. Kyprianou N, English HF, Isaacs JT. Programmed cell death during regression of PC-82 human prostate cancer following androgen ablation. Cancer Res 1990; 50: 3748–53

52. Colombel M, Symmans F, Gil S, et al. Detection of the apoptosis-suppressing oncoprotein bcl-2 in hormone-refractory human prostate cancers. Am J Pathol 1993; 143: 390–400

53. Kerr JFR, Winterford CM, Harmon BV. Apoptosis. Its significance in cancer and cancer therapy. Cancer 1994; 27: 2013–26

54. Hockenbery D, Nunez G, Milliman C, Schreiber RD, Korsmeyer SJ. Bcl-2 is an inner mitochondrial membrane protein that blocks programmed cell death. Nature 1990; 348: 334–6

55. Lu QL, Abel P, Foster CS, Lalani EN. bcl-2: role in epithelial differentiation and oncogenesis. Hum Pathol 1996; 27: 102–10

56. Lane DP. p53, guardian of the genome. Nature 1992; 358: 15–16

57. Kroemer G. The proto-oncogene Bcl-2 and its role in regulating apoptosis. Nature Med 1997; 3: 614–20

58. Bostwick DG. Prospective origins of prostate carcinoma. Prostatic intraepithelial neoplasia and atypical adenomatous hyperplasia. Cancer 1996; 78: 330–6

59. Bauer JJ, Sesterhenn IA, Mostofi FK, Mcleod DG, Srivastava S, Moul JE. Elevated levels of apoptosis regulator proteins p53 and bcl-2 are independent prognostic biomarkers in surgically treated clinically localised prostate cancer. J Urol 1996; 156: 1511–16

60. McDonnell TJ, Troncoso P, Brisbay SM, et al. Expression of the proto-oncogene bcl-2 in the prostate and its association with emergence of androgen-independent prostate cancer. Cancer Res 1992; 52: 6940–4

61. Apakama I, Robinson MC, Walter NM, et al. bcl-2 overexpression combined with p53 protein accumulation correlates with hormone-refractory prostate cancer. Br J Cancer 1996; 74: 1258–62

62. Krajewski M, Krajewski S, Epstein JI, et al. Immunohistochemical analysis of bcl-2, bax, bcl-X and mcl-1 expression in prostate cancers. Am J Pathol 1996; 148: 1567–76

63. Stattin P, Damber J-E, Karlberg L, Nordgren H, Bergh A. Bcl-2 immunoreactivity in prostate tumourigenesis in relation to prostatic intraepithelial neoplasia, grade,

hormonal status, metastatic growth and survival. Urol Res 1996; 24: 257–64

64. Vogelstein B, Kinzler KW. p53 function and dysfunction. Cell 1992; 70: 523–6

65. Levine AJ, Momand J, Finlay CA. The p53 tumour suppressor gene. Nature 1991; 351: 453–6

66. Mellon K, Thompson S, Charlton RG, et al. p53, c-erbB-2 and the epidermal growth factor receptor in the benign and malignant prostate. J Urol 1992; 147: 496–9

67. Thomas DJ, Robinson M, King P, et al. p53 expression and clinical outcome in prostate cancer. Br J Urol 1993; 72: 778–81

68. Visakorpi T, Kallioniemi OP, Heikkinen A, Koivula T, Isola J. Small subgroup of aggressive, highly proliferative prostatic carcinomas defined by p53 accumulation. J Natl Cancer Inst 1992; 84: 883–7

69. Aprikian AG, Sarkis AS, Fair WR, Zhang ZF, Fuks Z, Cordon-Cardo C. Immunohistochemical determination of p53 protein nuclear accumulation in prostatic adenocarcinoma. J Urol 1994; 151: 1276–80

70. Kallakury BV, Figge J, Ross JS, Fisher HA, Figge HL, Jennings TA. Association of p53 immunoreactivity with high Gleason tumor grade in prostatic adenocarcinoma. Hum Pathol 1994; 25: 92–7

71. Heidenberg HB, Sesterhenn JP, Gaddipati JP, et al. Alteration of the tumour suppressor gene p53 in a high fraction of hormone refractory prostate cancer. J Urol 1995; 154: 414–21

72. Navone NM, Troncoso P, Pisters LL, et al. p53 protein accumulation and gene mutation in the progression of human prostate carcinoma. J Natl Cancer Inst 1993; 85: 1657–69

73. Humphrey PA, Swanson PE. Immunoreactive p53 protein in high-grade prostatic intraepithelial neoplasia. Pathol Res Practice 1995; 191: 881–7

74. Miyashita T, Reed JC. Tumor suppressor p53 is a direct transcriptional activator of the human bax gene. Cell 1995; 80: 293–9

75. Moul JW, Bettencourt M-C, Sesterhenn IA, et al. Protein expression of p53, bcl-2 and KI-67 (MIB-1) as prognostic biomarkers in patients with surgically treated, clinically localized prostate cancer. Surgery 1996; 120: 159–66

76. Weidner N, Carroll PR, Flax J, Blumenfield W, Folfman J. Tumour angiogenesis correlates with metastasis in invasive prostate carcinoma. Am J Pathol 1993; 143: 401–9

77. Silberman MA, Partin AW, Veltri RW, Epstein JI.

Tumour angiogenesis correlates with progression after radical prostatectomy but not with pathologic stage in Gleason sum 5 to 7 adenocarcinoma of the prostate. Cancer 1997; 79: 772–9

78. Ferrer FA, Miller LJ, Andrawis RI, et al. Vascular endothelial growth factor (VEGF) expression in human prostate cancer: in situ and in vitro expression of VEGF by human prostate cancer cells. J Urol 1997; 157: 2329–33

79. Byrne RL, Leung H, Neal DE. Peptide growth factors in the prostate as mediators of stromal epithelial interaction. Br J Urol 1996; 77(5): 627–33

80. Urist MR. Bone formation by autoinduction. Science 1965; 150: 893–9

81. Hamdy FC, Autzen P, Wilson Horne CH, Robinson MC, Neal DE, Robson CN. Immunolocalization and mRNA expression of bone morphogenetic protein-6 in human benign and malignant prostate tissue. Cancer Res 1997; 57: 4427–31

82. Basilico C, Moscatelli D. The FGF family of growth factors and oncogenes. Adv Cancer Res 1992; 59: 115–65

83. Leung HY, Hughes CM, Kloppel G, Williamson RCN, Lemoine NR. Expression and functional activity of fibroblast growth factors and their receptors in human pancreatic cancer. Int J Oncol 1994; 4: 1219–23

84. Story MT. Regulation of prostate growth by fibroblast growth factors. World J Urol 1995; 13: 297–305

85. Leung HY, Mehta P, Gray LB, Collins AT, Robson CN, Neal DE. Keratinocyte growth factor expression in hormone-insensitive prostate cancer. Oncogene 1997; 15: 1115–20

86. Tanaka A, Miyamoto K, Matsuo H, Matsumoto K, Yoshida H. Human androgen-induced growth factor in prostate and breast cancer cells: its molecular cloning and growth properties. FEBS Lett 1995; 363: 226–30

87. Yoneda T, Sasaki A, Mundy GR. Osteolytic bone metastasis in breast cancer. Breast Cancer Res Treat 1994; 32: 73–84

88. Jones JI, Clemmons DR. Insulin-like growth factors and their binding proteins: biological actions. Endocrine Rev 1995; 16: 3–34

89. Kanety H, Madjar Y, Dagan Y, et al. Serum insulin-like growth factor-binding protein-2 (IGFBP-2) is increased and IGFBP-3 is decreased in patients with prostate cancer: correlation with serum prostate-specific antigen. J Clin Endocrinol Metab 1993; 77: 229–33

90. Denmeade SR, Lin XS, Isaacs JT. Role of programmed (apoptotic) cell death during the progression and therapy for prostate cancer. Prostate 1996; 28: 251–65

91. Takeichi M. Cadherin cell adhesion receptors as a morphogenetic regulator. Science 1991; 251: 1451–5

92. Umbas R, Isaacs WB, Bringuier PB, et al. Decreased E-cadherin expression is associated with poor prognosis in patients with prostate cancer. Cancer Res 1994; 54: 3929–33

93. Gunthert U, Stauder R, Mayer B, Terpe H, Finke L, Friedrichs K. Are CD44 variant isoforms involved in human tumour progression? Cancer Surveys 1995; 24: 19–42

94. Kallakury BVS, Yang F, Figge J, et al. Decreased levels of CD44 protein and mRNA in prostate carcinoma. Correlation with tumor grade and ploidy. Cancer 1996; 78: 1461–9

95. Cattoretti G, Becker MHG, Key G, Duchrow M, Schluter CG, Gerdes J. Monoclonal antibodies against recombinant parts of Ki-67 antigen detect proliferating cells in microwave-processed formalin-fixed paraffin sections. J Pathol 1992; 168: 357–63

96. Noordzij MA, van der Kwast TH, van Steenbrugge GJ, van Weerden WM, Oomen MH, Schröder FH. Determination of Li-67 in formalin-fixed, paraffin-embedded prostatic cancer tissues. Prostate 1995; 27: 154–9

97. Adolfsson J. Prognostic value of deoxyribonucleic acid content in prostate cancer: a review of current results. Int J Cancer 1994; 58: 211–16

98. Persons DL, Takai K, Gibney DJ, Katzmann JA, Lieber MM, Jenkins RB. Comparison of fluorescence in situ hybridisation with flow cytometry and static image analysis in ploidy analysis of paraffin-embedded prostate adenocarcinoma. Hum Pathol 1994; 25: 678–83

99. O'Malley B. The steroid receptor superfamily: more excitement predicted for the future. Mol Endocrinol 1990; 4: 363–9

100. Brolin J, Skoog L, Elman P. Immunohistochemistry and biochemistry in detection of androgen, progesterone, and estrogen receptors in benign and malignant human prostatic tissue. Prostate 1992; 20: 281–95

101. Masai M, Sumiya H, Akimoto S, et al. Immunohistochemical study of androgen receptor in benign hyperplastic and cancerous human prostates. Prostate 1990; 17: 293–300

102. Visakapori T, Hyytinen E, Koivisto P, et al. In vivo amplification of the androgen receptor gene and

progression of human prostate cancer. Nature Genetics 1995; 9: 401–6

103. Carter BS, Beaty TH, Steinberg GD, Childs B, Walsh PC. Mendelian inheritance of familial prostate cancer. Proc Natl Acad Sci (USA) 1992; 89: 3367–71

104. Liotta LA, Tryggvason K, Garbisa S, Hart I, Foltz CM, Shafie S. Metastatic potential correlates with enzymatic degradation of basement membrane collagen. Nature 1980; 284: 67–8

105. Liotta LA. Tumor invasion and metastases. Role of the extracellular matrix. Rhoads Memorial Award Lecture. Cancer Res 1986; 46: 1–7

106. Hamdy FC, Fadlon EJ, Cottam DW, et al. Matrix metalloproteinase-9 expression in human prostatic adenocarcinoma and benign prostatic hyperplasia. Br J Cancer 1994; 69: 177–82

107. Wood M, Fudge K, Mohler JL, et al. In situ hybridization studies of metalloproteinases 2 and 9, and TIMP-1 and TIMP-2 expression in human prostate cancer. Clin Exp Metastasis 1997; 15: 246–58

108. Still K, Robson C, Neal DE, Hamdy FC. The ratio of tissue matrix metalloproteinase-2 (MMP-2) to tissue inhibitor of matrix metalloproteinase (TIMP-2) is increased in high grade prostate cancer. J Urol 1997; 157: 25A

109. Bates TS, Armstrong J, Perry A, Gingell C. Increased expression of membrane-type matrix metalloproteinase in malignant prostate compared with paired benign tissue and specimens of benign prostatic hyperplasia. J Urol 1996; 155: 515A

110. Kaighn ME. Establishment and characterization of a human prostatic carcinoma cell line (PC-3). Invest Urol 1979; 17: 16–23

111. Stone KR, Mickey DD, Wunderli H et al. Isolation of a human prostate carcinoma cell line (DU-145). Int J Cancer 1978; 21: 274–81

112. Horoszewicz JS, Leong SS, Kawinski E, et al. LNCaP model of tumor prostatic carcinoma. Cancer Res 1983; 43: 1809–18

113. Buttyan R, Slawin K. Rodent models for targeted oncogenesis of the prostate gland. Cancer Metastasis Rev 1993; 12: 11–19

114. Pugh TD, Chang C, Uemura H, Weindruch R. Prostatic localization of spontaneous early invasive carcinoma in Lobund–Wistar rats. Cancer Res 1994; 54: 5766–70

115. Royai R, Lange PH, Vessella R. Preclinical models of prostate cancer. Semin Oncol 1996; 23: 35–40

116. Klein KA, Reiter RE, Redula J, et al. Progression of metastatic human prostate cancer to androgen independence in immunodeficient SCID mice. Nature Med 1997; 3: 402–8

Testis cancer

20

M. C. Parkinson and S. J. Harland

Introduction

The incidence of testis cancer continues to rise in most countries of the Western world and the reason for this is unknown. Denmark, which has the highest national prevalence, has seen a steady increase from 3 to 9/100 000 person years between 1945 and 1990 [1]. In six countries around the Baltic Sea, the annual increase between the early post-war period and 1990 varied from 2.3% in Sweden to 5.2% in the former East Germany [2]. Notable then are populations in which the incidence of testis cancer has not increased. These include North American Blacks, for whom the incidence is low (1 per 100 000), and Switzerland, where it is high (6 per 100 000) [3].

These rapid changes in the incidence of testis cancer are a persuasive argument for environmental factors being a major cause in its development. In fact, analysis of the data from the Baltic countries shows that birth cohort is a stronger determinant of testis cancer prevalence than time period [3]. It was of particular interest when it was shown that the upward trend in incidence by year of birth was interrupted during the war years in Denmark [1], a finding that was subsequently found to be true of Norway and Sweden also, but not of the former East Germany, Finland or Poland [3] (Figure 20.1). The implication was that if it was the wartime conditions that affected the testis cancer incidence in the early 1940s' cohorts, these conditions must have been operating in the very first few years of life, if not in utero.

The age distribution for testis cancer is unique (Figure 20.2). The sharp rise in incidence after the onset of puberty indicates the importance of factors that become operative at this time in tumour development. For the steep fall in the incidence curve after the mid-thirties two explanations are offered. The first is that all those testis tumours that have been initiated prior to adolescence progress during adolescent and adult life until there are none left (Figure 20.3a). Alternatively, testicular tumours may be initiated by an adolescence-specific factor (e.g. rapid testicular growth) and present after a limited interval afterwards (Figure 20.3b). Both epidemiological and histopathological studies might shed light on this issue (see below).

Epidemiology

Testicular maldescent

The association of testicular maldescent with testis cancer is well established. Although only 1–2% of cryptorchid boys develop testis cancer, the relative risk for the condition is increased, a figure of 4.7 being typical [4]. The question of whether early correction of maldescent can prevent tumour development is one that may have a bearing on the age of tumour initiation. Comparison of the age of correction for a population of cryptorchids who had developed testis cancer with a population which had not, led to the conclusion that early correction was ineffective in this regard [5]. Two large recent case-control studies – one in Denmark [6], the other in the UK [7] – have provided persuasive evidence that the reverse is the case (Table 20.1). The data shown

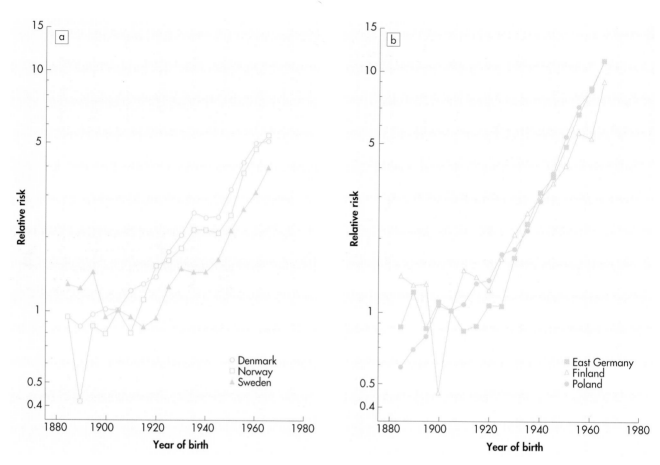

Figure 20.1 *(a, b) Relative risk of developing testicular cancer by country and birth cohort using men from between 1900 and 1909 as the reference. (Taken from Bergstrom et al, (1996) [2].)*

Table 20.1 Two large case-control studies comparing the age of correction of cryptorchidism with testis cancer incidence

	Denmark [6]			UK [7]		
	Cases (%) (n = 514)	Controls (%) (n = 720)	Odds ratio[1]	Cases (%) (n = 794)	Controls (%) (n = 794)	Odds ratio[1]
Treated or persisting cryptorchidism	6.6	1.8	3.6 (1.8–6.9)	8.2	2.1	3.8 (2.2–6.5)
Bilateral	2.1	0.4	4.9 (1.3–18.1)			
Unilateral	4.1	1.4	2.9 (1.3–6.3)			
Age at treatment (years)						
0–9	0.4	0.3	1.1 (0.2–8.2)	0.8	1.3	0.6 (0.2–1.7)
10–14	3.1	1.0	2.9 (1.2–7.1)	2.9	0.4	7.7 (2.3–26)
15+	1.4	1.4	3.5 (0.9–14)	0.6	0	∞ (1.2–∞)
Persisting	1.8	0.1	14.4 (1.8–115)	1.5	0.5	3 (0.97–9.3)

[1] 95% confidence interval.
∞ = infinity.

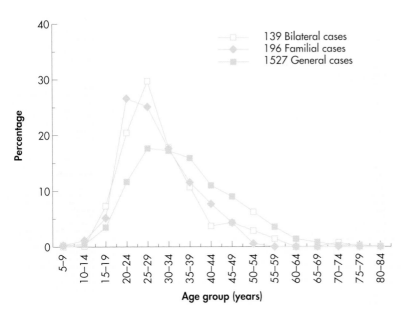

Figure 20.2 *Distribution of age of presentation of 1527 general cases of testicular germ cell cancer (Pugh, 1976 [73]), together with 139 bilateral cases (first tumour) and 196 familial cases. (Reproduced from Nicholson and Harland, 1995 [22].)*

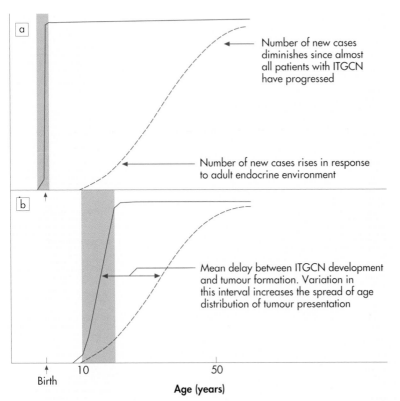

Figure 20.3 *Two hypotheses to account for the age distribution of testis cancer. (a) Intratubular germ cell neoplasia develops in utero (shaded). (b) Intratubular germ cell neoplasia develops in adolescence.*

suggest that there are biological events that occur in an undescended testis between the ages of 10 and 14 which can cause subsequent tumour development.

Other factors

Favouring the importance of environmental factors during adolescence
The recent British and Danish studies both found significant associations between young age of onset of puberty and testis cancer. The difference in testis cancer incidence between the oldest and youngest age groups for onset of puberty was 1.5–2.0-fold, depending on the pubertal indicator used. Other studies [6, 8] have also suggested a protective effect of late puberty. The onset of puberty in men is gradual and memory of the age at which it occurs is often poor. Furthermore, early onset of puberty brings forward the years at risk for testicular cancer, so confounding results can be obtained if a disproportionate number of younger-age tumours is collected. Nevertheless, the fall in age of onset of puberty that has been seen over the last century has been dramatic. Accurate figures for boys are not available, but in girls the fall has been from a mean age of 16.5 in 1885 to 13.4 years in 1965 [9]. The time frame seems to correspond to the observed increase in testicular cancer incidence and makes the age of onset of puberty a good candidate for further study.

Intensive physical exercise (over 15 hours per week at the age of 20) has been shown to be associated with protection from testicular cancer (35% less compared with a no-exercise group). Similarly, a high number of hours seated during the day was strongly associated with an increased risk of testis cancer [7]. This effect was seen even after correction for social class. It is therefore possible that a reduction in the amount of activity associated with certain occupations over the course of the last century (e.g. as a result of mechanisation) could be related to the change in testis cancer incidence that has been seen during this time.

The same study also found that increased sexual activity, using 20 years as the reference age, was slightly but significantly associated with an increased risk of testis cancer.

Favouring the importance of the intrauterine environment
Being a later sibling – i.e. being the fourth or fifth child in a family – is associated with a lower risk of testis cancer [7]. It has been suggested that this reflects differences in maternal physiology between early and late pregnancies.

The use of exogenous oestrogens during early pregnancy was fairly common in the USA in the 1940s and 1950s. Three studies have related their usage to testis cancer incidence (Table 20.2). All three studies show a trend in favour of oestrogen exposure in the cases, though only one shows a significant difference. In some cases, the exposure amounted to a single injection given as a pregnancy test. The history of exposure depended on the mother's memory of it. The possibility has been raised that this may have been subject to recall bias, given the publicity associated with the link between oestrogens and cancer [10].

Oestrogen exposure in pregnancy has been thought to be the link between testicular maldescent, testis cancer, low birth weight and an absence of acne in later years [11]. The recent European case-control studies

Table 20.2 Exposure of mothers of testis cancer patients and of controls to oestrogens during pregnancy

Author	Cases	Controls	Relative risk
Henderson *et al.* (1979) [122]	6/78	1/78	5 ($p = 0.11$)
Shottenfeld *et al.* (1980) [123]	11/190	3/141[1]	2.6 ($p > 0.10$)
Depue *et al.* (1983) [11]	9/97	2/105	8 ($p = 0.02$)

[1] Only 48% of cases had neighbourhood controls.

have made no contribution to this question because so few mothers were exposed. However, no relationship between acne and testis cancer was found [12].

The discovery that certain water pollutants can act as weak oestrogens has led to the hypothesis that these may be the cause both of the increase in testis cancer incidence and of the apparent decline in sperm density in semen in male populations [13]. The relationship between intrauterine exposure to exogenous oestrogens is unproven, however, and at the time of writing, exposure to environmental oestrogens has yet to be related to either low sperm density in humans or testicular cancer.

Hereditary factors

Studies on migrating populations have suggested the importance of genetic factors in determining susceptibility to testis cancer. Thus, both in Africa and the USA, Black populations have a low prevalence. Again, in the USA, those of North European descent ('Protestants') have a higher prevalence than those of Southern European descent ('Catholics'), reflecting the situation on the eastern side of the Atlantic. It is of interest that the UK Testicular Cancer Study Group found the two strongest associations with testis cancer were having a brother (relative risk 8) and having a father (relative risk 4) with the condition. However, a positive family history is not common in testis cancer, first-degree relatives being affected in only 1.0–2.8% of cases [14]. Furthermore, it is rare, unlike other types of familial cancer, for there to be more than two cases in a family [15, 16].

The paradox of a strong genetic influence on the development of testicular cancer but infrequent positive family histories may have been explained by studies on bilateral testicular cancer. Prolonged follow-up of testis cancer patients [17–19] has found that 5% of cases develop a tumour of the contralateral testis – a figure identical to the prevalence of contralateral intratubular germ cell neoplasia at the time of first presentation with testicular cancer [20, 21]. This is a much higher incidence than would be expected from chance alone. Analogy with bilateral tumours of other paired organs, such as retinoblastoma and Wilms' tumour, suggests that they are all of hereditary origin, i.e. that a susceptibility is carried in the germ-line of

these patients, as is the case in patients with familial disease.

Familial retinoblastoma is carried as a dominant gene with high penetrance: 50% of the offspring of an affected parent would carry the predisposition, which would give rise to tumour development in nearly all and bilateral disease in the majority. Familial testis cancer stands in marked contrast to this. Not only is it rare for the offspring of familial cases to be affected, but bilateral disease in familial cases is uncommon, probably in the region of 14% [16, 22].

If one makes the assumption that all bilateral cases (5% of all cases) are of hereditary origin and that these represent only 14% of the hereditary cases, the conclusion is reached that 33% of all cases are of hereditary origin [22]. The similarity in age distribution between hereditary cases and bilateral cases (see Figure 20.2) is evidence that the underlying assumption is correct. From the prevalence of testis cancer and the known risk to fathers and brothers of cases, the best-fit genetic model is one in which the inherited susceptibility is carried as a recessive gene, and an individual who is homozygous for this susceptibility has a 45% chance of developing a tumour [22]. This model is conjectural, but a subsequent segregation analysis on a large population of Norwegian and Swedish patients arrived at one very similar to it [23] (Table 20.3).

The contribution heredity makes to the increase in testis cancer incidence is almost nil: there is no suggestion that the genetic make-up of the populations in question has altered appreciably over the last 100 years. It would seem likely, however, that the penetrance of the genotype has increased during this time.

A search for the testis cancer susceptibility gene has so far been unsuccessful. Linkage analysis has been performed using testis cancer families. Whereas an earlier report described three genomic areas of high interest [24], work on further families has failed to confirm them as sites likely to carry a testis cancer gene, and no other strong candidate regions have emerged [25]. Cytogenetic analysis has not been helpful in testicular cancer as a result of the high frequency of chromosomal abnormalities. The commonest finding is the presence of the isochromosome i(12p), present in 80% of cases. In fact, fluorescent labelling of the short arm of chromosome 12 shows that, even

Table 20.3 Hereditary testicular cancer: two analyses compared

Authors	Nicholson and Harland (1995) [22]	Heimdal et al. (1997) [23]
Source of information	British Testicular Tumour Panel Danish and German testis biopsy series [20, 21] Published case reports	978 testis cancer patients treated in Oslo and Lund
Major gene effect	Assumed	Favoured by analysis
Proportion of general cases attributable to genotype (%)	33	19 (proband generation); higher in parental generation
Type of inheritance	Recessive	Recessive
Risk to homozygotes (%)	45	43
Gene frequency (%)	5	3.8

Taken from Giwercman et al. (1993) [48].

in those tumours that do not have the isochromosome, material from 12p is over-represented [26]. Despite the universal abnormalities in the short arm of chromosome 12 in testicular cancer, no consistent break point has been identified that might lead to the discovery of a cancer-inducing or cancer-suppressing gene. Among the genes mapped to 12p is that which encodes cyclin D2, a positive regulator of cell cycle progression. This gene was found to be deregulated in a panel of germ cell tumour cell lines [27].

Intratubular germ cell neoplasia (ITGCN)

Also known as carcinoma in situ, ITGCN is very commonly found in testes containing a germ cell tumour. Cytological abnormalities involving spermatogonia in tubules adjacent to such tumours were recognised by Wilms in 1896 [28]. But the suggestion that these atypical cells were a form of pre-invasive malignancy was made by Skakkebaek in 1972 [29] when he noted that two infertile men who developed germ cell tumours had had atypical germ cells in their preceding biopsies. This relationship was supported by extensive retrospective reviews of archival testicular biopsies from the infertile population associated with patient follow-up [30, 31]. Subsequently, the prevalence of intra-

tubular germ cell neoplasia in normal men and in various abnormal conditions was established (Table 20.4).

Table 20.4 The prevalence of intratubular germ cell neoplasia in various groups

	Prevalence (%)
General Danish population	<0.8
Cryptorchidism	2.3
Infertility	0.4–1.1
Contralateral testis in men with unilateral germ cell tumours	5.6
Androgen insensitivity	33 (4/12)
Gonadal dysgenesis	High (4/4)
Extragonadal germ cell tumours Retroperitoneal Mediastinal Central nervous system	42 Low (0/8) ? Low (0/2)

Taken from Giwercman et al. (1993) [48] and Daugaard et al. (1992) [124].

Morphology

In ITGCN, there are atypical germ cells situated at the periphery of the seminiferous tubules against a background of atrophy. Spermatogenesis is rarely seen in such tubules, although occasional malignant cells may be demonstrated immunocytochemically in tubules showing spermatogenesis, presumably reflecting 'Pagetoid spread' – i.e. along the plane of the basement membrane – as seen in the rete. The benign tubules within the biopsy are usually also the site of depressed spermatogenesis, intratubular germ cell neoplasia being associated with a Johnsen score of less than 4 [31]. The abnormal germ cells comprising ITGCN have ballooned clear cytoplasm (containing fat and glycogen) and a large hyperchromatic nucleus, which may show mitotic figures (infrequently seen in benign tubules). The diagnosis is best made on biopsies fixed in Stieve's, Cleland's or Bouin's fluid and stained with haematoxylin and eosin. Interpretation of biopsies fixed in formal saline is hampered by the diminution of nuclear detail. Immunocytochemical demonstration of placental alkaline phosphatase in a paranuclear and cytoplasmic membrane situation provides useful confirmation under these circumstances, but in rare cases is not detected [32]. Immunocytochemistry following Bouin's fixation is not reliable so, ideally, the biopsy tissue should be fixed in both Bouin's and formal saline.

Cytogenetic and staining characteristics

Further investigations of ITGCN established that it was aneuploid [33], with an average nuclear DNA content of about 4C [34] (i.e., twice that of a normal diploid cell). The high proliferative activity of this neoplasia is reflected in AgNOR counts per nucleus [35] and MIB-1 positivity [36]. A variety of immunocytochemical markers has been demonstrated in intratubular germ cell neoplasia, of which placental alkaline phosphatase is used in diagnostic histopathology [32]. In up to 60% of cases, p53 glycoprotein has been identified [37], but its significance is uncertain as p53 protein is expressed in elevated amounts in normal spermatogenesis. The data on p53 gene mutations are conflicting. On the one hand, they have been reported as absent from germ cell tumours [38]. On the other, mutations were found in intratubular germ cell neoplasia adjacent to 12 of 18 germ cell tumours, and in one instance an identical p53 mutation was identified in both the preinvasive and invasive tumour [39]. TRA-1-60, M2A and c-kit are of pathogenetic interest as they may also be found in normal fetal germ cells [40]. This may imply that ITGCN arises from fetal germ cells or that such fetal antigens are re-expressed in the neoplasia, arising postnatally. Ultrastructural studies also support similarity between intratubular germ cell neoplasia and germ cells in the early stage of differentiation [41]. A major difference between these two cell types is the limited development of ultrastructural cell contacts in the neoplasia. In this context, it is interesting to note that progression of intratubular germ cell neoplasia to invasive seminoma is marked by the loss of α3 integrin subunit expression [42].

Association with microlithiasis (microcalcification)

Intratubular concretions containing calcium phosphate may be seen in association with intratubular germ cell neoplasia. The significance of this observation has assumed clinical importance with the rise of ultrasonography. A recent study of 429 testicular biopsies identified microlithiasis in 39% of the 36 specimens showing neoplasia and in 2% of the 429 non-malignant testicular disorders [43]. Two series describe the presence of a germ cell tumour in association with microlithiasis in 17 out of 42 and 6 out of 16 cases [44, 45]. Testicular biopsies were not routinely performed in the patients without a tumour so it is not known what proportion contained ITGCN. The question of whether the incidental finding of testicular microlithiasis on ultrasound justifies a biopsy is at present unanswered.

Type of biopsy

The biopsy used in most studies has been the 'open biopsy' in which a 3-mm stab incision is made through the tunica. Needle biopsy of the testis using a Biopty gun has been used in Norway [46]. In a series of patients at high risk for ITGCN, the pick-up rates in 92 open and 93 needle biopsies were 12% and 15% respectively [31]. This seems surprising as needle biopsies are sometimes distorted and contain fewer tubules. Follow-up of this series will give useful data on the false-negative rates of the two biopsy techniques. A needle biopsy has the advantage that it can be performed under local anaesthetic and would be expected to cause less trauma to the gonads. Efforts to diagnose intratubular germ cell neoplasia on cytological features of seminal fluid have had some success in a research setting but are not used routinely [48].

Significance of the presence of intratubular germ cell neoplasia

Two series of infertile men with this ITGCN have both demonstrated that 50% of these patients developed an invasive germ cell tumour within five years of the biopsy. Patients followed beyond five years continued to develop invasive tumours [48, 49]. There are no data as yet to suggest that intratubular germ cell neoplasia may lie 'dormant' for decades, nor that it is a condition that only sometimes progresses to invasive tumour.

When patients with ITGCN of a testis contralateral to an established germ cell tumour have been managed by surveillance alone, the rate of tumour development has been identical to that seen in the infertile patients with the condition [20].

Significance of the absence of intratubular germ cell neoplasia on biopsy

An experimental approach to the question of the false-negative rate for testicular biopsies involved simulated biopsies on four orchidectomy specimens from infertile patients known to have ITGCN [50]. The results showed that neoplasia was detected on all 3-mm biopsies when 10% of the testicular volume was occupied by the preinvasive lesion. However, the diffuse nature of intratubular germ cell neoplasia in infertility (seen when orchidectomy was the treatment) contrasts with its focal distribution in orchidectomies performed for invasive germ cell tumour [51]. Thus, the validity of applying the findings in infertility studies to the biopsy of the atrophic contralateral gonad in men with germ cell tumours could be questioned.

Of greater value, perhaps, in providing information on the sensitivity of testis biopsy in detecting ITGCN are the several series of patients with biopsies negative for this condition that have been followed up from 3 to 35 years. The number of cases of germ cell tumour developing were 2 out of 718 [34], 1 out of 1500 [48], 3 out of 863 [49] and 3 out of 1853 [21].

A high-risk group for intratubular germ cell neoplasia of contralateral testis in testicular cancer

The overall prevalence of intratubular germ cell neoplasia of the contralateral testis in testicular cancer is 5% [20, 21], but within this population is a group of patients at particularly high risk. Two studies have now confirmed contralateral testicular atrophy and age at orchidectomy as independent risk factors for contralateral ITGCN [21, 31]. Thus, of 53 testis cancer patients who had a small (less than 12 ml) contralateral testis and who were aged 30 or less, 18 (34%) had a contralateral testis biopsy positive for intratubular germ cell neoplasia. Only 4 out of 59 (7%) with a small contralateral testis and aged over 30 had a positive biopsy. It is estimated that a policy of confining contralateral testicular biopsy to this very high-risk group, which comprises 6% of all testis cancer patients, would detect approximately 40% of all patients with contralateral intratubular germ cell neoplasia [31].

Sensitivity of intratubular germ cell neoplasia to radiotherapy and chemotherapy

There is good evidence that radiotherapy can destroy ITGCN. Repeat testicular biopsies carried out 24 months after administering 20 Gy in ten fractions for the condition showed only Sertoli cells present within tubules [52]. Most telling is the experience of the Christie Hospital, Manchester, where the practice was to include the contralateral testis in the field of radiation given as adjuvant therapy to stage 1 seminoma of testis. Of over 1000 patients treated, none developed a second tumour, whereas 30 to 50 would have been expected [53]. Testicular irradiation usually allows at least some preservation of Leydig cell function. Loss of libido is uncommon and may be dose related. Basal testosterone levels usually remain within normal limits, though luteinising hormone levels may be raised [52, 54]. The testosterone response to human chorionic gonadotrophin is usually impaired [52].

The efficacy of chemotherapy is much less certain. Testicular biopsies positive for both ITGCN and invasive tumour have been reported following platinum-based chemotherapy [55, 56]. In one series of orchidectomies performed a median of 22 weeks following such chemotherapy for metastatic testicular cancer, 8 out of 23 (35%) were positive for ITGCN [57]. Furthermore, in a large population of testis cancer patients, the proportion developing second tumours did not appear to be diminished amongst those who had received chemotherapy [19].

Age of onset of intratubular germ cell neoplasia

The age at which the morphological features constituting ITGCN can be commonly recognised is controversial. The question is of interest because of its pathogenetic significance. Furthermore, the value of performing a testicular biopsy to exclude ITGCN in younger age groups needs to be clarified.

In adults, clear information on the precursor relationship of ITGCN to invasive germ cell tumours and on the range of time intervals between these two lesions is available from testicular biopsies in the infertile population [28, 49, 58] and in patients with a contralateral germ cell tumour [20]. The fact that intratubular germ cell neoplasia in adults displays markers and some ultrastructural features seen in fetal germ cells has been interpreted as evidence that the neoplasia originates in the fetus. However, markers seen in the fetus may be displayed in adult tumours in the absence of intervening lesions (e.g. carcinoembryonic antigen in colon cancer). Furthermore, in contrast to the high incidence of ITGCN adjacent to adult germ cell tumours, it is the subject of only occasional case reports in childhood ones [59, 60] and was not identified morphologically or immunocytochemically in the orchidectomy specimens from pubertal germ cell tumour patients [61, 62]. Similarly, in a series of children and adolescents with intersex syndrome (known to be at high risk for developing invasive germ cell tumours) ITGCN was found in only 2 of 87 in the prepubertal age group but in 4 of 23 pubertal patients [63].

The sequential information available in adults relating intratubular germ cell neoplasia on biopsy to subsequent invasive germ cell tumour is rarely available in childhood [64]. In a review of biopsies from maldescended testes, ITGCN was only identified in the testis of a 16-year-old and not from biopsies taken from children aged 9, 10 and 14 years in whom germ cell tumours subsequently developed [65].

Diagnosis of germ cell tumours

The role of intraoperative cryostat section diagnosis

Unilateral testicular mass

Intraoperative frozen section diagnosis has a limited contribution to make to the management of a testicular mass as clinical diagnosis is usually sufficiently accurate to support a decision of orchidectomy. Testicular tumours frequently have a mixed morphology and, therefore, restricted sampling reduces the certainty with which the tumour type can be stated and opportunities for misinterpretation abound. For example, especially when normal anatomy is distorted, hyperkeratotic squamous epithelium may have originated from metaplasia in the epididymis or an encysted hydrocele, in addition to an area of differentiated teratoma. A chronic granulomatous inflammatory response may later prove to be within a seminoma. However, intraoperative confirmation of the neoplastic nature of a mass in a solitary testis may be valuable if the clinical findings are equivocal.

Bilateral testicular masses

There are rare instances of bilateral testicular swelling in which the diagnosis may be strongly suspected and intraoperative confirmation may preclude bilateral orchidectomy. Lymphoma, bilateral in 13–50% of cases, may be suspected clinically because lymphomas usually occur in men over 60 years of age, in contrast to the younger age group in whom germ cell tumours present [66, 67]. Hamartomas are seen in up to 25% of postpubertal juveniles and adults with androgen insensitivity. These may present a management problem in those patients raised as males, but in phenotypic females bilateral orchidectomy will be the treatment of choice after puberty [68]. The tumours associated with undiagnosed or inadequately treated adrenogenital syndrome may arise from Leydig cells, adrenal rests or pluripotential stromal cells stimulated by adrenocorticotrophic hormone and suppressed with adequate steroid replacement [69–71]. Papillary cystadenomas occur within the epididymis and efferent ducts associated with von Hippel–Lindau syndrome. These tumours are benign but their clear-celled nature may raise the possibility of metastatic renal parenchymal carcinoma, which also occurs in von Hippel–Lindau syndrome. Orchitis as a localised event or part of a systemic disorder occasionally causes diagnostic difficulty, for example in lepromatous leprosy [72].

Classification of testicular tumours and histological predictors of metastatic spread

Following orchidectomy for testicular tumour, the histopathological features of direct relevance to clinical management include the tumour cell type and its extent (stage), including vascular invasion. Up to the age of 60, germ cell tumour is the most frequent diagnosis, neoplasms arising from Sertoli or Leydig cells accounting for less than 5% of cases, and mesothe-lioma, rete carcinoma, metastases and intratesticular neoplasms of mesenchymal origin (e.g. leiomyoma) are rarities.

Nomenclature relating to germ cell tumours is governed by the two classifications [73, 74]. These systems have far more similarities than differences. Equivalence in nomenclature is easily demonstrated (Table 20.5) and synonyms are given in the most recent WHO publication on histological typing of testis tumours [75]. Disagreements on minutiae of histopathological detail have ceased to be clinically relevant. However, when interpreting publications, the most important difference to note is that the term 'teratoma' in the British classification is applied to all non-seminomatous tumours, but in the WHO system it is restricted to neoplasms composed entirely of differentiated somatic elements, which may be mature or immature. Both classifications have persisted predominantly as a means of communication. In therapeutic trials, their use enables the tumour populations in different studies to be compared.

The advent of immunocytochemistry enabled the cell of origin of the serum markers to be localised. Thus, human chorionic gonadotrophin may be seen most commonly in scattered solitary syncytiotropho-

Table 20.5 Classification of testicular germ cell tumours

British Testicular Tumour Panel and Registry [73]	World Health Organisation [74]

Seminoma
  Classical
  Spermatocytic
	Seminoma
	  Classical
	  Anaplastic
	  Spermatocytic

Teratoma differentiated (TD)
  Mature
  Immature
	Teratoma
	  Mature
	  Immature
	  With malignant transformation

Malignant teratoma intermediate (MTI)	Embryonal carcinoma and teratoma
Malignant teratoma undifferentiated (MTU)	Embryonal carcinoma
Malignant teratoma trophoblastic (MTT) Teratoma trophoblastic (pure form)	Choriocarcinoma ± teratoma, embryonal carcinoma Choriocarcinoma
Yolk sac tumour/orchioblastoma (predominantly a tumour of childhood)	Yolk sac tumour/embryonal carcinoma, infantile type

blasts in malignant teratoma intermediate, malignant teratoma undifferentiated or even seminoma. Although malignant teratoma trophoblastic (choriocarcinoma) produces high serum human chorionic gonadotrophin levels, this tumour type is a rare cause of elevation of this serum hormone. Alphafetoprotein was predominantly localised to yolk-sac tumour and it thus became apparent that this neoplasm, initially recognised in childhood, was not confined to this age group and was present within the morphological patterns previously assigned to areas of undifferentiated teratoma (embryonal carcinoma) in adult tumours. Occasionally, alphafetoprotein can be seen in immature gastrointestinal tract components of teratoma. Placental alkaline phosphatase, in addition to its presence in intratubular germ cell neoplasia, is common in seminoma, but the staining reaction and extent are not so marked in undifferentiated teratoma (embryonal carcinoma).

The WHO classification was always intended to be descriptive, whereas the British classification was based on the known course of certain tumour types and telescoped into groups according to patient survival in the era of orchidectomy and radiotherapy. Improvements in clinical staging and the success of cisplatin-based chemotherapy have completely changed the management and prognosis for patients with germ cell tumours. Following the operation of a high-surveillance regime for patients with stage I teratoma treated by orchidectomy, the subgroups of the British classification were associated with significantly different relapse-free rates on univariate analysis [76]. However, on multivariate analysis, the features predicting relapse that have stood the test of prospective studies with a reproducibility analysis are the presence of undifferentiated teratoma (embryonal carcinoma) and vascular invasion by tumour [77, 78]. Similarly, in studies of prognostic factors in metastatic germ cell tumours, trophoblastic teratoma was a significant prognostic factor on multivariate analysis [79], and the presence of undifferentiated and trophoblastic teratoma was associated with a significantly worse three-year survival rate on univariate analysis [80]. However, the prognostic features seen consistently and now incorporated into an international consensus classification reflect the volume and site of metastases. Thus, a large mediasti-

nal mass, degree of elevation of alphafetoprotein, human chorionic gonadotrophin and lactate dehydrogenase, and the presence of non-pulmonary visceral metastases are all poor prognostic factors [81].

Morphological prognostic features in seminoma are not uniformly accepted and their incorporation into clinical management varies. Some studies indicate the importance of vascular invasion as a predictor of relapse in stage I disease [82, 83] but this has not been a consistent finding [84, 85]. The indication that primary tumour size might be of prognostic value [82] has been confirmed in patients with stage I disease treated by orchidectomy and high surveillance [85].

Assessment of excised tumour masses post-chemotherapy

Following chemotherapy for metastatic non-seminomatous germ cell tumours, if markers are within normal limits but residual masses remain, resection is performed as a diagnostic and therapeutic procedure. Features related to the postoperative disease course include the number and site of metastases, the mediastinum being an adverse location [86, 87], and the completeness of resection as assessed intraoperatively [88–90]; the content of the mass, the presence of viable malignant germ cell tumour (undifferentiated teratoma/embryonal carcinoma, yolk-sac tumour and trophoblastic tumour) predict progressive disease [89–91].

In nine series, each reporting residual masses from more than 50 patients, malignant germ cell tumour components were found in 6–28% (mean 17%), fibrosis and necrosis only in 22–65% (mean 45%) and differentiated teratoma (plus or minus necrosis/fibrosis) in 22–57% (mean 36%) [90]. The two-year progression-free survival for patients whose masses include malignant germ cell tumour elements was 12.5%, compared with 88% in patients in whom these components were absent [90]. As decisions on further chemotherapy are based on the contents of the mass, non-operative predictors of morphology have been sought with a view to leaving necrotic masses in situ. It has been shown that shrinkage of the mass during chemotherapy to a size $\leq 1.5\,cm$, high serum lactic dehydrogenase and normal serum alphafetoprotein and human chorionic gonadotrophin levels pre-chemotherapy and the absence of differentiated teratoma from the primary are indicative of necrotic tissue only in the residual mass [92, 93].

Whether the morphological features of one resected mass can safely be assumed to reflect the findings at other sites remains controversial [90, 94–96].

Case reports draw attention to the development of non-germ cell tumour malignancies (e.g. sarcoma, adenocarcinoma and squamous carcinoma) in residual masses associated with a poor prognosis. Although these tumours were found in up to 6.6% of post-chemotherapy retroperitoneal lymph node dissections in 557 patients with testicular teratomas at the Indiana University Medical Center [97], they were not identified in sections from a series of 163 residual masses reviewed recently in the UK [90]. These differences may have occurred by chance or could reflect referral of malignancies to highly specialised centres.

Tumour markers

Testicular tumours have been strongly associated with the release of proteins into the plasma. Some of these, notably alphafetoprotein and human chorionic gonadotrophin, are found in only very low concentrations in the plasma of healthy adult males, and their presence in the context of a testicular tumour is strong evidence of the persistence or recurrence of viable tumour, hence they are considered to be tumour markers. Furthermore, although the capacity for a mass of given size to produce marker substances is very variable, fluctuations in marker levels within an individual usually reflect changes in the total body tumour mass. Marker substances can therefore be a sensitive measure of response to treatments.

The secretion of marker substances, in particular hormones, by tumours is often described as ectopic – that is, involving the expression of genes normally suppressed by the cell of origin. In the case of testicular tumours, the secretion of substances is frequently appropriate to the tissue present within the tumours. Thus, the presence of alphafetoprotein in the plasma usually implies the presence of yolk-sac elements within the tumour. The secretion of human chorionic gonadotrophin by a testicular tumour indicates the presence of syncitiotrophoblasts, most frequently as single cells and rarely associated with cytotrophoblast in trophoblastic teratoma (choriocarcinoma).

The sensitivity of tumour markers is proportional to the magnitude of the fluctuations that are seen. For a tumour composed of pure choriocarcinoma, it would not be unknown for a patient to present with a human chorionic gonadotrophin level in excess of 10^6 iu/l. At this stage, the patient may have 10^{12} cells of tumour, implying that the human chorionic gonadotrophin level will not return to normal until there are only 10^6 cells present. This would correspond to a viable tumour volume of $10\,mm^3$ [98].

Human chorionic gonadotrophin

Intact human chorionic gonadotrophin comprises an alpha (larger) and a beta subunit. The alpha subunit is identical to that of luteinising hormone, follicle-stimulating hormone and thyroid-stimulating hormone. Though it has 80% homology with the alpha subunit, the beta subunit is specific to human chorionic gonadotrophin and it is this which provides the epitope for modern radio-immunoassays for the hormone in serum. Free beta human chorionic gonadotrophin is also secreted but, as its clearance rate is high – 33 ml/min compared to 3.3 ml/min for intact human chorionic gonadotrophin – it usually contributes little to the measured level [99].

Elevations of serum human chorionic gonadotrophin are seen in 55% of non-seminomatous germ cell tumours, depending on the stage [100], and in 19% of seminomas [101]. Trophoblastic tumour is only likely to be present in the neoplasm when higher serum levels are found. The secretion of human chorionic gonadotrophin by a tumour of uncertain type is often considered to be evidence of a germ cell origin. It must be realised, however, that this hormone is secreted by other tumour types, notably colon, bladder and pancreatic cancers. Occasionally, it is secreted in inflammatory bowel disease.

In patients with localised seminoma of testis, production of human chorionic gonadotrophin is of no prognostic significance [101]. In patients with metastatic non-seminomatous germ cell tumours, prognosis worsens with increasing levels of the hormone. The prognostic significance of serum levels is shown in Table 20.6.

As the trophoblastic elements of testis tumours have a tendency to metastasise to brain, measurement of human chorionic gonadotrophin levels in the cerebrospinal fluid can be of value in the detection of this complication. The level is normally less than one-sixtieth of that of the plasma, except when the plasma level is falling rapidly [102].

Alphafetoprotein

Within a germ cell tumour of testis, it is the yolk-sac elements that are associated with alphafetoprotein production [103]. Raised serum levels of alphafetoprotein are found in 60% of non-seminomatous germ cell tumours patients [100].

Under physiological conditions, large amounts of alphafetoprotein are produced by the yolk sac and the liver during gestation. It is the major plasma protein in the fetus. Following birth, very little is produced, so that low 'adult' levels are reached within a few months. Liver disease can produce a modest elevation of plasma levels. Hepatocellular carcinoma and occasional gastrointestinal tumours can be associated with high levels. Few other tumours produce alphafetoprotein, so a raised level can be of diagnostic value in a patient with metastatic disease of unknown type. Although raised levels have, on rare occasions, been associated with pure seminoma [104], the treatment of metastatic seminoma with radiotherapy in the presence of a raised alphafetoprotein has been disastrous [105], suggesting that, in the majority of these cases, covert non-seminomatous germ cell tumour is also present.

In metastatic non-seminomatous germ cell tumours, very high levels of alphafetoprotein may be found. Prognosis relates to serum level (see Table 20.6).

Lactate dehydrogenase

A raised lactate dehydrogenase level is frequently found in advanced cancer. It is specific neither for testis cancer nor for neoplastic disease in general. Furthermore, unlike human chorionic gonadotrophin and alphafetoprotein, elevations greater than tenfold above normal are uncommon, so its sensitivity is low. Its interest in testis cancer is its very strong association with prognosis (Table 20.6).

Table 20.6 Prechemotherapy serum levels of tumour markers in metastatic non-seminomatous germ cell tumour (NSGCT): frequency and relation to prognosis

	Percentage of patients with metastatic NSGCT	Progression free at five years (%)	Survival at five years (%)
Alphafetoprotein (mg/ml)			
<1000	84	79	83
1000–10 000	12	59	68
>10 000	4	51	57
Human chorionic gonadotrophin (i.u./l)			
<5000	86	79	84
5000–50 000	7	59	66
>50 000	7	43	51
Lactate dehydrogenase (× ULNR)			
<1.5	67	84	88
1.5–10	32	63	69
>10	1	37	47

Taken from International Germ Cell Cancer Collaborative Group (1997) [81]. ULNR, upper limit of normal range.

Placental alkaline phosphatase

Malignant teratoma undifferentiated (embryonal carcinoma), seminoma and intratubular germ cell neoplasia all give a positive stain in histological sections for placental alkaline phosphatase. Modestly elevated serum levels are seen in over 50% of patients with metastatic seminoma [106]. However, this assay is neither sensitive nor specific – elevations are seen in smokers – and placental alkaline phosphatase levels are little used clinically.

The basis of the sensitivity of testicular tumour to DNA-damaging agents

The efficacy of both radiotherapy and cytotoxic chemotherapy in metastatic testicular neoplasia is well known. Seminoma metastatic to para-aortic nodes is usually cured with radiotherapy. Disease beyond this site is usually treated, as with the non-seminomatous germ cell tumours, with chemotherapy and this again usually produces long-term cure. Radiotherapy is seldom used in metastatic non-seminomatous germ cell tumour, as much because of the likelihood of latent disease outside the irradiated areas as because of its lack of efficacy against bulky tumour. The ability of moderate doses of radiotherapy to prevent the development of metastatic disease within an irradiated area is established, however [107].

New light has been shed on the reason for the exquisite sensitivity of germ cell tumours to genotoxic agents from studies on human testis cancer cell lines. Compared to bladder cell lines, a given concentration of etoposide produced a 16-fold loss of clonogenicity. The DNA damage produced showed a difference of only twofold, but testis cancer cell lines showed five times as much apoptosis as those from bladder tumours. When an equivalent frequency of strand breaks was produced, the testicular cell lines died more readily [108].

Normal tissues react to DNA damage by increasing the amount of p53 glycoprotein in cells. This induces the transcription of other proteins, notably Waf-1 and Mdm-2. Waf-1 is a potent inhibitor of cyclin-dependent kinases [109, 110] and can cause cell cycle arrest in G1, i.e. before the phase of DNA synthesis. G1-arrested cells have the opportunity to recover from genotoxic damage. Alternatively, particularly when myc, myb or E2F is over-expressed, an elevated p53 expression may lead to apoptosis [111–113] (Figure 20.4).

Normal germ cells contain high levels of wild-type p53. Germ cell tumours are similar [37, 114] and do not have mutations in the p53 gene [115–117]. When germ cell tumour lines are exposed to etoposide, p53 protein is increased, but Waf-1 only modestly so, and apoptosis ensues [108]. Bladder carcinoma cell lines show two patterns of response. Either the p53 protein remains at a low level, possibly because of the pres-

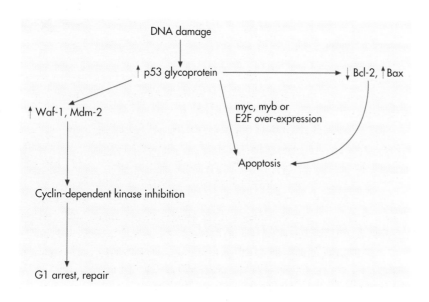

Figure 20.4 Pathways for repair or apoptosis following DNA damage.

ence of a *p53* mutation, or p53 induction takes place and the associated Waf-1 induction causes G1 arrest. The sensitivity of germ cell tumour to genotoxic agents is therefore associated with the apoptotic response to genotoxic damage. This in turn is in part attributed to the high levels of wild-type p53, the absence of *p53* mutations and only a modest level of Waf-1 induction.

Germ cell tumour cell lines have higher levels of the apoptosis-promoting proteins Bax than bladder cancer cell lines and lower levels of the suppressor of apoptosis, Bcl-2 [108]. The Bax:Bcl-2 ratio may be of importance in determining whether the response to cell damage is apoptosis or repair. The role of p53 in affecting this ratio in germ cell tumours is uncertain. Whereas, in certain cells, p53 has been shown to up-regulate Bax and to down-regulate Bcl-2 [118–120] and Bax up-regulation has been observed following geno-toxic damage [121], perturbations of the Bax:Bcl-2 ratio were not seen in the germ cell tumour lines following etoposide exposure [108].

References

1. Moller H. Clues to the aetiology of testicular germ cell tumours from descriptive epidemiology. Eur Urol 1993; 23: 8–15

2. Bergstrom R, Adami HO, Mohner M, *et al.* Increase in testicular cancer incidence in six European countries: a birth cohort phenomenon. J Natl Cancer Inst 1996; 88: 727–33

3. Ekbom A, Akre O. Increasing incidence of testis cancer: a birth cohort effect. In: Rajpert-De Meyts E, Grigor KM, Skakkebaek NE (eds) Neoplastic transformation of testicular germ cells. APMIS 1998; 106: in press

4. Giwercman A, Grindsted J, Hansen B, *et al.* Testicular cancer risk in boys with maldescended testis: a cohort study. J Urol 1987; 138: 1214–16

5. Pike MC, Chilvers C, Peckham MJ. Effect of age at orchidopexy or risk of testicular cancer. Lancet 1986; (May 31): 1246–8

6. Moller H, Skakkebaek NE. Risks of testicular cancer and cryptorchidism in relation to socio-economic status and related factors: case control studies in Denmark. Int J Cancer 1996; 7: 264–74

7. Forman D, Pike MC, Davey G, *et al.* Aetiology of testicular cancer – association with congenital abnormalities,

8. Swerdlow AJ, Huttly SR, Smith PG. Testis cancer: post-natal hormone factors, sexual behaviour and fertility. Int J Cancer 1989; 43: 549–53

9. Tanner JM. Trend towards earlier menarche in London, Oslo, Copenhagen, The Netherlands and Hungary. Nature 1973; 243: 96–7

10. Senturia Y. The epidemiology of testicular cancer. Br J Urol 1987; 60: 285–91

11. Depue RH, Pike MC, Henderson BE. Estrogen exposure during gestation and the risk of cancer of the testis. J Natl Cancer Inst 1983; 71: 1151–5

12. Chilvers CED, Forman D, Oliver RTD, *et al.* Social behavioural and medical factors in the aetiology of testicular cancer – results from the UK study. Br J Cancer 1994; 70: 513–20

13. Carlsen E, Giwercman A, Keiding N, Skakkebaek NE. Evidence for decreasing quality of semen during past 50 years. Br Med J 1992; 305: 609–13

14. Dieckmann K-P, Pichlmeier U. The prevalence of familial testicular cancer. Cancer 1997; 80: 1954–60

15. Forman D, Oliver RTD, Brett AR, *et al.* Familial testicular cancer: a report of the UK family register, estimation of risk and an HLA Class 1 sib-pair analysis. Br J Cancer 1992; 65: 255–62

16. Heimdal K, Olsson H, Tretli S, *et al.* Familial testicular cancer in Norway and Southern Sweden. Br J Cancer 1996; 73: 964–9

17. Osterlind A, Berthelsen JG, Abildgaard N, *et al.* Risk of bilateral testicular germ cell cancer in Denmark: 1960–1984. J Natl Cancer Inst 1991; 83: 1391–5

18. Colls BM, Harvey VJ, Skelton L, *et al.* Bilateral germ cell testicular tumours in New Zealand: experience in Auckland and Christchurch 1978–1994. J Clin Oncol 1996; 14: 2061–5

19. Hoff Wanderas E, Fossa SD, Tretli S. Risk of a second germ cell cancer in 2201 Norwegian male patients. Br J Cancer 1997; 33: 244–52

20. Von der Maase H, Rorth M, Walbom-Jorgensen S, *et al.* Carcinoma in situ of contralateral testis in patients with testicular germ cell cancer: study of 27 cases in 500 patients. Br Med J 1986; 293: 1398–401

21. Dieckmann K-P, Loy V. Prevalence of contralateral testicular intraepithelial neoplasia in patients with testicular germ cell neoplasms. J Clin Oncol 1996; 14: 3126–32

22. Nicholson PW, Harland SJ. Inheritance and testicular cancer. Br J Cancer 1995; 71: 421–6

23. Heimdal K, Olsson H, Tretli S, *et al.* A segregation

analysis of testicular cancer based on Norwegian and Swedish families. Br J Cancer 1997; 75: 1084–7

24. Leahy MG, Tonko S, Moses JH, et al. Candidate regions for a testicular cancer susceptibility gene. Hum Mol Genet 1995; 4: 1551–5

25. Rapley E, Bishop T, for the International Testis Cancer Linkage Consortium. Candidate regions for testis cancer susceptibility genes. In: Rajpert-De Meyts E, Grigor KM, Skakkebaek NE. (eds), Neoplastic transformation of testicular germ cells. APMIS 1988; 106: in press

26. Guerts van Kessel A, Suijkerbuijk RF, Sinke RJ, et al. Molecular cytogenetics of human germ cell tumours: i(12p) and related chromosomal abnormalities. Eur Urol 1993; 23: 23–9

27. Chaganti RSK, Houldsworth J. The cytogenetic theory of the pathogenesis of human adult male germ cell tumours. In: Rajpert-De Meyts E, Grigor KM, Skakkebaek NE (eds), Neoplastic transformation of testicular germ cells. APMIS 1998; 106: in press

28. Sigg C, Hedinger C. Atypical germ cells in testicular biopsy in male sterility. Int J Androl 1981; Suppl. 4: 163–71

29. Skakkebaek NE. Possible carcinoma in situ of the testis. Lancet 1972; 2: 516–17

30. Pryor JP, Cameron KM, Chilton CP, et al. Carcinoma in situ in testicular biopsies from men presenting with infertility. Br J Urol 1983; 55: 780–4

31. Harland SJ, Cook PA, Fossa SD, et al. Intratubular germ cell neoplasia of the contralateral testis in testicular cancer: defining a high risk group. J Urol 1998; 160: 1353–7

32. Jacobsen GK, Norgaard-Pedersen B. Placental alkaline phosphatase in testicular germ cell tumours and in carcinoma in situ of the testis. Acta Pathol Microbiol Scand Sect. A 1984; 92: 323–9

33. Moller J, Skakkebaek NE. Microspectrophotometric DNA measurements of carcinoma in situ germ cells in the testis. Int J Androl 1981; Suppl. 4: 211–21

34. Nistal M, Codesal J, Paniagua R. Carcinoma in situ of the testis in infertile men. A histological, immunocytochemical and cytophotometric study of DNA content. J Pathol 1989; 159: 205–10

35. Moller J, Lauke H, Hartmann M. The value of the AgNOR staining method in identifying carcinoma in situ testis. Pathol Res Pract 1994; 120: 429–35

36. Ball RY, Sandison A, Areas AM, et al. DNA ploidy and proliferation fraction in classical seminoma and intratubular germ cell neoplasia. J Urol Pathol 1998; 78: 141–55

37. Bartkova J, Bartek J, Lukas J, et al. p53 protein alterations in human testicular cancer including pre-invasive intratubular germ cell neoplasia. Int J Cancer 1991; 49: 196–202

38. Rukstalis DB. Molecular mechanisms of testicular carcinogenesis. World J Urol 1996; 14: 347–52

39. Kuczyk MA, Serth J, Bokemeyer C, et al. Alterations of the p53 tumour suppressor gene in carcinoma in situ of the testis. Cancer 1996; 78: 1958–66

40. Jorgensen N, Rajpert-De Meyts E, Graem N, et al. Expression of imunohistochemical markers for testicular carcinoma in situ by normal human foetal germ cells. Lab Invest 1995; 72: 223–31

41. Gondos B. Ultrastructure of developing and malignant germ cells. Eur Urol 1993; 23: 68–75

42. Timmer A, Oosterhuis JW, Koops HS, Sleijfer DT, Szabo BG, Timens W. The tumour micro-environment: possible role of integrins and the extracellular matrix in tumour biological behaviour of intratubular germ cell neoplasia and testicular seminomas. Am J Pathol 1994; 144: 1035–44

43. Kang J-L, Rajpert-De Meyts W, Giwercmann A, Skakkebaek NE. The association of testicular carcinoma in situ with intratubular microcalcifications. J Urol Pathol 1994; 2: 235–42

44. Backus ML, Mack LA, Middleton WD, et al. Testicular microlithiasis: imaging appearances and pathological correlation. Radiology 1994; 192: 781–5

45. Hobarth K, Szabo N, Klingher HC, Kratzik C. Sonographic appearance of testicular microlithiasis. Eur Urol 1993; 24: 251–5

46. Heikkila R, Heilo A, Stenning AE, Fossa SD. Testicular ultrasonography and 18G Biopty biopsy for clinically undetected cancer or carcinoma in situ in patients with germ cell tumours. Br J Urol 1993; 71: 214–16

47. Harland SJ, Nicholson PW. Implications of a hereditary model for testis cancer. In: Appleyard I, Harnden P, Joffe JK (eds) Germ cell tumours IV. John Libbey, 1998:19–27

48. Giwercman A, von der Maase H, Skakkebaek NE. Epidemiological and clinical aspects of carcinoma in situ of the testis. Eur Urol 1993; 23: 104–14

49. Bettocchi C, Coker C, Deacon J, et al. A review of testicular intratubular germ cell neoplasia in infertile men. J Androl 1994; 15: 145–65

50. Berthelsen JG, Skakkebaek NE. Distribution of carcinoma in situ in testes from infertile men. Int J Androl 1981; Suppl. 4: 172–84

51. Loy V, Wigand I, Dieckmann K-P. Incidence and distri-

bution of carcinoma in situ in testis removed for germ cell tumour: possible inadequacy of random testicular biopsies in detecting the condition. Histopathology 1990; 16: 198–200

52. Giwercman A, von der Maase H, Berthelsen JG, Rorth M, Skakkebaek NE. Localised irradiation of testes with carcinoma in situ: effects on Leydig cell function and eradication of malignant germ cells in 3 patients. J Clin Endocrin Metab 1991; 73: 596–603

53. Read G. Carcinoma in situ of the contralateral testis. Br Med J 1987; 294: 121

54. Shalet SM. Effect of irradiation treatment on gonadal function in men treated for germ cell cancer. European Urol 1993; 23: 148–52

55. Fossa SD, Aass N. Cisplatin-based chemotherapy does not eliminate the risk of secondary testicular cancer. Br J Urol 1989; 63: 531–4

56. Von der Maase H, Meinecke B, Skakkebaek NE. Residual carcinoma in situ of contralateral testis after chemotherapy. Lancet 1988; i: 477–8

57. Bottomley D, Fisher C, Hendry WF, Horwich A. Persistent carcinoma in situ of the testis after chemotherapy for advanced testicular germ cell tumours. Br J Urol 1990; 66: 420–4

58. Skakkebaek NE, Berthelsen JG, Visfeldt J. Clinical aspects of testicular carcinoma in situ. Int J Androl 1981; Suppl. 4: 153–62

59. Hu LM, Phillipson SH. Intratubular germ cell neoplasia in infantile yolk sac tumour: verificiation by tandem repeat sequence in-situ hybridization. Diagn Mol Pathol 1992; 1: 118–28

60. Stamp IM, Barlebo H, Rix M, Jacobsen GK. Intratubular germ cell neoplasia in an infantile testis with immature teratoma. Histopathology 1993; 22: 69–72

61. Manivel JC, Simonton S, Wold LE, Dehner LP. Absence of intratubular germ cell neoplasia in testicular yolk sac tumours in children. Arch Pathol Lab Med 1988; 112: 641–5

62. Soosay GN, Bobrow L, Happerfield L, Parkinson MC. Morphology and immunohistochemistry of carcinoma in situ adjacent to testicular germ cell tumours in adults and children: implications for histogenesis. Histopathology 1991; 19: 537–44

63. Ramani P, Yeung CK, Habeebu SSM. Testicular intratubular germ cell neoplasia in children and adolescents with intersex. Am J Surg Pathol 1993; 17: 1124–33

64. Moller J, Skakkebaek NE, Nielsen OH, Graem N. Cryptorchidism and testis cancer. Atypical infantile germ cells followed by carcinoma in situ and invasive carcinoma in adulthood. Cancer 1984; 54: 629–34

65. Parkinson MC, Swerdlow AJ, Pike MC. Carcinoma in situ in boys with cryptorchidism: when can it be detected? Br J Urol 1994; 73: 431–5

66. Duncan PR, Checa F, Gowing NFC, McElwain TJ, Peckham MJ. Extranodal non-Hodgkin's lymphoma presenting in the testicle. Cancer 1980; 45: 1578–84

67. Turner RR, Colby TV, MacKintosh FR. Testicular lymphomas: a clinico-pathologic study of 35 cases. Cancer 1981; 48: 2095–102

68. Rutgers JL, Scully RE. Pathology of the testis in intersex syndromes. Semin Diagnostic Pathol 1987; 4: 275–91

69. Witten FR, O'Brien BP, Sewell CW, Wheatley JK. Bilateral clear cell papillary cystadenoma of the epididymes presenting as infertility: an early manifestation of von Hippel–Landau's syndrome. J Urol 1985; 133: 1062–4

70. Rutgers JL, Young RH, Scully RE. The testicular 'tumour' of the adreno-genital syndrome. Am J Surg Pathol 1988; 12: 503–13

71. Knudsen JL, Savage A, Mobb GE. The testicular 'tumour' of adreno-genital syndrome – a persistent diagnostic pitfall. Histopathology 1991; 19: 468–70

72. Akhtar M, Ali MA, Mackey DM. Lepromatous leprosy presenting as orchitis. Am J Clin Pathol 1980; 73: 712–15

73. Pugh RCB. Testicular tumours – introduction. In: Pugh RCB (ed) Pathology of the testis. Oxford: Blackwell Scientific Publications, 1976: 139–159

74. Mostofi FK, Sobin LH. Histological typing of testis tumours. International histological classification of tumours, No. 16. Geneva: World Health Organisation, 1977

75. Mostofi FK, Sesterhenn IA, in collaboration with Sobin AH and pathologists in nine countries. World Health Organisation International Histological Classification of Tumours. Histological typing of testis tumours. Second edition. Berlin: Springer Verlag, 1998

76. Freedman LS, Parkinson MC, Jones WG, et al. Histopathology and the prediction of relapse of patients with stage I testicular teratoma treated by orchidectomy alone. Lancet 1987; ii: 294–8

77. Read G, Stenning SP, Cullen MH, et al. Medical Research Council prospective study of surveillance for stage I testicular teratoma. J Clin Oncol 1992; 10: 1762–8

78. Cullen MH, Stenning SP, Parkinson MC, *et al.* Short course adjuvant chemotherapy in high risk stage I non-seminomatous germ cell tumours of the testis: a Medical Research Council report. J Clin Oncol 1996; 14: 1106–13

79. Stoter G, Sylvester R, Sleijfer DT, *et al.* Multivariate analysis of prognostic factors in patients with disseminated non-seminomatous testicular cancer: results from a European Organisation for Research on Treatment of Cancer multi-institutional phase III study. Cancer Res 1987; 47: 2714–18

80. Mead GM, Stenning SP, Parkinson MC, *et al.* The second Medical Research Council study of prognostic factors in non-seminomatous germ cell tumours. J Clin Oncol 1992; 10: 85–94

81. International Germ Cell Cancer Collaborative Group. International germ cell consensus classification: a prognostic factor-based staging system for metastatic germ cell cancers. J Clin Oncol 1997; 15: 594–603

82. Marks LB, Rutgers JL, Shipley WU, *et al.* Testicular seminoma: clinical and pathological features that may predict para-aortic lymph node metastases. J Urol 1990; 143: 524–7

83. Horwich A, Alsanjari N, Ahern R, *et al.* Surveillance following orchidectomy for stage I testicular seminoma. Br J Cancer 1992; 65: 775–8

84. Hoeltl W, Kosak D, Pont J, *et al.* Testicular cancer: prognostic implications of vascular invasion. J Urol 1987; 137: 683–5

85. Jacobsen GK, von der Maase H, Specht L, *et al.* Histopathological features of stage I seminoma treated with orchidectomy only. J Urol Pathology 1995; 3: 85–94

86. Loehrer PJ, Hui S, Clark S, *et al.* Teratoma following cisplatin-based combination chemotherapy for non-seminomatous germ cell tumours: a clinico-pathological correlation. J Urol 1986; 135: 1183–9

87. Steyerberg EW, Keizer HJ, Zwartendijk J, *et al.* Prognosis after resection of residual masses following chemotherapy for metastatic non-seminomatous testicular cancer: a multivariate analysis. Br J Cancer 1993; 68: 195–200

88. Hendry WF, Ahern RP, Hetherington JW, *et al.* Para-aortic lymphadenectomy after chemotherapy for metastatic non-seminomatous germ cell tumours: prognostic value and therapeutic benefit. Br J Urol 1993; 71: 208–13

89. Gerl A, Clemm C, Schmeller N, *et al.* Outcome analysis after post-chemotherapy surgery in patients with non-seminomatous germ cell tumours. Ann Oncol 1995; 6: 483–8

90. Stenning SP, Parkinson MC, Fisher C, *et al.* Residual masses post-chemotherapy for germ cell tumour: content, clinical features and prognosis. Cancer 1998; 83: 1409–19

91. Hendry WF. Decision-making in abdominal surgery following chemotherapy for testicular cancer. Eur J Cancer 1995; 31A: 649–50

92. Toner GC, Panicek DM, Heelan RJ, *et al.* Adjunctive surgery after chemotherapy for non-seminomatous germ cell tumours: recommendations for patient selection. J Clin Oncol 1990; 8: 1683–94

93. Steyerberg EW, Keizer HJ, Stoter G, Habbena JDF. Predictors of residual mass histology following chemotherapy for metastatic non-seminomatous testicular cancer: a quantitative overview of 996 resections. Eur J Cancer 1994; 30A: 1231–9

94. Gerl A, Clemm C, Schmeller N, *et al.* Sequential resection of residual abdominal and thoracic masses after chemotherapy for metastatic non-seminomatous germ cell tumour. Br J Cancer 1994; 70: 960–5

95. Brenner PC, Herr HW, Morse MJ, *et al.* Simultaneous retroperitoneal, thoracic and cervical resection of post-chemotherapy residual masses in patients with metastatic non-seminomatous germ cell tumours of the testis. J Clin Oncol 1996; 14: 1765–9

96. Steyerberg EW, Keizer HJ, Messemer JE. Residual pulmonary masses after chemotherapy for metastatic non-seminomatous germ cell tumour prediction of histology. Cancer 1997; 79: 345–55

97. Little JS, Foster RS, Ulbright TM, *et al.* Unusual neoplasms detected in testis cancer patients undergoing post-chemotherapy retroperitoneal lymphadenectomy. J Urol 1994; 152: 1144–9

98. Bagshawe KD, Rustin GDS. Circulating tumour markers. In: Peckham M, Pinedo HM, Veronesi U (eds) Oxford textbook of oncology. Vol. 1. Oxford: Oxford Medical Publications, 1995: 412–20

99. Wehmann RE, Nisula BC. Metabolic and renal clearance rates of purified human chorionic gonadotrophin. J Clin Invest 1981; 68: 184–93

100. Rustin GJS, Vogelzang NJ, Sleijfer DT, Nisselbaum SN. Consensus statement as circulating tumour markers and staging of patient with germ cell tumours. In: Prostate cancer and testicular cancer, EORTC Genitourinary Group Monograph 7. New York: AR Liss, 1990

101. Schwartz BF, Auman R, Peretsman SS, *et al.* Prognos-

tic value of BHCG and local tumour invasion in stage I seminoma of the testis. J Surg Oncol 1996; 61: 131–3

102. Bagshawe KD, Harland S. Immunodiagnosis and monitoring of gonadotrophin producing metastases in the central nervous system. Cancer 1976; 38: 112–18

103. Teilum G, Albrechtsen R, Norgaard-Pedersen B. Immunofluorescent localization of alpha-fetoprotein synthesis in endodermal sinus tumor (yolk sac tumor). Acta Pathol Microbiol Scand 1974; 82A: 586–8

104. Oliver RTD. A comparison of the biology and prognosis of seminoma and non-seminoma. In: Horwich A (ed) Testicular cancer, investigation and management. Chapman and Hall Medical, 1991: 51–63

105. Lange PH, Nochomovitz LE, Rosai J, et al. Serum alpha-fetoprotein and human chorionic gonadotrophin in patients with seminoma. J Urol 1980; 124: 472–8

106. Lange PH, Millan JL, Stigbrand T, et al. Placental alkaline phosphatase as a tumor marker for seminoma. Cancer Res 1982; 42: 3244–7

107. Rorth M, Jacobsen GJ, von der Maase H, et al. Surveillance alone versus radiotherapy after orchidectomy for clinical stage I non-seminomatous testicular cancer. J Clin Oncol 1991; 12: 1543–7

108. Chresta CM, Masters JR, Hickman JA. Hypersensitivity of human testicular tumours to etoposide-induced apoptosis is associated with functional p53 and a high Bax:Bcl-2 ratio. Cancer Res 1996; 56: 1834–41

109. El Deiry WS, Harper JW, O'Connor PM, et al. WAFI/CIPI is induced in p53-mediated G_1 arrest and apoptosis. Cancer Res 1994; 54: 1169–74

110. Canman CE, Gilmer TM, Coutts SB, Kastan MB. Growth factor modulation of p53-mediated growth arrest versus apoptosis. Genes Dev 1995; 9: 600–11

111. Wagner AJ, Kokontis JM, Hay N. Myc-mediated apoptosis requires wild-type p53 in a manner independent of cell cycle arrest and the ability of p53 to induce p21wafl/cipl. Genes Dev 1994; 8: 2817–30

112. Lin D, Fiscella M, O'Connor PM, et al. Constitutive expression of B-myb can bypass p53-induced Wafl/Cip1-mediated G_1 arrest. Proc Natl Acad Sci USA 1994; 91: 10079–83

113. Wu X, Levine AJ. p53 and E2F-1 cooperate to mediate apoptosis. Proc Natl Acad Sci USA 1994; 91: 3602–6

114. Bartek J, Bartkova J, Vojtesek B, et al. Aberrant expression of the p53 oncoprotein is a common feature of a wide spectrum of human malignancies. Oncogene 1991; 6: 1699–703

115. Peng HQ, Hogg D, Malkin D, et al. Mutations of the p53 gene do not occur in testis cancer. Cancer Res 1993; 53: 3574–8

116. Heimdal K, Lothe RA, Lystad S, et al. No germline TP53 mutations detected in familial and bilateral testicular cancer. Genes Chromosomes Cancer 1993; 6: 92–7

117. Fleischhacker M, Strohmeyer T, Imai Y, Slamon DJ, Koeffler HP. Mutations of the p53 gene are not detectable in human testicular tumours. Mod Pathol 1994; 7: 435–9

118. Miyashita T, Harigai M, Hanada M, Reed JC. Identification of a p53-dependent negative response element in the Bcl-2 gene. Cancer Res 1994; 54: 3131–5

119. Miyashita T, Krajewski S, Krajewska M, et al. Tumour suppressor p53 is a regulator of Bcl-2 and bax gene expression in vitro and in vivo. Oncogene 1994; 9: 1799–805

120. Selvakumaran M, Lin HK, Miyashita T, et al. Immediate early up-regulation of bax expression by p53 but not TGF β1: a paradigm for distinct apoptotic pathways. Oncogene 1994; 9: 1791–8

121. Zhan Q, Fan S, Bae I, et al. Induction of bax by genotoxic stress in human cells corelates with normal p53 status and apoptosis. Oncogene 1994; 9: 3743–51

122. Henderson BE, Benton B, Jing J, et al. Risk factors for cancer of the testis in young men. Int J Cancer 1979; 23: 598–602

123. Shottenfeld D, Warshauer ME, Sherlock S. The epidemiology of testicular cancer in young adults. Am J Epidemiol 1980; 112: 232–46

124. Daugaard G, Rorth M, von der Maase H, Skakkebaek NE. Management of extragonadal germ cell tumours and the significance of bilateral testicular biopsies. Ann Oncol 1992; 3: 283–9

Principles of radiotherapy

21

G. M. Duchesne

The use of ionising radiation to treat cancer followed quickly after its discovery at the turn of the century, but for several decades it was used empirically, with little understanding of its effects on normal tissues or cancer cells, or of how to optimise its delivery. Study of the biological effects of radiation and the development of sophisticated physical techniques now provide a treatment modality firmly based on scientific principles.

Types of ionising radiation

Radiation used in clinical practice to treat malignant disease has its effect through the ionisation of molecules it contacts within the cell, and thus is called ionising radiation (in distinction to ultraviolet light, for example, which is non-ionising). The majority of treatments use high-energy X-ray photons, generated by orthovoltage X-ray machines or linear accelerators. The energies used to generate the X-ray beams range from 100 kilovolts (kV) to 15–20 megavolts (MV). The higher the energy of the beam, the more penetrating it is, as the photons are less readily stopped in the superficial layers of tissue. Treatment of deep-seated tumours such as bladder and prostate within the pelvis is commonly undertaken at energies of 8 MV or above. The term deep X-ray therapy (DXR), which is mistakenly applied to all types of radiotherapy, uses an energy of 250 kV, and was the maximum available until the development of linear accelerators; it has an effective penetration of only 3–4 cm, and deposits a significant radiation dose in the skin. The

linear accelerator technology in effect hitches the electrons generated by the cathode on to radio waves, accelerating them to high energies by increasing the wave frequency, with energies in the megavoltage range when they hit the tungsten target. This emits X-ray beams that penetrate 10 cm or more and spare skin. Megavoltage photons can also be generated through the decay of radioactive isotopes, when they are known as gamma rays; cobalt 60 is commonly used in cancer therapy, producing a beam with two components, each of energy of just over 1 MV.

Other types of radiation are also used in external beam radiotherapy (or teletherapy). The electron beam from an X-ray generator can be used directly by bypassing the tungsten target. As electrons are negatively charged, they stop rapidly in the tissues, and provide a beam with a well-defined cut-off, which is used to avoid critical underlying tissues. Heavy nuclear particles, either uncharged such as neutrons, or charged such as protons, amongst others, are also available. They have distinct physical properties that can be manipulated to provide very specific dose distributions, and biological effects that produce high levels of cell kill. In most circumstances, however, their use is still regarded as experimental, as the equipment needed to generate heavy particles is prohibitively expensive and, with few exceptions, does not provide a significant improvement in therapeutic ratio, and therefore clinical advantage, over the use of standard techniques.

Radio-isotopes are used not only in teletherapy but also in brachytherapy, when they are in close contact with the treated tissue. The isotopes may be solid and inserted as either temporary or permanent implants into the tumour, emitting gamma radiation, electrons or nucleons as they decay. Iridium-192 is commonly used as a temporary implant, and iodine-125 seeds as a permanent implant. 'Liquid' isotopes such as iodine-131 or strontium-89 can be administered systemically, and have the advantage of tissue-specific uptake (iodine to the thyroid, strontium to areas of bone turnover, as it is handled like calcium). Radio-isotopes also have the advantage of giving a very localised high dose, which falls off rapidly from the source following the inverse square law (reducing the dose to normal tissues), but they cannot easily be used to treat large volumes and require careful protection procedures.

Interaction of radiation with matter

When ionising radiation passes through a cell, it may go straight through without 'touching' a molecule, the chances of contact depending on the amount of energy in the photon or associated with the particle: the lower the energy, the more likely a collision is to occur. If a molecule is encountered, the radiation gives up energy by ejecting electrons from the atoms in the molecule, which therefore become charged or ionised, or by raising others to higher energy levels (excitation), a process lasting nanoseconds. These events lead to the breakage of chemical bonds and the formation of highly unstable free radicals. At this stage, the free radicals can be inactivated by combination with, for example, sulphydryl molecules, or the damage may be fixed, by oxygen or similar active compounds, to produce chemically stable changes.

The abundant water molecule is that most frequently encountered; this is split into hydroxyl radicals and hydrated electrons, themselves both highly reactive. Other molecules within the cell may then be ionised in turn, or they may be hit directly by the primary radiation. Alteration of macromolecular structure may affect protein function, but it is the interaction with the DNA that is the critical event. Changes in chemical structure may lead to genetic mutation (underlying the process of radiation carcinogenesis), or to breakage of one or both of the DNA strands. A single-strand break may be recog-

nised and repaired, but if several ionisations occur in close proximity to each other, a double-strand break may be induced; this is thought to be the lethal lesion, resulting in cell kill.

Determinants of radiosensitivity

While the physical characteristics of the radiation beam determine in part the effect on the biological material it encounters, there are a number of features relating to the cells themselves that influence their response. Clinical radiotherapy schedules have evolved empirically to make maximum use of the small differences between normal and malignant cells, and the underlying biological processes are only now being clarified with the advent of modern molecular biology approaches.

Classical radiobiology teaching promoted the 'four Rs' of radiation response [1], repair, reoxygenation, reassortment and repopulation, to which was added a fifth a decade ago, intrinsic radiosensitivity. Much of the early radiobiology work was undertaken on yeast systems, but developing tissue culture techniques allowed the immortalisation and growth of mammalian cell lines, from which much of our understanding stems. The gold standard for the measurement of radiation response is the clonogenic cell survival assay, in which the ability of a single cell to survive the radiation insult and proliferate to form a clone is assayed. Molecular techniques have subsequently dissected the whole cell response and are beginning to clarify the molecular events involved.

Recovery from radiation damage
After the initial induction of damage to the DNA, the cell may respond by recognising the damaged area and attempting its repair. The presence of the ability to recover viability following a radiation insult was recognised by Elkind [2], who demonstrated that the survival of cells treated with a single dose of radiation was lower than that of cells for which the same total dose was divided into two fractions separated by a period of hours. To achieve the same cell kill with a fractionated dose required the use of a higher total dose, suggesting that the cells were able to recover

from some of the damage induced by the initial exposure. Depending on the mathematical model used to describe the experimental data, when the survival of cells exposed to increasing radiation doses is plotted on a logarithmic scale, there appears to be a 'shoulder' at low radiation doses at which cell kill is less per unit dose increment than at higher dose increments (Figure 21.1). The conclusion was that cells are able to recover from low doses of radiation, and that the split-dose experiment of Elkind was allowing reconstitution of the shoulder between fractions, and thus recovery. Giving a second fraction immediately after the first abolishes the shoulder effect, but if it is given after recovery, the shape of the curve is repeated (Figure 21.2).

The length of time between fractions is important; there appears to be an initial rapid component, and maximal recovery appears complete between four and six hours (although survival is not 100%, meaning

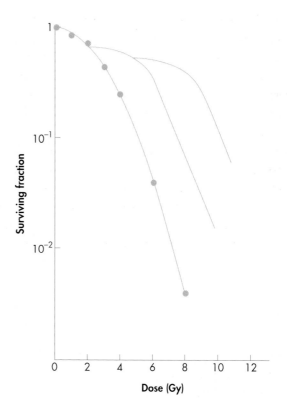

Figure 21.2 *Split-dose recovery from radiation damage. If a radiation dose is given in two fractions (for example of 2 Gy each) rather than a single larger fraction (e.g. 4 Gy), the resulting final cell kill is reduced. Provided a minimum of four hours elapses between exposures, the cell recovers in part from the damage, and the 'shoulder' of the survival curve is reconstituted. In a multifraction treatment course, this event is repeated; if normal tissue recovery is more efficient than in malignant cells, therapeutic gain results.*

that not all damage can be repaired). This has been termed recovery from sublethal damage. Recovery may also be demonstrated if cells are held in plateau phase after irradiation before being allowed to proliferate; this would seem to give the cells time to overcome some of the inflicted damage before having to enter the cell cycle. This is called potentially lethal damage, as it would only be expressed if the cell proceeded immediately into cycle after irradiation.

The ability of mammalian cells to recover from radiation damage is also dependent on the rate at which ionisation events occur within the cell. In the same way that two events spatially close to each other in the DNA may lead to a double-strand break and cell kill, temporal proximity of lesions is important. If two events happen within a short time frame, there may not be time to repair the first before the second

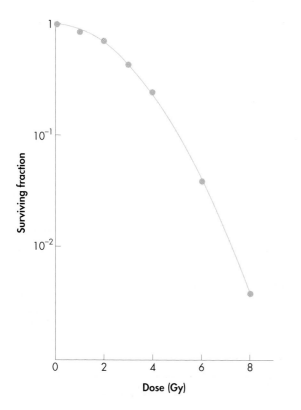

Figure 21.1 *Clonogenic cell survival curve following radiation. A single-cell suspension is prepared from an irradiated cell population; surviving cells form colonies, and the numbers formed relative to untreated controls are plotted as the surviving fraction at each dose. A typical surviving fraction at 2 Gy would be 0.6, with higher doses producing rapidly increasing cell kill.*

appears, converting what would be two independent single-strand breaks into the lethal double lesion. This is readily demonstrated by lowering of the dose rate given to experimental cultures, which allows increasing cell survival for equivalent total doses [3]. At low enough dose rates, the repair capacity of the cells

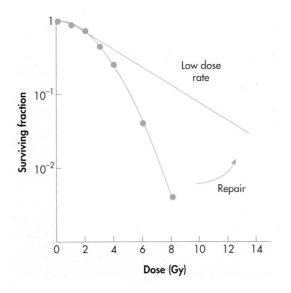

Figure 21.3 *Lowering the rate at which radiation is delivered to the cell allows some of the induced damage to be repaired as the radiation is delivered, with improved levels of cell survival. The bendy or curvilinear characteristic of the survival curve disappears, as cell kill resulting from reparable damage is prevented. However, even at very low dose rates, some damage is not repaired, represented by the linear low dose-rate survival response.*

accommodates all accessible or reparable damage; there is still cell kill, which is thought to result from irreparable damage (shown in Figure 21.3).

What is involved in the recovery process? It has long been attributed to the process of DNA repair, but until recently little has been known about the mechanism of repair of damage from ionising radiation in mammalian cells. Recent work has identified a number of genes in yeast systems involved in DNA repair. Analysis of X-ray-sensitive mutant mammalian cell lines has shown defects in genes homologous with the yeast genes, and when the defects are corrected the normal cellular capacity to repair DNA damage is restored. The process is probably one of excision repair, which involves recognition of the damaged segment of DNA, its isolation and excision, and reconstitution of integrity by the insertion of new nucleotides against the complementary strand by DNA polymerase; a likely schema is illustrated in Figure 21.4. The identification of mammalian DNA repair enzymes is an area of intense current activity; some of the enzymes involved in mammalian cell systems are shown in Table 21.1, and are discussed in more detail later.

To date, our knowledge of the recovery process has determined the minimum safe interval between radiation fractions to allow maximal healing in the normal tissues, obviously important when schedules using more than one fraction per day are prescribed. We also

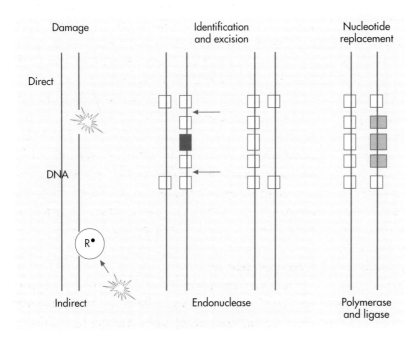

Figure 21.4 *Damage to DNA can be either by direct ionisation of the base molecules, or indirectly through ionisation of water molecules, which causes secondary damage to the DNA. After recognition of the damaged sequence, these bases are excised and new ones inserted against the template of the remaining strand. Double strand breaks, unless the ends overlap (sticky), cannot be repaired in this way.*

Table 21.1 Mammalian DNA repair enzymes

Name	Mechanism	Comment
Rodent homologues		
XRCC1	Single strand break repair	CHO mutant EM9
	Activates DNA ligase III	
XRCC2	Double strand break rejoining	irs-1
XRCC3	Single strand break	
XRCC4	Double strand break. V(D)J recombination	XR-1
XRCC5	Double strand break. Ku80 ⎫ Heterodimer	xrs-5 and 6, sxi-3 and 2
XRCC6	Double strand break. Ku70 ⎬ binds to double strand break ends	sxi-1
XRCC7	Double strand break. Catalytic subunit of DNA-dependent protein kinase	scid1
XRCC8	Chromosomal stability	
Yeast homologues		
RAD6/HHR6	Post-replication repair	
RAD 51 ⎫	Double strand break repair	
52 ⎬	Meiotic recombination	
54 ⎭		
DNA	Single strand break and double strand break, replication	
ligase I	Form part of protein complex involved in repair	Uncertain human role
ligase II ⎫	Closely related ?Meiotic	
ligase III ⎬	?Base excision	Proliferating cells
ligase IV ⎭		
Poly (ADP ribose) polymerase	Levels rise in response to broken DNA strands. ? Damage recognition	
AP endonuclease	Damage excision	

' See text for abbreviations.

know that the extent to which a cell can deal with radiation damage differs between rapidly proliferating normal tissues and tumours, on the one hand, and the slowly proliferating normal tissues on the other. Some of these differences may be related to differences in the capacity to repair damage, at least at higher fractional doses. Acute-reacting tissues and tumours tend to have survival curves that are nearly exponential at higher doses, whereas, for late-reacting tissues, the survival curve at higher doses is much 'bendier', meaning that the amount of cell kill increases to a greater extent for each dose increment, meaning in turn an increased sensitivity to high fractional doses. Conversely, the use of decreasing fraction sizes rapidly increases the survival capacity (and presumably the repair ability) of the late-reacting tissues, with less dramatic effects for the tumour, increasing the therapeutic ratio. This concept is discussed further in the section on fractionation and normal tissue toxicity (see page 404).

These processes can be described in mathematical terms. Many cell survival data points are best fitted by a survival curve that has a linear (α) component of cell kill dominant at low doses and a quadratic component (β) in which the cell kill increases as the square of the dose. Late-reacting tissues have a more predominant β component than rapidly proliferating cells, either normal or tumour. Examples of survival curves with high and low β values are shown in Figure 21.5; a high β value confers a rapidly increasng amount of cell kill with increasing dose. Overall cell kill will be a balance between the linear component, thought to represent damage that is not repairable, and the quadratic component, which may be repaired.

Reoxygenation

Tumours larger than a few millimetres in size rely on neovascularisation for their further growth, and stimulate angiogenesis from the surrounding capillaries.

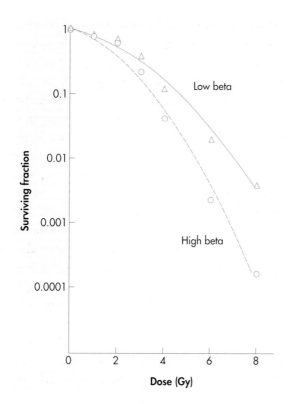

Figure 21.5 *The ability to repair 'sublethal' radiation damage varies between cell types. In some, this ability is rapidly overwhelmed with increasing doses, and these cell types will show higher levels of cell kill at higher fractional doses than those in which damage repair is less critical. Late-reacting tissues such as lung and spinal cord typically have high beta values and sensitivity to high doses per fraction.*

These tumour vessels are often fragile and collapsible, with little arterial tone, and this, together with a deranged growth pattern of stroma and tumour cells alike, leads to areas of hypoxia within tumours. Opening and closing of tumour vasculature is a dynamic process [4], leading to transient hypoxia, but the presence of oxygen in the few nanoseconds following ionisation is essential for the chemical fixation of radiation damage. Hypoxic cells are therefore protected from such damage.

The effects of oxygen and hypoxia can be demonstrated experimentally in mice bearing transplantable tumours and in cultured cell lines. Hypoxia is achieved either by clamping the tumour feeding vessels or by equilibrating tissue cultures in an oxygen-free environment prior to radiation. Subsequent clonogenic cell survival assay will show that the dose of radiation required to achieve the same cell kill under hypoxic as under oxygenated conditions is in

the order of two to three times greater [5]. Figure 21.6 illustrates the effects on clonogenic cell survival: the oxygen enhancement ratio (the ratio of isoeffective doses for cell kill) is 2.26.

The proportion of hypoxic cells within solid tumours may vary from a few per cent to the majority, depending on the tumour type. Although a dynamic process, the hypoxic proportion is thought to remain relatively constant within a given tumour. Immediately after a radiation exposure, the remaining viable cells are likely to be hypoxic, as cell kill will be predominantly of the oxygenated cell population. Over the following hours, reoxygenation occurs and the proportion of hypoxic cells returns to the baseline. The next exposure will have the same effect, but will kill some of the cells previously protected through hypoxia but which are now oxygenated. Over a prolonged fractionation schedule it is likely that most cells will receive at least a few exposures while in the oxygenated state.

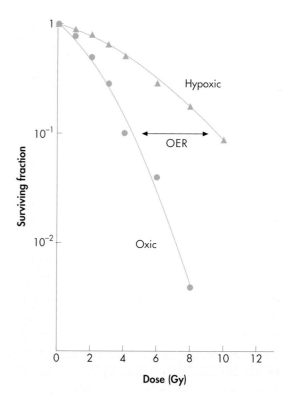

Figure 21.6 *The presence of oxygen at the time of ionisation fixes the initial damage, but in its absence the molecular events may be rapidly reversed, leading to increased cell survival. The oxygen enhancement ratio (OER) is the ratio of hypoxic to oxic dose required to achieve the same level of cell kill, and is typically around 2.5.*

Knowledge of the oxygen effect was one of the early biological observations to be exploited for therapeutic gain, but with unfortunately limited success. Several approaches have been adopted, all of which, with hindsight, would produce gains of a size difficult to detect in the clinical trials that were undertaken. The classic radiosensitisers are small molecules that diffuse readily through tissue and that mimic oxygen in damage fixation, but that are not metabolised and can therefore persist in the cell and obviate the need for the physical presence of oxygen. The nitroimidazoles such as misonidazole were first studied but had dose-limiting neurotoxicity at therapeutic concentrations. As such, they could be used with only a few fractions out of a radical treatment regimen and, not surprisingly, little benefit was demonstrated. Studies are continuing on subsequent generations of sensitisers, with reasonable grounds for optimism. Hyperbaric oxygen (at double atmospheric pressure) has been used to increase the physical perfusion of oxygen into hypoxic tissues, but is physically cumbersome and hazardous, and cannot be employed realistically on a large scale. The use of heavy particles such as neutrons bypasses the need for oxygen to be present for damage fixation; on the whole, clinical studies with neutrons have shown increased local tumour control at the expense of increased normal tissue toxicity, with little enhancement of therapeutic ratio.

More recently, the very presence of tumour hypoxia has been studied as a means of obtaining differential cytotoxicity between normal and tumour cells. There are several drugs that are non-toxic in an oxygenated environment and require activation in a hypoxic environment to become cytotoxic – the so-called bioreductive drugs [6]. There are also data that suggest that some cancer cells may have specific cytochrome P450 systems not commonly found in normal cells that may activate these drugs, providing another means of differential toxicity. This is an area of great experimental interest currently, but it is too early to interpret the clinical data.

Reassortment

Cellular sensitivity to radiation depends on the cell cycle status in two ways. Firstly, the DNA damage caused by radiation, although inflicted at the time of exposure, is frequently not revealed or expressed until the cell attempts to replicate its DNA prior to mitotic division. Cells that are out of cycle (G0) or cycling very slowly will not express damage immediately. Most tumour cells, however, are rapidly dividing, with potential cell cycle times of around 24 hours. In these, the timing between radiation fractions may be critical to the amount of cell kill obtained, as the sensitivity varies by at least twofold through the cycle. This is the second way that cellular sensitivity to radiation is dependent on cycle status. Cells are most sensitive to radiation in G2 and mitosis, slightly less so in G1, and become progressively radioresistant as the synthetic S phase progresses. The relative ratios of dose required to achieve equal cell kill in the different phases are illustrated in Figure 21.7.

Given the differing sensitivities, a single exposure to radiation will eliminate the sensitive cells and leave the more resistant cells as the majority of the surviving population. This in effect synchronises the residual cells with a surviving cohort in S phase. During subsequent hours, this cohort will move into G2 and M, at which time they will gain sensitivity. This is unfortunately almost impossible to exploit clinically as it is not possible to calculate or derive the cell cycle times in an individual tumour to predict when the sensitive phase will occur. In addition, the synchronisation is only partial, and the effect lessens as members of the surviving cohort progress through to mitosis at different rates.

Repopulation

A subject of increasing awareness and concern, the repopulation of tumour cells during the duration of a fractionated treatment course is one in which an understanding of the biological process can be exploited for clinical gain. For empirical reasons, including machine output and availability, numerous different fractionation schedules have been developed, using different total doses and different overall treatment times, which provide the same level of local tumour control. Schedules extending over six weeks or more include a higher total dose given in a number of smaller fractions compared with those given over three or four weeks, in which fraction size is larger and

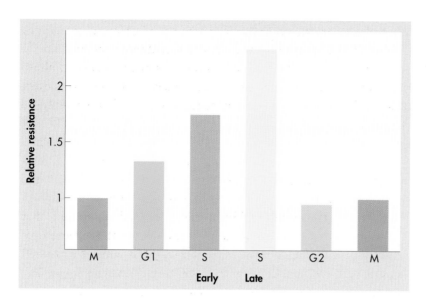

Figure 21.7 *Cells vary in their radiosensitivity according to their phase in the cell cycle, being most sensitive in G2 and M, and with resistance increasing as they enter the DNA synthetic phase.*

total dose lower. The possible advantages of using smaller fraction sizes are discussed below when considering normal tissue toxicity, but the difference in total dose required to achieve tumour control raises an interesting question: does the tumour continue to grow during a course of fractionated radiotherapy?

There are experimental data to suggest that the surviving irradiated cells at first experience cell cycle delay (presumably to allow DNA repair), but then recommence the mitotic cycle, and after several days the rate of cell division exceeds that prior to irradiation, succeeding in repopulating the tumour cell numbers [7]. This phenomenon of accelerated repopulation is also suspected in clinical practice. From published series in head and neck cancer and other tumour sites [8], it is possible to calculate the TCD50 (the radiation dose required to achieve local control in 50% of tumours) for different fractionation schedules. Until approximately three weeks of treatment have elapsed, little increase in TCD50 is noted (Figure 21.8). Prolonging treatment times beyond three weeks requires a rapid increase in the total dose delivered to achieve the same local control, suggesting that some of the dose is 'wasted' in overcoming the effects of emerging and accelerated tumour cell repopulation. Potential tumour-doubling times under these circumstances may be as short as three days. Assuming that the average radiation fraction dose of 2 Gy kills 50% of surviving cells, 0.6 Gy of radiation may be wasted each day in keeping pace with repopulation. Several

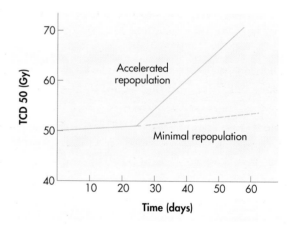

Figure 21.8 *Cell repopulation rates in untreated tumours are slow, but, under optimal circumstances, doubling times may be a short as three days. Under the stimulus of cytotoxic cell kill, tumour cells begin to divide rapidly, and this is reflected by the need to increase total doses to achieve equivalent tumour control rates as overall treatment times are prolonged.*

retrospective studies also suggest that unscheduled gaps in treatment (for example over Christmas) lead to reduced local control rates unless dose compensation is prescribed.

Efforts are being made to identify those tumour types in which accelerated repopulation is a clinical problem; these probably include all squamous carcinomas of the head and neck, carcinoma of the cervix and transitional cell carcinoma of the bladder, with prostatic carcinoma being relatively slowly proliferating. It is possible to calculate tumour potential doubling times as an indication of the capacity to repopulate rapidly, using the DNA-binding properties of BUDR, injected into the patient prior to tumour biopsy, and analysing the cell cycle distribution using a fluorescent anti-BUDR antibody and a FACS scanner. This has yet to become routinely available, and suffers from being labour intensive and from the possibility of the biopsy being unrepresentative of the tumour as a whole. It may, however, provide a useful tool to identify those patients who might benefit from a shortened or accelerated treatment schedule.

Clinical trials are underway for a number of tumour sites for which there are theoretical data to suggest that accelerated repopulation may be a significant factor in failure to achieve local tumour control. Rather than increase the total tumour dose to compensate for repopulation, with a corresponding effect on the normal tissues, multiple fractions of radiation per day may be used, which allows a roughly equivalent total dose to be delivered in a much shorter overall time period. The most compressed schedule yet evaluated [9] is CHART (continuous hyperfractionated accelerated radiotherapy) in which radical treatment doses are given over 12 days, treating three times a day and over weekends. Randomised data show a significant increase in local control in primary bronchial carcinoma, and a suggestion of benefit in head and neck cancer. The need to maintain an interfraction interval of at least six hours to allow maximal normal tissue recovery, and the prolonged working week make the routine application of CHART logistically difficult, and modifications are being developed for more routine use. It is nonetheless gratifying to see the scientific predictions being borne out in clinical practice, and better means of identifying those tumours (rather than patients) most likely to respond to this approach may make its use more acceptable because of significant clinical gain.

Normal tissue toxicity

It is self-evident that the maximum radiation dose that can be used to attempt to sterilise a tumour is limited by the tolerance of the surrounding normal tissues. Recent technological advances in diagnostic and planning systems have improved tumour localisation greatly and allow accurate beam direction, which can minimise the amount of normal tissue included in the target volume. It is never possible, however, to eliminate normal tissue completely, and inevitably treatment to a radical curative dose will involve some toxicity.

Normal tissues can be divided into two types, depending on the time of onset of the radiation reaction, which relates directly to the rate at which the stem cell population is dividing. Although radiation damages the DNA at the time a cell is exposed, that damage is not usually expressed until the cell attempts to enter mitosis, when it dies. (Only a minority of cell types undergo interphase programmed cell death – apoptosis.) Tissues that are constantly renewing and in which the stem cells are in cycle – namely, skin, mucosa, hair and bone marrow – will express radiation damage relatively soon after exposure. As the stem cell population becomes depleted, the integrity of the tissue it maintains is lost, and the reaction appears. For skin, erythema, dry and moist desquamation, and skin breakdown occur in an orderly progression, starting about ten days to two weeks after the start of a course of treatment and increasing in severity depending on dose. The effects on mucosa may appear more rapidly as the mucosal cells have a shorter cell cycle time and, similarly, the effects on marrow and other dividing tissues appear at a time reflecting their speed of cell division. When a treatment course ends, provided there are sufficient remaining normal stem cells, they can repopulate and restore integrity and function, again with healing occurring at a rate relative to the cell cycle time.

By contrast, in fully differentiated tissues there is no renewable cell compartment; the injured cells may die months or years after the radiation insult, are not replaced as they die, and the tissue expresses damage permanently. All tissues may also be damaged by late effects of radiation on the vasculature, inducing endarteritis obliterans in smaller vessels and damaging the blood supply. Damage to late-reacting tissues may be devastating because it is permanent, but also because good function is critical in many of these organs. Spinal cord damage, for example, results in demyelination [10] and paraplegia; lung damage leads to fibrosis; kidney irradiation may cause renal failure and hypertension. In planning radiotherapy, it is essential to keep the volumes of these normal tissues and the doses they receive to a minimum. There is a fine balance between giving the best possible chance of cure (the highest possible radiation dose) and exceeding normal tissue tolerance; with a curative treatment, the maximum doses prescribed are those that are unlikely to cause serious late side-effects (those requiring intervention) in more than 2–3% of patients.

There is a second fundamental difference between acute-reacting or early-reacting tissues and the late-reacting ones: the changing response of the tissues with change in fraction size. As described in the section on recovery from radiation damage, one component of cell kill increases with the square of the radiation dose, thought to be the component that the cell can repair if radiation is given in small doses, but which is overwhelmed at higher doses. This component (β) is usually larger in the late-reacting tissues, so that if fractional dose is increased, the level of cell kill increases rapidly. The use of small fraction sizes, or hyperfractionation, allows relative sparing of the late-reacting tissues as tumours tend to behave as acute reactors. The reasons for the differences are not clear.

In clinical practice, hyperfractionation of a radical dose schedule generally requires the use of multiple fractions per day to avoid prolongation of the overall treatment time. The improvement in therapeutic ratio gained by a reduction in fraction size can be used either to reduce normal tissue toxicity while maintaining equivalent tumour control, or to dose escalate (with the hope of increasing local control) while keeping a constant rate of complications. Pilot studies of the latter approach, with dose escalation up to 84 Gy for carcinoma of the bladder, have been reported to improve local control and survival, but more studies are needed to confirm the validity of this approach.

Molecular radiobiology

DNA damage

The lesions inflicted on DNA by ionising radiation are single-strand and double-strand breaks, the latter being thought to be the lethal lesion. The presence of strand breaks can be detected using a variety of experimental techniques, including neutral and alkaline elution of DNA, which alter conformation and allow small DNA fragments to be eluted by filtration, whilst intact strands are not. There has been much debate as to whether variations in cellular sensitivity can be attributed to differences in the amount of initial damage inflicted, and the experimental data obtained using such assays suggest that variation in the amount of damage is critical for some cell lines, but not for others. Interpretation may be clouded by possible differences in the type of critical lesion inflicted; a double-strand break in which the two ends overlap (sticky) is less likely to be lethal than one in which there is no overlap (blunt). Clusters of ionisations occurring together (locally multiply damaged sites) may be particularly difficult for a cell to cope with.

It is also suggested that not all damage to different parts of the genome is equally as effective in causing cell kill. Damage to thymine bases occurs more commonly in replicating than in quiescent DNA, and DNA protein cross-links, which may impede function, are also more common in actively transcribing regions. It is also likely that certain genes are more vulnerable to radiation insult than others, and damage in these will be more critical for cell survival than damage in some other areas [11].

Repair of DNA damage

Intense research activity over the last few years has allowed the identification of a number of enzymes and genes involved in mammalian DNA repair [12]. Many such enzymes and genes have been identified because of striking homology with yeast repair genes, for example *HHR6* (human homologue to the yeast gene *RAD6*), which is involved in post-replication repair of DNA damage. Other genes have been identified in rodent strains exhibiting particular sensitivity to ionising radiation. The use of cross-complementation techniques – in which DNA from one cell type is transfected into a deficient line, which will lose its sensitive phenotype if the gene involved has been replaced by the normal allele through transfection – has identified a number of genes implicated in repair. More are being identified, and the picture is rapidly increasing in complexity. Table 21.1 includes a number of the genes whose activity has been identified with reasonable certainty.

The X-ray cross-complementing (XRCC) genes have been studied in a number of sensitive rodent mutants. Scid (severe combined immune deficiency) mice have an autosomal recessive mutation which impairs both V(D)J recombination and DSB repair. Two other XRCC genes, 5 and 6, produce proteins that are components of the Ku antigen complex, deficient in xrs (X-ray sensitive) and sxi mice. Together with the product of XRCC7, which is a catalytic subunit of this DNA-dependent protein kinase, the Ku antigen is an essential component of the recombination repair pathway. Others in this group are involved in single-strand break repair. The analysis of genes involved in the nucleotide excision repair pathway has shown a strong resemblance between genes from yeast and humans, suggesting a functional conservation of DNA repair. While several human homologues to the yeast RAD repair genes have now been identified, their functions are as yet generally unknown. Another group of genes involved in repair is the DNA ligase group, of which DNA ligase I is the major ligase in proliferating cells and is strongly implicated in DNA replication and repair. Mutations in this gene have been identified in fibroblasts isolated from an immunodeficient patient who also exhibited sensitivity to sunlight.

The classic clinical syndrome associated with hypersensitivity to ionising radiation is ataxia telangiectasia, in which patients develop a number of abnormalities, including cerebellar degeneration and telangiectasis, but are also cancer prone because of defective DNA repair [13]. Although a rare autosomal recessive syndrome, ataxia telangiectasia has received an enormous amount of attention, firstly, because the heterozygous population appears to have an increased cancer risk, and, secondly, because the syndrome provides a means to study abnormal radiosensitivity in human cells. Ataxia telangiectasia cells, for example, are known to lack the normal radiation-induced delay in transition from G1 to S phase in the cell cycle, and they may also exhibit increased conversion of double strand breaks to chromosome breaks, implicating defects in recombinational repair. The gene has recently been identified [14], and is likely to be a critical regulator of many important cellular processes. The ATM protein has strong similarity to the cell signal proteins phosphoinositol-3 kinases, which mediate a number of growth factor responses. Another part of the protein has homology to yeast DNA repair proteins, providing a possible explanation for the sensitivity to ionising radiation. Several complementation groups had previously been identified in ataxia telangiectasia families, which had suggested that several mutant genes might contribute to the clinical syndrome; it is more likely that these represent different mutations within the one gene.

p53 and ionising radiation

Cell death through apoptosis is now widely recognised as a normal cellular response to environmental insult [15]. Numerous genes are involved in the regulation of the cell cycle, of which p53 has received most attention. Known as the 'guardian of the genome', it stops a cell from entering the cell cycle if DNA damage is detected, to prevent replication of the damage, and apoptosis is initiated if the damage is incompatible with repair. Although many cells do not show apoptosis, this mode of cell death can be triggered by some types of DNA damage caused by ionising radiation. This process may be disrupted in malignancy in several ways. One of the common late mutations in malignant cells is mutation of p53, which increases its cellular stability but prevents its normal activity. This promotes longevity of the cell, and also removes one mechanism by which radiation-damaged cells succumb, producing radiation resistance [16]. Another acquired mechanism that may block the normal apoptotic response is seen with over-expression of the bcl-2 oncogene (initially described in lymphoma but subsequently identified in many solid tumours), which prevents radiation-induced apoptosis. This may be particularly important in prostate cancer as increased bcl-2 expression is found in androgen-insensitive cells compared with their sensitive counterparts.

References

1. Withers HR. The four Rs of radiotherapy. Adv Radiat Biol 1975; 5: 241–7

2. Elkind MM, Sutton H. Radiation response of mammalian cells grown in culture. I. Repair of X-ray damage in surviving Chinese hamster cells. Radiat Res 1960; 13: 566–93

3. Steel GG, Down J, Peacock JH, Stephens TC. Dose–rate effects and the repair of radiation damage. Int J Radiat Biol 1986; 61: 479–87

4. Chaplin DJ, Durand E, Olive PL. Acute hypoxia in tumours: implication for modifiers of radiation effects. Int J Radiat Oncol Biol Phys 1986; 12: 1279–82

5. Wright EA, Howard-Flanders P. The influence of oxygen on the radiosensitivity of mammalian tissues. Acta Radiol 1957; 48: 26–32

6. Stratford IJ, Adams EG, Bremner JC, et al. Manipulation and exploitation of the tumour environment for therapeutic benefit. Int J Radiat Biol 1994; 65: 85–94

7. Begg AC. Prediction of repopulation rates and radiosensitivity of human tumours. Int J Radiat Biol 1994; 65: 103–8

8. Bentzen SM, Thames HD. Clinical evidence for tumor clonogen regeneration: interpretations of the data. Radiother Oncol 1991; 22: 161–6

9. Saunders MI. Fractionation and dose in thoracic radiotherapy. Lung Cancer 1994; 10 (Suppl 1): 245–52

10. Ang KK, Price RE, Stephens LC, et al. The tolerance of primate spinal cord to re-irradiation. Int J Radiat Oncol Biol Phys 1993; 25: 459–64

11. Powell S, McMillan TJ. DNA damage and repair following treatment with ionising radiation. Radiother Oncol 1990; 19: 95–108

12. McMillan TJ, Peacock JH. Molecular determinants of radiosensitivity in mammalian cells. Int J Radiat Biol 1994; 65: 49–56

13. Taylor AMR, Byrd PJ, McConville CM, Thacker S. Genetic and cellular features of ataxia telangiectasia. Int J Radiat Biol 1994; 65: 65–70

14. Savitsky K, Bar-Shira A, Gilad S, et al. A single ataxia telangiectasia gene with a product similar to PI-3 kinase. Science 1995; 269: 1749–53

15. D'Amico AV, McKenna WG. Apoptosis and a re-investigation of the biologic basis for cancer therapy. Radiother Oncol 1994; 33: 3–10

16. Lowe SW, Bodis S, McClatchey A, et al. p53 status and the efficacy of cancer therapy in vivo. Science 1994; 266: 801–10

Further reading

G. Gordon Steel. Basic clinical radiobiology. London: Edward Arnold, 1993

Embryology

22

D. F. M. Thomas

Introduction

Embryology provides the key to understanding the congenital anomalies and inherited disorders encountered in urological practice. Supplemented by additional information from scanning electron microscopy and immunocytochemistry, 'conventional' embryology provides us with a detailed picture of the developmental anatomy of the embryo and fetus. Now, equipped with the powerful new research methods of molecular biology, notably polymerase chain reaction and fluorescent in-situ hybridisation, researchers are in a position to study the genetic mechanisms regulating this complex and tightly ordered anatomical sequence. In addition to the task of mapping and sequencing genes, research is underway to isolate the many gene products responsible for implementing the genetic 'programme' encoded on DNA at a cellular and molecular level. The successful culture of pluripotent embryonic stem cells has been reported recently [1]. This exciting breakthrough may ultimately pave the way to the use of a wide range of human cells for tissue reconstruction or regenerative repair. Advances in the new science of developmental biology will create new opportunities for the diagnosis, prevention and possible treatment of inherited disorders and genetically determined anomalies of the genitourinary system. But these opportunities will be inevitably accompanied by new responsibilities and ethical dilemmas. Much of this chapter is devoted to a practical, clinically orientated account of developmental anatomy, but it would be incomplete without some consideration of genetics and the rapidly advancing field of developmental biology.

Fertilisation and early development of the human embryo

Human gestation spans the period from fertilisation to birth – an average of 38 weeks. Obstetricians conventionally subdivide pregnancy into three, three-month trimesters. Embryogenesis, the formation of organs and systems, occurs principally between the third and tenth week. Subsequent development throughout the rest of fetal life is characterised by the processes of differentiation, branching, maturation and growth.

Fertilisation is defined by fusion of the nuclear material of the fertilising spermatozoa and the definitive oocyte. The process of gametogenesis, whereby spermatozoa and oocytes develop from their germ cell precursors, is considered below. In males, spermatogenesis is a continuing process initiated at puberty. In contrast, the initial phases of female gametogenesis occur in fetal life, and primary oocytes remain dormant in the prophase of the first meiotic division until the onset of puberty. During each ovulatory cycle, under the influence of follicle-stimulating hormone, a small number of primary oocytes resume meitoic activity, but of these, only one usually progresses to maturity as a Graafian follicle. At the mid-point of the menstrual cycle, the primary oocyte destined for ovulation transforms into a secondary oocyte by proceeding into the remaining phases of the long-arrested first meiotic division. Protected by the zona pellucida, the secondary oocyte is extruded from the surface of the ovary, from where it is drawn into the reproductive tract by the fimbriae of the Fallopian tube. Of an ejaculate totalling perhaps 40–100 million spermatozoa, only a few hundred are destined to complete the journey up the female reproductive canal to come into potential contact with the ovulated oocyte.

Penetration by the fertilising spermatozoon of the zona pellucida surrounding the secondary oocyte triggers the second meiotic division, which results in the formation of the definitive oocyte and an aggregate of non-functional DNA known as a polar body.

The normal human karyotype comprises a total of 23 pairs of chromosomes, i.e. 22 pairs of autosomes and one pair of sex chromosomes, either XX (female) or XY (male). As a result of the two meiotic divisions, each gamete (the spermatozoon or definitive oocyte) carries only half the normal complement of chromosomes, i.e. 22 unpaired autosomes and either an X or Y sex chromosome. Fusion of the haploid nuclei of the two gametes at the time of fertilisation imparts diploid status (i.e. 22 pairs of autosomes plus two sex chromosomes) to the nucleus of the fertilised zygote. From the time of fertilisation, the journey down the Fallopian tube to the site of implantation in the primed uterine endometrium takes five to six days (Figure 22.1). During this journey, the fertilised zygote undergoes a series of cell divisions termed cleavage. By the fourth day, sequential cleavage has created a 32-cell embryo, classically likened to a berry (hence the Latin-derived description 'morula'). Further cell division is accompanied by structural differentiation and the formation of a sphere-like blastocyst. It is at this stage in development that the embryo implants into the uterine endometrium, six days after fertilisation.

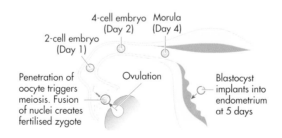

Figure 22.1 *Key stages in the five to six days from fertilisation to implantation.*

Chromosomal abnormalities: clinical considerations

A detailed account of the pathogenesis and clinical manifestations of chromosomal abnormalities arising during gametogenesis and cleavage is beyond the scope of this chapter. Major chromosomal abnormalities are common, but most result in the death of the embryo and spontaneous abortion at an early stage in pregnancy. The most serious chromosomal abnormalities consistent with survival to term are the trisomies, notably trisomy 21 – Down's syndrome. The trisomy state occurs when an additional chromosome or portion of a chromosome becomes incorporated into the nucleus of a gamete by non-disjunction or translocation. Non-disjunction refers to the faulty separation of a pair of chromosomes during meiotic or mitotic cell division. In translocation, paired chromosomes separate completely but one of the pair, or a fragment thereof, becomes inadvertently attached to another unrelated chromosome and is thus retained within the haploid nucleus. Non-disjunction of the X and Y sex chromosomes during gametogenesis accounts for a number of genetically determined syndromes, notably Turner's syndrome (45 X0 karyotype) and Klinefelter's syndrome (47 XXY). Not surprisingly, the gross genetic imbalance created by the presence of so much additional replicated DNA within the zygote nucleus is reflected in profound disturbances of embryogenesis across a number of systems, including the genitourinary tract. The incidence of coexistent renal anomalies ranges from approximately 5% in Down's syndrome (trisomy 21) to 75% in Turner's syndrome (45 X0) (Table 22.1).

Non-disjunction and translocation anomalies are not confined to gametogenesis, but can also arise during the early mitotic cell divisions in the process of cleavage. In the resulting state, termed mosaicism, the embryonic tissues contain a varying ratio of chromosomally normal and abnormal cells, depending on the phase of cleavage at which non-disjunction occurred, e.g. two-cell, four-cell, eight-cell embryo etc. Abnormalities of the sex chromosomes are often found in mosaic form. True hermaphroditism can be explained on this basis. Affected individuals possess both ovarian (XX) and testicular (XY) tissue, coexisting in

Table 22.1 Chromosome defects associated with urinary tract anomalies

Chromosome defect or syndrome	Frequency (%)	Genito-urinary anomalies
Turner's syndrome 45X	60–80	Horseshoe kidney Duplication
Trisomy 18 (Edwards' syndrome)	70	Horseshoe kidney Renal ectopia Duplication Hydronephrosis
Trisomy 13 (Patau syndrome)	60–80	Cystic kidney Hydronephrosis Horseshoe kidney Ureteric duplication
4p (Wolf–Hirschorn syndrome)	33	Hypospadias Cystic kidney Hydronephrosis
Trisomy 21 (Down's syndrome)	3–7	Renal agenesis Horseshoe kidney

streak-like ovotestes. Gonadal mesenchyme carrying a Y chromosome differentiates as testicular tissue, whereas tissue derived from the original population of non-Y embryonic cells differentiates passively down the female (ovarian) pathway. Karyotypes show a varied pattern including 45 X/46 XY, 46 XX/ 47 XXY, etc. Turner's syndrome and Klinefelter's syndrome are often associated with mosaic karyotypes.

Implantation and early embryonic development

On the fifth or sixth day after fertilisation, having journeyed down the Fallopian tube, the blastocyst implants into the endometrium of the uterine cavity – which has been primed by progesterone. Over the ensuing ten days, two cavities are formed within the spherical mass of rapidly proliferating embryonic cells. The embryonic disc, from which the embryo itself originates, develops in the three-layered interface between the amniotic cavity and definitive yolk sac. The amniotic surface of the trilaminar embryonic disc gives rise to the ectodermal tissues of the embryo, whereas the endodermal derivatives originate from the yolk sac-derived surface. The intraembryonic mesoderm is formed by the inpouring of cells on the amniotic surface of the disc via the primitive streak (Figure 22.2). The layer of intraembryonic mesoderm created by the inpouring process soon subdivides into three components, i.e. paraxial mesoderm, intermediate mesoderm and lateral plate mesoderm. It is from this intermediate mesoderm that much of the genitourinary tract is ultimately derived. The third and fourth weeks of gestation are dominated by the processes of segmentation and somite formation that characterise all vertebrate embryogenesis. At this stage, folding of the expanding embryonic disc imparts recognisable shape to the growing embryo.

Embryology of the upper urinary tract

The kidneys are derived from the caudal zones of the paired columns of intermediate mesoderm flanking the midline. The emergence of the metanephros, the

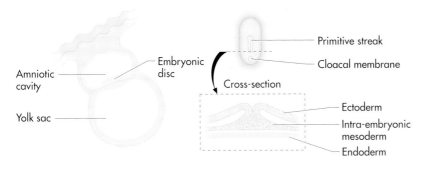

Figure 22.2 *The embryonic disc at 16 days. Inpouring of cells at the primitive streak creates the intra-embryonic mesoderm from which the genitourinary tract is formed.*

precursor of the definitive kidney, is preceded by the formation of the pronephros and mesonephros – primitive kidney-like structures. During the fourth week of gestation, the primitive pronephros appears in the cervical portion of the intermediate mesoderm but rapidly undergoes regression. Later in the fourth week, nephron-like tubular structures appear in the mid-section of intermediate mesoderm – the mesonephros (Figure 22.3a). Concurrently, condensations of mesenchyme lying lateral to the developing mesonephros become the mesonephric ducts. These advance caudally to fuse with the cloaca (the terminal portion of hindgut destined to give rise to the bladder by the process of subdivision). Canalisation of the mesonephric duct creates a patent excretory unit, which is believed to function briefly by producing very small quantities of urine. The beginning of the fifth week sees the appearance of the ureteric buds (Figure 22.3b), arising from the most distal portion of the paired mesonephric ducts. At around 32 days, the advancing ureteric bud makes contact with the metanephros and the interactive process of nephrogenesis commences (Figure 22.4). During the sixth to ninth week, the lobulated embryonic kidneys ascend up the posterior abdominal wall from their caudal sites of origin to their definitive lumbar position.

Nephrogenesis

The process whereby nephron units are created within the embryonic and fetal kidney spans a period of approximately 30 weeks, from the sixth to the thirty sixth week of gestation. The ureteric bud and the metanephric mesenchyme each make specific contributions to the definitive structure of the kidney. Sequential branching of the ureteric bud gives rise to the renal pelvis, the major calices, the minor calices and the collecting ducts. Within the metanephric mesenchyme, differentiating cells aggregate to form the glomeruli, convoluted tubules and loop of Henle. At around the tenth week, the distal convoluted tubules (derived from metanephric mesenchyme) establish continuity with the collecting ducts (of ureteric bud origin) to establish functional excretory units. Branching and budding of the ureteric bud derivatives cease at around 15 weeks but, within the fetal renal cortex, new generations of nephrons continue to appear until the cessation of nephrogenesis at 36 weeks. The process of tubular differentiation within the metanephric mesenchyme is initiated by contact with the ureteric bud. Similarly, proliferative budding and branching of the ureteric bud tissues are dependent upon induction by the metanephric mesenchyme. When grown in tissue culture in isolation, neither of these embryonic tissues has the capacity to differentiate into nephron-like structures. However, when cultured together, nephrogenesis is observed. The identity of the gene products responsible for mediating the cell to cell signalling at a molecular level is being extensively studied in tissue culture, organ culture and genetically engineered transgenic mice. The following have been shown to play a role in regulating nephrogenesis [2]:

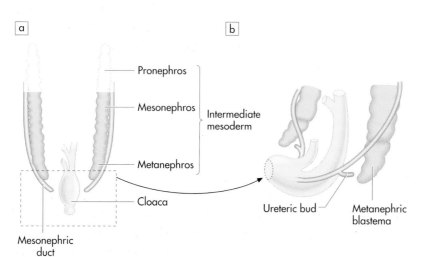

Figure 22.3 *(a) Following the regression of the pronephros, the mesonephros assumes prominence before the emergence of the metanephros as the definitive embryonic kidney. (b) At around 28 days, the ureteric buds appear and advance towards the metanephric mesenchyme.*

Pronephros

Mesonephros

Intermediate mesoderm

Metanephros

Cloaca

Mesonephric duct

Ureteric bud

Metanephric blastema

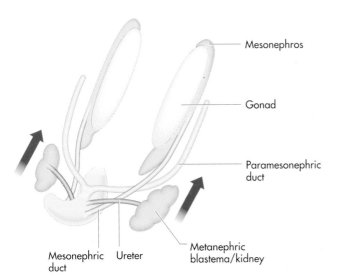

Mesonephros

Gonad

Paramesonephric duct

Mesonephric duct   Ureter   Metanephric blastema/kidney

Figure 22.4 Five to seven weeks: penetration of the metanephric mesenchyme promotes nephrogenesis by a process of mutual induction. Mesonephric tissues support the development of the embryonic gonads in the genital ridges. The paramesonephric ducts develop in the mesenchyme adjacent to the mesonephric ducts.

growth factors, e.g. fibroblast growth factor 2, glial cell line-derived neurotrophic factor: substances such as tumour necrosis factor α act as negative growth factors by promoting apoptosis (programmed cell death);

transcription factors: these are DNA-binding proteins that regulate gene expression, e.g. WT1 protein;

adhesion molecules responsible for cell to cell adhesion and cell to matrix adhesion, e.g. laminins and integrins.

Congenital renal malformations: clinical considerations

Four broad morphological categories can be defined:

1. renal agenesis – total absence of the kidney;
2. renal dysplasia – a kidney is present, although it is often abnormal in size: the internal architecture is disordered and the histological appearances typically include areas of immature, primitive, 'undifferentiated' tubules and the inappropriate presence of tissues such as cartilage and fibromuscular tissue within the renal parenchyma;
3. cyst formation;

4. gross developmental anomalies, e.g. duplication, horseshoe kidney, pelvic kidney.

Ureteric duplication is readily explained on the basis of bifurcation of the ureteric bud [3]. Depending on the level of the original bifurcation, the duplication may be complete or incomplete. In cases of complete ureteric duplication, the upper pole ureter paradoxically joins the urinary tract more distally than the lower pole ureter. This anatomical pattern (described by the Mayer Weigert law) occurs when the Müllerian duct separates from the embryonic ureter and its terminal portion descends towards the primitive posterior urethra (with a tendency to take the upper pole ureter with it). Gross renal anomalies such as horseshoe kidney, pelvic kidney and crossed ectopia date from the period of ascent, during which embryonic kidneys may fuse (horseshoe kidney), cross the midline (crossed fused ectopia) or fail to ascend (pelvic kidney).

Pathogenesis of renal malformations

Various mechanisms or aetiological insults have been invoked to explain the patterns of renal malformations described above. The adult and infant forms of polycystic renal disease provide the most convincing examples of genetically determined structural renal disease. Genetic factors have also been implicated in the aetiology of renal agenesis, vesicoureteric reflux and upper tract duplication. In the majority of instances, however, renal malformations are believed to occur on a sporadic basis. Malformations of the upper tract may be the result of an intrinsic abnormality of the metanephros, defects of the ureteric bud, or exposure of the embryonic or fetal kidney to the mechanical effects of obstruction or reflux.

Embryology of the lower urinary tract (bladder and urethra)

The bladder and urethra originate from the anterior portion of the cloaca, the common terminal section of hindgut into which the mesonephric ducts and embryonic ureters drain. The cloaca also contributes the urogenital sinus – which in turn contributes to the vagina. Between the fourth and sixth weeks of gestation, the urorectal septum descends in a shutter-like fashion to subdivide the cloaca into the urogenital canal anteriorly and the anorectal canal posteriorly (Figure 22.5). The process of compartmentalisation initiated by the urorectal septum is aided by the lateral in-growth of the folds of Rathke. When the bladder is taking shape in the upper portion of the urogenital canal, the points of entry of the ureter and mesonephric ducts begin to separate (Figure 22.6). As the distance between them increases, the mesonephric ducts descend caudally to open into the developing posterior urethra. In contrast, the ureters retain their original position with respect to the developing bladder. Although the triangular plate of mesoderm enclosing the ureteric orifices and openings of the mesonephric ducts is covered by the endodermal lining of the urogenital canal, its outline is retained as the trigone. The most distal (perineal) portion of the urogenital canal gives rise to the entire length of the female urethra and to the posterior urethra in the male. The anterior portion of the male urethra is created by closure of the urogenital groove, described below. The allantois, an elongated diverticulum, protruding from the dome of the fetal bladder into the umbilicus, is gradually obliterated but persists as the median umbilical ligament.

Clinical considerations

Failed or incomplete descent of the urorectal septum results in a spectrum of anomalies ranging from urogenital sinus to a complete persistent cloaca [4]. The aetiology of bladder exstrophy and epispadias is incompletely understood, but these anomalies are believed to reflect underlying defects of the cloacal membrane. Persistence of all or part of the allantois gives rise to the various urachal abnormalities.

Functional development of the fetal urinary tract

From the ninth or tenth week of gestation, fetal urine is excreted into the amniotic cavity. Initially, the composition of fetal urine closely resembles that of plasma filtrate. In intrauterine life, the excretory and homeostatic functions of the kidney are fulfilled by the placenta and the principal role of the fetal kidneys is to contribute urine to amniotic fluid. The volume of amniotic fluid reaches its maximum of around

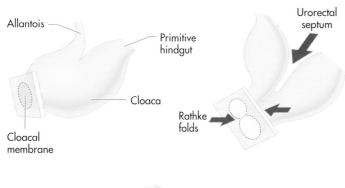

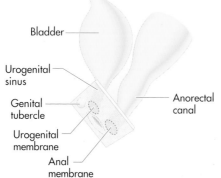

Figure 22.5 *Descent of the urorectal septum between four and six weeks divides the cloaca into an anterior urogenital compartment, the precursor of the bladder, urethra, prostate and distal vagina, and a posterior anorectal canal.*

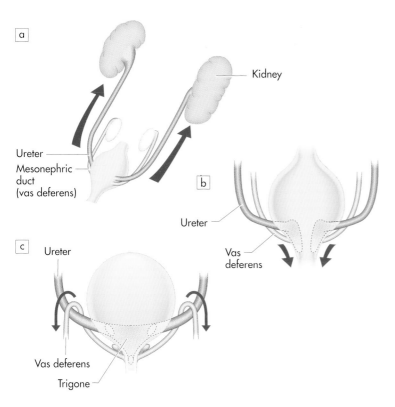

Figure 22.6 *(a) and (b) Although the ureters maintain their position in relation to the developing bladder, the mesonephric ducts are drawn distally to enter the proximal urethra. (c) Testicular descent causes the mesonephric ducts (vasa deferentia) to loop over the ureters.*

1000 ml at 38 weeks' gestation – at which point fetal urine comprises 90% of the amniotic fluid. As well as providing a protective fluid environment for the fetus, amniotic fluid plays a vital role in fetal lung development. When fetal urine output is reduced, as a result of either renal agenesis or infravesical obstruction, the resulting oligohydramnios is associated with pulmonary hypoplasia. Moulding or compression deformities can be produced by the compressive effect of the surrounding uterus.

Genital tracts

The internal and external genitalia of both sexes are formed from identical embryonic precursors and it is only from the sixth week onwards that differences begin to appear. In both sexes, the formation of the gonads and genital tracts is initiated by the migration of primordial germ cells from the base of the yolk sac, across the coelomic cavity to condensations of mesenchyme flanking the midline of the lumbar region of the embryo (Figure 22.7). The arrival of the primordial germ cells in these zones of mesenchyme stimulates the formation of the paired genital ridges. By a

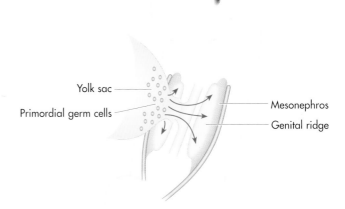

Figure 22.7 *Migration of the primordial germ cells from the yolk sac across the coelomic cavity to colonise the mesoderm of the genital ridges during the fifth week.*

process of mutual induction (analogous to nephrogenesis), the interaction of the germ cells and surrounding mesenchyme results in the formation of the primitive sex cords within the embryonic gonad. It is around this time that a second pair of potential genital ducts (the paramesonephric ducts) makes its appearance. Derived from condensations of coelomic epithelium and lying lateral to the mesonephric ducts, these ducts fuse distally at their point of attachment to the urogenital canal. From the sixth week onwards, the paths of male and female differentiation diverge.

Female

Unless the genetic information carried by the testis-determining gene (SRY) is present, the gonads and genital tract of the embryo are programmed to differentiate down a female pathway. The primitive sex cords degenerate but secondary sex cords derived from genital ridge mesoderm enclose the primordial germ cells to form the primitive follicles. In contrast to male gametogenesis, which does not commence until

puberty, in a female the first half of this process, the transition from primordial germ cell to primary oocyte, is completed in the fetal ovary. During fetal life, the primary oocytes undergo the first phase of meiosis before entering a long phase of arrested division, which only resumes again after puberty (Figure 22.8). Without the influence of testosterone, the mesonephric ducts regress (with the exception of vestigial remnants of the epoophoron and paroophoron and Gartner's cysts). The paramesonephric ducts persist and develop to become the Fallopian tubes. Their merged distal portions give rise to the uterus and upper two-thirds of the vagina (Figure 22.9). At their point of attachment to the urogenital sinus, the fused tips of the paramesonephric ducts

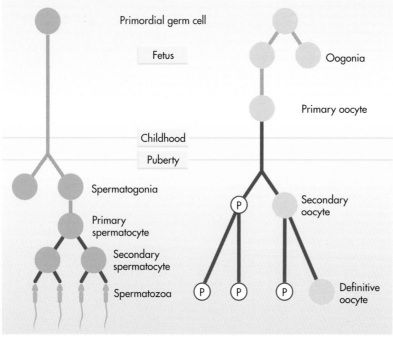

Figure 22.8 Gametogenesis. Mitotic division of the primordial germ cells in the male embryo is suppressed by the Sertoli cells of the embryonic germinal epithelium. Gametogenesis recommences at puberty. The gametes (spermatozoa) are the product of two meiotic divisions, i.e. primary spermatocyte to secondary spermatocyte and secondary spermatocyte to spermatozoa. Immediately after the second meiotic division, the immature haploid gametes are termed spermatids. The morphological maturation to spermatozoa occurs during passage through the seminiferous epithelium into the lumen of the seminiferous tubule. In the female, the initial phases of gametogenesis occur in the first five months of fetal life. Primary oocytes remain in arrested meiotic division until meiosis recommences in the maturing Graafian follicle. The two meiotic divisions culminate in the production of a single definitive oocyte and three polar bodies (P).

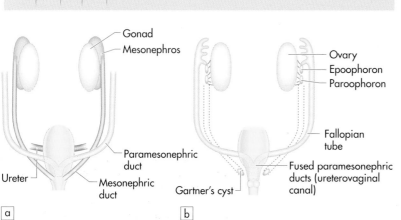

Figure 22.9 (a) The genital tract of both male and female embryos remains in the same undifferentiated state until the sixth week of gestation. (b) Paramesonephric duct derivatives in the female embryo.

induce a condensation of tissue – the sinuvaginal bulb. Downward growth of the sinuvaginal bulb in the direction of the fetal perineum between the tenth and twentieth weeks has the effect of separating the vagina from the urethra. The vagina is initially represented by a solid plate of paramesonephric tissue, but a lumen develops before the twentieth week. The distal third of the vagina is derived from the urogenital sinus (endoderm), whereas the introitus and external genitalia are ectodermal in origin (Figure 22.10).

External genitalia

The external genitalia of the embryo and fetus are 'programmed' to differentiate down a female pathway unless exposed to androgenic stimulation. Thus, the genital tubercle forms the clitoris, the urogenital sinus contributes the vestibule of the vagina, the urogenital folds evolve into the labia minora, and the labioscrotal folds persist as the labia majora.

Male

Although many aspects of the male differentiation pathway are mediated by 'downstream' genes, the process is initiated by a single testis-determining gene (SRY) located on the Y chromosome [5]. It is believed that the testis-determining factor encoded on this gene stimulates the medullary sex cords of the embryonic gonad to differentiate into secretory Sertoli cells. From the seventh week onwards, the Sertoli cells secrete a glycoprotein – anti-Müllerian hormone or Müllerian-inhibiting substance – which switches differentiation down the male pathway. At least three key functions have been ascribed to Müllerian-inhibiting substance [6]:

it causes regression of the paramesonephric ducts: with the exception of vestigial remnants (the appendix testis and the utriculus), the paramesonephric ducts disappear completely in the male;

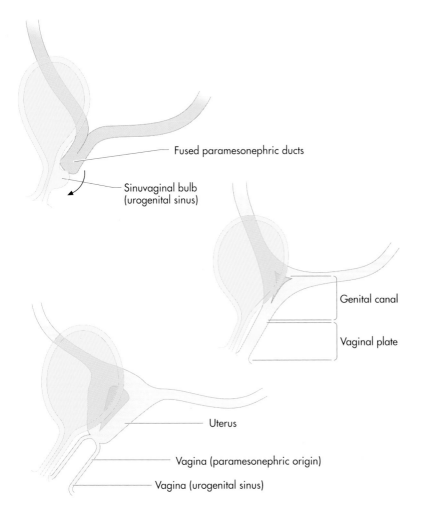

Fused paramesonephric ducts

Sinuvaginal bulb (urogenital sinus)

Genital canal

Vaginal plate

Uterus

Vagina (paramesonephric origin)

Vagina (urogenital sinus)

Figure 22.10 *Development of the lower female genital tract between 10 and 20 weeks. Migration of the sinuvaginal bulb towards the fetal perineum results in formation and elongation of the vaginal plate and separation of the vagina from the urethra.*

it stimulates the production of testosterone by the Leydig cells of the embryonic testis from the ninth week of gestation;

it induces the first stage of testicular descent by its action on the gubernaculum, which anchors the testis in the vicinity of the developing inguinal canal.

Further division of the primordial germ cells is inhibited in the male embryonic gonad, and the subsequent steps in gametogenesis are only resumed again at puberty. Regression of the paramesonephric ducts in response to Müllerian-inhibiting substance is accompanied by the development of mesonephric duct derivatives under the influence of testosterone secreted by the fetal testis (Figure 22.11a). In a process spanning the eighth to twelfth weeks of gestation, the mesonephric ducts give rise to the epididymis and rete testis, vas deferens, ejaculatory ducts and seminal vesicles (Figure 22.11b). Within the testis, the seminiferous tubules take their origin from the primitive sex cords of the genital ridge mesoderm.

The development of the prostate gland [7] provides another example of reciprocal induction. At around the twelfth week, in response to androgenic stimulation, a condensation of mesenchyme in the fetal pelvis induces the outgrowth of endodermal buds on the adjacent region of the developing urethra. Interestingly, in the experimental setting, transitional epithelium from the adult rat can be induced to differentiate into prostatic glandular epithelium when cultured in contact with the appropriate embryonic mesenchyme. In normal fetal development, however, the endodermal proliferation and branching that give rise to the ducts and glandular acini of the prostate gland are switched off after the fifteenth week of gestation. The glandular tissue of the prostate is derived from urethral (urogenital sinus) endoderm, the capsule and smooth muscle are mesenchymal in origin, whereas the mesonephric ducts form the intraprostatic vas deferens and ejaculatory ducts.

External genitalia (Figure 22.12)

Prior to the compartmentalisation of the cloaca into the urogenital and anorectal canals between the sixth and seventh weeks, the primitive perineum consists of little more than the cloacal membrane and genital tubercle. Separation of the cloaca into the urogenital canal and anorectal canal is accompanied by subdivision of the cloacal membrane into the urogenital membrane anteriorly and the anal membrane posteriorly. Urogenital folds surround the urogenital membrane, flanked by the labioscrotal folds. From the seventh week onwards, the urogenital sinus advances onto the perineum anteriorly and onto the penis as the urethral groove. Ingrowth of the urethral groove creates a solid urethral plate, which subsequently canalises to form the definitive urethra. The differentiation of the male external genitalia is dependent, firstly, upon the enzymatic conversion of testosterone to dihydrotestosterone and, secondly, on the presence of the appropriate receptors in the target tissues. During the twelfth to fourteenth week, exposed to increasing androgenic stimulation, the external genitalia begin to adopt a distinctively male configuration. Closure of the urethra is complete by around fifteen weeks, the terminal portion being formed by ingrowth of ectoderm from the tip of the glans.

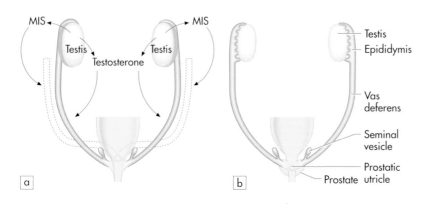

Figure 22.11 *(a) Differentiation of male internal genitalia. Secretion of Müllerian-inhibiting substance (MIS) by pre-Sertoli cells induces regression of the paramesonephric ducts between eight and ten weeks. (b) MIS also stimulates the embryonic Leydig cells to secrete testosterone, which in turn stimulates the mesonephric ducts to differentiate into the definitive male internal genitalia.*

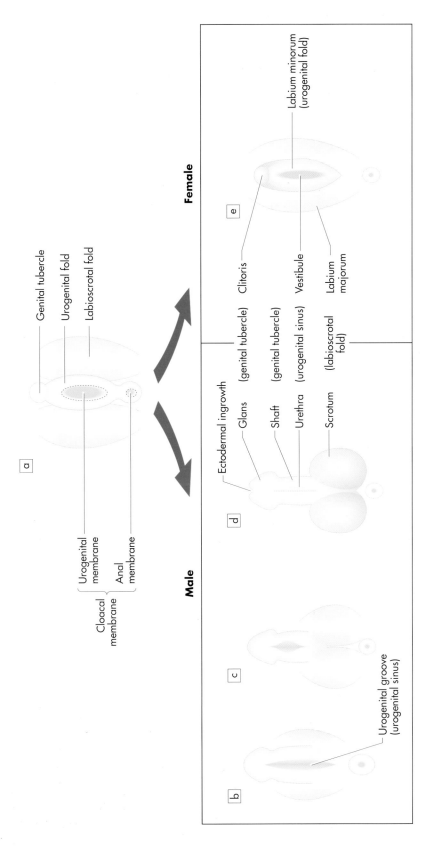

Figure 22.12 (a) Undifferentiated precursors of male and female external genitalia. (b), (c) and (d) Androgen (testosterone-derived dihydrotestosterone) induced differentiation of the male external genitalia between 12 and 16 weeks. (e) In the absence of androgenic stimulation, the external genitalia are programmed to differentiate along a female pathway.

The testis

As described above, the fetal testis originates from the interaction of primordial germ cells, the mesenchyme of the genital ridge and mesonephric duct derivatives. Testicular descent occurs in two phases, the first prompted by Müllerian-inhibiting substance, the second under the stimulus of testosterone. In both phases, the endocrine influences are mediated via the gubernaculum. Between the eighth and fifteenth weeks, the cord-like gubernaculum extending down from the testis enlarges at its distal end in the region of the labio-scrotal swellings (Figure 22.13a). Because the length of the gubernaculum remains relatively fixed during a period of active fetal growth, the effect is to anchor the testis in the region of the future inguinal canal (Figure 22.13b). The second, more active, phase of testicular descent is delayed until the twenty-fifth to thirtieth week of gestation when testosterone causes the gubernaculum to shrink and contract – thus guiding the testis down the inguinal canal into its final scrotal position (Figure 22.13c). On its route of descent, the testis is preceded by a sac-like protrusion of peritoneum, the processus vaginalis, which normally closes spontaneously prior to delivery or in the early months of life.

Genital anomalies: clinical considerations

Defects occurring in the development of the paramesonephric duct system result in a variety of clinical manifestations. The occurrence of unilateral renal agenesis in conjunction with complete absence of the ipsilateral paramesonephric duct derivatives points to a fundamental defect at the level of the original intermediate mesoderm.

Congenital absence or atresia of the vagina is a rare anomaly. Total agenesis (Rokitansky syndrome) is thought to result from failure of the paramesonephric ducts to make contact with the urogenital sinus.

Virilisation of the external genitalia in the 46 XX female with congenital adrenal hyperplasia accounts

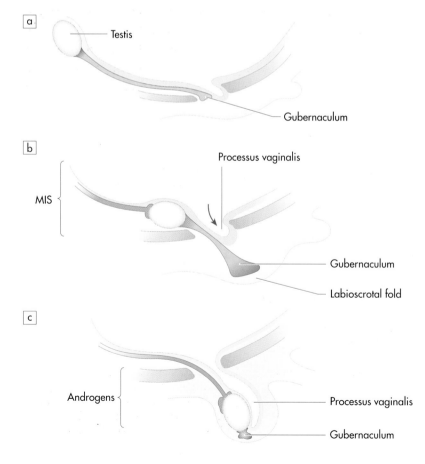

Figure 22.13 (a) Formation of the gubernaculum. (b) 10–15 weeks: enlargement of the caudal end of the gubernaculum (in response to Müllerian-inhibiting substance) anchors the fetal testis at the developing inguinal canal. (c) 25–30 weeks: testosterone-induced second stage of testicular descent.

for 80% of infants with ambiguous genitalia [8]. In these patients, the internal reproductive tract develops normally along female lines but the external genitalia differentiate down a male pathway under the influence of high levels of circulating androgens of adrenal origin. In androgen-insensitivity syndrome (testicular feminisation syndrome), the external genitalia of 46 XY males fail to virilise despite the production of Müllerian-inhibiting substance and testosterone by the fetal testes. The explanation lies in a genetically determined peripheral receptor insensitivity to dihydrotestosterone.

Incomplete closure of the urethral groove accounts for moderate and severe forms of hypospadias, whilst distal (glanular) hypospadias probably represents failure of ectodermal ingrowth from the glanular tip. Although severe hypospadias, particularly when associated with cryptorchidism and an enlarged utriculus (Müllerian remnant), is probably the manifestation of a more generalised virilisation defect, attempts to identify a specific endocrinopathy in such cases have generally proved unrewarding.

Congenital disorders of the testis and its descent are common. Cryptorchidism affects between 1% and 2% of the male infant population [9]. In the rare, genetically determined syndrome of Müllerian-inhibiting substance deficiency, intra-abdominal testes are found in association with persistent paramesonephric duct structures including Fallopian tubes and uterus. Virilisation defects (e.g. androgen-insensitivity syndrome and 5-α-reductase deficiency) account for some cases and cryptorchidism also forms a well-recognised component of many syndromes. Although simple mechanical factors provide the most obvious explanation for unilateral cryptorchidism, the reported finding of histological abnormalities in the contralateral descended testis suggests that endocrinopathy may also play a role in unilateral cryptorchidism. The presence of a blind-ending vas and spermatic vessels in most cases of testicular 'agenesis' is widely interpreted as evidence of intrauterine testicular torsion rather than a defect of embryogenesis.

The genetic basis of genitourinary malformations

Malformations of the urinary and genital tracts are estimated to account for one-third of all congenital anomalies. Although most are believed to represent sporadic, i.e. 'one-off', anomalies resulting from defective embryogenesis or faulty development in fetal life, the importance of genetic factors is being increasingly recognised (Table 22.2). Moreover, in

Table 22.2 The genetic basis of common urinary tract abnormalities

Adult polycystic kidney disease	Autosomal dominant	Chromosome 16p Chromosome 4
'Infantile' polycystic kidney disease	Autosomal recessive	
Vesico-ureteric reflux	Autosomal dominant, variable penetrance and expression	(Pax-2 gene in renal–coloboma syndrome)
Renal agenesis	Various, i.e. autosomal dominant, recessive and X-linked patterns identified	
Ureteric duplication	Autosomal dominant – variable penetrance and expression	
Pelvi-ureteric junction obstruction	When familial behaves as autosomal dominant	Documented familial incidence as isolated anomaly or pelvi-ureteric junction obstruction in association with specific syndromes (e.g. Schinzel Gideon and Johanson Blizzard syndromes)

conditions with a well-established inherited aetiology, molecular biology is beginning to identify the faulty chromosome(s) and pinpoint the site(s) of mutation. Genitourinary malformations are most commonly inherited as autosomal traits of variable penetrance and expression.

The current state of knowledge suggests that few renal anomalies will prove to be the consequence of a single gene mutation (although some such conditions have been documented). In general, the complex process of embryogenesis reflects the regulated, sequential expression of a number of genes. Where genitourinary anomalies constitute one part of a recognised syndrome, it is likely that the affected gene (or genes) encodes for gene products that play a fundamental molecular role in the regulation and development of a number of systems. For example, the *KAL* gene implicated in X-linked Kalmann's syndrome (microphallus, renal agenesis, anosmia) is known to code for an adhesion molecule implicated in the migration of olfactory neurons in the brain and also in the process of nephrogenesis. Other examples include renal–coloboma syndrome (vesicoureteric reflux and the ophthalmic anomaly, coloboma) [10], which has been attributed to a mutation of the *PAX-2* gene encoding for a transcription factor. A detailed account of this exciting and rapidly expanding field is beyond the scope of this chapter. It is already apparent, however, that research in genetics and molecular biology is destined to make a major contribution to our understanding of the normal and abnormal development of the urinary and genital tracts.

References

1. Thomson JA, Itskovitz-Eldor J, Shapiro SS, Waknitz MA, Swiergiel JJ, *et al*. Embryonic stem cell lines derived from human blastocysts. Science 1998; 282: 1145–7

2. Wolfe AS. Molecular control of nephrogenesis. British Journal of Urology 1998; 81 (Suppl. 2): 1–7

3. Stephens FD, Smith DE, Hutson J. Congenital anomalies of the urinary and genital tracts. Oxford: Isis Medical Media Ltd, 1996, pp 222–34

4. Thomas DFM. Cloacal malformations: embryology, anatomy and principles of management. In: Spitz *et al.* (eds) Progress in Paediatric Surgery. Berlin, Heidelberg: Springer-Verlag, 1989, Vol. 23, pp 135–43

5. Larsen WJ. The search for the testis-determining factor. In: Larsen WJ (ed) Human Embryology. Edinburgh: Churchill Livingstone, 1993: pp 276–9

6. Hutson JM, Terada M, Baiyun Z, Williams MPL. Normal testicular descent and the aetiology of cryptorchidism. Advances in Anatomy, Embryology and Cell Biology 132. Berlin: Springer, 1996, pp 8–6

7. McNeal JE. Anatomy and embryology. In: Fitzpatrick JM, Kane RJ (eds) The Prostate. Edinburgh: Churchill Livingstone, 1989, pp 3–9

8. Whitaker RH, Williams DM. Post-natal investigation and management of genital intersex anomalies. In: Thomas DFM (ed) Urological Disease in the Fetus and Infant. Oxford: Butterworth Heinemann,1997, pp 279–92

9. John Radcliffe Cryptorchidism Study Group. Cryptorchidism: a prospective study of 7,500 consecutive male births, 1984–8. Archives of Disease in Childhood 1992; 67: 892–9

10. Feather S, Woolf AS, Gordon, Risdon RA, Verrier-Jones K. Vesicoureteric reflux – is it all in the genes? Lancet 1996; 348: 725–8

Intersex

23

M. O. Savage and C. Sultan

Introduction

Intersex states are characterised by an abnormality in the formation of the internal or external genital structures. This is usually due to a defect, frequently genetically determined, in the process of fetal sexual differentiation. Many intersex states are associated with an ambiguous appearance of the external genitalia resulting in disturbance of the balanced psychological and physical make-up of an individual, to which normal genital development is the key.

During the past two decades, the study of intersex disorders moved towards the biochemical and molecular identification of the defects that cause them. If such an aetiological approach is to be used, a fundamental understanding of normal sexual differentiation, as described in the previous chapter, is required. This provides the basis for the classification, investigation and management of patients with intersex states.

Classification of intersex states

The classification that has stood the test of time and forms the basis of clinical assessment and management depends on gonadal morphology (Table 23.1). Female pseudohermaphroditism describes genital ambiguity resulting from abnormal virilisation of the female with normal ovaries. The male counterpart – male pseudohermaphroditism – is the result of incomplete virilisation of the male with differentiated testes. Thirdly, the true hermaphrodite possesses both ovarian and testicular tissue.

Table 23.1 Classification of intersex states

Female pseudohermaphrodite: virilisation of genetic female with ovaries
Male pseudohermaphrodite: incomplete virilisation of genetic male with testes
True hermaphrodite: individual with ovarian and testicular tissue

Female pseudohermaphroditism

Female pseudohermaphrodites have 46XX karyotypes with normal ovaries and Müllerian structures, but the external genitalia are virilised. The aetiology of female pseudohermaphroditism is given in Table 23.2. The degree of genital ambiguity can range from enlargement of the clitoris or fusion of the posterior labia to a completely male appearance (Figure 23.1), depending on the timing of androgen production and the concentration of androgens in the fetal circulation. Virilisation may be caused by excessive production of either fetal or maternal androgens.

Virilisation by fetal androgens

Congenital adrenal hyperplasia
The commonest cause of ambiguous genitalia in the newborn female is a recessively inherited enzyme defect of cortisol synthesis, with diversion of intermediates to androgen production [1]. A reduction in

Table 23.2 Aetiology of female pseudohermaphroditism

Virilisation of fetal androgens
  Congenital adrenal hyperplasia
    21α-Hydroxylase deficiency
    11β-Hydroxylase deficiency
    3β-Hydroxysteroid dehydrogenase deficiency
  Other causes of fetal androgen overproduction
    Fetal adrenal adenoma
    Nodular adrenal hyperplasia
    Persistent fetal adrenal in preterm infants

Fetal virilisation by maternal androgens
  Ovarian tumours
  Adrenal tumours
  Aromatase deficiency: oestrogen synthetic defect

Iatrogenic fetal virilisation
  Testosterone and progestins

Female pseudohermaphroditism with associated congenital malformations

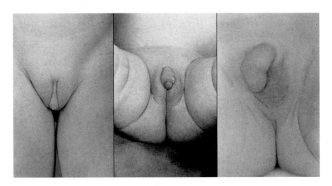

Figure 23.1 *Variation in degree of virilisation in three female infants with 21α-hydroxylase deficiency.*

steroid 21α-hydroxylase or absence of 11β-hydroxylase or 3β-hydroxysteroid dehydrogenase can be the cause of congenital adrenal hyperplasia. In the absence of, or when there is a lowered potential for, cortisol production, there are high adrenocorticotrophic hormone levels, leading to adrenal hyperplasia and excess androgen production.

21α-Hydroxylase deficiency

In classical 21α-hydroxylase deficiency, high plasma concentrations of androgens, due to the diversion of the precursors early in gestation, cause virilisation of the external genitalia of the 46XX female fetus. This deficiency is the most common cause of female pseudohermaphroditism. About 75% of patients with classic 21α-hydroxylase deficiency do not correctly synthesise aldosterone, which induces a potentially fatal salt-wasting state [1].

In this form of congenital adrenal hyperplasia, 17α-hydroxyprogesterone is not effectively converted to 11-deoxycortisol in the pathway of cortisol synthesis. The classical form of 21α-hydroxylase deficiency has a frequency estimated at 1 in 14000 live births. The definitive test to make the diagnosis is a standard adrenocorticotrophic hormone stimulation test and measurement of plasma 17α-hydroxyprogesterone. A variant of 21α-hydroxylase deficiency, due to a milder defect, is the non-classical form of the disease. Affected females do not present neonatal genital ambiguity, but develop other signs of androgen excess such as hirsutism.

Prenatal diagnosis is important to identify a fetus affected by the enzyme deficiency. In this way, genital ambiguity in affected females can be improved or prevented by early dexamethasone treatment to the pregnant mother [2]. This prenatal diagnosis can be hormonal, by the measurement of amniotic fluid 17α-hydroxyprogesterone levels, or genetic after chorionic villus sampling at nine to ten weeks of gestation. Early prenatal diagnosis and treatment of 21α-hydroxylase deficiency may thus spare the newborn female the consequences of genital ambiguity, sex misassignment, and gender confusion.

11β-Hydroxylase deficiency

Female newborns usually present with signs of androgen excess such as masculinisation of the external genitalia [3]. Patients may also develop signs and symptoms of aldosterone deficiency and a small percentage develop hypertension rather than mineralocorticoid deficiency.

This enzyme deficiency, which fails to convert 11-deoxycortisol to cortisol, is the second most common cause of congenital adrenal hyperplasia and results in a hypertensive form of the disease [4]. Humans have two isoenzymes with 11β-hydroxylase activity that are required for cortisol and aldosterone synthesis respectively. CYP11B1, which presents the 11β-hydroxylase activity, is regulated by adrenocorticotrophic hormone; CYP11B2, which presents the aldosterone synthetase activity, is regulated by angiotensin II. Moreover, in addition to the 11β-hydroxylase activity, the latter enzyme has 18-hydroxylase and 18-oxidase activities and can thus synthesise aldosterone from deoxycorticosterone.

Deficiency of 11β-hydroxylase results from mutations in the *CYP11B1* gene. All mutations identified in patients with the classical form abolish enzymatic activity [5]. However, there is no consistent correlation between the severity of hypertension and the degree of virilisation in individuals with the same homozygous mutation. The treatment of affected children with hydrocortisone achieves a number of goals; while feminising genitoplasty must be performed at 6–12 months of age.

3β-Hydroxysteroid dehydrogenase deficiency

The complete form of 3β-hydroxysteroid dehydrogenase deficiency results in partially virilised genitalia in genetic females, whereas a partial form results in adolescent hyperandrogenism. Salt losing is present when the deficiency is complete. Elevated secretion of pregnenolone and 17α-pregnenolone is characteristic of this form of congenital adrenal hyperplasia [6]. Hydrocortisone and salt-retaining hormone replacement therapy are needed.

Oestrogen synthetic defect: aromatase deficiency

Aromatase deficiency within placental syncytiotrophoblasts is responsible for impaired or absent conversion of fetal and maternal androgens to oestrogens. It subsequently leads to the development of signs of maternal hyperandrogenism (acne, hirsutism) during the second half of pregnancy. Exposure of the female fetus to this androgen excess also causes virilisation of the infant, with severe ambiguous genitalia at birth. Micropenis hypospadias and posterior labioscrotal fusion may be present. At puberty, affected females present with pubertal failure, hypergonadotrophic hypogonadism and virilisation similar to that observed in polycystic ovary syndrome. In aromatase deficiency, oestrogen levels are exceedingly low. In both sexes, it leads to delayed bone age and tall stature.

Several mutations within the *P450 arom* gene have been described in the past few years [7]. The descriptions of aromatase deficiency in males and females provide new insights into the physiological roles of oestrogens in pregnancy, puberty and bone maturation and into the sex steroid-gonadotrophin feedback mechanism in the male.

Virilisation by maternal androgens

Virilisation of the external genitalia by a maternal ovarian or adrenal androgen-secreting tumour is a rare but well-recognised cause of female pseudohermaphroditism. The degree of virilisation may be striking. In a recent report and review of the literature [8], the diagnosis of female pseudohermaphroditism and the causative maternal adrenal tumour (Figure 23.2) were confirmed only when the patient, having been brought up as a boy, started to feminise at puberty.

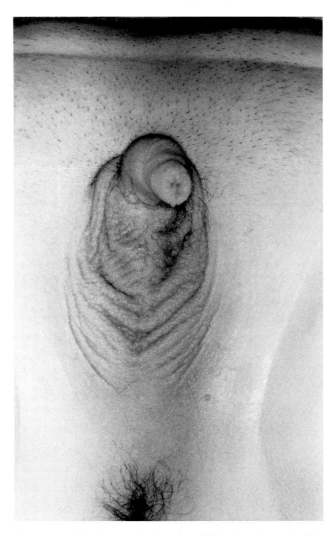

Figure 23.2 *Virilisation of a female 46XX infant during fetal life by a maternal androgen-secreting adrenal adenoma.*

Other causes of fetal virilisation

Female pseudohermaphroditism due to administration of progestogen preparations to the mother was recognised about 30 years ago. A number of dysmorphic childhood syndromes may also be associated with virilised female genitalia [9].

Male pseudohermaphroditism

Male pseudohermaphroditism arises as a result of a disturbance of normal male genital development in patients with testes and a 46XY karyotype (Table 23.3). The genital anomaly can vary from apparently female external genitalia to male external genitalia with a small penis or perineal hypospadias. Male sexual differentiation, as described in the previous chapter, is brought about by a number of interrelated mechanisms, and failure of any of these may lead to incomplete virilisation.

Abnormalities of sex differentiation

After sex determination, the events of male sex differentiation take two pathways [10]: one inhibitory, i.e. the regression of the Müllerian ducts by action of

Table 23.3 Aetiology of male pseudohermaphroditism

Impaired Leydig cell activity
    Inborn errors of testosterone biosynthesis
        Congenital lipoid adrenal hyperplasia
        3β-Hydroxysteroid dehydrogenase deficiency
        17α-Hydroxylase deficiency
        17,20-Desmolase deficiency
    Leydig cell hypoplasia: luteinising hormone receptor defect

Androgen-insensitivity syndromes
    Complete androgen insensitivity
    Partial androgen insensitivity
    5α-reductase deficiency

Incomplete differentiation of testes with deficient testosterone and anti-Müllerian hormone production
    XY gonadal dysgenesis
    Mixed gonadal dysgenesis

Other forms
    Iatrogenic male pseudohermophroditism
    Associated with other congenital anomalies
    Persistent Müllerian structures

the anti-Müllerian hormone, and the other stimulatory, which requires the two androgens, testosterone and 5α-dihydrotestosterone, and a functional androgen receptor very early in embryogenesis. It is clearly demonstrated that androgens are essential for virilisation of Wolffian duct structures, the urogenital sinus and the genital tubercle. In the urogenital sinus and the genital tubercle, testosterone is converted to 5α-dihydrotestosterone by 5α-reductase. Testosterone or 5α-dihydrotestosterone binds to a nuclear receptor to stimulate protein synthesis.

Molecular cloning and genetic, biochemical and pharmacological approaches have provided strong support for the existence of at least two steroid 5α-reductase enzymes in humans (designated as types 1 and 2 to reflect the chronological order in which the genes were isolated) [11]. Molecular genetic evidence, such as gene deletions and point mutations, demonstrated that the 5α-reductase 2 gene is the morbid locus for 5α-reductase deficiency.

The androgen receptor belongs to the subfamily of steroid hormone receptors within a larger family of nuclear proteins that activates target gene transcription through the same hormone response elements. As a member of the nuclear receptor family (Figure 23.3), the androgen receptor contains an NH_2-terminal region, which is variable in length and has a role in transcriptional activation, a central cysteine-rich DNA-binding domain, and a carboxy-terminal ligand-binding domain [12].

Although the two physiologically active androgens, testosterone and 5α-dihydrotestosterone, interact directly with the androgen receptor and mediate hormonal responses, conversion of testosterone to the more potent agonist 5α-dihydrotestosterone in certain tissues is required for the androgen action to occur. This requirement is particularly clear during male sexual development, when formation of 5α-dihydrotestosterone is mandatory for virilisation of external genitalia and development of the prostate. Virilisation of the Wolffian duct structures is, however, thought to be mediated by testosterone. The actions of androgens on the target cell occur via the classical steroid receptor pathway (Figure 23.4) [12]. After the binding of the androgen to its receptor, a hyperphosphorylation of the N-terminal domain of

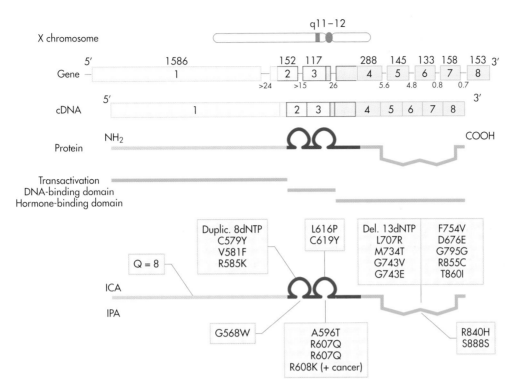

Figure 23.3 Schematic representation of the androgen receptor gene, and protein organisation (top). Androgen receptor abnormalities (from personal experience). The single amino acid letter code is used (bottom).

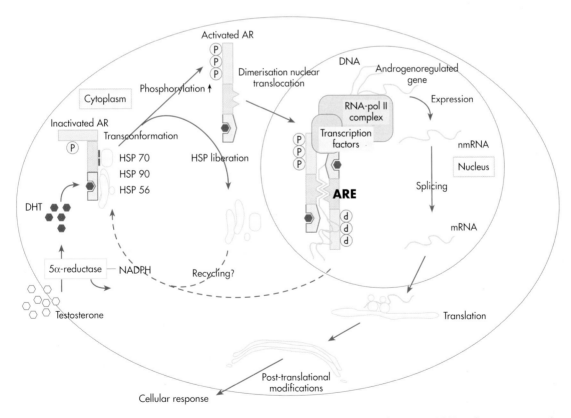

Figure 23.4 Schematic representation of androgen action in the target cell. HSP, heat shock protein; ARE, androgen response element; DHT, 5α-dihydrotestosterone; AR, androgen receptor.

the protein is observed. The androgen-activated receptor complex migrates to the nucleus and interacts as a homodimer with the androgen responsive-elements of target genes and their flanking DNA [13]. The mechanism by which the receptor regulates gene transcription probably involves N-terminal sequences of the protein, but the molecular details of this activation process remain to be elucidated. Protein–protein interactions, probably with other transcription factors, may occur near the transcription start site of the gene. Both promoter and host cell specificities appear to influence the requirement for the N-terminal domain in transcriptional activation, suggesting that this region interacts with cell-specific transcription factors.

Defects of testis development

XY gonadal dysgenesis

Y-linked XY gonadal dysgenesis

XY complete gonadal dysgenesis (Swyer syndrome)
The syndrome of pure gonadal dysgenesis is characterised by the presence of bilateral streak gonads in phenotypic females with sexual infantilism and XY karyotype. Most individuals come to medical attention in their mid-teens or later for evaluation of problems related to lack of ovarian function. Most of the patients do not present with sex chromosome structural abnormalities but some sporadic cases exist with a deletion in the short arm of the Y (Yp) or a 46 XXp resulting from translocation of an extra fragment of Xp on an otherwise normal Y chromosome. Gene abnormalities of SRY such as deletion and point mutations have been described in only 10 to 15% of the patients; the majority of the point mutations are located in the HMG box of the SRY gene (Figure 23.5).

The management of patients with pure gonadal dysgenesis is similar to Turner's syndrome in that long-term oestrogen therapy should be instituted at the expected time of puberty. Neoplastic transformation of the dysgenetic gonads is likely to occur in patients with XY pure gonadal dysgenesis making routine gonadectomy mandatory.

Mixed gonadal dysgenesis
Mixed gonadal dysgenesis is characterised by a unilateral testis (often intra-abdominal), a contalateral streak gonad, persistent Müllerian duct structures, and is associated with varying degrees of inadequate masculinisation [14]. The most common karyotype is 45XO/46XY, but other mosaics have been reported with a structurally abnormal or normal Y chromosome. Features of Turner's syndrome may be present (Figure 23.6).

Patients with mixed gonadal dysgenesis are at increased risk for gonadal (and Wilms') tumour. It is recommended that they should be reared as females. This allows for the removal of the gonads and avoidance of their malignant potential. As males, they would be infertile.

Dysgenetic male pseudohermaphroditism
This denomination encompasses wide heterogeneity and refers to a group of patients presenting with bilateral dysgenetic testes, persistent Müllerian structures,

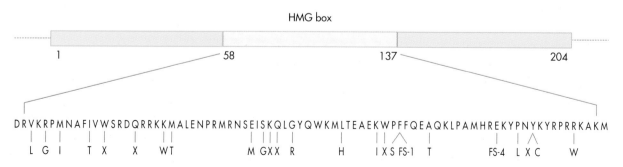

Figure 23.5 *Sex-reversing mutations in the SRY gene. X indicates termination codon and FS indicates frameshift mutation. The number (9n) of base pairs deleted causing frameshift is indicated as FS-n.*

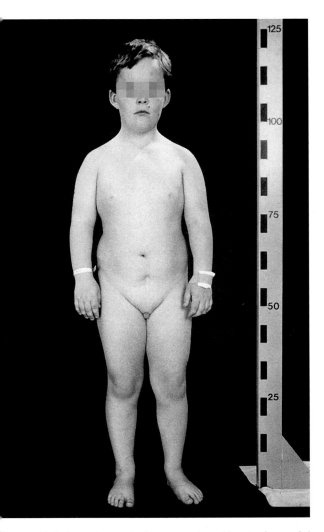

Figure 23.6 A patient, raised as a male, with mixed gonadal dysgenesis associated with a 45XO/46XY karyotype. Note the broad chest and incomplete virilisation.

cryptorchidism and inadequate virilisation [15]. Because the uterus is frequently present, the sex of rearing is often female, and gonadectomy is recommended. These patients should be screened routinely for tumour formation.

X-linked 46XY gonadal dysgenesis

Sex reversal in 46XY patients with a duplication of the short arm of the X chromosome suggested the existence of a gene in the X chromosome, named DSS (dosage-sensitive sex reversal), which when present in two copies can override the effect of the Y chromosome [16]. In the 160-kb stretch within the Xp21 region containing the DSS locus and also the locus for congenital adrenal hypoplasia, the first, and only, gene

isolated is DAX-1. DAX-1 encodes a nuclear receptor related to steroidogenic factor 1, which has been shown in homozygous knock-out studies to result in the absence of gonads in both sexes. The close embryological relationship between adrenals and gonads, and their shared steroidogenic properties, support the hypothesis that DAX-1 might be both the DSS and the gene responsible for congenital adrenal hypoplasia. In fact, mutations of DAX-1 [17] do not affect testis development and no mutation has been described in XY females.

Autosomal-linked 46XY gonadal dysgenesis

Another gene has been isolated that also appears to exert its effects on sex determination in a dose-sensitive fashion. This gene, SOX-9 (SRY box-related sequence), maps to the locus known as SRA1 on chromosome 17, which is associated with campomelic dysplasia and sometimes gonadal dysgenesis. SOX-9 belongs to the same family of HMG proteins as SRY. Despite similarities, it does not seem that SOX-9 and SRY would compete with each other on a target site because it is a reduction of SOX-9 expression [18] that leads to sex reversal from male to female.

True hermaphroditism

True hermaphroditism is defined as the simultaneous presence of testicular and ovarian tissue in a single individual in either the same or opposite gonads [19] (Table 23.4). Both the external genitalia and the internal duct structures of true hermaphrodites display gradations between male and female. The initial manifestations are ambiguous genitalia in 90% of cases or, more rarely, isolated clitoromegaly or penile hypospadias. Two-thirds of true hermaphrodites are raised as males. Among those raised as females, most will have clitoromegaly. Virtually all patients have a urogenital sinus, and in most cases a uterus is present.

The most common peripheral karyotype is 46XX but mosaicisms are observed (XX, XY). The SRY gene is present in 10–30% of patients, suggesting that true hermaphroditism is a heterogeneous condition in terms of its genetic background. The most important aspect of the management of true hermaphrodites is

Table 23.4 Gonadal distribution in 384 cases of true hermaphroditism

Type of distribution		Number of patients	Percentage
Gonad on one side	Gonad on opposite side		
Ovary	Testis	113	29.5
Ovotestis	Ovary	114	29.7
Ovotestis	Ovotestis	79	20.6
Ovotestis	Testis	40	10.4
Ovotestis	Unknown	15	3.9
Ovotestis	Variations	23	5.9

From van Niekerk (1981) [19].

gender assignment. Such decisions should be based upon the adequacy of the phallus and findings at laparotomy. True hermaphrodites have the potential for fertility.

XX males

These patients with no genital ambiguity develop gynaecomastia at puberty. Although they present some degree of testosterone deficiency and impaired spermatogenesis, they differ from patients with the latter in that they are not tall and show no impairment of intelligence [20]. The SRY gene is present in some XX males. Others, however, have no demonstrable Y sequences. Management of XX males is similar to that for Klinefelter's syndrome.

Leydig cell hypoplasia

Leydig cell hypoplasia is a form of pseudohermaphroditism in which Leydig cell differentiation and testosterone production are impaired. The phenotype is female, although Müllerian structures are absent. Inhibiting mutations in the sixth transmembrane domain of the luteinising hormone-receptor have recently been reported in these patients [21].

Inborn errors of testosterone biosynthesis

These rare disorders (Figure 23.7) lead to defective testosterone secretion during the critical period of fetal sexual differentiation. The result is inadequate

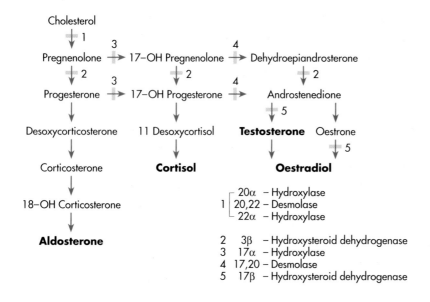

Figure 23.7 Enzyme defects in testosterone biosynthesis.

estosterone secretion, either locally to virilise the Wolffian ducts or peripherally to virilise the external genitalia. Lack of virilisation may be severe and many patients are raised as female. The synthesis of anti-Müllerian hormone, being a glycoprotein rather than a steroid, is unaffected. When the enzyme deficiency is situated early in the biosynthetic pathway, adrenal steroid synthesis may also be impaired. These disorders are rare and are described here only briefly as a number of reviews are available [22, 23].

Congenital lipoid adrenal hyperplasia

Congenital lipoid adrenal hyperplasia is a rare disease, characterised by a defect in the synthesis of the three classes of steroid hormones, and resulting in severe salt wasting and female phenotype. No mutation, in humans, has been found thus far in the gene encoding for P450scc, the first candidate gene, nor in the various proteins involved in the cholesterol transport, such as SCP-2. Recently, the gene responsible for this disease has been cloned and validated by the demonstration of a non-sense mutation [24]. It encodes for a protein named StAR (steroidogeneic acute regulatory protein), probably responsible for the transport of cholesterol to the inner membrane of mitchondria, and thus to the P450scc enzyme complex.

17α-Hydroxylase deficiency

Defects in P450c17 lead to a male pseudohermaphroditism with various degrees of ambiguous genitalia, most often a severe form, frequently diagnosed at puberty, associating female phenotype and hypertension. Cytochrome P450c17 catalyses the transformation of progesterone and pregnenolone into 17α-hydroxyprogesterone and 17α-hydroxypregnenolone and then into dehydroepiandrosterone and Δ4-androstenedione.

The gene encoding for this enzyme complex, the CYP17 gene, is located on chromosome 10q24-25. Several different mutations have been reported in the CYP17 gene, leading to either the complete or partial form of the disease [25, 26].

3β-Hydroxysteroid dehydrogenase deficiency

Defects in 3β-hydroxysteroid dehydrogenase synthesis result in 46XY individuals with male pseudo-hermaphroditism sometimes associated with salt wasting in the classical form [27]. The 3β-hydroxysteroid dehydrogenase enzyme is responsible for the conversion of Δ5 (3β-OH) steroids into Δ4 (3-ceto) steroids. Two different cDNAs have been identified: type 1 in placenta, and type II in gonads and adrenal glands. The two genes are located on chromosome 1p13.

Almost 15 mutations of the type II 3β-hydroxysteroid dehydrogenase enzyme have been reported to date, but no mutations of type I have been found. This can explain the virilisation that occurs in 46XX subjects, because of a peripheral, non-steroidogenic conversion of elevated testosterone precursors. A non-classical form of 3β-hydroxysteroid dehydrogenase deficiency has been described, characterised by a late-onset and less severe form of the disease. The clinical diagnosis of this form is not easy, and its existence remains controversial because no mutations of the gene have been found.

17β-Hydroxysteroid dehydrogenase deficiency

17β-Hydroxysteroid dehydrogenase deficiency is a rare cause of male pseudohermaphroditism. The typical subject is a 46XY male born with female external genitalia, testes located in the inguinal canals or labia majora, who virilises at the time of puberty (Figure 23.8), associated with elevated levels of androstenedione contrasting with low or normal levels of testosterone. Two characteristics of the disorder are particularly puzzling: the defect in virilisation and the deficiency in testosterone synthesis that are usually more complete during embryogenesis than in later life, and the well-differentiated Wolffian duct structures.

17β-Hydroxysteroid dehydrogenase converts Δ4-androstenedione into testosterone and dehydroepiandrosterone into androstenediol. It also acts on the interconversion of oestradiol and oestrone. This is a key enzyme leading to active androgenic compounds, and the only one of the steroidogenic pathways whose action is reversible. Four different enzymes, with tissue-specific expression, encoded by four different genes have been identified. The 17β-hydroxysteroid dehydrogenase type 1 has a peripheral activity and a specificity toward oestrogens. The 17β-hydroxysteroid dehydrogenase type 2 enzyme

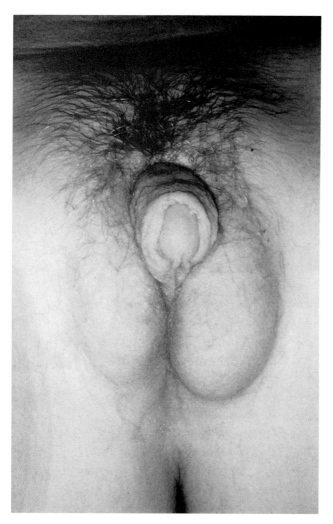

Figure 23.8 *Genital virilisation at puberty of a 46XY patient with 17-β hydroxysteroid dehydrogenase deficiency who has been raised as a female. (With kind permission of Dr DB Grant.)*

is mainly of placental origin and acts on both androgens and oestrogens. The 17β-hydroxysteroid dehydrogenase type 3 enzyme has a specific testicular expression and functions with NADPH as cofactor (in contrast to the two former enzymes that utilise NADH). Finally, abnormalities of the type 3 enzyme are responsible for the 17β-hydroxysteroid dehydrogenase deficiency.

Among the gene alterations, mis-sense and non-sense mutations, splice junction abnormalities and a small deletion that resulted in a frame shift have been described [28]. Affected newborns are considered female, but the sex of rearing of the patients remains questionable: the choice of sex will be influenced by the social group. The authors believe that, during

infancy or childhood, because the female sex of rearing is maintained, an orchidectomy should be carried out. If the diagnosis is not made prior to puberty, a gender change to male is acceptable [29].

Androgen-insensitivity syndromes
(Table 23.5)

5α-Reductase deficiency

Several investigators have reported a wide clinical, biological and biochemical spectrum associated with genetic heterogeneity in 5α-reductase deficiency. Patients with this disorder are characterised at birth by the presence of a pseudovagina, a urogenital sinus, and testes in the inguinal canals, labia or scrotum in all cases. The clinical presentation can range from almost normal female structures to a clear-cut male phenotype with hypospadias, and normally virilised Wolffian structures that terminate in the vagina. An important characteristic of 5α-reductase deficiency is the virilisation of the external genitalia that occurs at puberty (Figure 23.9) together with the acquisition of male gender identity in patients raised as female [30].

The characteristic endocrine features of 5α-reductase deficiency are normal to high male levels of testosterone and low levels of 5α-dihydrotestosterone, elevation in the ratio of testosterone to 5α-dihydrotestosterone in adulthood and after stimulation with human chorionic gonadotrophin in childhood, and elevated ratios of urinary 5β-metabolites to 5α-metabolites of androgen and C21-steroids.

From a biochemical point of view, the decrease in 5α-reductase activity in genital skin fibroblasts supports the diagnosis of 5α-reductase deficiency, but enzymatic activity is sometimes in the normal range. The decreased activity in sonicated cell extracts at acidic pH provides strong evidence that the mutation results in a loss of type 2 enzyme activity.

Isolation and sequencing of the cDNA encoding the 5α-reductase type 2 provide the molecular tools for the definition of the gene abnormalities responsible for 5α-reductase deficiency. To date, only three gene deletions have been described. Indeed, when a sequence alteration is identified, it is usually a point mutation, which vary greatly and are found through-

Table 23.5 Clinical phenotype of androgen-insensitivity states

	5α-Reductase deficiency	Androgen receptor disorders		
		Complete	Partial	Mild
External genitalia	Predominantly female	Female	Ambiguous	Male
Wolffian structures	Male	Absent	Hypoplastic male	Male
Urogenital sinus	Female	Female	Rudimentary male	Male
Breast	Male	Female	Gynaecomastia	± Gynaecomastia
Sexual orientation	Female–male	Female	Male–female	Male

out the gene. The standard methods of molecular genetic analysis have so far revealed two non-sense mutations, one splicing defect, and 24 mis-sense mutations [11, 31, 32].

The management of 5α-reductase deficiency is primarily dependent upon the phenotypic findings and gender at the time of diagnosis. Given the severe defect of the external genitalia (Figure 23.10), most newborns are raised as female. Gonadectomy should be performed early to prevent masculinisation, together with vaginoplasty and clitoral reduction. If the diagnosis is made at puberty, one can consider raising the patient as male. The administration of supraphysiological doses of testosterone or local application of

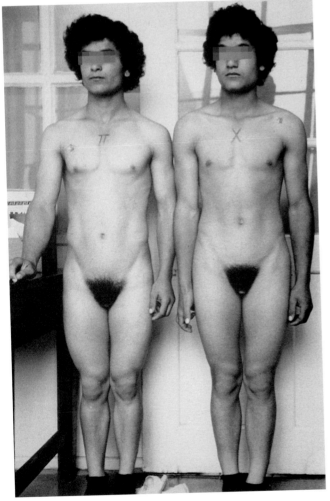

Figure 23.9 *Two Greek Cypriot brothers with 5α-reductase deficiency.*

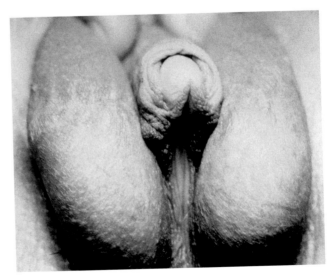

Figure 23.10 *External genitalia of a pubertal patient with 5α-reductase deficiency. Note that the phallus remains small.*

5α-dihydrotestosterone cream results in some long-term enhancement of virilisation [33].

Complete androgen insensitivity

This form of androgen insensitivity is characterised by an unambiguous female phenotype with a blind vaginal pouch and no uterus. In some cases, an under-development of the clitoris and labia minora may be observed. At puberty, breast development is normal or augmented, contrasting with absent or scanty axillary and pubic hair in the majority of cases. Individuals with complete androgen insensitivity come to medical attention either during infancy because of an inguinal hernia, or during puberty with primary amenorrhoea.

Partial androgen insensitivity

This covers a wide spectrum of clinical phenotypes, from patients with essentially female phenotype with limited virilisation such as mild clitoromegaly and/or a slight degree of posterior labial fusion, to infertile individuals who had normal responsiveness during fetal life and thus an unequivocally male phenotype with azoospermia. A X-linked pattern of inheritance may be identified (Figure 23.11). The diagnosis may be made in infancy when the child presents with ambiguous genitalia, perineal hypospadias and palpable testes (Figure 23.12). At puberty, virilisation and/or feminisation may occur, depending upon the degree of androgen resistance.

Since the androgen receptor gene was cloned, molecular biology techniques have made it possible to identify mutations within the gene from patients with different phenotypes of androgen insensitivity [34]. Such techniques include restriction fragment length polymorphism analysis and enzymatic amplification of the various exons of the gene to detect large-scale changes in the gene structure. Screening procedures with sequencing of the gene allow identification of subtle changes responsible for mis-sense or non-sense mutations.

Androgen receptor gene alterations may be classified into two groups, according to the DNA and mRNA alterations: (1) loss or gain of genomic information, such as macrodeletions and microdeletions and base-pair insertions; and (2) point mutations, responsible for non-sense, mis-sense and splice-site mutations. A wide variety of molecular defects may underlie the clinical and biochemical heterogeneity of the androgen-insensitivity syndrome. Moreover, the same mutation can be associated with different phenotypes, even within the same family. Markedly different molecular defects (major deletion, premature termination, single amino acid substitution in the protein) can also produce the same phenotype. The screening of carriers and prenatal diagnosis of androgen insensitivity in high-risk families are impossible unless the mutation has been identified. Thereafter, sequencing of the suspected exon of the 46XX proband or the 46XY fetus ascertains whether the affected chromosome is being carried [35].

The treatment of patients with complete androgen-insensitivity syndrome relates primarily to the optional timing of gonadectomy. The authors normally perform gonadectomy before puberty and prescribe oestrogen replacement as necessary. The management of patients with partial androgen-insensitivity syndrome must be individualised from the degree of genital ambiguity, the growth response of the penile size to a supraphysiological dose of testosterone, and the type of androgen receptor mutation. Although certain androgen receptor defects may

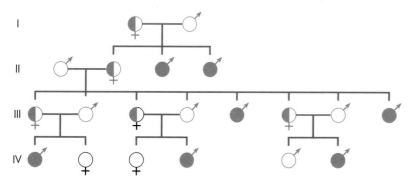

Figure 23.11 Pedigree of a family with X-linked partial androgen-insensitivity syndrome.

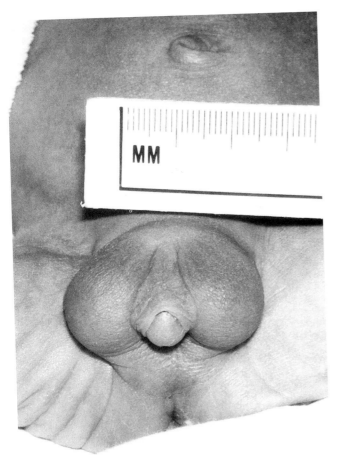

Figure 23.12 External genitalia of a male pseudohermaphrodite infant with partial androgen insensitivity.

be amenable to androgen therapy, multiple reconstruction of the external genitalia and azoospermia are good arguments in favour of a female sex of rearing.

Persistent Müllerian duct syndrome

Persistent Müllerian duct syndrome is usually discovered at surgery performed for cryptorchidism and/or hernia. It is a rare form of familial male pseudohermaphroditism, characterised by the persistence of the uterus and the fallopian tubes in 46XY phenotypic males, and is due to defects in the synthesis or action of anti-Müllerian hormone.

To date, one homozygous mutation of the anti-Müllerian hormone receptor has been described in an anti-Müllerian hormone-positive patient out of 21 such patients [36]. This splice mutation generated two abnormal mRNAs, one missing the second exon required for ligand binding and the second coding for

an abnormal protein due to an amino acid substitution followed by the insertion of four amino acids. The treatment of persistent Müllerian duct syndrome is relatively straightforward in that all patients are phenotypic male and require orchidopexy.

Clinical and laboratory assessment of patients with intersex states

The assessment of patients with intersex states may be considered from the point of view of the paediatrician assessing an infant with ambiguous genitalia. The same principles apply to the older child or adult. It must be emphasised that the general appearance of the external genitalia, although important in deciding the appropriate gender for the child, is of very little help in defining the aetiology of the disorder.

Clinical assessment

The principles of clinical assessment are shown in Table 23.6. A history of a similar disorder in other family members may shed light on the likely diagnosis: many of these conditions are genetically determined. Examination for other anomalies that could point to a dysmorphic syndrome known to be associated with abnormal genital development is also relevant. The most important aspect of the examination, however, is careful palpation of the gonads.

Table 23.6 Patient with intersex state: clinical assessment

Family history, general examination for dysmorphic features
Examination of external genitalia
  No gonads palpable
    Female pseudohermaphrodite: congenital adrenal hyperplasia (21α-hydroxylase deficiency)
    Male pseudohermaphrodite
  One gonad palpable
    Abnormal gonadal differentiation
    Mixed gonadal dysgenesis (XO/XY)
    True hermaphroditism
  Two gonads palpable
    Male pseudohermaphrodite
    Impaired testosterone biosynthesis
    Androgen receptor defect
    5α-Reductase deficiency
    True hermaphroditism

If *no gonads are palpable*, the most likely diagnosis is female pseudohermaphroditism due to congenital adrenal hyperplasia, and this is virtually certain if symptoms of salt loss develop. Other possible disorders are true hermaphroditism or male pseudohermaphroditism with intra-abdominal gonads. When *both gonads are palpable* in the scrotum or labial folds, the patient is likely to be a male pseudohermaphrodite, and measurement of plasma androgens will indicate whether the aetiology is a testicular or peripheral defect. A true hermaphrodite with bilateral ovotestes may also present in this way. The presence of only *one palpable gonad* or asymmetry of the perineum is suggestive of mixed gonadal dysgenesis or true hermaphroditism with asymmetrical gonads.

Laboratory assessment

A similar scheme may be devised as a guide to confirming the aetiology biochemically (Table 23.7). In all intersex patients, a karyotype is indicated. If *no gonads are palpable*, determination of plasma 17α-hydroxyprogesterone will confirm or exclude 21α-hydroxylase deficiency. In 11β-hydroxylase deficiency, the plasma 11-deoxycortisol concentration is elevated.

The infant with *two palpable gonads* needs a human chorionic gonadotrophin stimulation test to assess testicular androgen secretion. Numerous human chorionic gonadotrophin regimens exist, of which two examples are 1000 iu daily for three days or a single injection of 1500 iu/m^2 body surface area [37]. Basal and post-stimulatory concentrations of testosterone, 5α-dihydrotestosterone and androstenedione should distinguish a disorder of testosterone biosynthesis from a syndrome of androgen insensitivity. Molecular analysis of the androgen receptor gene may identify a mutation.

If *one gonad is palpable*, gonadal biopsy may be helpful, particularly if ovarian tissue is suspected. Pelvic ultrasonography or exploratory laparotomy for the identification of internal genital structures may also be indicated. In any patient with incomplete virilisation, urethrography should be performed to identify a vaginal cavity communicating posteriorly with the urethra.

Medical management

Choice of gender

Parents are usually shocked to learn that there is doubt as to the sex of their child; they are often under the impression that the child may grow up to be neither male nor female. They often press for an early answer as to the infant's sex. Temptation to give a provisional opinion should be avoided until the nature of the disorder is known and an informed answer can be given. In the newborn, the decision as to the appropriate sex of rearing is based mainly on the appearance of the external genitalia and on the likely pattern of secondary sexual development at puberty. This decision should be taken jointly by the paediatric endocrinologist, the urologist and the parents, making use of the clinical, biochemical, cytogenetic and radiological features of the individual case. The gender should be assigned as soon as possible after birth; however, in some cases of severe ambiguity, there is a case for waiting to assess the effect of early treatment with depot testosterone (25–50 mg at monthly intervals) on phallic growth as a guide to androgen responsiveness. The karyotype has no direct bearing on the sex of rearing.

Virilised female infants with congenital adrenal hyperplasia should in general be raised as female. XY males with severe genital ambiguity due to deficient testosterone biosynthesis or androgen insensitivity are also probably best raised as females. The demonstration of absent androgen binding in cultured geni-

Table 23.7 Patient with intersex state: laboratory assessment

No gonads palpable
  Karyotype, plasma 17-hydroxyprogesterone,
  11-deoxycortisol
One gonad palpable
  Karyotype, human chorionic gonadotrophin test,
  gonadal biopsy, pelvic ultrasonography, laparotomy
Two gonads palpable
  Karyotype, human chorionic gonadotrophin test (1000
  units daily × 3), plasma testosterone,
  dihydrotestosterone, dehydroepiandrosterone,
  androstenedione on days 0 and 4
In-vitro androgen-binding studies
Molecular analysis
Sinography

tal fibroblasts would add weight to this argument in the latter category. Other factors favouring female assignment are the presence of a vaginal pouch with an XO cell line. However, ethnic considerations, which usually favour male gender assignment, may be overriding.

The concept that, once established, gender identity and role are more or less fixed has now been questioned by the studies of Imperato-McGinley et al. [38]. Although a change of gender may be extremely difficult, the possibility of gender conversion should be viewed with an open mind in the case of individual subjects who, because of spontaneous virilisation or feminisation at puberty, find existence in their original gender intolerable.

Gender identity in intersex patients

Sex hormone therapy

Long-term treatment with androgens to increase phallic growth in early childhood has rightly fallen into disrepute because of the inevitable acceleration of bone maturation, which leads to loss of ultimate growth potential. While standard testosterone treatment is effective for inducing pubertal development in males with androgen-responsive syndromes, it is of limited value in patients with androgen insensitivity. Induction of full masculinisation in these patients is still very unsatisfactory. It has, however, been demonstrated that some further virilisation in adult patients may be effectively induced using supraphysiological doses of depot testosterone, i.e. 500 mg weekly [33]. Effects, which were slow to appear, were specifically seen on penile length and facial body hair growth.

In a number of intersex disorders, gender identity, i.e. the gender in which the patient perceives him or herself, appears relatively unequivocal. For example, the female patient with virilisation of the external genitalia, as in congenital adrenal hyperplasia, usually develops a predominantly female gender identity, although a number of androgen-dependent behaviour traits may be noticeable. This suggests that fetal androgen exposure influences subsequent behaviour. In complete androgen insensitivity, however, there is apparently no conflict of gender identity or role, both

being unequivocally female. Patients with partial androgen insensitivity present a more complex picture. Such patients, assigned and raised as males, have been compared with those assigned and raised as females. Those raised as boys are said to have developed male gender identity but, as their pubertal development was incomplete, they had difficulty in establishing a male gender role. In contrast, those raised as females developed a female gender identity and role.

Recent studies of patients with 5α-reductase deficiency have rekindled the controversy of biological versus psychological origins of gender identity. Exposure to testosterone prenatally and during puberty appears to have a strong influence in converting female to male gender identity. However, no prospective studies have been performed, and the affected subjects may have been influenced by social pressures to assume a male role.

References

1. New MI. Steroid 21-hydroxylase deficiency (congenital adrenal hyperplasia). Am J Med 1995; 98 (SIA): 2S–8S
2. Speicer PW, New MI. Prenatal diagnosis and treatment of congenital adrenal hyperplasia. J Paed Endocrinol 1994; 7: 183–191
3. Rösler A, Lieberman E. Enzymatic defects of steroidogenesis: 11β-hydroxylase deficiency congenital adrenal hyperplasia. In: New MO, Levine M (eds) Adrenal diseases in childhood. Basel: Karger, 1984:47–71
4. Hughes IA, Arisaka O, Perry LA, Honour JW. Early diagnosis of 11β-hydroxylase deficiency in two siblings confirmed by analysis of a novel steroid metabolite in newborn urine. Acta Endocrinol 1986; 111: 349–354
5. White PC, Curnow KM, Paseo L. Disorders of steroid 11β-hydroxylase isozymes. Endocr Rev 1994; 15: 421–38
6. Zhang L, Sakkal-Alkaddour H, Chang YT, Yang X, Pang S. A new compound heterozygous frameshift mutation in the type II 3β-hydoxysteroid dehydrogenase (3β-HSD) gene causes salt-wasting 3β-HSD deficiency congenital adrenal hyperplasia. J Clin Endocrinol 1996; 81: 291–5
7. Morishima A, Grumbach MM, Simpson ER, Fisher C, Qin K. Aromatase deficiency in male and female siblings caused by a novel mutation and the physiological role of oestrogens. J Clin Endocrinol Metab 1995; 80: 3689–98

8. Kirk JMW, Perry LA, Shand WS, Kirby RS, Besser GM, Savage MO. Female pseudohermaphroditism due to a maternal adreno-cortical tumour. J Clin Endocrinol Metab 1990; 70: 1280–4

9. Rimoin DL, Schimke RN. Genetic disorders of the endocrine glands. St Louis: CV Mosby, 1971

10. Sultan C, Lobaccaro JM, Lumbroso S, et al. Molecular aspects of sex differentiation applications in pathological conditions. In: Bergada C, Moguilevsky JA (eds) Frontiers in endocrinology. Puberty: basic and clinical aspects. Rome: Serono Symposia Publications, 1995: 21–35

11. Wilson JD, Griffen JE, Russell DW. Steroid 5α-reductase 2 deficiency. Endocr Rev 1993; 14: 577–93

12. Brinkman AO. Steroid hormone receptors: activators of gene transcription. J Pediatr Endocrinol 1994; 7: 275–82

13. Lobaccaro JM, Poujol N, Chiche L, Lumbroso S, Brown TR, Sultan C. Molecular modeling and in vitro investigations of the human androgen receptor DNA-binding domain: application for the study of two mutations. Mol Cell Endocrinol 1996; 116: 137–47

14. Robboy SJ, Miller T, Donahoe PK, et al. Dysgenesis of testicular and streak gonads in the syndrome of mixed gonadal dysgenesis: perspective derived from a clinopathologic analysis of twenty-one cases. Hum Pathol 1982; 13: 700–16

15. Rajfer J, Walsh PC. Mixed gonadal dysgenesis – dysgenetic male pseudohermaphroditism. Pediatr Acta Endocrinol 1981; 8: 105–15

16. Bardoni B, Zanaria E, Guioli G, et al. A dosage sensitive locus at chromosome Xp21 is involved in male to female sex reversal. Nat Genet 1994; 7: 497–501

17. Muscatelli F, Strom TM, Walker AP, et al. Mutations in the DAX-1 gene give rise to both X-linked adrenal congenital hypoplasia and hypogonadotrophic hypogonadism. Nature 1994; 372: 672–6

18. Wagner T, Wirth J, Meyer J, et al. Autosomal sex reversal and campomelic-dysplasia are caused by mutations in and around the SRY-related gene SOX-9. Cell 1994; 79: 160–4

19. Van Niekerk WA. True hermaphroditism. Pediatr Adol Endocrinol 1981; 8: 80–99

20. Wachtel SS, Bard J. The XX testis. Pediatr Adol Endocrinol 1981; 8: 116–32

21. Kremer H, Kraaij R, Toledo SPA, et al. Male pseudohermaphroditism due to a homozygous missense mutation of the luteinizing hormone receptor gene. Nat Genet 1995; 9: 160–4

22. New MI, Josso N. Disorders of gonadal differentiation and congenital adrenal hyperplasia. Endocrinol Metab Clin North Am 1988; 17: 333–366

23. Forest MG. Inborn errors of testosterone biosynthesis. Pediatr Adol Endocrinol 1981; 8: 133–55

24. Lin D, Sugawara T, Staruss JF III, et al. Role of steroidogenic acute regulatory protein in adrenal and gonadal steroidogenesis. Science 1995; 267: 1828–31

25. Yanase T, Simpson ER, Waterman MR. 17 alpha-hydroxylase/17, 20-lyase deficiency – from clinical investigation to molecular definition. Endocr Rev 1991; 12: 91–108

26. Morel Y, Mbarki F, Portrat S. Génétique des pseudohermaphrodisms masculins par anomalies de la synthèse de la testostérone. In: Chaussain JL, Roger M (eds) Les ambiguïtés sexuelles. Paris: SEPE, 1995; 53–75

27. Martin F, Perheentupa , Aldercreutz E. Plasma and urinary androgens in a pubertal boy with 3β-hydroxysteroid with hypertension due to a 17α-hydroxylation deficiency. Clin Endocrinol 1976; 5: 53–9

28. Andersson S, Geissler WM, Wu L, et al. Molecular genetics and pathophysiology of 17β-hydroxysteroid dehdrogenase 3 deficiency. J Clin Endocrinol Metab 1996; 81: 130–6

29. Gross DJ, Landau H, Kohn G, et al. Male pseudohermaphroditism due to 17β-hydroxysteroid dehydrogenase deficiency – a report of 3 cases. Clin Endocrinol 1985; 23: 439–44

30. Savage MO, Preece MA, Jeffcoate SL, et al. Familial male pseudohermaphroditism due to deficiency of 5α-reductase. Clin Endocrinol 1980; 12: 397–406

31. Jenkins EP, Andersson S, Imperato-McGinley J, Wilson JD, Russell DW. Genetic and pharmacological evidence for more than one human steroid 5α-reductase. J Clin Invest 1991; 89: 293–300

32. Boudon C, Lumbroso S, Lobaccaro JM, et al. Molecular study of the 5 alpha-reductase type 2 gene in three European families with 5 alpha-reductase deficiency. J Clin Endocrinol Metab 1995; 80: 2149–53

33. Price P, Wass JAH, Griffin JE, et al. High dose androgen therapy in male pseudohermaphroditism due to 5α-reductase deficiency and disorders of the androgen receptor. J Clin Invest 1984; 74: 1496–508

34. Quigley CA, Debellis A, Marschke KB, Elawady MK, Wilson EM, French FA. Androgen receptor defects: historical, clinical, and molecular perspectives. Endocrine Rev 1995; 16: 327–32

35. Lumbroso S, Lobaccaro JM, Belon C, Boulot P,

Amram S, Sultan C. Molecular prenatal exclusion of Reifenstein syndrome. Eur J Endocrinol 1994; 130: 327–32

36. Imbeaud S, Faure E, Lamarre I, *et al.* Insensitivity to anti-Müllerian hormone due to a mutation in the human anti-Müllerian hormone receptor. Nat Genet 1995; 11: 382–8

37. Smals AGH, Gerlag FFM, Pieters GFF, Drayer JIM, Benraad TJ, Kloppenborg PWC. Leydig cell responsive-

ness to single and repeated human chorionic gonadotrophin administration. J Clin Endocrinol Metab 1979; 49: 12–14

38. Imperato-McGinley J, Peterson RE, Gautier T, Sturla E. Male pseudohermaphroditism secondary to 5α-reductase deficiency. A model for the role of androgen in both the development of the male phenotype and the evolution of a male gender identity. J Steroid Biochem 1979; 11: 637–45

Immunology

24

A. C. Cunningham and J. A. Kirby

Introduction

The immune system is one of the largest and most complex organs in the body. Its primary roles are the inactivation of potentially pathogenic micro-organisms and viruses, the prevention of infestation by potential parasites, and the suppression of tumours. Effective functioning of the immune system is dependent upon the availability of an effective and flexible arsenal with which to fight infection. The power of immune 'effector' mechanisms is well demonstrated by the damage associated with immuno-pathologies seen in diseases such as glomerulo-nephritis, rheumatoid arthritis and the extreme vigour of acute allograft rejection. The morbidity associated with genetic or induced immunodeficiency is also indicative of the importance of immune function. Clearly, sensitive, though reliable, mechanisms must exist to regulate the numerous functions of the normal immune system.

The objective of this chapter is to describe the function and regulation of the major components of the immune system. The chapter concludes with a specific discussion of immunological examples drawn from the fields of clinical transplantation and cancer immunobiology.

Innate immunity

Non-specific barriers to infection are the first obstacles a pathogen must overcome to achieve successful invasion of its host. These barriers are not acquired, do not change, and allow the specific immune system time to mount a response. The innate system of immune defence is therefore fast acting but relatively non-specific and non-adaptive. It consists of physical and biochemical barriers such as the skin, mucus, acid in the stomach and lysozyme in many secretions, which all help to prevent the entry of micro-organisms into the body.

A battery of complex mechanisms designed to eliminate microbes that have penetrated normal body tissues also exists. These mechanisms include cellular components of the reticuloendothelial system, such as phagocytic mononuclear and polymorphonuclear leucocytes, natural killer cells, alternative-pathway activation of the complement system, and a range of acute-phase inflammatory mediators.

Phagocytes

Phagocytes engulf and digest micro-organisms and particles that are harmful to the body. Cells in this category fall into several subpopulations but are all derived from common stem cells within the bone marrow.

Neutrophils are generally the first cellular components to respond to tissue injury. They migrate from the blood across the endothelium and into the tissues within seconds of the recognition of a chemotactic stimulus. These stimuli may be chemicals specifically produced by bacteria, factors produced by damaged body cells, or peptides produced during the activation of complement.

Other phagocytic cells include tissue macrophages such as mesangial cells in the kidney, Küpffer cells in the liver, alveolar macrophages in the lung, histiocytes in connective tissue and microglial cells in the nervous system. Macrophages are highly phagocytic and contain numerous lysosomes and endocytic vesicles. They possess an enhanced antimicrobicidal capacity following activation.

Phagocytes are also capable of secreting soluble agents able non-specifically to damage cells and pathogens within the micro-environment. The most active of these factors are oxygen radicals, which are produced during the 'respiratory burst' that follows cell activation [1].

Natural killer cells

Natural killer cells are frequently termed large granular lymphocytes on the basis of their morphology. Though reportedly related to cytotoxic T lymphocytes, they have no specific antigen receptor and are characterised on the basis of their unrestricted cytotoxic function in vitro. The physiological role of these cells remains unclear, but they are thought to play a role in tumour immunity. Many tumours have defective genes, or defective genetic regulation, which cause a lowering of the expression of major histocompatibility (MHC) antigens (see section p. 439). This reduces the classical immunogenicity of these cells but appears to enhance their susceptibility to natural killer cell-mediated cytolysis. Recent work has demonstrated that normal expression of class I MHC antigens elicits a strong negative signal to natural killer cells preventing the lysis of healthy cells [2, 3].

Natural killer cells are also thought to limit the early stages of infection by certain viruses. For example, patients with defective natural killer cells frequently suffer severe infection by viruses such as cytomegalovirus.

Alternative pathway of complement activation

The complement system consists of up to 20 serum proteins that are involved in two interrelated enzyme cascades termed the 'classical' and the 'alternative' pathways. The end result of these cascades is the generation of a 'membrane attack complex', which forms a potentially lethal membrane pore and a series of pro-inflammatory mediators. The alternative pathway may be activated directly but non-specifically by bacterial cell wall components, e.g. lipopolysaccharide. Its products bind directly to the bacterial cell wall (Figure 24.1) [4].

Inflammatory mediators

The innate immune system's vast cocktail of pro-inflammatory substances can directly damage, or induce cells to damage, invading pathogens. The C3a and C5a peptides released during complement activation possess wide-ranging capabilities, including the promotion of smooth muscle contraction, the retraction of endothelial cells, and the release of histamine by mast cells. Furthermore, these peptides stimulate the chemotaxis and activation of phagocytic leucocytes. These cells carry C3b receptors on their surface and are able to bind specifically to C3b-coated microorganisms prior to phagocytosis.

Other active peptides, including Hageman factor and fibrinopeptides, are released during blood clotting and increase local vascular permeability and the recruitment of phagocytes. Acute-phase proteins, for example C-reactive protein, are produced during infection and increase alternative pathway complement activation and phagocyte activity. Interferons are produced by virally infected cells and protect other cells from infection by the stimulation of mechanisms that prevent viral replication. The above-mentioned substances represent only a selection from the plethora of inflammatory mediators currently known to exist.

Adaptive immunity

The adaptive immune system has evolved to provide a versatile defence mechanism against infectious pathogens. The innate immune system is able to hold pathogens at bay for a time, but infectious microorganisms rapidly evolve to bypass these defences. Each process of adaptive immunity is dependent on the function of lymphocytes and is characterised by an escalating response with a high degree of specificity. Furthermore, adaptive responses are characterised by immunological memory, which enables a more vigorous reaction following secondary exposure to a specific agent.

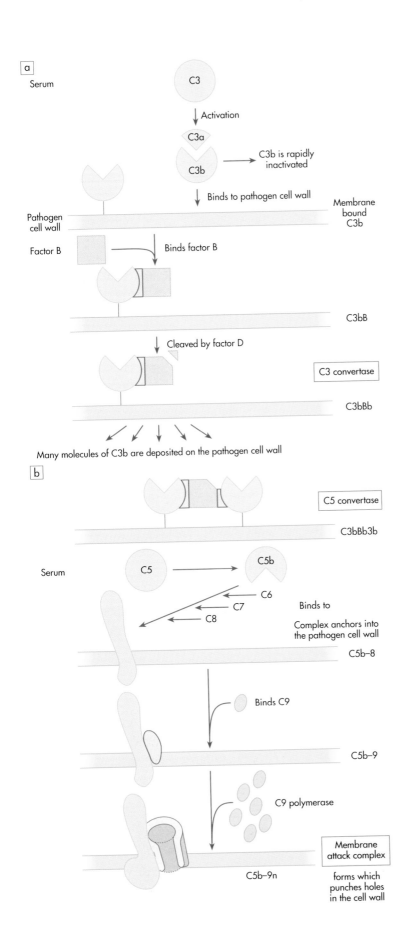

Figure 24.1 *The alternative pathway of complement activation. (a) C3 activation. (b) Lytic pathway.*

Resting lymphocytes are small mononuclear cells with little cytoplasm. However, following exposure to an antigen, a small proportion of antigen-specific cells expand rapidly and begin to divide. This process of clonal expansion is an essential feature of adaptive immunity. Lymphocytes may be divided functionally into T and B cells.

T lymphocytes and cellular immunity

The T cell precursor is generated within the bone marrow but migrates to the thymus before maturing and developing the ability to recognise foreign antigen. Each newly formed T cell expresses numerous copies of an identical T cell antigen receptor. However, the receptor on each different T cell varies in sequence and antigen specificity. This seemingly random variability enables at least a few cells within the total T cell population to respond to antigens on any given pathogen. Following antigen encounter, these few cells divide to generate a sufficient number of responsive cells to mount a useful immune response. Estimates show that a single antigen-specific T cell can proliferate to generate a clone of over 1000 identical cells. This mechanism is termed clonal selection.

In recent years, the process by which maturing T cells generate their enormous receptor diversity has been determined. The receptor is a heterodimer and, for more than 90% of the cells, consists of an α and a β chain. Each chain is composed of a variable region, a constant region, a transmembrane region and a cytoplasmic tail. The initial genomic sequence of DNA encoding each chain contains a large number of possible variable sequences followed by multiple diversity and joining sequences. Each mature chain is produced after a genetic rearrangement process that involves extensive deletion of genomic DNA and the resplicing of single, variable, joining and diversity regions. It has been estimated that this process can yield a total of 10^{17} different $\alpha\beta$ T cell receptors [5].

A proportion of T cells, particularly those found close to the epithelial cells of the mucosa (including the genitourinary tract), express an alternative form of the T cell antigen receptor. This consists of a γ and δ chain heterodimer. The function of these $\gamma\delta$ T cells is not clear. They appear to be less variable than $\alpha\beta$ T

cells, and are thought to represent an older, more primitive lineage [6].

Receptors expressed by each T cell are generated by a random process and it is therefore likely that some newly formed cells will recognise antigens produced by healthy, or 'self', body cells. The capacity to discriminate between self and non-self, and to prevent a response to self, is vital for normal immune function. This important requirement is fulfilled by the thymus, which is essential for the generation of T cell self-tolerance. Equally essential to normal immune function is the thymus' other function – to provide a micro-environment suitable for T cell maturation.

Thymic tolerance

T cell function is regulated by the affinity of the antigen receptor for a given ligand. The T cell will only be activated by interaction with an antigen if the affinity is sufficiently high. Essentially, the thymus selects newly formed cells that show no more than a low affinity for all self antigens but deletes any cell bearing receptors that recognise self antigens with a dangerously high affinity. It has been estimated that only 3% of newly formed T cells survive this selection process and escape the thymus to join the recirculating pool.

T cell recirculation

T lymphocytes that have not encountered their specific antigen, and are therefore naïve, migrate from the circulation across specialised high endothelial venules to secondary lymphoid sites such as the spleen, lymph nodes, and Peyer's patches in the genitourinary tract. These sites provide the ideal environment for contact with foreign antigens, and enable antigen-specific clonal expansion and the generation of effector/memory subsets. If a naïve lymphocyte is not activated after 10–20 hours, it recirculates from the lymph node, through the lymphatic system and back into the blood at the thoracic duct. However, during an immune response, the blood flow through a lymph node rises dramatically and increases the number of lymphocytes within the node. Non-specific resting cells leave the node followed, after three or four days, by a large number of activated antigen-specific T lymphocytes. These cells recirculate to the site of primary inflammation and to local lymphoid tissues. Finally, after a week or so, small, long-lived memory cells begin to leave the lymph node to join the recirculating pool. It has been estimated for adults that almost 50% of recirculating T lymphocytes are memory cells. These memory cells migrate differently from naïve T lymphocytes and recirculate through the peripheral tissue where they first encountered their specific antigen (e.g. the skin, genitourinary, gastrointestinal or respiratory system) [7, 8].

Major histocompatibility antigens
Human cells can express two classes of MHC antigen. The class I antigens are expressed constitutively on most cells, whereas the class II antigens are generally induced by stimulation with pro-inflammatory cytokines such as interferon-γ or tumour necrosis factor-α. Class II MHC antigens are generally only expressed constitutively by specialised cells of the immune system that are adapted for antigen presentation (e.g. dendritic cells). MHC molecules are specialised glycoproteins that bind a diverse array of peptides and present them as T cell ligands.

Resolution of the structure of the MHC antigens (Figure 24.2) has been one of the most significant advances in immunology during the past few years [9, 10]. Class I and class II MHC antigens have a similar three-dimensional structure but a different subunit structure. Class I MHC consists of a transmembrane α-chain that has three domains and a non-covalently attached β2-microglobulin. Class II MHC is a heterodimer of two transmembranous glycoproteins. A remarkable feature of these molecules is the prominent groove on their membrane-distal surface, which is always occupied by short peptide sequences. Class I MHC molecules typically contain nine amino-acid peptides, whereas class II molecules can accommodate much larger peptides of up to 25 amino acid residues.

The genes encoding MHC antigens are extremely polymorphic within the human population. This polymorphism is generally restricted to the region of the groove and allows different forms of the MHC molecule to bind different families of short peptides. Table 24.1 contains the number of polymorphisms for the human class I (HLA-A, HLA-B and HLA-C) and class II (HLA-DR, HLA-DP and HLA-DQ) MHC alleles.

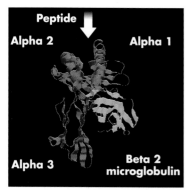

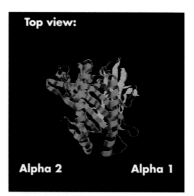

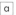

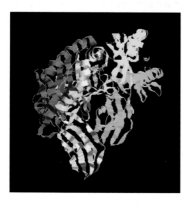

Figure 24.2 Crystal structure of (a) class I and (b) class II MHC antigens. These structures were obtained from the Database of Immunological Structures (http://histo.cryst.bbk.ac.uk/WWW Files/structures.html).

Table 24.1 Number of serologically identified polymorphic variants of human MHC antigens

MHC	Class I			Class II		
Name	HLA-A	HLA-B	HLA-C	HLA-DR	HLA-DP	HLA-DQ
Number of alleles	28	61	10	26	9	6

A complete list of HLA alleles is available at http://www.anthonynolan.com/HIG/nomenc.html.

T cell antigens

The T lymphocyte antigen receptor can only recognise short peptide 'epitopes' bound in the groove of MHC antigens. Evidence suggests that the T cell receptor interacts simultaneously with the MHC molecule and the peptide. In general, peptides from intracellular proteins are loaded into class I molecules and peptides from phagocytosed extracellular proteins are loaded into class II antigens.

T cell self-tolerance is vital given the inability of MHC molecules to discriminate between loading peptides from normal self proteins and peptides from, for example, a pathogenic organism. The lymphocyte is only activated when the T cell receptor binds to an MHC–peptide complex with an affinity greater than a triggering level. Thus, thymic deletion of all T cells that recognise MHC–self peptide complexes with an affinity above this level will produce cells that can only reach the required affinity by interaction with complexes formed with non-self peptides.

Helper or CD4$^+$ T lymphocytes

Approximately 60% of human peripheral T lymphocytes express the CD4 antigen on their cell surface. This antigen binds to a domain on the class II MHC antigen during interaction between the T cell receptor

and the class II MHC–peptide complex. Formation of this complex plays an important role in T cell activation and has an additional implication for the immune response. As class II MHC antigens primarily form complexes with peptides derived from extracellular proteins, it follows that CD4$^+$ T cells are activated, albeit indirectly, by extracellular antigens (Figure 24.3).

It is now clear that CD4$^+$ T cells are responsible for the regulation of most phases of the adaptive immune response. These cells are generally not directly cytotoxic, but produce a range of soluble mediators, or cytokines, able to affect other cells in the local environment. For this reason, they are often termed helper cells. Recent studies of individual clones of activated helper cells have shown that they can be divided functionally into at least two subpopulations. These are termed Th1 and Th2 cell types and are distinguished from each other by the range of cytokines they produce [12, 13].

The Th1 lymphocyte subpopulation appears to direct delayed-type hypersensitivity reactions by the production of cytokines such as interferon-γ (IFN-γ), interleukin-2 (IL-2), interleukin-12 (IL-12) and tumour necrosis factor-β (TNF-β). These factors enhance the local recruitment and activation of phagocytes and

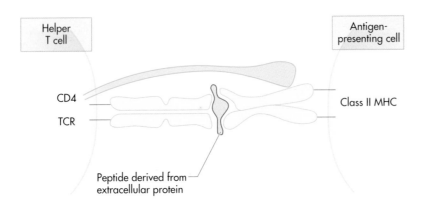

Figure 24.3 *The presentation of antigen to CD4$^+$ T cells.*

stimulate the division of antigen-specific lymphocytes, including the CD8[+] cytotoxic cells described in the next section.

The Th2 subpopulation produces a range of cytokines that are involved in antibody responses mediated by B lymphocytes and in mast cell proliferation, eosinophilia and granuloma formation. These cytokines include IL-3, IL-4, IL-5 and IL-10. Significantly, IL-4 stimulates B cells to produce the IgE class of antibody, and these antibodies are involved in the release of histamine by degranulating mast cells.

Th1 and Th2 cells are mutually regulated. The IFN-γ produced by Th1 cells inhibits the activity of Th2 cells, whereas the IL-4 and IL-10 produced by Th2 cells inhibit Th1 lymphocytes (Figure 24.4) [14].

Cytotoxic or CD8[+] T lymphocytes

Approximately 40% of peripheral T lymphocytes express the CD8 antigen. This molecule binds to a domain on the class I MHC antigen during interaction between the T cell receptor and the class I MHC–peptide complex. The formation of this complex plays an important role in the activation of CD8[+] T cells. As class I MHC antigens primarily form complexes with peptides derived from intracellular proteins, it follows that CD8[+] T cells are activated by intracellular antigens (Figure 24.5).

The CD8[+] lymphocyte subpopulation fulfils two roles. Its primary role is its involvement in the process of antigen-specific target cell lysis followed by cytokine secretion. Following activation, the CD8[+] T cell differentiates from a resting, or precursor, state to form a cytotoxic effector cell. This cell efficiently kills target cells that express the specific class I MHC–peptide complex. The direct lytic process involves lymphocyte degranulation and the secretion of agents including perforin, which forms pores in the target cell membrane. However, recent studies have shown cytotoxic T cells can also induce the fragmentation of DNA within the target cell by a process termed apoptosis.

The ability of CD8[+] cytotoxic cells to lyse target cells containing non-self proteins is consistent with their involvement in the prevention of the spread of viruses by killing virally infected cells. Virally infected cells are recognised by the cytotoxic lymphocyte because non-self viral peptides are expressed in the peptide-binding groove of their class I MHC antigens.

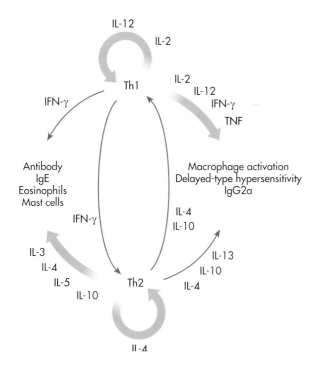

Figure 24.4 *The function and regulation of Th1 and Th2 helper T cells. Positive regulation by cytokines (broad arrows); negative regulation by cytokines (fine arrows).*

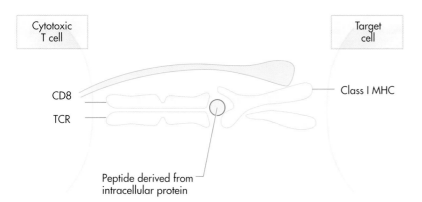

Figure 24.5 *The presentation of antigen to CD8[+] T cells.*

A similar mechanism may allow cytotoxic cells to kill class I MHC antigen-expressing tumour cells that produce novel tumour-associated antigens (see the section on tumour immunology, p. 450).

B lymphocytes and humoral immunity

In humans, B cells constitute approximately 10% of the circulating lymphocytes and are produced within the bone marrow. Resting B cells are morphologically similar to T cells despite being functionally distinct from them. B cells use a membrane-bound form of immunoglobulin to recognise antigen. The receptor can also be secreted as an immunoglobulin molecule or antibody following B cell activation. Like T cells, B cells also have a clonal specificity for antigen, with each activated cell producing soluble immunoglobulins with a single specificity. B cells also express class II MHC antigens constitutively, and can therefore present foreign peptide to T cells.

Immunoglobulins

The immunoglobulins (Igs), or antibodies, are a group of five glycoproteins that are divided into five classes, termed IgM, IgG, IgA, IgD and IgE. These classes differ from each other in structure and molecular weight but their functions are broadly similar. One portion of the molecule, the variable region, binds to a specific site on an antigen, whereas the constant region may interact with, and regulate the function of, additional components of the immune system such as complement, phagocytes or cytotoxic cells. Unlike the T cell receptor, immunoglobulins are not restricted to peptide binding and are able to bind efficiently to carbohydrates, nucleic acids, proteins and a range of chemical and biochemical compounds.

Approximately 10% of the total immunoglobulin pool consists of IgM, which is a large, pentameric structure normally restricted to the blood. After primary infection, IgM is the first immunoglobulin produced by antigen-specific B cells. It has a low affinity for antigen but the multivalency confers a relatively high avidity of overall binding. IgM is able to activate complement efficiently. Activated helper T cells, particularly of the Th2 phenotype, produce cytokines able to stimulate B cells to class-switch from production of IgM to IgG. This smaller immunoglobulin makes up about 75% of the immunoglobulin pool, can diffuse more rapidly than IgM and, in addition to the activation of complement, can bind to a range of cellular components of the innate immune system.

IgA makes up about 15% of the total immunoglobulin pool and is generally restricted to mucosal sites. It is present in colostrum, saliva and tears. Nearly all the IgD is associated with antigen recognition on the surface of B cells, whereas IgE is found on the surface of mast cells.

Immunoglobulin diversity

The diversity of immunoglobulin specificities is generated by genetic splicing in a manner analogous to that of the rearrangement of the genes encoding the T cell antigen receptor. In the case of human immunoglobulins, it has been estimated that this process can produce up to 10^{11} different immunoglobulin molecules. However, unlike the T cell, B cells supplement this process by rearranging immunoglobulin genes after antigen recognition by 'somatic hypermutation'. The mutated B cells which, coincidentally, have a higher affinity for the antigen than the original clone, survive. The overall immunoglobulin response tends to become more specific as the immunoglobulins produced by the mutant cells possess an increased affinity for their antigen. This process is termed affinity maturation [15].

Classical pathway of complement activation

The classical pathway of complement is activated by the interaction between subunit q of the complement C1 complex with the constant region of IgM or IgG molecules bound to their specific antigen. The activated C1 complex initiates the classical pathway of complement activation, in which classical C3 and C5 convertase are produced (Figure 24.6). Beyond this point, both the alternative and classical pathways are identical and cause cell damage in a similar way (see Figure 24.1b) [4].

Opsonisation

Many human leucocytes express one or more of three classes of Fc receptor for domains on the constant region of IgG molecules. These cells include mononuclear phagocytes, neutrophils, eosinophils and natural

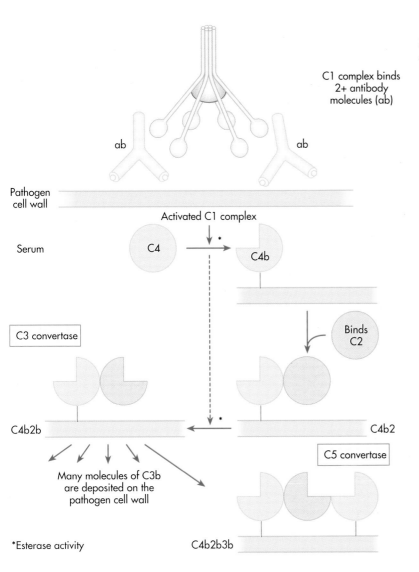

C1 complex binds
2+ antibody
molecules (ab)

ab   ab

Pathogen
cell wall

Activated C1 complex

Serum   C4   C4b

C3 convertase

Binds
C2

C4b2b   C4b2

C5 convertase

Many molecules of C3b
are deposited on the
pathogen cell wall

*Esterase activity   C4b2b3b

Figure 24.6 *The classical pathway of complement activation.*

killer cells. These Fc receptors enable the leucocytes to recognise antibody-coated antigens by a process known as opsonisation. This greatly enhances the efficiency of phagocytosis and increases the specificity of cellular elements of the innate immune response.

Antibody-dependent cell-mediated cytotoxicity
Many natural killer cells express a relatively low-affinity Fc receptor for IgG. This receptor enables these cells to bind to IgG-coated targets and triggers a process that results in target cell lysis. As the receptor has a low IgG affinity, it binds aggregated IgG more readily than monomeric immunoglobulin in the plasma. This appears to prevent the inappropriate activation of natural killer cells in the blood.

Adhesion molecules

A series of specialised adhesion and signalling molecules is involved in the migration of leucocytes across vascular endothelium and into body tissues and also in the regulation of T lymphocyte activation [16].

Ligands and receptors
Three main families of molecules are involved in binding and supporting the migration of leucocytes. These are the selectins and members of the integrin and immunoglobulin superfamilies. The involvement of selectins is mainly restricted to an initial low-affinity interaction typified by leucocyte 'rolling' across the vascular endothelium. Members of the other two

families are of importance during leucocyte stimulation, tight adhesion to endothelium, and extravasation into tissues.

Selectins

The three members of the selectin family are designated L-selectin, E-selectin and P-selectin after the lymphocyte, endothelial cell and platelet on which they were respectively identified. These molecules contain three structural regions and a cytoplasmic tail. The N-terminal domain is closely related to calcium-dependent lectins, whereas the central domain shares characteristics with an epidermal growth factor sequence. The third domain contains a number of repeating sequences homologous to a sequence found in proteins that regulate the activity of complement.

Each selectin is thought to possess the ability to bind to a number of carbohydrate ligands.

Integrins

Integrins are a superfamily of transmembrane glycoproteins consisting of non-covalently linked α and, generally smaller, β subunits. They are widely expressed by cells of the body and are usually grouped by virtue of their common β chains into eight subfamilies. At least 14 discrete α subunits have been identified and it is clear that a given α chain may associate with more than one β chain (Table 24.2). The extracellular portion of the α chain contains three or four sites that bind divalent cations essential for integrin function. Both chains generally have short cytoplasmic regions able to interact with the cytoskeleton

Table 24.2 The integrin family

Integrin	β subunit	Other names	α subunit	Other common names	Ligands
VLA-1	β1	CD29	α_1	CD49a	Laminin (collagen)
VLA-2		or VLAβ	α_2	CD49b	Collagen (laminin)
VLA-3		or gpIIa	α_3	CD29c	Fibronectin, laminin, collagen
VLA-4			**α_4**	**CD49d**	**VCAM-1, fibronectin**
VLA-5			α_5	CD49e	Fibronectin
VLA-6			α_6	CD49f	Laminin
$\beta 1\alpha_7$			α_7		Laminin
$\beta 1\alpha_8$			α_8		
$\beta 1\alpha_V$			α_V	CD51	Fibronectin
LFA-1	**β2**	**CD18**	**α_L**	**CD11a**	**ICAM-1, ICAM-2, ICAM-3**
Mac-1			**α_M**	**CD11b**	**ICAM-1, C3bi, fibrinogen**
p150, 95			**α_X**	**CD11c**	**C3bi**
CD41a	β3	CD61	αIIb	CD41	Fibrinogen, fibronectin, vitronectin, Von Willebrand factor
$\beta 3\alpha_V$		or gpIIIa	α_V	CD51	As above + thrombospondin
$\beta 4\alpha_6$	β4		α_6	CD49f	Laminin
$\beta 5\alpha_V$	β5	β_x, β_s	α_V	CD51	Vitronectin, fibronectin
$\beta 6\alpha_V$	β6		α_V	CD51	Fibronectin
LPAM-1	**β7**	**βp**	**α4**	**CD49d**	**VCAM-1, MadCam1, fibronectin**
CD103			**αe**		**E-cadherin**
$\beta 8\alpha_V$	β8	α_V		CD51	

Elements in bold print are of particular importance for leucocyte adhesion.

and these may be phosphorylated. Phosphorylation is often associated with cell activation and can enhance the affinity of adhesion to the ligand (inside-out signalling) [17].

Integrins play a key role in both cell–cell and cell–matrix adhesion. They bind to components of the extracellular matrix such as collagen, fibronectin, laminin and vitronectin. Some integrins have affinity for specific peptide domains such as the well-characterised arginine-glycine-aspartic acid sequence, which is present on a number of extracellular matrix components. Three subfamilies of integrins are of particular importance for leucocyte adhesion. These include a member of the β1 family of 'very late antigens', VLA-4 ($α_4β1$), β2 integrins termed the leucocyte cell adhesion molecules (LCAM; $α_Lβ2$, $α_Mβ2$ and $α_Xβ2$) and β7 integrins ($α_4β7$ and $α_eβ7$).

The β1 integrin VLA-4 is expressed by many mononuclear leucocytes and binds to the immunoglobulin superfamily member vascular cell adhesion molecule-1 (VCAM-1) in addition to fibronectin. The β2 subfamily is restricted to cells of the leucocyte lineage and includes lymphocyte function-associated antigen-1 (LFA-1) and Mac-1, which both serve to anchor leucocytes to cells that express intercellular adhesion molecule-1 (ICAM-1). The β7 family is expressed by mucosal lymphocytes. The $α_4β7$ integrin has recently been demonstrated to be the gut-homing receptor, enabling gut-trophic lymphocytes to enter the Peyers' patches. The $α_eβ7$ (CD103) integrin is expressed by nearly all lamina propria lymphocytes in the gut, and by approximately 50% of intraepithelial lymphocytes [18].

Immunoglobulin superfamily members
ICAM-1 is a large transmembrane glycoprotein bearing five domains containing the folded β sheet characteristic of immunoglobulins. The molecule is expressed constitutively by endothelial cells but is significantly up-regulated by stimulation with IL-1, TNF-α and IFN-γ. The cytokines TNF-α and IFN-γ also induce and up-regulate the expression of ICAM-1 on a range of parenchymal cells including fibroblasts and epithelial cells in the skin, lung and liver. This process enhances the adhesion of β2 integrin-expressing leucocytes.

Structural studies have shown that VCAM-1 contains seven immunoglobulin domains. The first and fourth of these regions are homologous and function during lymphocyte adhesion. VCAM-1 is constitutively expressed on endothelial cells at a low level, but expression is up-regulated within 12 hours and then maintained at high levels by stimulation with the cytokines IL-1 and TNF-α. Immunocytochemical studies have also demonstrated the presence of VCAM-1 on a variety of non-vascular cells, including renal epithelial cells, neural cells, and the synovial cells of inflamed joints [19].

Co-stimulation

Ligation of a T cell receptor with its specific MHC–peptide ligand is insufficient to activate the T cell. This observation has generated the two-signal hypothesis for lymphocyte activation. Signal one is defined as interaction with specific MHC and peptide, and signal two is a non-specific co-stimulatory signal.

Studies have indicated that the T cell antigen receptor has only a very modest affinity for its specific MHC–peptide ligand. This has been estimated as between 1×10^{-5}M and 5×10^{-5}M, which is considerably lower than the value for a typical IgG molecule, which is of the order of 1×10^{-9}M. This affinity is too low to allow stable conjugates to form between T cell receptors and the 210 to 340 specific MHC–peptide ligands required for lymphocyte activation [20]. The multiplicity of antigen-independent adhesion molecule interactions play a vital role in stabilising the T cell and antigen-presenting cell complex sufficiently to allow T cell receptor signal transduction to take place. This adhesion is rapidly increased following T cell receptor ligation by an increase in the affinity of LFA-1 (inside-out signalling) [21].

Appropriate ligation of the lymphocyte adhesion molecules LFA-1 and VLA-4 is known to generate co-stimulatory signals able to augment lymphocyte activation. Furthermore, monoclonal antibodies specific for LFA-1 have been shown to stimulate the proliferation of resting lymphocytes. Adhesive interactions between the T cell-surface molecule CD28 and members of the B7 ligand family (CD80, CD86) on antigen-presenting cells are also known to generate a signal important for the activation of antigen-specific T cells.

Expression of the B7 family of ligands is restricted to a small group of specialised mononuclear cells including dendritic cells and B lymphocytes. Antigen presentation in the absence of satisfactory co-stimulatory signal transduction may even produce stable lymphocyte hyporeactivity. Indeed, the therapeutic elimination of CD28 signalling by the blockade of B7 molecules with the soluble receptor-like construct CTLA4-Ig has resulted in partial cardiac allograft tolerance in a murine model [22].

Examples of clinical immunology

Acute allograft rejection

The extreme vigour of allograft rejection can be explained by the process termed alloreactivity. Although mature T lymphocytes have been selected in the thymus for specific tolerance of all potential self MHC antigen–self peptide complexes, the cells have not been selected for tolerance of the subtly different MHC molecule–peptide complexes expressed on the surface of donor cells. It has been estimated that up to 2% of all recipient T cells may respond to the allogeneic MHC molecules expressed by graft tissues. Furthermore, as this situation reflects an artificial cross-reaction, a significant proportion of the responsive lymphocytes is present as memory cells, which facilitate the rapid initiation of the rejection response [23, 24].

It is not clinically feasible to match the organ donor and recipient for identical MHC antigens, given the enormous polymorphism of MHC alleles (see Table 24.1). Consequently, it has been necessary to develop drugs to suppress the immune response. One of the most successful immunosuppressive drugs in use today is cyclosporin A. This cyclic peptide blockades the production of IL-2 during T cell activation. The function of this cytokine is best illustrated by its original name, which was 'T cell growth factor'. Without IL-2, the graft-specific lymphocytes are unable to divide and cannot initiate the rejection response [25].

Cancer immunotherapy

The prospects for successful cancer immunotherapy are dependent on the capability of T cells in the recognition of tumour antigens. During the 1950s, some chemically induced tumours were shown to express specific, 'non-self' antigens that allowed sensitised animals to reject transplanted tumour cells. More recent studies have shown that T lymphocytes are able to recognise tumour-derived peptides complexed in the groove of MHC molecules.

A range of tumour-specific antigens has been detected including the MAGE family (MAGE-1), which is found in 37% of human melanomas, a smaller proportion of other tumours, and no normal tissues except the immunologically privileged testis [26]. Peptides from MAGE-1 associate with the class I molecules HLA-A1 and HLA-Cw16 and can be recognised by cytotoxic lymphocytes. The related molecule MAGE-3 is associated with a greater proportion of cancers and yields immunogenic peptides that complex with HLA-A1 and HLA-A2. Studies have demonstrated that up to 35% of transitional bladder cancers express MAGE antigens, with the proportion increasing to 61% of invasive tumours. Further tumour-associated proteins have been identified, including BAGE, and GAGE-1 and GAGE-2, which also yield peptides that can be recognised by cytotoxic T lymphocytes and are expressed by between 10% and 20% of bladder cancers. In addition to the identification of proteins expressed by a range of cancer cells, tumours also express unique peptide epitopes derived from mutated genes. Recent work has identified such mutations in murine cancers, which yield peptides recognisable by both CD8 + CTL and CD4 + 'helper' T lymphocytes.

Lack of B7 molecule expression by the cells of most solid tumours may explain the inability of the immune system to reject even those tumours that express recognisable complexes of MHC antigen and tumour-derived non-self peptide. Engagement of the T cell receptor in the absence of co-stimulation can induce a state of T cell unresponsiveness, termed anergy. This process would serve to stabilise immunological hyporesponsiveness to tumour cells. Several groups have shown that T cells can respond to tumour cells after transfection with B7. Models studied include murine melanoma, sarcoma, lymphoma, colon, carcinoma and mastocytoma. The manipulation of lymphocyte co-stimulation will undoubtedly llow the development of novel and highly specific methods for the immunotherapy of cancer.

Acknowledgements

The authors wish to thank Dr Sam Hamilton for her critical review of the manuscript.

References

1. Allen LAH, Aderem A. Mechanisms of innate immunity. Curr Opin Immunol 1996; 8: 36–40

2. Ljunggren H-G, Karre K. In search of the missing self: MHC molecules and NK recognition. Immunol Today 1990: 11: 237–44

3. Gumperz JE, Parham P. The enigma of the natural killer cell. Nature 1995; 378: 245–8

4. Reid KBM. The complement system. In: Hames BD, Glover DM (eds) Frontiers in molecular biology, Vol. 9. Molecular immunology. Oxford: IRL Press, 1996: 326–82

5. Davis MM, Chien Y-H. T cell antigen receptor genes. In: Hames BD, Glover DM (eds) Frontiers in molecular biology, Vol. 9. Molecular immunology. Oxford: IRL Press, 1996: 101–31

6. Lundqvist C, Baranov V, Hammarstrom S, et al. Intraepithelial lymphocytes. Evidence for regional specialisation and extrathymic T cell maturation in the human gut epithelium. Int Immunol 1995; 7: 1473–87

7. Picker LJ, Treer JR, Ferguson-Darnell B, et al. Control of lymphocyte recirculation in man. I Differential regulation of the peripheral lymph node homing receptor L-selectin on T cells during the memory to virgin transition. J Immunol 1993; 150: 1105–21

8. Picker LJ, Treer JR, Ferguson-Darnell B, et al. Control of lymphocyte recirculation in man. II Differential regulation of the cutaneous lymphocyte associated antigen, a tissue selective homing receptor for skin homing cells. J Immunol 1993; 150: 1122–36

9. Bjorkman PJ, Saper MA, Samroui B, et al. Structure of the human class I histocompatibility antigen HLA-A2. Nature 1987; 329: 506–18

10. Brown JK, Jardetzky TS, Gorga JC, et al. Three-dimensional structure of the human class II histocompatibility antigen HLA-DR1. Nature 1993; 364: 33–9

11. Bodmer JG, Albert ED, Bodmer WF, et al. Nomenclature for factors of the HLA system 1991. Immunogenetics 1992; 36: 135–48

12. Mossman TR, Coffman RL. Th1 and Th2 cells: different patterns of lymphocyte secretion lead to the different functional properties. Ann Rev Immunol 1989; 7: 145–73

13. Romagnani S. Human Th1 and Th2 subsets: doubt no more. Immunol Today 1991; 12: 256–7

14. Carter LL, Dutton RW. Type 1 and type 2: a fundamental dichotomy for all T cell subsets. Curr Opin Immunol 1996; 8: 336–42

15. Max EE. Immunoglobulins: molecular genetics. In: Paul WE (ed) Fundamental immunology. 3rd edition. New York: Raven Press, 1993: 315–82

16. Springer TA. Adhesion receptors of the immune system. Nature 1990; 346: 425–34

17. Hynes RO. Integrins: versatility, modulation, and signalling in cell adhesion. Cell 1992; 69: 11–25

18. Berlin C, Berg EL, Briskin MJ, et al. Alpha-4, beta-7 integrin mediates lymphocyte binding to the mucosal vascular addressin MadCam-1. Cell 1993; 74: 185–95

19. Lin Y, Kirby JA, Browell DA, et al. Renal allograft rejection: expression and function of VCAM-1 on tubular epithelial cells. Clin Exp Immunol 1993; 92: 145–51

20. Valitutti S, Muller S, Cella M, et al. Serial triggering of many T-cell receptors by a few peptide–MHC complexes. Nature 1995; 375: 148–51

21. Dustin ML, Springer TA. T cell receptor cross-linking transiently stimulates adhesiveness through LFA-1. Nature 1989; 341: 619–24

22. Baliga P, Chavin KD, Qin L, et al. CTLA4-Ig prolongs allograft survival while suppressing cell-mediated immunity. Transplantation 1994; 58: 1082–90

23. Lechler RI, Lombardi G, Batchelor JR. The molecular basis of alloreactivity. Immunol Today 1990; 11: 83–8

24. Lombardi G, Sidhu S, Daly M, et al. Are primary alloresponses truly primary? Int Immunol 1990; 2: 9–13

25. Schreiber SL, Crabtree GR. The mechanism of action of cyclosporin A and FK506. Immunol Today 1992; 13: 136–42

26. Patard JJ, Brasseur F, Gil-Diez S et al. Expression of MAGE genes in transitional cell carcinomas of the urinary bladder. Int J Cancer 1995; 64: 60–4

S. N. Venn and A. R. Mundy

Two types of tissue transfer are common in urology, firstly, the use of skin and buccal or bladder mucosa for urethral reconstruction and, secondly, the use of bowel for bladder reconstruction. The three factors that require some consideration in relation to the subject of tissue transfer in these contexts are the general subject of wound healing, the use of grafts and flaps, and the consequences of incorporating bowel into the urinary tract.

Wound healing

This is the replacement of destroyed tissue by living tissue. In certain reptiles, it includes the ability to replace a tail or limb. This occurs due to the ability of cells to dedifferentiate and then redifferentiate, which does not occur in human adults. Healing in adults is limited to the fibrous obliteration of dead space and limited regeneration. In the embryo, scarless healing has been noted and this is currently the focus of intense research [1].

Healing consists of:

1. contraction,
2. replacement of lost tissue by:
   - regeneration – the closest found in adults is repair of bone and cartilage; or
   - repair – replacing lost tissue with granulation tissue to form a scar.

Contraction

This is an important process to reduce the size of the scar. The cell responsible is the myofibroblast [2], which is a type of fibroblast that has the ability to contract, as demonstrated by the inhibition of contraction by smooth muscle antagonists. The degree of contraction is inversely related to the amount of dermal collagen present, so deep wounds contract a lot and superficial abrasions contract very little. Equally, wounds closed with a split skin graft contract, whereas those covered with full-thickness grafts do not. Other factors that inhibit wound contraction are ionising radiation and glucocorticoids.

Granulation

There are three phases to the formation of granulation tissue. They do not occur in isolation, but overlap.

1. Inflammation. Cells are stimulated by the injury. Damaged endothelial cells increase their expression of adhesion molecules that attract circulating white cells, which then accumulate at the site of injury both by direct leakage and by transmigration and extravasation, and these in turn produce further compounds such as complement C5a and leukotriene B4, which cause a further influx of inflammatory cells. The accumulation of inflammatory cells is potentiated by the local increased vascular permeability and vasodilatation.
2. Demolition. Dead tissue and polymorphs liberate autosomal enzymes. Initially, the predominant white blood cell is the neutrophil but, with time, macrophages come to predominate and it is these

cells rather than neutrophils that have a critical role in normal wound healing. Both types of cells are necessary to remove bacteria and other debris from the wound, but macrophages are primarily responsible for secreting the chemical mediators necessary for normal wound healing, and whereas healing can occur in the absence of neutrophils, it cannot occur in the absence of macrophages.

Macrophages are derived from circulating blood monocytes and increase in the wounded area at a steady rate until they predominate after about three days [3]. Accumulating macrophages secrete various growth factors, as do the haemostatic cells that precede them, particularly platelets. Platelet-derived growth factor and epidermal growth factor, in particular, stimulate the accumulation and proliferation of fibroblasts derived from the surrounding wound, which migrate into the fibrin mesh where they proliferate and secrete collagen [4].

3. Organisation. The first capillary loops appear at day three.

Vascularisation: buds of endothelial cells arise from existing capillaries. These vessels have 'gaps' between cells that allow leakage. This process is mediated by angiogenic factors such as fibroblast growth factor and transforming growth factor [5]. The accompanying fibroblast cells form collagen around these vessels. Initially, the collagen is type III but, as it matures, is it converted to type I. The immature vessels develop into a capillary network. The early granulation tissue is highly vascular.

Maturation and devascularisation: between about three weeks from the time of injury and two years, the wound matures. The wound swelling subsides as the watery glycosaminoglycans are re-absorbed, and the tensile strength of the wound increases as collagen deposition becomes more organised. There is both synthesis of collagen and degradation initially, so that there is no net increase in collagen but the collagen is increasingly cross-linked, which strengthens its load-bearing characteristics. Whilst this is taking place, fibroblasts begin to

disappear, and many of the capillary network formed during the angiogenic response regress and disappear. The scar becomes correspondingly paler in appearance as it becomes less vascular, and it becomes softer and more supple as the fibroblastic response regresses.

Healing of skin wounds

Wounds are classically described as healing by primary or secondary intention. The processes that occur are essentially the same and involve the following:

1. Vasoconstriction. The initial response to injury is a transient vasoconstriction of the injured vessel to reduce the bleeding. During this period, the coagulation system is activated to seal the severed vessels before the initial vasoconstrictive phase is followed by vasodilatation five to ten minutes later. Coagulation is activated by the extravasation of blood and the exposure of subendothelial collagen through both the extrinsic and intrinsic cascades. Both trigger a common pathway, which leads to the conversion of prothrombin to thrombin, which in turn cleaves plasma fibrinogen enzymatically to form fibrin, and this combines with activated platelets to form a clot. Platelets are activated both by the exposure of subendothelial collagen and by the clotting mechanism, and the activated platelets accumulate at the site of tissue injury to stabilise the fibrin clot, augment the coagulation cascade and thus prevent further exsanguination. The clot that is interposed between the edges of a primarily closed wound consists of a mixture of biologically active molecules and cells within the fibrin mesh. This fibrin mesh serves as a temporary scaffold, holding the two wound edges together while further cellular ingrowth occurs and while fibrin is replaced by collagen over the next few weeks.
2. Acute inflammatory response.
3. Epithelial covering, usually within 24 hours.
4. Organisation.

These last three processes have been described above. Healing by secondary intention (where the wound edges are widely separated) differs in two respects.

1. Epithelialisation occurs from the basal cells of the epidermis at the margins of the wound. These cells lose their attachment to the basement membrane and send out cytoplasmic projections, becoming flatter as they do so. As they change, they become more like phagocytes in appearance. Within a day or two of injury, the basal cells show mitosis at an increasing rate and continue to replicate until the defect is covered. When coverage is complete and the epidermis (or other epithelium) has reconstituted itself, the basal cells regain their normal appearance and synthesise their own basement membrane constituents.

2. Contraction plays a far more important role in healing by secondary intention. Animal models have demonstrated contraction of up to 80% [6]. However, the pathological process involved in contraction is the same.

Complications of wound healing

Complications include infection, wound dehiscence, excessive granulation, keloid, pigmentation, pain, weak scars, circatrisation, implantation cyst and neoplasia. Factors influencing healing are listed in Table 25.1.

Grafts and flaps

Most surgical trainees gain their first experience of grafting in the use of thin split skin grafts to cover a granulating open wound. The open wound, which is secreting collagen and actively generating small new

Table 25.1 Factors influencing wound healing

Local factors	Poor blood supply
	Adhesion to underlying structures
	Direction of wound
	Infection/foreign body
	Movement
	Drying
	Neoplasia
General	Age
	Nutrition (protein, vitamin C, zinc)
	Hormones
	Temperature

vessels, is covered by a nutrient-rich layer of serum, from which the thin split skin graft gains its nutrition by a process known as 'imbibition'. This is sufficient to nourish a split skin graft for a day or two but to nourish it beyond that time, as well as to fix it and incorporate it into the healing wound, there must be a link-up between the capillary bed on the undersurface of the graft and the developing capillaries in the open wound, together with interlinking of collagen, and this process is known as 'inosculation'. During the 48 hours of imbibition and the 48 hours of inosculation, the graft must be immobilised and, if it is immobilised and the host bed is well vascularised, then the graft will 'take'. At the end of 96 hours, blood flow into the graft should be established. Eventually, lymphatics will grow in as well.

Immobilisation in this context should not be taken to mean simply pressure, although the 'tie-over' dressing commonly used for immobilising a small skin graft clearly produces some pressure. The intention, though, is to immobilise the graft. Pressure sufficient to inhibit the formation of small haematomas and seromas would probably be sufficient to impair blood flow in the host bed [7, 8].

Thus far, we have been considering the simple split skin graft, and at this stage we should draw attention to the difference between grafts and flaps. A graft is tissue transferred from a donor site to a recipient site without a blood supply, whereas a flap is tissue that is transferred from a donor site with its own blood supply intact, although one type of flap is the free flap, in which tissue is transferred with its blood supply disconnected and then reconnected by mean of microvascular surgery at the recipient site. In urology we are principally concerned with split-thickness skin grafts, full-thickness skin grafts, buccal mucosal grafts, bladder epithelial grafts and flaps of local genital skin for urethral reconstruction. In addition, the urologist may wish to use a dermal graft for the correction of Peyronie's disease, and some have used a graft of tunica vaginalis for this purpose [9, 10].

Other than the use of genital skin flaps for urethral reconstruction, simpler advancement, rotation and transposition flaps are commonly used for wound closure, although we do not often think of them as such, except in the specific case of the Z-plasty. Less commonly, flaps may be used for perineal and genital reconstruction and in this way a simple scrotal flap may be used to cover a perineal defect, or the infinitely more complex radial or ulnar forearm flap may be transferred by microvascular techniques for phalloplasty [11].

Grafts

Skin has an epidermal layer and a dermal layer, under which lies a subcutaneous, fatty layer. At the interface between the dermis and the subcutaneous layer is the subdermal plexus, which is fed from deeper segmental vessels and which in turn feeds the dermal and epidermal layers above through a second, more superficial, plexus within the dermis itself, called the intradermal plexus (Figure 25.1). The outermost layer of the epidermis is the cornified layer, and the inner layer – the epidermis proper – contains the skin appendages, some of which extend into the dermal layer. The principal skin appendages are the sweat glands, sebaceous glands and hair follicles, and in urological practice it is worth noting that the glans and prepuce in the male and the skin of the labia minora

and introitus in the female are free of skin appendages. The same areas also have skin in which the dermis is thin. The dermis consists of the more superficial 'papillary' or 'adventitial' dermis and the deeper 'reticular' dermis. The papillary dermis has a fairly constant thickness, and fibroblasts and capillaries predominate. The deeper reticular dermis is thicker but more variable and here collagen and elastin predominate. The subdermal plexus lies on the deep aspect of the reticular dermis, and the intradermal plexus lies between the reticular and the papillary dermis.

A full-thickness skin graft includes both the epidermis and the dermis with the vessels of the subdermal plexus exposed on its undersurface, and it is to these vessels that the new vessels developing within the host bed must connect by inosculation. Full-thickness skin grafts, because of their high content of dermal collagen, contract very little during healing and tend to give the most satisfactory long-term results as a consequence, but there are two problems associated with their use. Firstly, the amount of suitable skin is restricted and, secondly, the subdermal plexus is less

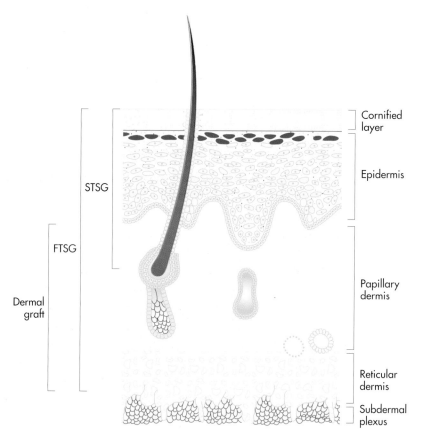

Figure 25.1 Cross-sectional diagram of the skin. STSG, split-thickness skin graft; FTSG, full-thickness skin graft.

extensive than the intradermal plexus and, because of this and also because the graft is relatively thick, it is only slowly revascularised and takes only under the most favourable conditions.

The split-thickness skin graft contains the epidermis and a portion of the adventitial dermis with the vessels of the intradermal plexus exposed on its undersurface. The graft is thinner and the vessels of the intradermal plexus are more plentiful and so a split-thickness graft is more likely to take, and will do so under less favourable circumstances than a full-thickness skin graft. On the other hand, because there is less dermal collagen, a split-thickness graft tends to contract and, lacking the collagen and elastin of the reticular dermis, the graft tends to be more brittle and fragile than a full-thickness graft.

Bladder epithelial grafts and buccal mucosal grafts are harvested and behave as full-thickness grafts. Bladder epithelium has the disadvantage that it is very prone to desiccation, which leads to hypertrophic changes when, for example, it is used at the urethral meatus [12]. Buccal mucosa is far more resistant to desiccation, and there is the additional advantage that it is easier to open the mouth than the bladder, although this advantage is offset by the greater amount of bladder mucosa available than buccal mucosa. The particular advantages of buccal mucosa are its thickness and toughness (which contrast markedly with the thinness and fragility of bladder epithelium), and the density of the intradermal and subdermal plexuses [13].

Grafts were the first sort of tissue to be used for urethral reconstruction but fell into disfavour because of their unpredictability until just recently, with the advent of buccal mucosal grafting for so-called 'patch' urethroplasty of strictures that are too long for excision and end-to-end anastomosis [14]. Until then, grafts had become virtually restricted to the use of meshed split-skin grafts for the salvage repair of extensive urethral strictures [15]. This is a technique that is only rarely indicated nowadays. A free preputial skin graft might be used by specialist resconstructive surgeons for anterior urethroplasty, particularly for hypospadias repair, but grafting had become almost entirely superseded by the use of flaps for hypospadias repair and for urethroplasty in the penile urethra, largely under the influence of Duckett [16].

Preputial and postauricular full-thickness skin grafts are now being used more frequently again, particularly for the two-stage reconstruction of the penile urethra [17]. Postauricular full-thickness skin grafts have a particularly rich subdermal plexus and, although the amount of tissue is relatively restricted, the take is far more predictable than with other extragenital skin. Thus, preputial or postauricular full-thickness skin grafts may be used to reconstruct the anterior urethra, usually in two stages, and buccal mucosal grafts, which behave as full-thickness grafts, may be used for the repair of more proximal urethral strictures. Buccal mucosal grafts and bladder epithelial grafts have also been used as tube grafts in the anterior urethra [18]. Only in extreme cases, for extensive urethral salvage procedures, is split-thickness skin used, and then only after it has been meshed, as described by Schreiter [19].

Flaps

Flaps consist of skin, muscle, bone, fascia, omentum, intestine or combinations of these, but in urology we are principally concerned with skin flaps for urethral and genital reconstruction, omental flaps to help support vesico-vaginal fistula closure, and intestinal flaps for bladder reconstruction.

Flaps may be classified in two ways [7, 8]. Firstly, according to their method of elevation, into peninsular flaps, in which the base of the flap remains in continuity; island flaps, in which the flap is only in continuity through the arteriovenous pedicle; and free flaps, in which all continuity of the flap is interrupted but the vascularity is re-established at the recipient site. The second way of classifying flaps is by vascular classification (Figure 25.2), which distinguishes between: random flaps, in which there is no identifiable arteriovenous pedicle and survival is dependent entirely on the dermal and intradermal plexuses; axial flaps, which have an identifiable artery and vein entering through the base; and two special forms of axial flap known as myocutaneous and the fasciocutaneous flaps. Random flaps are restricted in use by a length to width ratio whereas axial flaps are not, being restricted in length only by the nature of the feeder vessels. A peninsular flap may be either a random or an axial flap, but island flaps are all axial

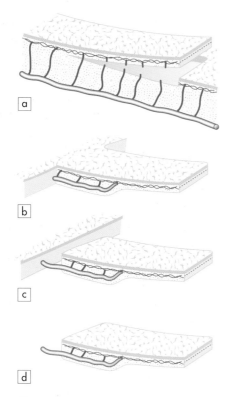

Figure 25.2 *Diagrammatic representation of: (a) a random penin-sular flap; (b) an axial peninsular flap; (c) an axial island flap; and (d) a free microvascular flap.*

flaps. Peninsular flaps are used for advancement, rota-tion and transposition but are relatively restricted in scope. Axial island flaps have a much greater range of application. Island flaps are somewhat fragile and have to be handled with care as the vascular pedicle pro-vides both structural and vascular continuity – with such a fragile structure that vascular continuity is threatened unless great care is taken. Sometimes, how-ever, the continuity of an island flap is maintained through a muscle or fascial flap, giving rise to the two particular forms of axial flap referred to above. In the myocutaneous flap, the arteriovenous pedicle is within the muscle itself and the skin island (or 'paddle') retains its attachment to the muscle. Examples include gracilis and rectus abdominis muscle flaps, both of which have applications in urology [20, 21]. Similarly, the fasciocutaneous flap transmits the arteriovenous pedicle in close relation to a defined layer of fascia to which the skin paddle is attached. In both the myocu-taneous and the fasciocutaneous flaps, the muscle and fascia, respectively, support and protect the arterio-nous pedicle, making the flap more robust.

Free flaps, to be transferred by microvascular anas-tomoses to the recipient site, can be elevated as axial cutaneous, axial myocutaneous, or axial fasciocuta-neous flaps and are the most versatile flaps of all because they can be transferred anywhere. The limi-tations in their use are firstly technical – they are dif-ficult to learn how to perform – and they tend to leave large donor sites that may leave ugly scars [22], although this is usually more than offset by a satis-factory end result from the flap itself. Most flaps are mobilised with a defined sensory nerve to provide sensibility to the flap. The best example of the use of a free flap in urology is the radial or ulnar forearm flap used for phalloplasty [11]. The radial artery flap is easier to raise but has considerable donor-site mor-bidity because the many tendons in the forearm are exposed and, even if these can be covered, the donor site leaves an unsightly scar. The ulnar forearm flap exposes fewer, if any, tendons and the donor site is more easily concealed and has the additional advan-tage that the skin on the ulnar side of the forearm is much less hirsute, but the flap is more difficult to raise. Both flaps are innervated by the lateral and medial antibrachial cutaneous nerves, which are eas-ily identified and mobilised with the flap to provide sensibility.

Gracilis and rectus myocutaneous flaps have also been used for phallic reconstruction, but are more commonly used for covering large skin defects in and around the groins and perineum. The gracilis muscle can also be used purely as a muscle flap for filling dead space and holding suture lines apart, in the same way that the labial fat pad and omentum are used.

Intestinal flaps in bladder reconstruction

There are more urologists using bowel for bladder reconstruction or replacement by continent or con-duit urinary diversion than there are urologists using skin for urethral reconstruction. Bowel is always car-ried on its blood supply and, as long as there is no undue tension on the vascular pedicle, the bowel heals well in its new circumstances and ischaemia is rare, except when the bowel and its blood supply are com-promised by previous radiotherapy. The purpose of this section is not to discuss the more technical aspects related to mobilising gut segments for use in the urinary tract, but to discuss the metabolic, infective, histological and other consequences of incorporating the gut into the urinary tract. Such matters have been extensively studied by certain groups in experimental models [23] and the clinical consequences have been extensively scrutinised by other groups in humans, but it is still not yet clear how we should apply the theoretical knowledge gleaned from such studies in clinical practice as that knowledge is currently very incomplete.

Bowel has been used in urology for many years and this has engendered an attitude that it can be freely deployed within the urinary tract without significant consequence. On the other hand, intestine was never meant to serve either as a conduit for urine or as a storage vessel for it, and a more likely explanation for the fact that it appears to be capable of being used freely without complication is that in most circumstances only a small section of bowel is incorporated and, in most patients in whom such procedures are performed, there are compensatory mechanisms to deal with any adverse consequences that might otherwise result. Furthermore, many of these patients have only a short life expectancy, as when an ileal conduit or substitution cystoplasty is used after cystectomy for bladder cancer, and the short duration of use in a patient who is expected to die before long in any case might lead one to overlook consequences that might be apparent in younger patients with longer to live.

Even with this proviso, it was recognised many years ago that patients with uretero-sigmoidostomy were prone to the specific metabolic problem of hyperchloraemic acidosis from the absorption of urinary constituents by the colon [24], and prone also to the development of tumours at the site of implantation of the ureters into the colon [25]. For these reasons, uretero-sigmoidostomy fell into relative disuse some years ago, although it is undergoing something of a resurrection at present [26].

Other than the consequences of incorporating a segment of gut into the urinary tract, there may be consequences from removing it from its natural situation. In practice, the only problem that commonly arises is a degree of bowel dysfunction [27], although it is not clear whether this arises because the bowel has been removed or because the functional status quo has been disturbed by the process of bowel preparation and the starvation associated with the perioperative period and the time that it takes thereafter for normal function to be restored. There is, in any case, a strong association between detrusor instability and the irritable bowel syndrome [28] and neuropathic bowel and neuropathic bladder dysfunction [29] and it is these two groups that are most prone to notice disturbance of bowel function after augmentation cystoplasty. Bowel dysfunction is far less commonly noted after substitution cystoplasty for conditions such as bladder cancer.

Removal of the terminal ileum or of the ileocaecal valve can interfere with the absorption of bile salts [30] and lead to bacterial colonisation of the terminal ileum, both of which may give rise to diarrhoea. For this reason, the terminal ileum is avoided whenever possible during such surgery. There has been concern that the removal of the terminal ileum can give rise to vitamin B12 deficiency and other forms of anaemia, but these rarely seem to occur in practice. It is not clear how much ileum has to be removed from the intestinal tract before bile acid malabsorption is sufficiently severe to cause malabsorption of fat and fat-soluble vitamins, but malnutrition and steatorrhoea are rarely, if ever, seen in clinical practice. Such problems might occur, and diarrhoea undoubtedly does occur in people who have had enterocystoplasty, ileal conduit diversion or continent diversion after previous bowel excision or when the bowel is diseased or deficient in any other way.

Removing the right side of the colon may cause diarrhoea, although this does not seem to be a long-term problem. Removal of the sigmoid colon may be a problem in neuropathic patients in whom the sigmoid colon is an important storage organ, but it does not usually cause bowel problems otherwise.

In short, other than in those with previously abnormal bowel, problems rarely arise from taking the bowel out of continuity, and all we need really consider are the problems that arise from incorporating it into the urinary tract.

The consequences of incorporating the bowel into the urinary tract

The first point to make is that bowel continues to behave like bowel even when it is in the urinary tract and has been there for many years. It continues to produce mucus – the only overt abnormality that most patients are aware of – and it continues to secrete and absorb just as it does in its natural situation. There is a tendency for both the ileal and colonic epithelium to atrophy with time [31], and it is not clear whether this represents the consequence of loss of the normal stimulation that it receives during faecal transport in its normal situation or whether, alternatively, it represents some toxic effect of urine. However, the atrophy is less when the intestine is in contact with urine than when it is not in contact with anything at all, so it appears that urine tends to maintain ileal integrity, if anything, albeit less so than does the faecal stream. The atrophic appearance is therefore likely to represent a true, albeit partial, atrophy rather than a toxic effect.

Metabolic changes

The principal metabolic abnormality is a tendency to a respiratory-compensated metabolic acidosis, usually of mild degree [32]. This may influence bone metabolism to a sufficient degree to cause demineralisation of the skeleton in growing children [33]. Changes otherwise tend to be subtle, particularly, it is thought, if renal function is normal. Thus, only young patients are prone to any sort of problems in most circumstances.

Why people seem to suffer less from metabolic acidosis these days with a substituted intestinal bladder than they used to suffer with a uretero-sigmoidostomy is almost certainly related, at least in part, to the recurrent sepsis that they also suffered with refluxing uretero-sigmoidostomies [34].

The nature and severity of the electrolyte anomalies that patients can suffer from depend on the segment of bowel used in the urinary tract. If stomach is used, hypochloraemic metabolic alkalosis can occur. This is rarely significant in the presence of normal renal function, but may be when renal function is severely limited.

When jejunum is used, hyponatraemic hyperchloraemic hyperkalaemic metabolic acidosis occurs and this is both common and potentially serious, resulting in lethargy, nausea, vomiting, dehydration, muscular weakness and an elevated body temperature and, if uncorrected, death. This is the so-called 'jejunal conduit syndrome' [35].

If ileum or colon is used, hyperchloraemic acidosis may occur. The reported incidence varies and to a certain extent depends on how it is looked for. If the plasma chloride level is the parameter used to make the diagnosis, then about 15% of patients suffer; if arterial blood gas analysis is performed, then a respiratory-compensated metabolic acidosis is found far more commonly – indeed, in the majority [32]. The mechanism of the metabolic acidosis when ileum or colon is interposed in the urinary tract is not entirely clear. What is known is largely derived from the work of McDougall and co-workers [36].

Water transport across the intestinal epithelium normally follows its osmotic gradient and is dependent upon the permeability of the intercellular junctions of the luminal cells. If these junctions are tight, there is very little leakage; when they are not so tight, water follows its osmotic gradients. Generally, the tightness of the intercellular junctions increases the further down the intestinal tract the segment is taken from. Stomach is very leaky, but there are bidirectional fluxes that cancel each other out. Jejunum is leaky and jejunal conduits lose large amounts of water. Ileum is better but is still somewhat leaky. Colon is the most efficient segment of gut because its intercellular junctions are tighter, and colon segments therefore have a much lower tendency to lose water.

Most electrolyte shifts in the gut are transcellular, although paracellular movement of ions does occur. Furthermore, most electrolyte movements in one direction are coupled with movement of other electrolytes in the opposite direction. Thus, when sodium is absorbed, hydrogen is excreted and when chloride is absorbed, bicarbonate is excreted. Under certain circumstances, these transport processes can be reversed.

Sodium absorption is much the same in the ileum and in the colon and, in general, ileum absorbs less chloride but more potassium than colon. In neither ileal nor colonic segments is either sodium or potassium loss a problem, although in extreme metabolic acidosis, hypokalaemia can occur, as can hypocalcaemia and hypomagnesaemia.

The mechanism for the development of hyperchloraemic acidosis appears to be primarily because of ammonia absorption. Ammonium ions may dissociate into ammonia and hydrogen, in which case the ammonia diffuses into the cell and the hydrogen ion is actively absorbed in exchange for sodium. Alternatively, ammonium may be absorbed as a substitute for potassium through potassium channels. Either way, ammonium enters the ileal or colonic luminal cell and this is balanced by chloride absorption in exchange for bicarbonate secretion. Thus, ammonium and chloride are absorbed, causing hyperchloraemic acidosis, and bicarbonate is lost.

When hypokalaemia does occur it is usually in uretero-sigmoidostomy [37] or as a result of osmotic diuresis. Hypocalcaemia is usually due to bone demineralisation. Hypomagnesaemia may be associated with hypocalcaemia but is more commonly due to nutritional depletion or renal wasting.

In most patients, this metabolic acidosis is of little consequence, but in growing children it may be a particular problem as it appears to cause a reduction in growth potential [38]. Children with intestine incorporated into the urinary tract are more prone to orthopaedic problems and pathological fractures and there is a tendency for them to drop off the growth curve that they were previously following. Exactly why acidosis should lead to skeletal demineralisation in growing children and not in anybody else is not clear, but post-menopausal women who might also be prone to skeletal demineralisation do not show this abnormality after enterocystoplasty or urinary intestinal diversion.

Again, the mechanism by which acidosis causes demineralisation of the skeleton is not clear, but chronic acidosis is buffered predominantly by muscle protein and by bone. In bone, in chronic metabolic acidosis, hydrogen ions are buffered in exchange for calcium. The main buffer is thought to be bicarbonate or carbonate derived from skeletal carbon dioxide stores, and the utilisation of this buffer system is accompanied by an efflux not only of calcium but of divalent phosphate as well, due to dissolution of the mineral phase. Calcium efflux is dependent on the bicarbonate concentration as well as on the pH, and compensated chronic metabolic acidosis, in which there is a systemically reduced bicarbonate concentration, will have an adverse effect on skeletal mineralisation even though the pH is within the normal range because of the compensation mechanism.

It should again be emphasised that it is growing children who are vulnerable to skeletal demineralisation in this way. Once the skeleton has reached maturity, it appears to be resistant to this mechanism. In practice, it means that growing children should have any identifiable metabolic acidosis corrected, but in adults it need not be corrected if it is asymptomatic [33].

It is frequently reported that patients with renal function below a certain level should not undergo any form of enterocystoplasty or urinary intestinal diversion because metabolic problems are far more likely. Although frequently reported, there is little evidence to support this except in uretero-sigmoidostomy patients who have continuing faecal reflux to contend with as well as hyperchloraemic acidosis. In practice, most patients with impaired renal function undergoing enterocystoplasty or urinary diversion have an obstructive nephropathy, either due to frank outflow obstruction at sphincter level or to high intravesical pressure. If these two problems are eliminated by enterocystoplasty, whatever the level of renal function, there will be at least a temporary stabilisation, if not an overt improvement in renal function, and this usually amounts to a window of 18 months to two years before intrinsic renal disease causes further deterioration in renal function on the downward slope to renal replacement therapy.

Urinary infection and malignant transformation

Bacterial colonisation of the urinary tract is very common after bowel interposition. Although one or two authors report sterile urine in their patients, the majority of surgeons find that the urine is usually, if not always, colonised.

Very often this is with a mixed growth of bacteria and less than the usual 100 000 organisms per ml associated with a 'classic' urinary infection. Not only is this bacteriuria common, there is also an increased incidence of both local and systemic infection in such patients. Average reported figures are that 80% of patients suffer bacteriuria [39] with a diverse bacterial flora and that 15% of patients will suffer acute pyelonephritis at some stage [40]. The highest incidence appears to be during the first year. This incidence is higher than in those who are on clean, intermittent self-catheterisation with a normal bladder [38].

Unlike urothelium, bowel does not attempt to sterilise its luminal content. When bowel is distended it becomes relatively ischaemic and the mucosal barrier preventing bacterial translocation from mucosa to blood is disrupted. Urine from a substitute bladder is less bacteriostatic because the concentration of urea is lower and the pH higher than in normal urine. These three points probably account for the increased incidence of infection in such patients.

This infection is difficult, if not impossible, to eliminate and most patients suffer asymptomatic bacteriuria even if they are completely unaware of it. Although asymptomatic, it may be nonetheless important in the long run as there is a theoretical link between infection and cancer.

Patients with uretero-sigmoidostomy were noted to have an incidence of cancer at the uretero-intestinal anastomosis of between 6% and 29%, with a mean of 11% [25]. Generally speaking, there is a lag time of 10 to 20 years between the surgery and the development of the tumour. These tumours are extremely aggressive and one-third of patients die from them. They appear to be adenocarcinomas in the main, although other histological types have been reported. Overall, this represents a 500-fold increase in the incidence of tumours in the sigmoid colon in this patient group, and it has been reported that, in patients diverted by this means before the age of 25, the increased risk is 7000-fold [41].

The aetiology of these tumours is not clear. Presumably, as most are adenocarcinomas, they arise in intestinal epithelium adjacent to the anastomosis, although adenocarcinoma has been shown to arise from transitional epithelium exposed to faeces in experimental animals [42]. Furthermore, histological assessment of the ureters in patients with uretero-

sigmoidostomies shows a high incidence of dysplasia as judged by biopsies or surgical specimens from close to the anastomosis [43]. Stewart suggested that these tumours arose as a result of the conversion of nitrates and secondary amines in the urine into nitrosamines due to the action of faecal bacteria [44]. Nitrosamines are known carcinogens and certainly patients with uretero-sigmoidostomies show high concentrations of nitrosamines in the faecal/urinary slurry that they pass.

Patients with enterocystoplasties or urinary diversions show dysplastic changes, and malignant change has been reported, albeit infrequently [45]. Most patients show chronic inflammatory changes in their bladder on biopsy, and nitrosamines are present in the urine, in this case produced by the bacteriuria that they have rather than by exposure to faeces. The greater the degree of the bacteriuria, the greater degree of the pyuria associated with it, the higher the nitrosamine levels in the urine and the higher the incidence of histological changes, which in some instances would be classified as premalignant if they were found in the bowel in its natural situation. Such changes include keratinising squamous metaplasia and transitional epithelial mucin distribution – changes similar to the alterations in colonic mucin secretion demonstrated in patients with uretero-sigmoidostomy.

Other factors have been suggested for the development of these tumours, including superoxide radicals and epidermal growth factor receptor proliferation, induced by the urothelial–colonic juxtaposition. Whatever the cause, there seems to be little doubt that some patients, at least, will develop tumours in the long run. Patients should therefore not be lost to follow-up so that such tumours can be detected at the earliest possible moment.

Stones

Patients with ileal conduits were found to have a 20% incidence of renal calculus formation if followed for more than 20 years [38]. Up to one-third of patients with Kock pouches were found to have stones in their pouch, in this instance related to non-resorbable staples. More recently, stones have been noted in the absence of foreign material in patients with diversions and orthotopic substitutions and these have been attributed to acid renal tubule fluid, an increased excretion of calcium, a high incidence of infection with urease-producing bacteria, as well as to the presence of mucus and almost universal bacteriuria.

However, it should be noted that patients with ileal conduits and with orthotopic substitution cystoplasties who empty spontaneously have a low incidence of stone formation. An orthotopic substitution that has to be emptied by clean, intermittent self-catheterisation has a higher incidence. But the highest incidence of all occurs in patients with continent diversions being emptied by clean, intermittent self-catheterisation – generally from the top of the bladder, rather than from the bottom – suggesting that stagnation is the most important factor, with mucus presumably acting as a nidus and bacterial colonisation as the catalyst.

Other problems

It has already been noted, when discussing metabolic abnormalities, that the primary abnormality leading to acidosis is the increased absorption of ammonia. This ammonia is normally converted into urea by the liver. If the liver is in any way abnormal, then hyper-ammonaemic encephalophathy may result [46], and is particularly common in patients with chronic liver disease such as cirrhosis. The hepatic reserve to clear ammonia in this way is great, so this is not a common problem unless liver disease is fairly advanced.

Certain drugs may be absorbed from the urine when bowel is interposed, and phenytoin [47] and certain antimetabolites such as methotrexate [48] have been reported to reach toxic levels in such patients.

Perhaps more importantly, glucose can be reabsorbed from the urine in diabetic patients and control of their diabetes may be made more difficult as a result [49].

References

1. Adzick NS, Harrison MR. The fetal surgery experience. In: Adzick NS, Longaker MT (eds) Fetal wound healing. New York: Elsevier, 1992: 1–23

2. Skalli O, Gabbiani G. The biology of the myofibroblast relationship to wound contraction and fibrocontractive disease. In: Clark RAF, Henson PM (eds) The molecular and cellular biology of wound healing. New York: Plenum Press, 1988: 373

3. Stewart RJ, Duley JA, Dewdney J, et al. Wound fibroblast and macrophage II. Their origin studied in the human after bone marrow transplantation. Br J Surg 1981; 68(2): 129–31

4. Kingsnorth AN, Slavin J. Peptide growth factors and wound healing. Br J Surg 1991; 78: 1286–90

5. Furcht LT. Critical factors controlling angiogenesis: cell products, cell matrix and growth factors. Lab Inv 1986; 55: 505–9

6. Blair GH, Slome D, Walter JB. Review of experimental investigations on wound healing. In: Ross JP (ed) British surgical practice: surgical progress. London: Butterworth, 1961

7. Converse JM, McCarthy JG, Brauer RO, Ballentyne DL. Transplantation of skin. Grafts and flaps. In: Reconstructive plastic surgery, Vol. 1, 2nd edition. Philadelphia: WB Saunders, 1977: 152–82

8. Grabb WC, Smith JW. Plastic surgery, 2nd edition. Boston: Little Brown, 1973: 1–122

9. Devine CJ Jr, Horton CE. Surgical treatment of Peyronie's disease with dermal graft. J Urol 1989; 142: 1223–6

10. Perlmutter AD, Montgomery BT, Steinhardt G. Tunica vaginalis free graft for the correction of chordee. J Urol 1985; 134: 311–13

11. Gilbert DA, Horton CE, Terzis J, Devine CJ Jr, Winslow BH, Devine P. New concepts in phallic reconstruction. Ann Plast Surg 1987; 18: 128–36

12. Ehrlich RM, Reda EF, Koyle MA, et al. Complications of bladder mucosal graft. J Urol 1989; 142: 626–7

13. Baskin LS, Duckett JW. Mucosal grafts in hypospadias and stricture management. AUA Update Series 1994; XIII, 34: 270–5

14. Burger RA, Muller SC, El-Damanhoury H, Tschakaloff A, Riedmiller H, Hohenfellner R. The buccal mucosal graft for urethral reconstruction: a preliminary report. J Urol 1992; 147: 662–4

15. Horton CE, Devine CJ Jr. A one stage repair of hypospadias cripples. Plast Reconstr Surg 1970; 45: 425–30

16. Duckett JW. The island flap technique for hypospadias repair. Urol Clin N Am 1981; 8: 503–11

17. Morehouse DD. Current indications and technique of two stage repair for membraneous urethral strictures. Urol Clin N Am 1989; 16: 325–8

18. Mundy AR. Results and complications of urethroplasty and its future. Br J Urol 1993; 71: 322–5

19. Schreiter F, Noll F. Meshgraft urethroplasty using split thickness skin graft of foreskin. J Urol 1989; 142: 1223–6

20. McCraw J, Massey F, Shaiklin K, Horton C. Vaginal reconstruction with gracilis myocutaneous flaps. Plast Reconstr Surg 1976; 58: 176–83

21. Sadore RC, Jordan GH, Sagher U, et al. Use of the rectus abdominis muscle flap in secondary reconstruction of extrophy-epispadias. Clin Plast Surg 1988; 15: 393–7

22. Taylor GI, Daniel RK. The anatomy of several free flap donor sites. Plast Reconstr Surg 1975; 56: 243–53

23. Koch MO, McDougal WS, Thompson CO. Mechanisms of solute transport following urinary diversion through intestinal segments: an experimental study with rats. J Urol 1991; 146: 1390

24. Fern DO, Odel HM. Electrolyte pattern of the blood after bilateral ureterosigmoidostomy. JAMA 1949; 142: 634–41

25. Zabbo A, Kay R. Ureterosigmoidostomy and bladder extrophy: a long-term follow-up. J Urol 1986; 136: 396

26. Fisch M, Wammack R, Muller SC, Hohenfellner R. The Mainz 11 (sigma rectum pouch). J Urol 1993; 149: 258–63

27. Singh G, Thomas DG. Bowel problems after enterocystoplasty. Br J Urol 1997; 79: 328–32

28. Whorwell PJ, Lupton EW, Erdiran D, Wilson K. Bladder smooth muscle dysfunction in patients with irritable bowel syndrome. Gut 1986; 27: 1014–17

29. Spirnak SP, Caldamone AA. Ureterosigmoidostomy. Urol Clin North Am 1986; 13: 285

30. Durrans D, Wujanto R, Carrol RN, Torrance HD. Bile acid malabsorption: a complication of conduit surgery. Br J Urol 1989; 64: 485–8

31. Dean AM, Woodhouse CRJ, Parkinson MC. Histological changes in ileal conduits. J Urol 1984; 132: 1108

32. Nurse DE, Mundy AR. Metabolic complications of cystoplasty. Br J Urol 1989; 63: 165–70

33. Mundy AR, Nurse DE. Calcium balance, growth and skeletal mineralisation in patients with cystoplasties. Br J Urol 1992; 69: 257–59

34. Wear JB Jr, Barquin OP. Ureterosigmoidostomy. Urology 1973; 1: 192

35. Klein EA, Montie JE, Montague DK, Kay R, Strafton RA. Jejunal conduit urinary diversion. J Urol 1989; 64: 412

36. Koch MO, McDougall WS, Thompson CO. Mechanisms of solute transport following urinary diversion through intestinal segments: an experimental study with rats. J Urol 1991; 146: 1390–4

37. Geist RW, Ansell JS. Total body potassium after ureteroileostomy. Surg Gynaec Obst 1961; 113: 585–9

38. McDougall WS, Koch MO. Impaired growth and development and urinary intestinal interposition. Trans Amer Ass Genito-Urin Surg 1991; 105: 3

39. Guinan PD, Moore RH, Neter E, Murphy GP. The bacteriology of ileal conduit urine in man. Surg Gynaec Obst 1972; 134: 78–82

40. Schwarz GR, Jeffs RD. Ileal conduit urinary diversion in children: computer analysis of follow-up from 2 to 16 years. J Urol 1975; 114: 285

41. Husmann DA, Spence HM. Current status of tumour of the bowel following ureterosigmoidostomy: a review. J Urol 1990; 144: 607–10

42. Aaronson IA, Constantinides CG, Sallie LP, Sinclair-Smith CC. Pathogenesis of adenocarcinoma complicating ureterosigmoidostomy. Experimental observations. Urology 1987; 29: 538

43. Aaronson IA, Sinclair-Smith CC. Dysplasia of ureteric epithelium: a source of adenocarcinoma in ureterosigmoidostomy? Z Kinderchir Grenzgeb 1984; 39: 364–7

44. Stewart M, Hill MJ, Pugh RCB, et al. The role of N-nitrosamine in carcinogenesis at the uretero-colic anastomosis. Br J Urol 1981; 53: 115–18

45. Filmer RB, Spencer JR. Malignancies in bladder, augmentations and intestinal conduits. J Urol 1990; 143: 671–8

46. McDermott WV Jr. Diversion of urine to the intestines as a factor in ammoniagenic coma. New Engl J Med 1957; 256: 460

47. Savarirayan F, Dixey GM. Synope following ureterosigmoidostomy. J Urol 1969; 101: 844–5

48. Bowyer GW, Davies TW. Methotrexate toxicity associated with an ileal conduit. Br J Urol 1987; 60: 592

49. Sridhar KN, Samuell CT, Woodhouse CRJ. Absorption of glucose from urinary conduits in diabetics and non-diabetics. Br Med J 1983; 287: 1327–9

Screening

26

N. J. R. George

Screening has been defined as the identification of unrecognised disease or defect by the application of tests, examinations or other procedures that can be applied rapidly. The process may be broadly divided into 'one-shot' screening exercises, and procedures applied to chronic diseases or conditions that may be repeated at intervals. The second category may be further subdivided into mass screening, selective screening and case finding. In the context of urological surgery, debate concerning screening programmes chiefly concerns the search for chronic disease, typically urological neoplasia, usually by means of case finding or, at best, selective screening programmes.

'One-shot' screening

One-off screening procedures are most frequently employed to detect defects typified by congenital malformation or inherited metabolic disorders, such as phenylketonuria and galactosaemia, for which treatment is available. Screening for disorders that are untreatable has been generally avoided (for information on the fundamentals of screening, see page 467) although this basic concept has recently been challenged [1]. Programmes involving sophisticated tests for rare diseases [2,3] may not, at a superficial glance, be cost-effective; however, the long-term costs of supporting the patient with undetected disease to adulthood may be the crucial factor in determining public health policy.

Screening for chronic diseases

Mass screening

Mass screening is the identification of preclinical disease within the population by procedures that have been carefully assessed and validated as part of public health policy.

Mass screening programmes demand a precise cost–benefit analysis, which will be closely linked to the ethical and cultural ethos of the country and government concerned. In general, programmes initiated by the departments of health in the Western world will address only health issues that are both common and, at least in part, preventable, such as heart disease or certain types of neoplasia. Within this politico-medical process, certain groups, such as young women with pathology, will inevitably attract more political support than other groups, such as older men with chronic disease.

Selective screening

In an attempt to boost the effectiveness of screening programmes in relation to cost, the specified test may be directed at selected groups within the overall population. In fact, nearly all programmes are selective in terms of age and sex, as is seen in the case of breast cancer screening, for which high-risk groups of women are targeted in terms of age and menopausal status.

Genetic and racial variables are further examples of factors that may be selectively targeted in screening programmes. Within urology, the risks of prostate cancer are known to be increased in certain families with a history of the disease, and epidemiological studies clearly demonstrate the differing racial incidence of the disease, both worldwide and, most dramatically, within the USA.

Selective screening may also be undertaken by targeting groups exposed to various industrial or social risks. The lifelong follow-up of workers from aniline dye factories and the association of various diseases with heavy smoking are examples of this type of selectivity.

Case finding

Case finding is widely interpreted as 'screening' by both the general public and the medical profession. In essence, case finding is no more than sporadic attempts by interested doctors and patients to detect disease or establish that disease is not present. As described below, chronic urological disease does not in general attain the criteria sufficient to support full public health screening programmes. In the absence of such programmes – often interpreted by critics as a 'lack of interest' on behalf of the Department of Health – case finding becomes the predominant mode of preclinical disease identification, usually widely, and often inaccurately, reported by both the lay and medical press. Case finding is, however, a genuine and valid attempt by concerned doctors and patients to solve a medical dilemma, but the process should not be confused with scientifically designed and validated mass screening programmes.

In this chapter, the issues and principles of screening are described in general terms. The process is then analysed with reference to the generally accepted criteria for screening, and finally the application of these principles to chronic urological disease is discussed.

Lifetime events and screening terminology

When mass screening programmes for chronic diseases are developed, it is common practice to describe episodes that occur during the patient's lifetime using an accepted terminology that describes and defines the evolving events up to the point of death. These lifetime periods may be illustrated as in Figure 26.1.

Assuming initial health, the first event is the initiation of a biological disease process. This continues until, in the absence of a screening programme, symptoms appear, leading to presentation and eventual clinical diagnosis.

The time from disease initiation to clinical diagnosis is defined as the total preclinical phase (TPCP) [4]. Clearly, the total preclinical phase is a theoretical concept, as the time at which the disease is initiated can never be known with certainty and, indeed, with reference to neoplasia, it is likely that multiple events are required to establish the cancerous process, making it almost impossible to define precisely the start time of the disease.

If a mass screening test has been developed for a disease, it becomes possible to detect its presence during the total preclinical phase. The period between the earliest time at which the disease is detectable by the test and the time at which clinical symptoms become

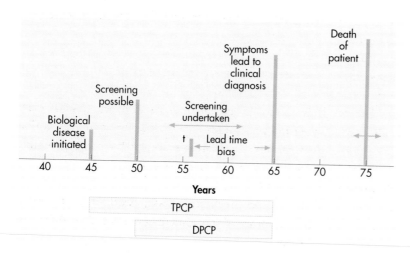

Figure 26.1 *Lifetime events and terminology of screening programmes. Depending on the sensitivity of the test, screening may be undertaken at any time t during the detectable preclinical phase (DPCP). Lead time bias is defined as the time between the initiation of the test and the time of symptomatic clinical presentation. The death of the patient may occur earlier or later, depending on whether the screening process is harmful or beneficial to the individual. TPCP, total preclinical phase.*

apparent is defined as the detectable preclinical phase (DPCP), also known as the 'sojourn time' [5]. Clearly, the length of the detectable preclinical phase depends on the sensitivity of the screening test and this is likely to be different for each disease under consideration. It is also apparent that different forms of screening tests for any one disease will be associated with different detectable preclinical phase times; thus, breast self-examination will have a shorter detectable preclinical phase than mammography, and digital rectal examination will have a shorter detectable preclinical phase than a prostate specific antigen screening test. Naturally, the effectiveness of any proposed mass screening programme will be determined by the ratio of the detectable to total preclinical phase – the longer the detectable phase, the more effective the programme. Occasionally, DPCP is mistakenly understood to stand for precancerous phase. This is misleading, as a variable portion of the correctly defined detectable phase may be related to invasive (i.e. not precancerous) yet asymptomatic cancerous growth. Thus, screening for diseases that have a significant invasive asymptomatic period during the detectable preclinical phase (perhaps diseases of the breast) is likely to be less effective than screening for diseases with extensive non-invasive periods during the detectable phase (perhaps diseases of the prostate).

The detection of disease during the detectable preclinical phase by the screening test itself results in difficulties when attempts are made to judge the effectiveness of any single programme. The time between the positive result of the screening test and the time at which clinical symptoms would have appeared is defined as the lead time bias. It will be evident that, if treatment for the disease is ineffective, the patient will die at the same point as he or she would have done had the disease originally been detected because of clinical symptoms. However, survival will apparently have been increased by the amount of time between the positive screening test and the clinical presentation, and thus it is necessary to account for lead time bias when assessing efficacy of screening for any particular disease [6]. For severe chronic disease such as cancer, the elimination of lead time bias is best achieved by randomised control trials of the screening programme, as described below.

The death of the patient is an event that is determined by the severity of the disease and the efficacy of treatment. As noted above, it is necessary to demonstrate that a screening programme results in prolonged survival after lead time bias and other distortions have been taken into account. It should not be forgotten that screening programmes may also lead to a shortening of the patient's life – if, for instance, death occurs due to septicaemia following transrectal biopsy for presumed prostate cancer suspected on the basis of a screening test, the programme (depending on the frequency of the complication) will be judged as being of questionable value with regard to the public health.

A further distortion that may be observed when mass screening for chronic disease is described is length bias [7]. In the case of neoplasia, different tumours grow at different rates and thus fast-growing cancers are characterised by a short detectable preclinical phase. A screening test undertaken during the detectable phase will, of necessity, detect more slow-growing cancers than fast-growing cancers (Figure 26.2), and thus the disease so detected will have a more favourable outcome than the disease detected by standard clinical tests. This length bias effect may be reduced by repeat screening but, once again, it can be seen that improved prognosis in the screening group may not necessarily be related to a real improvement in survival for the disease in question.

It is often difficult to persuade the general public – and occasionally the medical profession – that earlier detection of disease is not automatically associated with a better prognosis. Figures 26.1 and 26.2 illustrate well the complexity of the issues raised when mass screening is undertaken for chronic disease.

Fundamentals of screening

Before describing other issues concerned with mass screening programmes, it should be emphasised that there are certain situations in which it is not possible or necessary to offer a screening test.

If there is no preclinical phase, clearly it is not possible to offer a test that can detect that phase of disease.

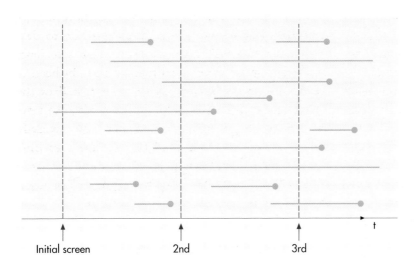

Figure 26.2 Length bias. Biologically active tumours develop and present more quickly than indolent tumours, which progress over long periods of time. Some tumours may never present clinically. Screening events (vertical dotted lines) automatically select a preponderance of the more indolent tumours. (——) Course of detectable preclinical disease; (●) time of clinical manifestation [20, 21].

Initial screen   2nd   3rd

If there is no possible treatment for the disease, conventional wisdom suggests that screening should not be offered as, by definition, no improvement in morbidity and mortality will be achieved. Interestingly, this principle has recently been questioned in relation to single-shot screening of the newborn for rare inherited disorders. Duchenne muscular dystrophy is an X-linked, lethal disorder of delayed onset with no effective treatment. It has been argued [8] that screening for the disease should be undertaken on the grounds that it would lessen parental distress by alerting them to the risks before the disease became apparent in their older children. Clearly, such a proposition raises highly complex ethical arguments that need to be carefully considered before any such programme could be adopted [1].

If it is possible to cure a disease when it presents clinically, there is no need to offer a screening test for the disease. Examples of neoplastic diseases that conform to this definition are clearly few and far between, but testicular tumour might be cited as an example of a curable cancer if efficiently detected in stage 1 by the patient himself.

Ethical considerations and attitudes to screening

It will be realised that, in a mass screening programme for disease, very different forces are at work, which depend on individual expectation of the enterprise. It is often assumed that satisfactory outcomes would, by definition, be acceptable to everybody concerned with the programme. To assess this matter, it is necessary to look at any screening programme from the point of view of both the Department of Health – 'the screener' – as well as the individual member of the general public – 'the screenee' – who is required to undertake the specified test.

The attitude and perspective of those offering a mass screening programme – usually the Department of Health – are principally influenced by their primary directive to improve the health of the nation as a whole. The screener does *not* promise or imply that every individual screened will be better off as a result of taking the test, although this point is rarely emphasised in the accompanying publicity, which suggests that 'screening must be good for you'. In this context, the death of a patient following prostatic biopsy (as noted above) would be an acceptable if regrettable incident were mass screening for prostate cancer to be established as a beneficial programme for the nation as a whole. The individual suffering disadvantage, which inevitably occurs in the best-validated screening programmes, will have a different perspective on the matter. The dichotomy between these two points of view is in part related to the generalised belief (noted above) that early diagnosis must be good – 'catch the disease early'. It is perhaps understandable how this entrenched view of health and disease may lead to disappointment, both for the screener [9] and for the screenee who suffers an adverse event following the screening test.

Cost issues are also a major factor for those considering ways of improving the public health. In developing countries, it would be by no means certain that screening for certain diseases would be of greater advantage to the population than money put into other aspects of public health such as water supplies, sewage systems etc. Within the Western world, cost–benefit analysis raises highly complex issues requiring scientific resolution, often in an atmosphere made obscure by the prominent opinions of vested interest groups. An example, discussed below, is the present controversy surrounding prostate cancer screening. Critical analysis of mortality figures clearly shows that this disease, compared to others affecting the younger male population, is a relatively insignificant problem, but these economic facts have failed to curtail the debate that is occupying a significant part of the medical and lay press at the present time.

The expectations and aspirations of those screened are very different. People selected by a programme or those who elect to go to their general practitioner naturally hope that disease will *not* be detected. Asymptomatic people who visit their practitioner do so in the expectation that they will be found to be healthy – what normal person would attend a physician in the expectation that cancer would be found? The screener is looking for disease, but the screenee expects a healthy outcome. These attitudes explain, in part, the problems that occur when a screening test 'goes wrong' – when the test either induces morbidity or reveals disease. Success or failure of the process is a value judgement based on point of view. In practice, of course, the vast majority of people who attend for screening tests are found to be negative (true negative – see below). When diseases are of low prevalence, a negative predictive value is both very accurate and very reassuring for the person concerned. A negative screening test for a rare but serious disease is, in fact, one of the greatest benefits that can accrue from a screening programme.

Ethical considerations in screening programmes are of major importance, both to health departments and to the population as a whole. Clinicians readily acknowledge ethical problems in routine medical practice but, in this case, the patients have almost invariably sought the help of the physician to deal with their disease. In the case of mass screening, selected people who consider themselves to be healthy have been approached by physicians on behalf of the Department of Health and asked to undertake tests that, as has been seen, will usually but not necessarily be of benefit to them. Initiation of the screening process deems that the ethical burden on the screener is as great or greater than that resting on colleagues in clinical medicine.

The validity of screening

Conventionally, the validity of screening is measured in terms of both the test or tests utilised in the procedure and the validity of the programme itself in its entirety. Each of these aspects may be measured by means of two indicators. Sensitivity relates to the positive identification of preclinical disease, and specificity is associated with the establishment of healthy people within the general population. Naturally, the validity of screening in terms of sensitivity and specificity can only be known if the true disease rate in the population is known: a follow-up diagnostic test is required to confirm or refute the result of the screening test.

The validity of screening tests

In terms of the test, sensitivity is defined as the percentage of people with a positive test amongst those who are later found to have the disease. Specificity is defined as the percentage of people screening negative amongst people who are genuinely free of disease. The relationship between the indicators and the presence or absence of disease is usually depicted as in Table 26.1. As noted above, the calculations demand that an independent diagnostic test is able to determine which members of the screened population have or do not have the disease itself. It has already been seen that the application of this diagnostic test may induce significant morbidity in individuals who are otherwise genuinely well. Sensitivity is the ratio between true positives and true positives with false negatives. Specificity is the ratio between true negatives and false positives with true negatives.

Table 26.1 Possible outcomes of screening examinations

Screening test result	Diagnosis	
	Disease present	Disease absent
Positive	a (True positive)	b (False positive)
Negative	c (False negative)	d (True negative)

Sensitivity = a/a + c; Specificity = d/b + d; Positive predictive value = a/a + b; Negative predictive value = d/c + d.

It is unusual for the screening test itself to demarcate exactly between those with and without disease. Almost invariably, the population groups (healthy and diseased) overlap considerably and thus variably specified test results will give rise to different levels of calculated sensitivity and specificity.

Conventionally, these difficulties are depicted by means of a bimodal graph, as illustrated in Figure 26.3. The screening test scale is shown on the horizontal axis, and the distribution of the healthy and diseased populations overlaps to a greater or lesser extent. The selection of different discriminant values of the test results (known as the 'cut-off point') demonstrates the inverse association between the sensitivity and specificity of the screening test. The selection of cut-off point A determines that the test will have high sensitivity and low specificity: all those with the disease will be identified by the test but a high proportion without disease will also be identified (false positive). Altering the cut-off point to B results in a test with low sensitivity but high specificity: a small number of people with the disease are missed (false negative), although the great majority of people without the disease are correctly identified as screen negative.

The selection of an appropriate cut-off point, and thus particular values of sensitivity and specificity, is a complex process involving considerable degrees of subjective judgement related to the disease in question. Some disorders, such as cervical cancer, can afford a high sensitivity for the screening test as diagnostic clinical confirmation is reliable and relatively inexpensive, whereas in others, high specificity would be of greater desirability. Value judgements concerning the disease in question, the cost of diagnostic tests and the place of the disease in society are required, and the results of such judgements will determine levels of false-positive and false-negative screening tests that will be tolerated.

Urologists well appreciate the affect a variable cut-off may have on the sensitivity and specificity of disease. Difficulties in calculating effective 'cut-offs' for prostate cancer 'screening' have been widely reported, and the advent of newer, more sophisticated prostate specific antigen tests ('free and bound') has not lessened the debate on the ideal discriminant value between benign and malignant disease.

A further attempt to refine and optimise values of sensitivity and specificity involves the construction of a receiver-operating characteristic curve. Such curves can be drawn if the screening test result is both quantitative and variable. Sensitivity on the vertical axis and 1 − specificity on the horizontal axis are plotted for a range of values (Figure 26.4) and the optimal point is that which lies furthest from the diagonal. Although, strictly speaking, receiver-operating characteristic curves are difficult to construct for subjective

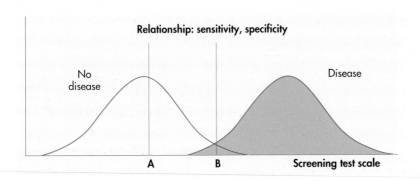

Figure 26.3 *Sensitivity and specificity of a screening test and the effect of variation of the cut-off value. A = High sensitivity, low specificity. B = Low sensitivity, high specificity.*

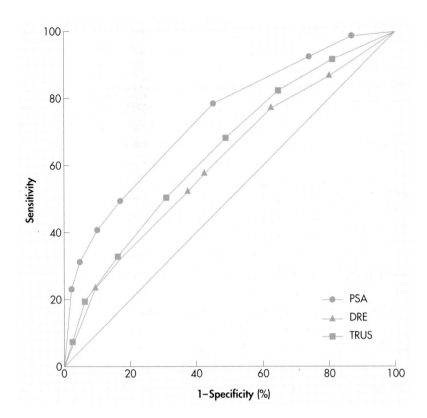

Figure 26.4 *Receiver–operator characteristic curve for serum prostate specific antigen (PSA) ●, transrectal ultrasonography (TRUS) ■ and digital rectal examination (DRE) ▲. (Data from reference Ellis et al. (1994) [10].)*

tests such as digital rectal examination, this form of analysis reinforces the impression that prostate specific antigen is the best predictor of the presence of prostatic carcinoma [10].

Checking the sensitivity of a test

The screening test has already been defined as a measurement that is able to identify disease in the detectable preclinical period. Unfortunately, because the true prevalence of disease during this stage must, by definition, be unknown, the sensitivity of the test cannot be calculated with certainty. To overcome this problem, screening tests are occasionally tested on populations with known clinical disease. Experience has shown, however, that this may be highly misleading in that the test may perform exceptionally well when offered such a relatively gross challenge but will perform indifferently in the true detectable preclinical phase screening situation. Thus, sensitivity and specificity may vary widely according to the stage of the disease.

A further theoretical approach to the problem of defining sensitivity might be to perform a diagnostic test on every person offered the screening test. Clearly, however, the morbidity of the diagnostic test applied to large numbers of asymptomatic people would preclude this approach on ethical grounds alone. The estimation of test sensitivity therefore rests imperfectly with the test itself and with the diagnostic measures that are subsequently undertaken to confirm or deny the presence of disease. The emergence of new clinical cases from a previously screened population, as well as information gathered from re-screening exercises (called, in cancer screening programmes, 'interval cancers'), eventually leads to a reasonable estimate of the sensitivity of a particular screening test. By contrast, the estimation of specificity is less problematical. As the ratio of people with disease to the general population is usually very low, an accurate estimation may be obtained by calculating those testing negative as a proportion of the sum of those with negative or false-positive tests.

The predictive value is an important measure of a screening test of interest to both the screener and the screened population (see Table 26.1). A positive predictive value is the proportion of those with preclinical disease relative to those with a positive screening test. A negative predictive value is the proportion of people who are healthy amongst the population with a negative test. Predictive values vary and relate not only to the validity of the test itself (see above), but to the prevalence of the disease in the general population. These effects are illustrated in Table 26.2. A high positive predictive value clearly indicates satisfactory test performance but, as disease prevalence declines, so does the positive predictive value, until, with a disease of low prevalence, only a very small percentage of those with a positive test actually have preclinical disease – 2% in the example given in Table 26.2. By contrast, under the same circumstances of low prevalence, a negative test clearly indicates that it is very unlikely indeed that the person has the disease. As stated above, this is an ideal result from the point of view of the screenee who has attended in the hope that his or her impression of good health will be supported by the test.

The effects of repeat screening

It might be expected that disease 'pick-up' rates would be maximal during the first screening exercise and reduced thereafter. Table 26.3 illustrates this effect for early studies involving programmes for cervix, breast and lung cancers. More recently, similar effects have been noted during 'screening' for prostate cancer in the USA, where the incidence of metastatic disease in bone has fallen steadily, perhaps indicating the detection of disease earlier in the detectable preclinical phase.

Programme validity

The performance of the screening test itself is naturally but one part of the overall efficacy of any particular screening programme. Other factors that will be crucial to the outcome of the enterprise include the screening request-response rate, the interval between screens, and the ability accurately to process those people found to be screen positive. Most recently in the UK, such problems have been vividly illustrated in the case of screening for cervical carcinoma. Allegedly, inexperience and underfunding of laboratories have led to significant doubts concerning the interpretation of large numbers of smear tests.

Table 26.2 The effect of preclinical prevalence of disease on positive and negative predictive values

Prevalence (%)		Predictive value (%)	
		Positive	Negative
10	(high)	68	99.4
1		16	99.9
0.1	(low)	2	99.99

Sensitivity: specificity: 95%

Table 26.3 The effect of repeat screening on the prevalence of disease

Cancer	Survey	Prevalence (per 10^3)	
		1st pass	2nd pass
Cervix	Females Age 20+ Rescreen <3 years	3.9	1.3
Breast	Females Age 20–64 Rescreen 1 year	2.7	1.5
Lung	Males Age 40–65 Rescreen 6 months	1.0	0.4

Abstracted from Christopherson (1966), Shapiro (1977) and Brett (1968) [22–24].

Clearly, the efficacy of a programme is no greater than the efficacy of its weakest link.

Overall, evaluation of a screening programme depends, therefore, not only on sensitivity and specificity indicators but on the entire screening infrastructure and, most particularly, on outcome measures as judged by objectives laid down at the commencement of the programme. Apart from these problems with infrastructure, resources, diagnostic quality control etc., it has been noted that screening programmes contain a degree of bias that may significantly affect outcome measures such that those persons identified with screen-positive disease will almost invariably survive longer than those detected using standard clinical criteria. Some of these biases have already been mentioned, but are restated to emphasise their importance in the overall evaluation of screening programmes.

Lead time bias is that proportion of the detectable preclinical phase by which survival will be increased even if the screening programme has no effect on disease mortality.

Length bias determines that the screening process will naturally select individuals with more indolent or biologically inactive disease. Length bias is most pronounced at the initial screen and is, in part, mitigated by subsequent screening.

Selection bias. Despite attempts to screen broad sections of the community, the process itself is inevitably voluntary and thus those who attend screening programmes are generally more interested in their own personal health than those who refuse. As stated above, these health-conscious people expect to be told that they do not have serious disease and, to this end, have usually spent their lives avoiding risk factors such as unhealthy diets and smoking. Additionally, even if these people are found to have disease, their attitude to personal health means that it is likely that they will have a better outcome from the disease than those who neglect themselves.

Overdiagnosis bias. A number of chronic conditions, particularly cancers, may have a semi-indolent phase that may not lead to clinical disease in the natural lifetime of the patient. Overdiagnosis of this form of disease – perhaps best illustrated by the case of prostate cancer – will again lead to false estimates of survival. This bias can be seen to be an extreme form of length bias, illustrated in Figure 26.2.

These forms of bias, acting individually and together, almost invariably mean that patients with screen-detected disease survive longer than those detected in the normal way. To eliminate effectively the combined influence of these factors requires a randomised controlled trial of the screening process itself [9]. The basic design for such a trial is illustrated in Figure 26.5. It can be seen that not only is the population randomly allocated to study or control group, but all cancers are followed whether screen detected or refusal detected. Although it is generally agreed that randomised trials offer the most objective test of a screening process, ethical issues may prevent the establishment of a formalised trial structure. Whereas such trials have been established for prostate cancer (see Chapter 27), these issues may cause significant problems in the case of diseases such as breast cancer for which randomisation to the control arm may meet with consumer resistance. To circumvent these problems, numerous complex methodologies have been proposed, the details of which are beyond the scope of this account.

Trial of screening

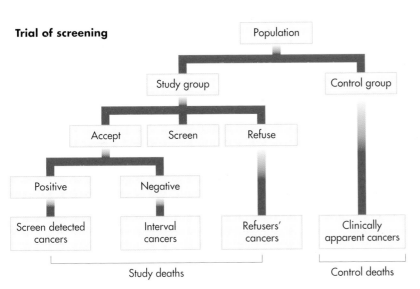

Figure 26.5 The ideal design of a randomised controlled trial to evaluate the benefits or otherwise of a screening programme. Refusers: people who refuse to undertake screening tests despite randomisation to the screening arm. Interval cancers: cancers arising by conventional clinical symptoms between screening tests.

Screening and the control of disease

Screening is but one method of controlling disease in the population. Others are prevention or the application of curative methods once the disease has become manifest. Of these options, screening is a relative newcomer and its role in the control of mass disease remains somewhat controversial. It is convenient to consider disease control in terms of both mass screening and selective screening.

Encouraged by successes in eliminating chronic inflammatory disease, health departments have turned their resources within the last 25 years towards an attempt to eradicate other chronic diseases such as cancer. However, inspection of mortality-reduction targets shows that screening is expected to contribute only a small proportion of the target total: it has gradually become clear that the complexities and problems involved in mass screening preclude the utilisation of this methodology as a significant means of disease control.

Several factors underlie this failure to achieve specified goals. The Wilson and Junger criteria (described below) dictate that the specified disease must be common and an important health problem. Yet careful analysis of mortality data (Figure 26.8) demonstrates clearly that this may often not be the case, despite public perception to the contrary. Currently, programmes are in place for cervical and breast cancer and certain aspects of cardiovascular disease (hypertension), although the organisation of programmes varies widely between countries and with time in any one country. There remain significant problems related to population compliance. No better example of the discrepancy between expectation and achievement is provided than by the prostate cancer 'screening' policy within the USA. Despite enormous publicity and guidelines provided by bodies such as the American Cancer Society, significant screening test take-up rates are to be found only within the white Anglo-Saxon population. Take-up within the black community is acknowledged to be extremely low and almost impossible to achieve, yet this is the single group identified by epidemiological studies as having the highest risk of prostate cancer mortality in the world. It is very clear that, in this group of people,

screening is almost useless as a method of disease control.

However, selective screening has been more successful at reducing disease rates in the last few decades. Targeting populations exposed to risk factors such as asbestos and tobacco has been, in part, successful in reducing disease due to these agents. Nevertheless, prevention strategies are at least as important as a means of disease control. Urine screening of workers who were in the past exposed to aniline dyes continues, but undoubtedly the main factor responsible for the reduction in industrial disease-related transitional cell carcinoma is the exclusion of the carcinogenic substances from the manufacturing process in the mid-1950s.

In summary, mass screening for chronic disease is effective as a means of disease control in certain carefully defined groups of patients. For the majority, however, other programmes of disease control are required. By contrast, 'single-shot' screening of the newborn is an effective method of disease containment that, even in the case of rare disease, may prove to be cost effective in the long term.

General principles relating to screening programmes

During the last 30 years, the general principles that underpin a successful screening programme have been analysed and refined. A broad consensus has emerged from individuals and international workshops [11, 12] regarding the criteria that should be met to establish a successful screening programme. Of these criteria, the most widely quoted at the present time are those published in the public health papers of the World Health Organisation [13] by Wilson and Junger (Table 26.4). It is instructive to discuss each individual principle in turn.

The condition should be an important health problem. Clearly, this statement refers to the point of view of the health department of the country concerned. Accurate mortality statistics (see Figures 26.8 and 26.9) will be required for that country, although these may well reveal that problems considered by

Table 26.4 Accepted criteria for successful population screening programmes

1. The condition sought should be an important health problem
2. The natural history of the condition should be adequately understood
3. There should be a detectable latent or preclinical stage
4. A test of suitable sensitivity and specificity should be available
5. There should be an accepted mode of treatment for patients discovered to have the disease
6. Adequate facilities for both diagnosis and treatment should be available
7. The tests must be acceptable to the population
8. The benefits should outweigh any adverse effects of screening
9. The cost of screening must be acceptable in relation to overall medical expenditure
10. Screening for chronic disease is an ongoing process requiring critical analysis and audit of results

From Wilson and Junger (1968) [13].

the general public to be of major importance may well not be significant in public health terms. Evidently, in the North West of England, cardiovascular disease is the pre-eminent public health problem, whereas in males, each organ-specific cancer site, with the possible exception of the lung, contributes little to the overall picture. For women, breast cancer assumes a significant position in the public health priority list, not only because of the numbers involved but because the disease affects younger women whose economic and social lives are important to the nation. By the same token, disorders tht affect older men – for example, colorectal and prostate tumours – score less heavily in terms of being an 'important health problem' in the eyes of the Department of Health. The controversy that surrounds prostate cancer screening at the present time is discussed further below.

The natural history of the condition should be adequately understood. It is naturally very important that the biological progress of the disease should be known with reasonable certainty. This matter is not always as simple as it might seem. In the case of 'single-shot' antenatal screening for hydronephrosis and urinary tract obstruction, significant numbers of babies with hydronephrosis were detected as the

sophistication of interuterine ultrasound increased. Subsequently, it became clear that physiological changes at and after birth restored many of these upper urinary tracts to normal and it was clear that the 'screening test' was overestimating the incidence of significant pathology in these children.

Prostate cancer provides the best example of a chronic condition whose natural history is incompletely understood. Evidence from well-known post-mortem studies from the 1950s indicates that the disease is extremely common in old age – men die 'with' rather than 'of' prostate cancer. The inability to distinguish indolent from aggressive cancers in younger men continues to generate heated debate.

There should be a detectable latent or preclinical stage. It has already been mentioned that it is impossible, by definition, to perform a screening test on a disease that does not have a detectable preclinical stage. Thus, whereas cervical dysplasia permits the consideration of effective programmes for cervical cancer, sputum cytology and chest X-ray have been found wanting in terms of their ability to reduce the mortality from lung cancer [9].

A test of suitable sensitivity and specificity should be available. The measures that describe the validity of any particular screening test have been described above and the difficulties of agreeing an acceptable cut-off point have been emphasised. This problem is particularly well illustrated by reference to prostate specific antigen and the ability of this marker to distinguish between benign and malignant prostate disease (Figure 26.6). Although 4 ng is generally accepted as an adequate cut-off, significant numbers of men with prostate specific antigen results under this value are found to have tumours, and some authorities argue that a lower cut-off, as illustrated, should be employed.

There should be an accepted mode of treatment for patients discovered to have the disease. The early diagnosis of an untreatable disease is, of course, not a cost-effective public health policy, although the debate surrounding such conditions as Duchenne muscular dystrophy has been noted. The proposed treatment should be effective in terms of reducing mortality, and the ideal methodology for the evaluation of screening programmes has been described.

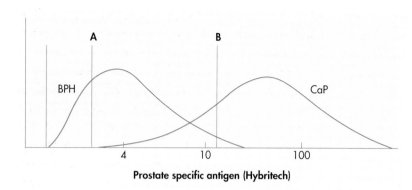

Figure 26.6 *Sensitivity and specificity as applied to prostate specific antigen testing. Conventionally, a cut-off of 4 ng is accepted as the best compromise, although significant numbers of cancers may be identified with prostate specific antigen values below that level. A = Theoretical ideal sensitivity, poor specificity. B = Good specificity, unacceptable sensitivity. BPH, benign prostatic hyperplasia; CaP, prostate cancer.*

Adequate facilities for diagnosis and treatment should be available. It is self-evident that there is no point in establishing an expensive screening process if facilities to confirm the diagnosis and confer treatment are not readily available.

The test must be acceptable to the population. The poor take-up rate in some screening programmes testifies to the fact that there is a limit to the discomfort that the public is willing to suffer in order to detect asymptomatic disease (from which, in any case, they believe they are not suffering). Mammography is not usually a comfortable procedure and there is no doubt that in North America the thought of a rectal examination and perhaps transrectal ultrasound is the primary reason for the poor attendance at screening sessions by certain segments of society. The paradoxical situation of the Afro-American in the USA has already been mentioned.

The benefits should outweigh any adverse effect of screening. 'Benefits' in this context are taken to refer to those as observed from the public health point of view. Clearly, from the individual standpoint, there may be significant morbidity (and, perhaps rarely, mortality) from a screening test and thus, personally, the individual would be unlikely to recognise any benefit. Judged overall, the benefits to the general population should outweigh the adverse effects within the same population, and outcome measures should indicate a real advantage to the screened populations, ideally in terms of increased survival times.

The cost of screening must be acceptable in relation to the overall medical expenditure. It has been emphasised that screening is but one part of health policy aimed at containing disease. Furthermore, disease contain-

ment is but one part of the overall medical strategy for the population and, as such, screening costs have to be considered side by side with all other claims on the health service purse.

Screening for chronic disease is an ongoing process requiring critical analysis and audit of results. Self-evidently, disease is an ever-present threat, emerging constantly during the life years of the population. Thus, effective screening programmes must be ongoing, as must continuing audit and evaluation of the process.

In general, the Wilson and Junger criteria [13] provide a very good framework for the discussion of disease as a matter of public health policy. The principles are naturally more applicable to some diseases than to others, and the opportunity is now taken to discuss screening programmes in terms of organ-based uropathology.

Screening for urological disease

'Single-shot' screening

Congenital abnormalities of the urogenital system are relatively common because such abnormalities are not invariably fatal for the fetus. Within the last 15 years, increasingly sophisticated ultrasound technology has been able to pick up urological abnormalities in utero with increasing confidence. Most normal fetal kidneys are visible before 20 weeks and hydronephrosis may be detectable as early as 16 weeks. Using such technology, the incidence of congenital renal abnormalities has been reported as approximately 1 in 800 live births [14], which compares favourably with 1 in 650 reported from autopsy series [15].

Good-quality pictures may be obtained of hydronephrosis and hydroureter when present (Figure 26.7). Although not all cases of simple hydronephrosis may need intervention after birth, the screening process undoubtedly identifies at-risk babies, allowing the paediatric service to concentrate its efforts in a cost-effective and efficient manner.

Screening for chronic urological disease

Screening programmes are understandably directed towards the eradication of serious chronic disease such as cancer (Table 26.5). Therefore, if such programmes are to be applied to the urogenital system, neoplastic disease is most likely to be the target of the enterprise. Serious chronic inflammatory disease such as tuberculosis is no longer a significant health problem from a screening point of view. However, as will be seen, in terms of numbers, urological cancers, with the possible exception of prostate, do not recommend themselves as ideal subjects for screening protocols.

Renal cancer

Although it is responsible for the most common open operation performed for urological malignancy, kidney cancer is relatively uncommon. This disease, ranking 11th within the UK, was responsible for approximately 1800 deaths in 1994 [16] and the cancer therefore cannot be viewed as a major health problem. Additionally, there is no obvious preclinical phase to detect: most early tumours are discovered by inciden-

tal ultrasound examination, which merely identifies relatively small, established cancers that have yet to bleed into the renal pelvis. A screening programme would therefore be inappropriate for this disease.

A form of selective screening might apply to those patients with von Hippel–Lindau disease, who have multiple abnormalities including a 30% incidence of renal cell carcinoma. However, the symptoms and signs of the disorder are so characteristic and the association with kidney cancer so strong that the term selective screening is unnecessary for what is, in effect, a practical clinical surveillance programme.

Bladder cancer

Although more common than kidney cancer, bladder cancer is again not a major public health problem, being responsible for 3% (5300) of all cancer deaths in 1994 [16]. Nevertheless, the debate continues in urological circles as to the diagnostic protocol that should follow the discovery of microscopic haematuria: it is accepted that bleeding usually arises not from a preclinical phase but from established urothelial tumour. Urine cytology is widely utilised as a diagnostic test in those patients who have been discovered to have haematuria, although it is acknowledged that significant false-negative results may occur, particularly in patients with well-differentiated transitional cell tumours. Carcinoma in situ is perhaps a genuine manifestation of the preclinical phase of invasive bladder cancer. Unfortunately, checking this condition against the Wilson and Junger criteria reveals that there is little hope of establishing an effective screening programme for the disease. Recent reports have

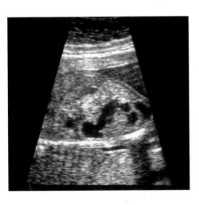

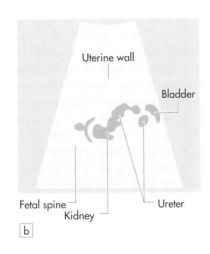

Uterine wall

Bladder

Fetal spine

Kidney

Ureter

Figures 26.7 (a) *Antenatal ultrasound of a fetus with hydronephrosis and hydroureter but a normal bladder.* (b) *Diagrammatic representation to illustrate the scan shown in* (a).

a

b

Table 26.5 The benefits and disadvantages of screening for cancer

Benefits	Disadvantages
Improved prognosis for some cases detected by screening	Longer morbidity for cases whose prognosis is unaltered
Less radical treatment needed to cure some cases	Overtreatment of borderline abnormalities
Reassurance for those with negative test results	False reassurance for those with false-negative results Unnecessary morbidity for those with false-positive results Hazard of screening test
Resource saving	Resource costs

From Prorok et al. (1984) [9].

demonstrated the efficacy of detecting bladder cancer by microsatellite analysis of urine DNA [17]. This approach clearly holds out hope for the future, but it should be noted that this work has adopted the questionable technique referred to earlier whereby a potential screening test is evaluated using patients with known clinical disease. As has been emphasised, the real test of such techniques will be when the procedure is applied to a true screening population.

Prostate cancer

Prostate cancer is widely heralded at the present time as being the second most common cause of UK cancer death in males, 9600 patients having died of the disease in 1994. However, from a public health point of view, these figures are relatively unimpressive. Figures 26.8 and 26.9 show that, taking the North West of England as an example and allowing for the disparity

in the data, prostate deaths only account for approximately 3–4% of the overall regional mortality. Furthermore, Cancer Research Campaign figures clearly show (Figure 26.10) that the great majority of these deaths occur in men over 65 years old (92%); thus, from a public health point of view, deaths from this disease in the 'high political impact' younger age group are a very small proportion of the overall health problem. On these grounds alone, mass screening could not be justified for this disease.

Nevertheless, there is at the present time tremendous public pressure on the Department of Health by both vested interest groups within the medical profession and the press generally, which identify with prominent public figures unfortunate enough to contract the disease. As a result of this publicity, extensive case finding is proceeding at the primary health care level, although the efficacy of these sporadic actions

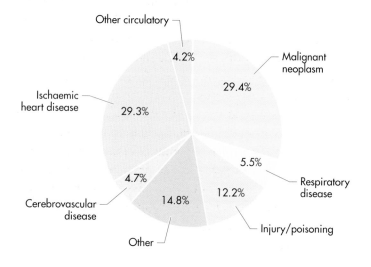

Figure 26.8 Disease-specific death rates for males (under 65 years) in North West England (1994). In public health terms, it is observed, when viewed in conjunction with Figure 26.9 that mortality due to cardiovascular-related disease far exceeds mortality due to any form of organ-specific cancer. (Data from the Centre for Cancer Epidemiology, University of Manchester, 1993 small area database, North West Regional Health Authority.)

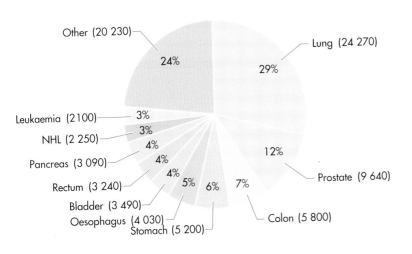

Figure 26.9 *The ten most common causes of cancer death in men in the UK (1994). (Total number of cancer deaths = 83 340.) Prostate deaths at any age constitute 12% of the whole. NHL, non-Hodgkin's lymphoma. (Data from Cancer Research Campaign Factsheet 3.2 (1995) [16].)*

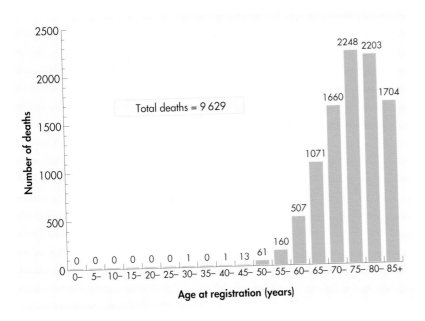

Figure 26.10 *Deaths by age from prostate cancer in the UK (1992): 743 of 9629 deaths (8%) occurred in men under 65 years, illustrating the relatively weak impact that the disease in younger men might make on public health policy. (Data from Cancer Research Campaign Factsheet 2.4 (1994) [25].)*

remains unproven. Nevertheless, relatively large numbers of younger men with biopsy-proven early prostate cancer are being identified and urologists are struggling to establish rational treatment protocols for the disease thus discovered. At the present time, as most of the Wilson and Junger criteria cannot be answered, both urologists and patients have had to settle for acknowledged over-treatment of detected disease [18].

Some laudable attempts have been made to determine whether or not a screening programme for early prostate cancer can influence mortality from the disease in the long term. The European Randomised Study of Screening for Prostate Carcinoma (ERSPC) is based in Rotterdam and has adopted the classical approach of a randomised clinical trial (see Chapter 27) to eliminate bias and evaluate the screening programme. Figure 26.11 depicts the screening algorithm for those randomised to the screening group. In this study, screening is by means of prostate specific antigen, rectal examination and transrectal ultrasound. So far, the reported cancer detection rate is 4.3%, and 91% of cancers by clinical staging are organ confined. In this study, receiver-operating characteristic analysis (see above) demonstrated that prostate specific antigen with rectal examination and the free/total prostate specific antigen ratio were significantly better predictors of a positive biopsy than prostate specific antigen alone [19].

This study also illustrates well the problem of establishing an appropriate prostate specific antigen cut-off value (see Figures 26.3 and 26.6). Figure 26.12 demonstrates the previously described reciprocal rela-

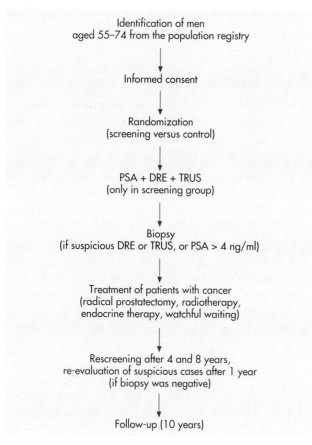

Figure 26.11 *Details of the Rotterdam randomised controlled trial of screening for prostate cancer [19]. PSA, prostate specific antigen; DRE, digital rectal examination; TRUS, transrectal ultrasonography.*

tion between sensitivity and specificity and it is clear that the optimal cut-off point is extremely difficult to ascertain. The authors conclude that the answer to this question can only be obtained by making a reasonable effort to detect all cancers in the population and by studying the long-term outcomes [19].

Selective screening for prostate cancer is widely practised for those members of the population with a familial history of the disease. Unfortunately, as noted above, Afro-Americans, who have a high incidence of the disease, are particularly reluctant to attend for screening programmes of any type. Individual case finding of compliant males seems to be the only possible solution to this dilemma.

Testis cancer

The rarity of this condition precludes a national screening effort, but all urologists will be aware of the importance of self-examination and self-referral in preventing the presentation of patients with advanced disease. The publicity about self-examination may be likened to that surrounding breast disease but, clearly, diagnostic confirmation and treatment are both easier and cheaper for cases of testis cancer, with the added benefit of excellent long-term outcome measures.

Glossary of terms

Incidence   The number of new cancer cases arising in a specified period of time.

Prevalence   The number of people with a history of cancer who are alive at any given time.

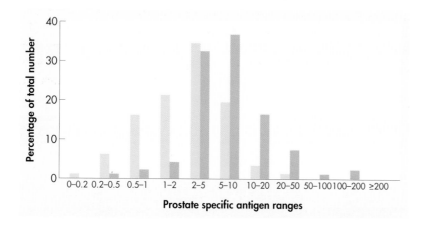

Figure 26.12 *Sensitivity, specificity and cut-off values illustrated using data obtained from the Rotterdam screening study [19]. The extraordinary difficulty of establishing a cut-off between health and disease can be appreciated.* ■ *No cancer (n = 786);* ■ *Cancer (n = 191).*

Sensitivity The proportion of people with a positive screening test amongst those with the disease.

Specificity The proportion of people with a negative test amongst those free from the disease.

Positive predictive value The proprtion of those with preclinical disease amongst those with a positive test.

Negative predictive value The proportion of those who are healthy amongst those with a negative test.

Lead time The interval between the time of detection by screening and the time at which the disease would have been diagnosed in the absence of screening.

Cut-off The point on the test scale that is associated with a particular combination of sensitivity and specificity.

References

1. Bowman JE. Screening new-born infants for Duchenne muscular dystrophy. Br Med J 1993; 306: 349

2. Bogart MH, Pandian MR, Jones OW. Abnormal maternal serum chorionic gonadotrophin levels in pregnancies with fetal chromosome abnormalities. Prenat Diagn 1987; 7: 623–30

3. Wald NJ, Cuckle HS, Densem JW, *et al.* Maternal serum screening for Down's syndrome in early pregnancy. Br Med J 1988; 297: 883–7

4. Cole P, Morrison AS. Basic issues in cancer screening. In: Miller AB (ed) UICC Technical Report Series, Vol. 40. Geneva: UICC, 1978: 7

5. Day NE, Walter SD. Simplified models for screening: estimation procedures from mass screening programmes. Biometrics 1984; 40: 1–7

6. Hutchison GB, Shapiro S. Lead time gain by diagnostic screening for breast cancer. J Natl Cancer Inst 1968; 41: 665–9

7. Feinleib M, Zelen M. Some pitfalls in the evaluation of screening programmes. Arch Environ Health 1969; 19: 412–7

8. Bradley DM, Parsons PE, Clarke AJ. Experience with screening new-borns for Duchenne muscular dystrophy in Wales. Br Med J 1993; 306: 357–60

9. Prorok PC, Chamberlin J, Day NE, *et al.* UICC Workshop on the Evaluation of Screening Programmes for Cancer. Int J Cancer 1984; 34: 1–4

10. Ellis WJ, Chetner MP, Preston SD, Brewer MK. Diagnosis of prostatic carcinoma: the yield of serum prostate specific antigen, digital rectal examination and transrectal ultrasonography. J Urol 1994; 152: 1520–5

11. Whitby LG. Screening for disease: definitions and criteria. Lancet 1974; 2: 819–21

12. Miller AB. Screening in cancer: a report of the UICC Workshop in Toronto. UICC Technical Report Series Vol. 40. Geneva: UICC, 1978

13. Wilson J, Junger G. Principles and practice of screening for disease. World Health Organisation Public Health Paper No. 34, Geneva: WHO, 1968

14. Thomas DFM, Whitaker RH. Prenatal diagnosis. In: Whitaker RH (ed) Current prospectives in paediatric urology. New York: Springer Verlag, 1989: 45–53

15. Ashleigh DJB, Mostofi FK. Renal agenesis and dysgenesis. J Urol 1960; 83: 211–30

16. CRC Factsheet 3.2. London: Cancer Research Campaign, 1995

17. Steiner G, Schoenberg MP, Linn JF, *et al.* Detection of bladder cancer recurrence by micro-satellite analysis of urine. Nature Med 1997; 3: 621–4

18. Schröder FH. To screen or not to screen. Br Med J 1993; 306: 407–8

19. Bangma CH, Rietbergen JBW, Schröder FH. Prostate specific antigen as a screening test – The Netherlands experience. Urol Clin N Am 1997; 24: 307–14

20. Prorok PC, Connor RJ, Baker SG. Statistical considerations in cancer screening programmes. Urol Clin N Am 1990; 17: 699–708

21. Prorok PC, Connor RJ. Screening for the early detection of cancer. Cancer Invest 1986; 4: 225–38

22. Christopherson WM. The control of cervix cancer. Acta Cytol 1966 10: 6–10

23. Shapiro S. Evidence on screening for breast cancer from a randomised trial. Cancer 1977; 39: 2772–82

24. Brett GZ. The value of lung cancer detection by 6 monthly chest radiographs. Thorax 1968; 23: 414–20

25. CRC Factsheet 2.4. London: Cancer Research Campaign, 1994

The design, construction and interpretation of clinical trials

27

J. A. Morris

Introduction

A clinical trial is defined as a medical experiment on a sample of patients to compare the effects of two or more treatments. The treatments could be, for example, different drugs or surgical techniques, and the measured effects might be symptom severity, recurrence of symptoms, recovery time or death. The results obtained from such a study are then used to make inferences about which treatment should be recommended for a more general population of patients.

Clinical trials are comparative, in that a group of patients given a new treatment is compared with a control group of similar patients receiving either a well-established treatment or no treatment (if no treatment has already been demonstrated to be effective). Furthermore, patients should be assigned randomly to the new or standard treatment to ensure an unbiased evaluation of the effect of the new treatment.

The randomised controlled trial is usually considered the most reliable method of conducting a clinical study.

Drug trials

The pharmaceutical industry defines four categories of trials: phases I, II, III and IV.

Phase I trials are essentially exploratory trials on healthy human volunteers. They are used to assess the frequency and degree of harmful side-effects (i.e. the toxicity of proposed therapy). Phase II trials deter-

mine the level of effectiveness of a particular treatment and further define the non-therapeutic effects (i.e. toxicity). These trials are carried out on patients and are used to decide whether the therapeutic effect of treatment is good enough to warrant further investigation. Phase III trials are definitive studies that are designed to compare a new treatment with an existing established treatment. They are often referred to by the general term 'clinical trials' because they involve the most comprehensive investigation of a new treatment. Phase IV trials are concerned with the monitoring of adverse effects after the drug has been approved for marketing and are basically long-term studies of morbidity and mortality.

In this chapter, only phase III trials (full-scale comparative studies) will be considered in detail, because it is this type of trial that most clinicians outside the pharmaceutical industry come across.

Early clinical trials

Treatment evaluation has been attempted as far back as prehistoric times, and there are various reports of studies being carried out in the seventeenth and eighteenth centuries.

An interesting description of a comparative trial of treatments for scurvy carried out in the mid-eighteenth century is given by Lind [1]. Twelve similar patients with scurvy were selected, and divided into six groups of two patients. Each group was given one of the following six treatments in addition to a common diet: a quart of cider a day, 25 gutts of elixir vitriol, two spoonfuls of vinegar, a course of sea water, a nutmeg, or two oranges and a lemon each day. The effects of treatment were evaluated at the end of six days. The men given the oranges and lemons were greatly recovered; one was fit for duty, and the other was appointed nurse to the rest of the sick. Nevertheless, the results of the study were not immediately acted upon. Lind recommended fruit and vegetables as only a secondary priority to 'pure dry air', and it took another 50 years before the British navy supplied lemon juice to its ships.

This study included many of the important aspects of a controlled trial. There was a homogeneous group of patients, equally divided into the various treatment groups, a good description of the differing treatment schedules, and a clear account of the outcome. However, properly conducted clinical trials were not carried out until the late 1940s. The first clinical trial with a properly randomised control group was for streptomycin in the treatment of pulmonary tuberculosis [2].

Protocols

An important starting point in designing a study is to write a study protocol. This is a formal document specifying how the clinical trial is to be conducted. It provides detailed information on the various components of the trial, including:

- aims and objectives
- patient selection
- trial design
- treatment schedules
- randomisation of patients
- main outcome measures
- required size of study
- planned statistical analysis
- protocol deviations
- adverse events
- patient consent.

It is, in essence, an operating manual giving clear instructions to the members of the clinical trial team as to how the study should be conducted. All clinicians and researchers involved in the study, including a statistician, should be consulted in writing the protocol. A detailed protocol often has to be submitted to ethical committees and funding bodies to provide evidence that the trial is well designed.

Trial design

There are two main types of design: parallel and cross-over. The simplest is the *parallel design*. Two groups of patients are given a different treatment regime over the same period of time. One group receives the new treatment and the other group, acting as the control, receives the standard or placebo treatment. Patients are randomised to one or other of the two groups. This design is most suitable for a study in which the treatment is expected to change the course of the disease and to make an appreciable difference to a patient's condition. The long-term effects of treatment can also be assessed using a parallel design study carrying on over a number of years.

The alternative design is the *cross-over* trial. In its simplest form, each patient receives two treatments, one after the other, and the order of treatments is chosen using a suitable randomisation method. Because an assessment of both treatments is made on each patient, a comparison of treatments is calculated 'within-patients'; that is, each patient acts as his or her own control. This allows a more precise comparison because the variability of an outcome measure for a patient recorded at different times will usually be less than that between different patients recorded at the same time. This means that smaller numbers of patients are required in cross-over trials. However, there are a number of disadvantages. A cross-over design is only viable if the evaluation of treatment involves measuring short-term relief of symptoms of a chronic condition. One problem with the design is that the effect of the first treatment may carry over to the second period and hence interfere with the effect of the second treatment. This *carry-over* effect will then bias any comparison between treatments. To overcome this problem, a *wash-out* period should be included between the first and second treatment periods in which no treatment is given. There may also be a greater number of patients who drop out of a cross-over study, simply because a much longer overall treatment period is required. Patients may drop out before receiving the second treatment.

For studies in which the treatment outcome is known fairly quickly, a *sequential design* is sometimes appropriate. This is a parallel group study in which patients are gradually recruited and the data are analysed after each new patient. The trial continues until either a clear difference between treatments emerges or it is considered unlikely that any difference will be shown. The advantage of this design is that the required sample size will be smaller than that of a simple parallel study if the difference between the two treatments is relatively large, and therefore fewer patients will receive the less beneficial treatment.

Random allocation

In a parallel design, the treatment given to each patient should be decided by chance – that is, by random allocation. There are various types of randomisation.

Simple randomisation gives equal probability for each patient to receive one of the treatments. If there are two treatments, labelled A and B, then a simple randomisation can be obtained by tossing a coin for each patient, allocating treatment A for heads and treatment B for tails. Alternatively, a table of random numbers can be used, with even numbers indicating treatment A and odd numbers indicating treatment B.

However, this does not ensure that at the end of recruitment, equal numbers of patients receive treatments A and B. This discrepancy can be substantive, particularly for large trials. One way to ensure that equal numbers of patients are allocated to the treatments is to use *blocked randomisation*. For every block or group of a specified number of patients, simple randomisation is used with the restriction that the block contains an equal allocation of patients. For example, if blocks of size 4 are specified, then a coin can be tossed to allocate the first two or three patients in each block. If the first two patients are allocated to treatment A, then, by default, the next two patients have to be allocated to treatment B. If the first two patients are allocated to treatment A and B respectively, then the third patient in the block is allocated by another toss of the coin. If this patient is allocated

to treatment B, then, by default, the fourth patient is allocated to treatment A, and so on.

It is important that the treatment groups in a randomised trial are similar with respect to relevant patient characteristics considered to be significant prognostic factors, for example age or severity of disease. *Stratified randomisation* can be used to guard against the possibility of imbalance of these prognostic factors between the different treatment groups. Each prognostic factor is categorised into two or more levels. As an example, suppose age and gender are the relevant factors, with age split into three categories – 'under 40 years', '40 to under 65 years' and '65 years and over'. These two factors define six patient types, or strata:

- male, age < 40
- male, age 40–< 65
- male, age 65 and over
- female, age < 40
- female, age 40–< 65
- female, age 65 and over.

For each of the patient strata, a separate blocked randomisation list is prepared. As a patient enters the trial, the stratum to which he or she belongs is identified and the treatment allocation is taken from the appropriate randomisation list. The strata should be reasonably low in number because there is a possibility of over-stratification, which may lead to an uneven distribution of patients over the defined strata (some strata may contain no patients at all), and may result in an imbalance in the prognostic factors between the treatment groups.

Note that in a cross-over design, the randomisation procedures outlined above are used to randomly allocate the order in which the patients receive the different treatments.

Non-random and systematic allocation

An alternative way of ensuring that the different treatment groups are similar with respect to prognostic factors is to use the *minimisation method*. This is a non-random procedure, but provides an acceptable method of allocating patients to treatment. It is particularly suitable for smaller studies with a few key patient characteristics known to be important prognostic factors. The allocation is not prepared in advance but is an ongoing process as patients are recruited. The first patient is given a treatment at random, but for subsequent patients the treatment which would give a better balance of prognostic factors across the treatment groups is determined. This is simply achieved by looking at the numbers of patients with similar prognostic factors who have already been allocated to one of the treatment groups. A weighted randomisation (in favour of the treatment which minimises the imbalance) is then used. The method of minimisation only requires a detailed record of the treatment allocations to be kept, which is constantly updated. It can be carried out manually, but is often implemented using a simple computer program.

Systematic allocation of subjects is sometimes used, but is not recommended. Examples of such methods are the alternate allocation of treatment to consecutive patients, or using a patient's date of birth to determine which treatment he or she should receive (e.g. those with even dates receiving treatment A, those with odd dates receiving treatment B). Although these procedures appear to lead to an unbiased allocation of treatment, it is possible for someone with prior knowledge of the assignment method to manipulate the system. For example, a clinician might be reluctant to enter a particular patient into the trial if he or she knows that the patient would be destined to receive a placebo.

Historical controls

Some researchers believe that a good control group to compare with current patients on a new treatment would comprise previous patients who had received the standard treatment. These patients are called historical or retrospective controls. The advantage of this approach is that all future patients can be given the new treatment, hence there is no need for randomisation of patients and a larger study size can be achieved. The main problem is that the use of the two groups of patients may not lead to a fair comparison.

There are many potential sources of bias, which cannot be discounted. Patients in the historical control group are likely to have less well-defined criteria for inclusion, may have come from a different source, and therefore may differ in the type and severity of disease. In addition, ancillary patient care may be much better for the current patients on the new treatment. Therefore, the use of historical controls is not recommended.

Blinding

It is essential to ensure that the patients randomly allocated to their respective treatments are treated in exactly the same way, otherwise bias may be introduced.

A *double-blind* trial is one in which both the clinician assessing the outcome of treatment and the patient are ignorant of the treatment allocation. This is feasible when, for example, the competing treatments are oral drug therapies. The differing tablets (including a placebo or dummy tablet if used) can be made to look and taste the same.

If it is impracticable to run a double-blind trial (for example if the competing treatments are different surgical procedures to which the clinician cannot be blinded), then the patient alone should be kept ignorant of the treatment. This would then be a *single-blind* trial.

The maximum degree of blindness that is possible should be used in a clinical trial.

Size of a trial

The number of subjects required in a study is an important consideration and depends on four different factors:

1. Response to the control/standard treatment, e.g. the expected percentage of patients showing relief from symptoms based on experience or previously published data, or the average peak flow rate.
2. Anticipated response to the new treatment.
3. Significance level (a). The quantity a is commonly referred to as the type I error, and is the probability of detecting a significant difference when the

treatments are really equally effective. It is usually set at 0.05. That is, a p value of 0.05 (a 5% significance level) is taken as the critical point at which a statistical comparison test of the data will show a significant difference.

4. Power $(1-\beta)$. This refers to the power of the study to detect a statistical difference between treatments of size equal to the expected response difference quoted above. The quantity β is commonly called the type II error, and is the probability of not detecting a significant difference between treatments when there really is a difference of this magnitude. In practice, a power of 80% is the lowest level considered acceptable.

The first two factors determine the size of the difference between the effects of the treatments regarded as important (usually denoted by δ). Detailed tables for sample size calculations are given in the book by Machin and Campbell [3]. Alternatively, specialised statistical computer software can be used to determine sample sizes for a wide range of trial designs.

Formulae are given below that correspond to a *two-sided significance level of 5%* and a *power of 80%*. The sample size calculations depend on whether the data are qualitative (e.g. percentages) or quantitative (e.g. continuous measures).

Comparison of proportions

To detect a difference in proportions, $\delta = p_1 - p_2$ (where p_1 is the proportion of successes expected on the standard treatment and p_2 is the proportion of successes on the new treatment), the number of subjects (n) in each group should be at least:

$$n = 7.85[p_1(1 - p_1) + p_2(1 - p_2)]/\delta^2 \qquad (1)$$

Example

In a comparative study of the benefits of radiotherapy versus surveillance in patients with stage I testicular cancer, the expected proportion of patients under surveillance who relapse is 0.25. The investigator believes that a reduction in relapse rate to 0.10 in the radiotherapy group would be clinically important. How many patients should be included in the study for a two-sided significance level of 0.05 and a power of 0.80?

From equation (1), with $p_1 = 0.25$, $p_2 = 0.10$ and $\delta = 0.15$, we obtain $n = 97$ in each of the groups, that is, 194 patients in total.

Comparison of means (unpaired data)

To detect a difference of size $\delta = m_1 - m_2$ (where m_1 and m_2 are the mean responses for the standard treatment and new treatment respectively), the number in each group should be at least:

$$n = 15.7\sigma^2/\delta^2 \qquad (2)$$

where σ is an estimate of the standard deviation of the response measure (assumed to be the same in both treatment groups).

Example

The effects of cimetidine and vitamin C on peak flow rate for patients with benign hypertrophy are to be compared in a randomised parallel trial. The clinician wishes to show a significant improvement of 5 ml/s or more in patients given cimetidine, and believes the standard deviation of peak flow rate in this group of patients will be about 10 ml/s. How many patients should the clinician recruit to the study for a 5% significance level and 80% power?

From equation (2), with $\sigma = 10$ and $\delta = 5$, we obtain $n = 63$ per group, that is, 126 patients in all.

Comparison of means (paired data, e.g. cross-over trial)

To detect a difference between treatments of size δ, and within-subject standard deviation σ_w, (i.e. the standard deviation of the paired difference between treatments), the number of subjects in each group should be at least:

$$n = 7.85\sigma_w^2/\delta^2 \qquad (3)$$

It is sometimes difficult to give a suitable value for the within-standard deviation σ_w. A rough approximation can be given by $\sqrt{2}\sigma$ (where σ is the standard deviation of the response measure).

Example

An investigator wishes to compare the effect of a drug having smooth muscle relaxant properties with a placebo on patients with idiopathic detrusor instability using a cross-over trial design. The investigator is looking for a difference in maximum voiding pressure of more than $10\,cmH_2O$ to be significant at the 0.05 level and with a power of 0.80. Previous studies have shown that in the absence of any drug effect, the standard deviation of within-subject maximum voiding pressure is $30\,cmH_2O$. How many patients should the investigator recruit?

From equation (3), with $\sigma_w = 30$ and $\delta = 10$, the investigator would require at least 71 patients in all.

It is important to recognise that studies in which the outcome measures are continuous (and have means as summary statistics) require fewer subjects than those in which the outcome is assessed as simply success or failure. An additional point to remember is that if a fair number of drop-outs is likely during the study, the calculated sample size should be increased accordingly.

Selection of subjects

If the results of a clinical trial are to be used to make general inferences, it is important that the patients included in the study form a representative sample of all patients with the particular disease. However, in practice, there are restrictions on the eligibility of patients to enter the trial and investigators are limited to patients for whom there is easy access (e.g. in-patients at their own hospital). In addition, it is usually advisable to ensure the variation in the outcome measure in the study group is kept reasonably low (so that the sample size required to show a significant difference between treatments is not prohibitively high), and therefore patients are restricted to those of, for example, a particular age group and severity of disease. It is important to realise that the results of the study will be less able to be generalised the more restrictions are made on the study patients.

Protocol deviations

There are a number of ways in which deviations from protocol can occur.

One instance is that in which ineligible patients are included in a trial. Such patients should be excluded from the analysis of the results of the study. The number of ineligible patients can be reduced by using a checklist for eligibility as every patient enters the study, prior to randomisation. Another problem occurs when patients do not adhere to their allocated treatment; that is, when they are non-compliant with treatment. This can be reduced, firstly, by ensuring that a detailed explanation of the treatment regime is given to each patient and, secondly, by having frequent checks during the course of treatment. The latter can be achieved by, for example, counting the number of remaining tablets the patient has or by blood/urine tests. The most extreme type of non-compliance occurs when a patient withdraws from the study. This is due either to patient refusal to carry on with the treatment (sometimes unavoidable if the patient moves away from the study area) or to a clinical decision that the treatment for this patient should be changed.

As a general rule, all eligible patients, including non-compliant patients, should be included in the analysis of the results where possible. This approach is sometimes referred to by the term 'analysis by intention to treat', and is considered to lead to a more valid comparison of treatments because it mimics what is likely to happen in clinical practice.

Pilot study

Before carrying out a definitive study involving a large number of subjects, it is sometimes prudent to run a small pilot study. This is used to estimate patient recruitment as well as the level and variability of the outcome measure. The latter information can then be used in the calculation of required sample size for the larger study. The pilot study can also show how questionnaires and assessment scales perform in practice, and whether the planned trial will run smoothly.

Multicentre trials

In some circumstances, it may not be feasible to carry out a trial at a single centre (i.e. one hospital or general practice surgery) because the number of eligible patients available over the study period will be too small. The involvement of a number of different centres in the study should be considered to increase the potential pool of patients. If the clinical trial includes patients and clinicians from a variety of centres, a more broad, representative set of patients will be attained and the results of the study will be more easily generalised. There are, however, a number of disadvantages to running a multicentre trial. A greater cost is involved because the number of staff working on the study and the administration is increased. It is also more difficult to ensure that the study protocol is followed exactly, and that the quality of the data is of a uniformly high standard.

Clinical versus statistical significance

If a clinical trial includes a large number of subjects, then even small differences can become statistically significant. For example, suppose in a trial assessing the effects of two drugs on the urinary composition of 1000 patients with enteric hyperoxaluria, the reduction in urinary oxalate excretion output was, on average, 0.01 mmol/24 h greater for one drug compared to the other and that this was found to be a statistically significant result. Because this is such a small difference, it would not be considered as clinically important or significant.

Alternatively, if a clinical trial includes only a small number of subjects, then quite large differences will not be statistically significant. For example, suppose the trial described above involved just ten patients and the difference in reduction in urinary oxalate excretion output was shown to be 0.15 mmol/24 h, but that this difference was not statistically significant. Because a reduction of this magnitude would be clinically important, the result should not be ignored; it provides evidence that a much larger study should be planned.

Guidelines for the critical appraisal of published clinical trial papers

Studies published in reputable journals are naturally thought to have a sound research basis, with credible results and reliable conclusions. However, this is a mistaken belief. Most journals do have a system of appraisal by independent referees and a number of journals use statisticians as referees, but many low-standard studies still manage to pass through the system and are published. The consequences of misleading results can be serious. A clinician may decide to switch to a new treatment for his or her patients when in actual fact the treatment does not actually have the beneficial effects extolled in the medical article. A researcher may employ time, effort and resources in a fruitless attempt to replicate a study finding. It is therefore important that medical researchers and clinicians are able critically to appraise a paper for themselves.

A summary of the relevant points that need to be considered when reading a clinical trial paper is given below. This closely follows the clinical trials checklist given in Gardner, Machin and Campbell [4]. The list was designed to help the statistical refereeing of papers submitted to the *British Medical Journal*. Note that studies must be judged on the information included in the published paper. A satisfactory answer to a question cannot be assumed if the relevant information is not given.

- *Objective of the study*. Are the aims and objectives of the trial sufficiently described?
- *Study design*. Was a parallel group or cross-over design used? Was the design appropriate for the type of disease and treatment studied? Is the study prospective (that is, a planned study with data to be collected) or retrospective (based on data already collected)? Were concurrent or historical controls used?
- *Criteria for subject eligibility*. Are the diagnostic criteria for entry into the trial specified and the exclusion criteria clearly stated? Are the criteria appropriate?
- *Source of subjects*. How were the subjects recruited? Were they, for example, all hospital

in-patients within a specific time frame or consecutive clinic attenders? Was sufficient information given about the health status of the subjects?

- *Treatments.* Were the treatments well defined? Are the treatment periods of reasonable length?
- *Randomisation.* Were the subjects randomly allocated to treatment? Is the exact method of randomisation (e.g. simple blocked randomisation using random number tables or stratified randomisation with age and severity of disease defining the strata) described? Is the practical way in which subjects were allocated to treatment (e.g. from a written schedule or sealed envelopes) described? Was there an acceptably short delay between allocation and commencement of treatment?
- *Blindness.* What degree of blindness was used (e.g. double blind, single blind)? How was this achieved? Was the maximum degree of blindness that is possible used in the study?
- *Outcome measures.* Were the outcome measures clearly defined? Are they appropriate? Were they accurately measured and recorded?
- *Prognostic factors.* Were data on important prognostic factors and other relevant patient characteristics recorded?
- *Sample size.* Does the paper report a pre-study calculation of required sample size? Is the study large enough to detect anything other than large (and perhaps unrealistic) differences in the effects of the treatments?
- *Follow-up.* Was there a clearly defined follow-up period? Was a high proportion of subjects followed-up? Did a high proportion of subjects complete their treatment?
- *Drop-outs.* Was the drop-out rate low? Were the drop-outs described for each treatment group separately? Was a comparison of relevant baseline characteristics made between those who dropped out and those who remained in the study?
- *Side-effects.* Were the side-effects of treatment reported?
- *Statistical analysis.* Is there an adequate description of all the statistical procedures used? Are the methods appropriate for the data? Were they applied correctly? If a parametric comparison test has been used (e.g. t-test), which requires the data to be Normally distributed, do the data really follow a Normal distribution? Have paired data (e.g. before and after treatment comparisons on the same group of patients) been analysed using an appropriate paired comparison test? Have multiple readings on one subject been treated incorrectly as independent observations? Were the prognostic variables adjusted for in the statistical analysis if there was a clinically significant difference between the treatment groups?

- *Presentation of results.* Is the statistical presentation of data satisfactory? Are the summary statistics given appropriate to the distribution of the data? Note that means and standard deviations should be given for Normally distributed data alone. Are graphs clearly labelled and do they have axes with an unchanging scale? Are confidence intervals presented for the main results?
- *Conclusions.* Are the conclusions drawn from the analysis of the data justified? Are the results of significance tests interpreted correctly? Is a causal relation erroneously implied from an observed association? Are findings wrongly extrapolated to a population of patients not represented in the study sample?

Further reading

A more detailed account of the design and statistical analysis of clinical trials is given by Pocock [5]. Readable introductions to the subject of clinical trials can also be found in Altman [6] and Campbell and Machin [7].

References

1. Lind J. A treatise of the scurvy. Edinburgh: Sands Murray & Cochran, 1753
2. Medical Research Council. Streptomycin treatment of pulmonary tuberculosis. Br Med J 1948; ii: 769–82

3. Machin D, Campbell MJ. Statistical tables for the design of clinical trials. Oxford: Blackwell Scientific Publications, 1987

4. Gardner MJ, Machin D, Campbell MJ. Use of checklists for the assessment of the statistical content of medical studies. Br Med J 1986; 292: 810–12

5. Pocock SJ. Clinical trials: a practical approach. Chichester: Wiley, 1983

6. Altman DG. Practical statistics for medical research. London: Chapman & Hall, 1991

7. Campbell MJ, Machin D. Medical statistics: a common-sense approach. Chichester: Wiley, 1993

Evidence-based medicine for urologists

28

M. Emberton

Few urologists will admit to not having felt some kind of emotional response when the term 'evidence-based medicine' was first heard or read. If pressed, urologists' responses are probably little different from those of other doctors. Some see it as just another addition to the long list of fashionable ways of thinking about clinical problems – general practitioner fundholding, quality assurance programmes, total quality management, clinical audit, and critical care pathways – and, typically, championed by a group of enthusiasts keen to promote their novel approach with something approximating evangelical zeal. A certain, but guarded, intellectual inquisitiveness in evidence-based medicine might be allowed – just enough to reasonably defend a position – but no more. For in the end, evidence-based medicine might be easily dismissed on the grounds that it states the very obvious, yet another term for describing what we already do. Responsible urologists, by definition, practise in a critical and careful way. They keep up to date, go to scientific meetings, discuss cases with their colleagues and give the best care they can to their patients. The question could be posed, 'Who are these people that insist on telling us what we should or should not be doing with men presenting with infertility, benign prostatic hyperplasia or early prostate cancer?' [1–3]. 'Surely, with our long specialist training and wealth of clinical experience, we must be best placed to decide what is best for our patients.'

Some urologists will feel increasingly uncomfortable with this position. They may experience guilt about the increasing pile of unread or even unopened journals in their offices. Over two million papers are

published in the peer-reviewed literature each year. Urologists will certainly have received numerous notices of new journals, relevant to their field of interest, which have been launched and which they are never likely even to see. They may have felt slight personal frustration at not really being able to get to grips with an important scientific paper because of the assumptions made, the complex design or way the results were analysed and expressed. They may have had the feeling that a recent afternoon spent leafing through some journals was wasted because most of the papers read described studies that were ridiculously small to be of any consequence, described patients who were quite distinct from their own, or were so badly conceived that they were forced to question the precise role of peer review and wonder what editorial discretion was all about. A recent computer literature search might have been equally frustrating: each time the search was altered by introducing a new key word, a different, often mutually exclusive, set of references was generated. All this on top of a nagging feeling that will not go away: just how effective is that new device that was introduced about a year ago? Do the benefits (which seem now to be not as dramatic as they at first appeared) really outweigh the harms (more patients seem to be presenting side-effects than they did at the beginning)?

If you are reading this at all, then the chances are that you will recognise some of the frustrations mentioned above. Although sceptical, you may want to know whether understanding what is meant by evidence-based medicine can help you make better clinical decisions. The answers to many of the clinical questions that we all ask are present in the medical literature, but they are not always easy to identify, locate, interpret or implement. Evidence-based medicine is all about searching, interpreting and implementing. This short chapter explains what is meant by evidence-based medicine and tries to say what it is not. The emphasis is on evidence-based medicine as applied to urology, and how it might be used to help in everyday clinical decision making. An appendix is provided, which should help direct the reader to sources of good-quality evidence, both paper based and electronic. If you see yourself (at least in part) as more of a sceptic than a believer, the author urges you to read on. The aim is to convince you that evidence-based medicine is not just a passing fad, but is an intellectual challenge that is as exacting and demanding as it is rewarding.

The case for evidence-based medicine

Urologists do not practise in a vacuum. The work they do is shaped by forces that are influencing the way that all clinicians practise. These forces are now universal. They do not depend on where you practise (developed versus underdeveloped countries), they do not depend on how you are paid (salaried versus fee for service), nor do they depend on how the health service is structured (nationally versus locally). There are, broadly, four forces that govern the way we practise medicine. The first is an overwhelming preoccupation with cost control. Second is the increasing trend for health care to be purchased for groups of people that can be easily defined: they might live in a particular area (health authority) or might be members of a particular organisation (a health insurance scheme). Thirdly, those groups who purchase health care are becoming increasingly accountable for their actions. As these groups become distanced from central government, their accountability will increase. The decisions purchasers make will need to be justified. The combination of the decentralisation of decision making and increasing accountability will result in a fourth force: a reduction in the freedom offered to clinicians to choose which patient will receive which treatment. It is likely that these rationing deci-

sions will be increasingly shared with the people that purchase health care. Also, although not yet apparent, the last of these forces will end in a realisation by the public, the media and politicians that decisions about rationing health care are becoming increasingly difficult. What is clear is that decisions on who should get what treatment should be explicit and based on the best available evidence. This is where evidence-based medicine can help. In the UK, urologists have seen the beginnings of change through the reforms undertaken in the National Health Service [4–5]. Urologists on both sides of the Atlantic have been sent a number of guidelines that state explicitly how common urological conditions should be managed in the future [3, 6]. Evidence-based medicine, or the conscientious, explicit and judicious use of current best evidence when making decisions about the care that patients receive, has been proposed as one solution to the the common problems of modern health care [7].

The forces described above that shape the way we all do our jobs are largely a response to increasingly scarce resources. Resources are only one of three factors that influence the way we treat patients. The other two are evidence and values or opinion. The two urologists with rather polarised opinions presented at the beginning of this chapter represent, in turn, a clinician who values opinion over evidence followed by a clinician who values evidence over opinion. It is the pressure on resources that will not permit opinion over evidence or presumed benefits over demonstrable benefits. Moreover, we can expect the pressure on resources to increase over the next decade. Individuals who become old will have greater expectations of what they might expect from a urologist compared with those who are already old: 75-year-old men will no longer accept mild lower urinary tract symptoms as a consequence of ageing. They will expect access to high-quality treatments (which might be new, more expensive technologies), and will be increasingly conversant with systems of redress if dissatisfied. The sector of society with greatest need will, in the future, make greater demands than in the past.

We can therefore expect that opinion will be forced to give way to high-quality evidence. There are plenty of examples in the medical literature that tell us that this is judicious – presumptions that were thought to be correct were shown not to be when put the test. The example, first used by Sackett, shows that biological plausibility might not necessarily be enough to predict an outcome [8]. Sackett cites two pieces of evidence: first, a study that showed that patients who had ventricular ectopic beats after myocardial infarction were more likely to die; second, that ventricular ectopic beats could be suppressed by certain drugs. It was presumed that administering these drugs would result in fewer deaths after myocardial infarction. This seemed reasonable, but when put to the test the presumption was shown to be wrong. Randomised controlled trials have since shown that the use of these drugs increased, rather than decreased, the risk of death in this group of patients [9]. As a result, the routine use of these drugs has been strongly discouraged. Good-quality evidence of this kind (appropriately designed and well-conducted studies) is available for many of the things that we clinicians do. Chalmers and his colleagues looked at 226 interventions carried out by obstetricians in the perinatal period. They found that there was evidence of reasonable quality available in about half; 20% were shown to confer some benefit to mothers or neonates; 30% were shown either to confer no benefit or, worse still, to do harm [10].

What evidence-based medicine involves

Sackett has described evidence-based medicine as a form of shorthand for five linked ideas [8], which he outlined as follows. First, the decisions we make on our wards and in our clinics should be based on the best patient, laboratory and population-based evidence. Second, the problem – rather than our habits – should determine where we get our evidence. Third, we need to be able to integrate epidemiological and biostatistical ways of thinking with those derived from pathophysiology and our own personal experience (use of numbers needed to diagnose or likelihood ratios to increase the power of diagnostic information, considering inception cohorts in making prognoses, incorporating meta-analyses of randomised controlled trials into decisions about therapy,

and introducing odds ratios into judgements about iatrogenic disease). Fourth, the conclusions of this search and critical appraisal of evidence are only worthwhile if they are translated into actions that affect patients directly. Fifth, we need continuously to evaluate our performance in applying these ideas. Sackett has summarised these five areas into a description of evidence-based medicine as a 'lifelong process of self-directed learning in which caring for patients creates the need for clinically important information about diagnosis, prognosis, therapy, decision analysis, cost utility analysis and other clinical and heath care issues.' In order to be able to do this, clinicians need to learn or refine some skills. These skills are outlined below, but readers wanting more detailed descriptions should refer to Sackett's book [11].

Asking the right questions

This is about formulating questions that have a reasonable chance of being answered [12]. It is an important first step because many hours might be wasted trying to get an answer to a question that is essentially unanswerable. At McMaster University in Canada, where medical students are taught an evidence-based approach to learning medicine, students are encouraged to construct or 'build' questions from 'knowledge gaps' that they become aware of when managing patients. The questions are constructed by first trying to classify the patient or the problem. In other words, one might ask, 'How would I describe a group of patients similar to the one I have just seen?' A concise description might be: fit men, less than 70 years with clinically localised prostate cancer. Once this classification has been made, the question of which cause/prognostic factor/treatment being considered arises. Would neoadjuvant hormonal cytoreduction be of benefit to this man prior to a radical treatment? This is then followed by consideration of any alternative intervention such as standard therapy alone. The final component of the question building addresses outcome. 'What can I hope to accomplish? Are the benefits of the intervention going to outweigh the risks?' Thus, the elements of question building proposed by advocates of evidence-based medicine are concerned with the patient or problem, the intervention, the comparator and the outcome [13]. This approach, rather than helping frame the perfect question, tends to help find the gaps in our knowledge that we are all too often aware of but too busy to do anything about.

Getting hold of the best evidence

This involves tracking down, with the greatest efficiency, the best evidence with which to answer the question posed. This means the best evidence *available* not the best evidence *possible*. In doing this, one should try to classify evidence into one of five broad categories. First (or grade one) evidence refers to systematic reviews of well-conducted randomised trials. This type of study will often contain a meta-analysis of relevant studies. This is the type of study one should aim to find and is becoming more common. Second (or grade two) evidence comes from a randomised controlled trial. If such a trial has not been conducted or was not possible, then grade three evidence should be sought. This group includes studies that were well designed but not randomised. These might include case control studies and prospective cohort studies. Other non-experimental or uncontrolled studies are labelled as grade four in terms of strength of evidence. These would include the multi-institutional prospectively collected case series. The final category, grade five, is given to expert opinion. Note, the single institution retrospective case series (probably the most commonly published surgical study) gets no category. As well as the many gaps in our knowledge (Figure 28.1), many areas of clinical urology have to rely on standards of evidence that lie between grades three to five.

Knowing where to look for evidence is half the battle. The dose of a particular drug is best found on the data sheet or from a formulary. But where the source is not so obvious, one needs to know how to look as well as where best to look. It is fair to say that, for most clinical questions, electronic media (which is periodically updated) is replacing written material for searching. Journals are still, and will continue to be, important in alerting clinicians to new important developments, much in the way that newspapers or magazines do. They also provide the reader with what Alan Bennett, the playwright, described as the 'lucky dip' component of learning: stumbling across an arti-

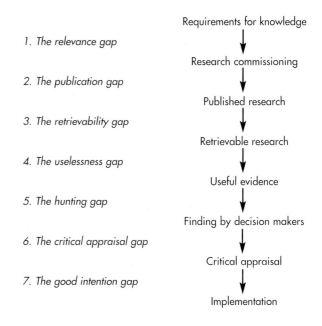

1. *The relevance gap*

2. *The publication gap*

3. *The retrievability gap*

4. *The uselessness gap*

5. *The hunting gap*

6. *The critical appraisal gap*

7. *The good intention gap*

Requirements for knowledge
↓
Research commissioning
↓
Published research
↓
Retrievable research
↓
Useful evidence
↓
Finding by decision makers
↓
Critical appraisal
↓
Implementation

Figure 28.1 *The evidence gaps. (Adapted from ref. [7]).*

cle on a subject of no immediate interest but which, on glancing through and on subsequent reading, proves either interesting or useful.

Electronic media have the advantage of being more accessible, better indexed, more up to date and probably cheaper than the paper alternative. Most importantly, electronic media are more easily kept up to date and can offer the searcher an almost infinite number of quickly accessible cross-references. In most hospitals, the medical libraries have become the evidence centres and, as a minimum, should now have access to the World Wide Web, access to bibliographic databases such as MEDLINE, EMBASE or the Cochrane Database of systematic reviews, a well-chosen selection of books and journals, arrangements for getting hold of original articles or published reports, and a good librarian or information manager who can teach/supervise clinicians about how best to use the resources. The main impediment to using such a centre is geography. If evidence is required in a meeting or a clinic, it is usually impractical to get up and leave. It will not be long before the electronic media will be available at the desk through terminals or via portable, handheld computers. A guide to electronic and other source is available in the appendix at the end of this chapter.

Critical appraisal

Many patients will be better than their doctors at finding information. Most of us have been faced with patients attending a clinic armed with pages and pages of output from several sources, the Internet being just one. Where we can help our information-seeking patients is in the critical appraisal of the literature. Critical appraisal involves asking two central questions: one, is this valid or close to the truth?; two, is this important or potentially useful (often called the 'so what' question)? The terms validity and importance need to be applied differently to different types of evidence. For example, if the validity of evidence regarding a new diagnostic test is being considered, the following questions need asking. Was the test compared against a gold standard? Was this done blindly and independently? Was the test evaluated on patients similar to those for which the test is intended? Was the reference standard applied regardless of the diagnostic test result? In other words, did the investigators forgo applying the reference standard in patients who had a negative result from the diagnostic test in question? For instance, men with negative sextant Tru-cut biopsies of the prostate are unlikely to undergo radical prostatectomy in order to determine whether they were truly free of prostate cancer (true negatives). In evaluating the test, in this case prostate biopsies, a group of men should be followed up in order to determine the proportion of patients truly free of the target disorder. Failure in any one of these three areas should encourage the reader to call into question the validity of the evidence.

Whether the evidence about a diagnostic test is important requires that another set of questions be asked. The first of these is one that clinicians must ask themselves. What, based on our own clinical experience, are the chances that the patient has the target disorder that we are testing for? These are known as prior or pre-test probabilities. Diagnostic tests that provide big differences between pre-test and post-test probabilities are likely to be useful diagnostic tests.

The next question refers to the ability of the test to distinguish between patients who have the target disorder and patients who do not. This relates to the specificity (the proportion of patients who have the target disorder who test positive) and sensitivity (the proportion of patients who do not have the target disease who test negative) of the test in question. From the specificity and sensitivity of a test, likelihood ratios, which are becoming the preferred expression, are derived [14]. One reason why likelihood ratios are preferred by devotees of evidence-based medicine is that they are not reliant on a test being positive or negative, as is the case with specificity and sensitivity. Different levels of a test result produce different changes from pre-test to post-test probabilities.

Although the above is a quick run through of how one might begin to assess the validity and importance of a paper reporting on a new diagnostic test, techniques of critical appraisal (each addressing validity and importance) need to be applied to other types of report. Papers on prognostic indicators, benefits or adverse effects of new treatments, and proposed guidelines all require a systematic approach so that the reader can decide whether or not to believe what is being said. Readers wanting details on how to become accomplished at critical appraisal should try David Sackett's book, *Clinical epidemiology: a basic science for clinical medicine*, or Trisha Greenalph's guide entitled *How to read a paper: the basics of evidence-based medicine*, details of which are given in the appendix. Sackett's well-written guide to critical appraisal was recently serialised in the *British Medical Journal* [15].

Applying evidence

Going to the trouble of finding evidence on a particular subject and deciding that it was both valid and important is not the end of it. We still have to apply evidence to a particular patient. Remember the mantra: evidence-based medicine must begin and end with patients. In order to apply evidence to a real patient, we need now to ask questions such as, 'Can I apply this *valid* and *important* evidence to a diagnostic test (such as free per cent prostate specific antigen) that I requested for my patient?' or 'Can I apply this *valid* and *important* evidence on the prognosis of the patient I saw yesterday in the clinic with superficial bladder cancer?' or 'Can I apply this *valid* and *important* evidence on treatment (e.g. BCG intravesical immunotherapy for carcinoma in situ of the bladder) for this patient?' or 'Can I apply this *valid* and *important* evidence on harm (e.g. the long-term complications of ileocystoplasty) for this patient?' These questions are even more relevant when looking at evidence produced by others, such as clinical guidelines, integrated care plans and quality improvement strategies.

Let us review ways in which we might apply evidence about treatment to an individual patient, a situation we commonly encounter. Sackett tells us to ask a series of questions when trying to decide whether evidence can be applied to a particular patient [11]. First, do the results apply to your patient? Rather than rejecting a trial because your patient does not fulfil its entry criteria, for this would exclude most patients we encounter, Sackett suggests we rephrase the question in the following way: 'Is my patient so different from those in the trial that the results cannot help me?' Patients may differ genetically, socially and medically. The problem with this is that each clinician's interpretation of this question will differ, as different degrees of biological plausibility are applied. We should be reassured that, historically, the main findings of well-conducted studies have been generally applicable to all patients if applying them made biological sense. There is considerably more risk in applying post-hoc subgroup analyses to our particular patient. There has been some notoriously spurious 'evidence' generated from subgroup analysis. That women receiving aspirin would not be protected from transient ischaemic attacks (as opposed to men) was eventually shown to be false when it was looked at prospectively. Equivalence of the treatment may also need to be questioned. Is the treatment under investigation similar to that available locally in terms of skills and resources?

Once direct applicability has been accepted, the second question needs to quantify the amount of benefit that the patient is likely to experience should the treatment be applied. This can be done in two, albeit related, ways: relative benefit and absolute benefit. The former is often expressed as an odds ratio. For a detailed account of how to calculate odds ratios, readers are referred to a statistics manual or the texts cited in the appendix. As a guide, an odds ratio of 1 shows that the treatment has no benefit; less than 1, the treatment has a benefit when compared to the control group; greater than 1, the treatment is less effective than the intervention applied to the control group.

Odds ratios are preferred to the relative risk, which tends to introduce a bias. Readers tend to interpret relative risks as more positive than they genuinely are – a bias called the framing effect. An alternative way of overcoming the framing effect is to calculate the absolute reduction in risk that a treatment will produce. This is an expression of absolute benefit and is most clearly expressed by using the number (of patients) needed to treat (NNT) in order to prevent one event. Put simply, NNTs are the reciprocal of the fraction of patients improved with active treatment minus the fraction improved in the control group. NNTs can summarise complex data remarkably simply and clearly. Some NNTs for cardiac interventions have been generated by the evidence-based medicine journal, *Bandolier* [16]. In order to prevent either one myocardial infarction or death in one year, 25 patients with unstable angina would need to take aspirin daily for one year. On the other hand, 500 healthy American doctors would have to take aspirin over the same period in order to prevent one myocardial infarction or death. As well as expressing the amount of effort that has to be expended in order to prevent a single event, NNTs can be applied to individual patients. This is done by dividing the NNT by the susceptibility of the particular patient to the outcome you want to prevent relative to the susceptibility in the control patients in the trial. If a patient's susceptibility is thought to be twice that of the control group, the NNT would be divided by 2.

Clearly, the decision of whether a man will undergo transurethral resection of the prostate will depend on more than the NNT. Factors such as patient choice, chance, costs and patient preferences are all part of medical or patient decision making. Evidence-based medicine practitioners have made considerable efforts to try to incorporate these important variables into treatment decisions. This is done by using decision analysis, which requires patients to place value on different disease states or outcomes. Decisions analyses are time consuming to conduct but particularly useful when good-quality evidence is missing.

Getting started with evidence-based medicine

The various ways in which evidence is found, appraised and applied will be of interest to most in that they formalise a process used by all clinicians much of the time. Although learning and applying evidence-based medicine will make it easier for clinicians to cope with many of the changes occurring in health care (Table 28.1), becoming an evidence-based

Table 28.1 How evidence-based medicine can help the clinician in a rapidly changing world

1. Time pressures
Meeting the reduction in junior doctors' hours of work has led many to focus on efficiency. Evidence-based medicine can be used to decide which time and resource intensive manoeuvres should be dropped and which should be saved.

2. Quality pressures
Purchasers of health care will increasingly demand that clinicians are indeed doing 'the right thing right'. Evidence-based medicine will identify clinical acts whose performance is consistent with quality care.

3. Team pressures
Increasingly, patients are managed by multidisciplinary teams. Evidence-based medicine provides a common language and rules of evidence by which urologists, oncologists and radiotherapists should be able to agree on who will do what to whom.

4. Teaching pressures
Learning evidence-based medicine is the same for undergraduates and postgraduates. It forms an ideal basis for continuous medical education.

5. Financial pressures
It is no longer sufficient to provide effective health care – it needs to be cost effective. Evidence-based medicine will identify those treatments that produce greater improvement in health per pound sterling or dollar spent.

6. Intellectual pressures
No-one wants to learn facts alone. Evidence-based medicine enables clinicians to keep up to date not only in their own and related fields, but also with the scientific framework within which to identify and answer priority questions about the effectiveness of the treatments they offer their patients.

Modified from Sackett *et al.* (1997) [11].

medicine practitioner requires some initial investment, and the learning of the specific techniques. One way of acquiring the necessary knowledge is to read one of the general texts on the subject. However, most find that applying the techniques of evidence-based medicine requires some kind of group work; relevant courses on evidence-based medicine are advertised quite regularly in the medical press. Alternatively, details of courses are held at the Department of Clinical Epidemiology and Biostatistics at McMaster University, Hamilton, Ontario, Canada, and on the World Wide Web site for the Centre for Evidence-Based Medicine in Oxford, United Kingdom: http://cebm.jr2.ox.ac.uk/. The courses have evolved from those held initially at McMaster University. They tend to be run as small groups, be problem based and centred on actual patients rather than idealised case scenarios. Typically, they last two or three days and should enable participants to be competent in the four key areas of evidence-based medicine outlined above: framing good questions; searching for the best evidence; critical appraisal; applying evidence to everyday practice. In addition, techniques of self-evaluation or self-audit are taught, thereby equipping the individual to make assessments about whether or not they are applying the techniques of evidence-based medicine optimally.

Appendix: Getting better information

Much of the information below was obtained from the very detailed list of sources in Muir Gray's excellent text on the subject [7].

Published evidence

Bibliographic databases

Primary research (original papers), literature reviews and systematic reviews can all be identified using electronic databases such as MEDLINE or EMBASE. MEDLINE is the National Library of Medicine's bibliographic database, which covers articles published in nearly 4000 biomedical journals since 1966. New journals are not usually included until a number of conditions have been satisfied, such as proof of an adequate peer review process. Once fulfilled, all issues will be represented. The EMBASE bibliographic database has been produced by Elsevier Science since 1974. It is particularly good for searches in the fields of pharmacology and therapeutics. EMBASE carries more European journals than MEDLINE. There is an increasing number of specialist bibliographic databases. Some of these specialise in nursing issues, others in health economics. HealthSTAR is typical of these. It has been produced since 1975 by the National Library of Medicine/American Hospital Association. It is strong on health services research, health economics and management issues. Many of the articles retrieved on a search conducted on HealthSTAR would not appear on an identical search on MEDLINE or EMBASE.

The Cochrane Library

The Cochrane Library, named after Archie Cochrane, one of the pioneers of evidence-based medicine, was formed in 1995. The library contains a number of databases in electronic format, which currently comprise: the Cochrane Database of Systematic Reviews (CDSR), prepared by an international network of people committed to preparing and disseminating high-quality systematic reviews; the York Database of Abstracts of Reviews of Effectiveness (DARE); the Cochrane Controlled Trials Register (CCTR), a useful source of ongoing but as yet unpublished research;

and the Cochrane Review Methodology Database (CRMD). Further information on the Cochrane Library can be obtained through Update Software, PO Box 696, Oxford, OX2 7YX, England; tel. (+44) (0)1865-513902; fax. (+44) (0)1865-516918; email: update@cochrane.co.uk; URL: http://update.co.uk/info.

NHS Centre for Reviews and Dissemination (CRD reports)

The CRD is based at the University of York. It receives commissions from the NHS Executive and Health Departments of Scotland, Wales and Northern Ireland. Through bulletins entitled 'Effectiveness Matters', summaries of high-quality systematic reviews are distributed free of charge to clinicians and other interested parties, including patients. 'Effectiveness Matters' tends to concentrate on the assessment of important new interventions. Its most recent publication is based on two separate systematic reviews and addresses prostate cancer screening [2]. More information on publications can be obtained by contacting CRD, University of York, York, YO1 5DD, England; tel. (+44) (0)1904-433648; fax. (+44) (0)1904 433661; email: revdis@york.ac.uk.

CRD, in association with the Nuffield Institute for Health at the University of Leeds and Churchill Livingstone, publishes bimonthly magazines on a variety of interventions. These again are distributed free of charge to interested clinicians. Two issues have addressed urological subjects; one addressed the management of subfertility [1], and the more recent issue addressed the management of prostate cancer [2].

Other reliable sources

Although using criteria less stringent than the reviews conducted by either CRD or the Cochrane Collaboration, useful reports can be obtained from the Development and Evaluation Committee of the Wessex Regional Health Authority (URL: http://cochrane. epi.bris.ac.uk/rd/) and from the NHS Research and Development Programmes, all of which have systematic reviews conducted as part of each initiative (URL: http://libsun1.jr2.ox.ac.uk/a-ordd/index.htm).

Electronic updates have been created in order to keep two recently published textbooks on evidence-based medicine current. The first of these, *Evidence based healthcare* by Muir Gray [7], is continuously updated in the Evidence-Based Healthcare Toolbox (http://www.ihs.ox.ac.uk/ebh.html). The second, *Evidence-based medicine*, by David Sackett and others [11], is also linked in the Toolbox.

Clinical standards advisory group reports
These documents, available through the Department of Health (London: HMSO), address variations in the quality and effectiveness of health care throughout England. The first was produced in 1993 and entitled, 'Access to and availability of specialist services'. No specific urological issues have been addressed since these reports were started.

Epidemiologically based needs assessment reviews
The NHS Executive's District Health Authority Project conducted a series of reviews aimed at assessing the need and demand for health care. These reports were intended to help purchasers plan local services. The reports have been put together in a document published by Radcliffe Medical Publications, Oxford [17]. Two from a total of 20 reports covered urological issues. One addressed the need for prostatectomy, the other the need for family planning, abortion and fertility services.

Journals of secondary publication
It seems likely that in the future we will see a new type of journal created, the task of which will be to sift through a number of sources of information in order to present edited highlights to a select readership. These journals may limit themselves to subject matter considered relevant to a particular group, such as urologists. Although essentially summarising papers that have been published elsewhere, they will be of interest to the reader on two counts: the time-consuming process of selection will have been taken care of and, more importantly, the reports will be accompanied by critical commentaries by experts. In urology, clinicians are alerted to articles of interest by a number of journals; *Current Opinion in Urology* (Current Science Ltd, London) is the best known of these, though it is rare for methodological issues to be highlighted and therefore is not strictly evidence based. Another type of journal, rather than limit itself to a certain subject area, defines its selection of papers to be summarised on methodological criteria alone. In November 1995, the BMJ Publishing Group, London (fax: (+44) (0)171 383 6402 or email: bmjsubs@dial.pipex.com), launched the journal *Evidence Based Medicine*, which reviews bimonthly over 70 international medical journals in order to identify key research papers that are considered by the editorial team to be both scientifically valid and relevant to general medical practice. The abstracts are restricted to one page and are accompanied by commentaries from experts. More recently, reports from *Evidence Based Medicine* have been compiled onto a CD ROM, together with the *American College of Physicians* (ACP) *Journal Club* (January 1991 onwards), called *Best Evidence*. The ACP *Journal Club* is available on CD ROM from the American College of Physicians, Independence Mall West, Sixth Street at Race, Philadelphia, PA19106, USA.

One journal, *Bandolier*, has taken secondary publication to new heights. Modern typesetting and a chatty, direct, no-nonsense style have proved very popular with both clinicians and purchasers of health care. The editors make a considerable effort to present the results of randomised clinical trials in ways that will mean something to clinicians. They avoid *p* values where possible, preferring confidence intervals or absolute risk reduction as summary statistics. Where possible, the editors try to calculate meaningful statistics such as numbers needed to treat (NNT) or numbers needed to diagnose (NND). Most health authorities make *Bandolier* available free of charge to health professionals working in the UK. Contact Andrew Moore, Pain Relief Unit, The Churchill, Oxford OX3 7LJ, England, or by email, andrew.moore%mailgate.jr2@ox.ac.uk, or via the Internet, http://www.jr2.ox.ac.uk/bandolier

Unpublished research
Finding out about what research is underway is now possible by using bibliographic databases produced by some of the funding bodies. Finding out about research that was conducted but not finished or abandoned for whatever reason is much more difficult. The databases that can help identify work in progress are as follows. First, the NHS Research and Development Programme keeps records of all funded projects. An

updated list is available from 1997. More details can be obtained by contacting Research and Development Directorate, NHS Executive, Quarry House, Leeds LS2 7UE, England.

The US National Library of Medicine, together with the Association for Health Services Research and the University of North Carolina, keeps an online facility that holds details of current research projects funded by both government agencies and private foundations in the USA (URL: http://www.nlm.gov or the National Library of Medicine, US Department of Health and Human Services, Public Health Service, National Institutes of Health, Bethseda, MD 20894, USA.

Textbooks on evidence-based medicine

Greenhalph T. How to read a paper: the basics of evidence based medicine, 1st edition. London: BMJ Publications, 1997

Muir Gray J. Evidence based health care: how to make health policy and management decisions. London: Churchill Livingstone, 1997

Sackett DL, Haynes RB, Guyatt GH, Tugwell P. Clinical epidemiology: a basic science for clinical medicine, 2nd edition. Boston: Little Brown, 1991

Sackett DL, Richardson W, Rosenberg W, Haynes R. Evidence-based medicine: how to practice and teach EBM. London: Churchill Livingstone, 1997

Although not in textbook form, a series entitled 'Users' guides to the medical literature' ran in the *Journal of the American Medical Association* from 1993 to 1995. The articles offer detailed accounts of how to interpret and apply different types of medical evidence to clinical situations. They are cited below.

Oxman A, Sackett D, Guyatt G. Users' guides to the medical literature. 1. How to get started. JAMA 1993; 270: 2093–5

Guyatt G, Sackett D, Cook D. Users' guides to the medical literature. 2. How to use an article about therapy or prevention. What were the results and how will they help me care for my patients? JAMA 1993; 270(21): 2598–601

Jaeschke R, Guyatt G, Sackett D. Users' guides to the medical literature. 3. How to use an article about a diagnostic test. Are the results of the study valid? Evidence Based Medicine Working Group. JAMA 1994; 271(5): 389–91

Levine M, Walter S, Lee H, Haines T, Holbrook A, Moyer

V. Users' guides to the medical literature. 4. How to use an article about harm. Evidence Based Medicine Working Group. JAMA 1994; 271(20): 1615–19

Laupacis M, Wells G, Richardson W, Tugwell P. Users' guides to the medical literature. 5. How to use an article about prognosis. Evidence Based Medicine Working Group. JAMA 1994; 272(3): 234–7

Jaeschke R, Guyatt G, Sackett D. Users' guides to the medical literature. 6. Are the results of the study valid? JAMA 1994; 271: 389–91

Richardson W, Detsky A. Users' guides to the medical literature. 7. How to use a clinical decision analysis. Are the results of the study valid? Evidence Based Medicine Working Group. JAMA 1995; 273(16): 1292–5

Hayward R, Wilson M, Tunis S, Bass E, Guyatt G. Users' guides to the medical literature. 8. How to use clinical practice guidelines. Are the recommendations valid? Evidence Based Medicine Working Group. JAMA 1995; 274(7): 570–4

Guyatt G, Sackett D, Sinclair J, Hayward R, Cook D, Cook R. Users' guides to the medical literature. 9. A method for grading health care recommendations. Evidence Based Medicine Working Group. JAMA 1995; 274(22): 1800–4

References

1. The management of sub-fertility. Effective Health Care 1992; 3: 1–23

2. Screening for prostate cancer. Effectiveness Matters 1997; 2(2): 1–4

3. Chamberlain J, Melia J, Moss S, Brown J. Report prepared for the Health Technology Assessment Panel of the NHS Executive on the diagnosis, management, treatment and costs of prostate cancer in England and Wales. Br J Urol 1997; 79(Suppl. 3): 1–32

4. Secretaries of State for Health, England, Wales, Northern Ireland and Scotland. Contracts for services and role of District Health Authorities. London: HMSO, 1989

5. Secretaries of State for Health, England, Wales, Northern Ireland and Scotland. Working for patients. London: HMSO, 1989

6. McConnell J, Barry M, Bruskewitz R, *et al*. Benign prostatic hyperplasia: diagnosis and treatment. Maryland: Agency for Healthcare Policy and Research, 1994

7. Muir Gray J. Evidence based health care: how to make health policy and management decisions. London: Churchill Livingstone, 1997

8. Sackett D, Rosenberg W. The need for evidence based medicine. J R Soc Med 1995; 88: 620–4

9. Echt D, Liebsen S, Mitchell B. Mortality and morbidity in patients receiving encainide, flecainide, or placebo: the cardiac arrhythmia suppression trial. N Engl J Med 1991; 324: 781–8

10. Chalmers I, Enkin M, Keirse M. Effective care in pregnancy and child birth. Oxford: Oxford University Press, 1989: 1471–6

11. Sackett D, Richardson W, Rosenberg W, Haynes R. Evidence-based medicine: how to practice and teach EBM. London: Churchill Livingstone, 1997

12. Oxman A, Sackett D, Guyatt G. Users guide to the medical literature: 1. How to get started. JAMA 1993; 270: 2093–5

13. Richardson W, Wilson M, Nishikawa J, Hayward R. The well built clinical question: a key to evidence based decisions. ACP J Club 1995; A12–13

14. Jaeschke R, Guyatt G, Sackett D. Users guide to the medical literature. 6. Are the results of the study valid? JAMA 1994; 271: 389–91

15. Greenhalph T. Statistics for the non-statistician (1): different types of data need different statistical tests. Br Med J 1997; 315: 364–6

16. Moore A, McQuay H, Muir Gray J. NNTs for some cardiac interventions. Bandolier 1995; 17: 7

17. Stevens A, Raftery J. Health care needs assessments: the epidemiologically based needs assessment reviews. Oxford: Radcliffe Medical Publications, 1994

Index

G

R